PHARMACEUTICAL DOSAGE FORMS

PHARMACEUTICAL DOSAGE FORMS

Tablets

SECOND EDITION, REVISED AND EXPANDED

In Three Volumes
VOLUME 2

EDITED BY

Herbert A. Lieberman

H. H. Lieberman Associates, Inc.
Consultant Services
Livingston, New Jersey

Leon Lachman

Lachman Consultant Services
Westbury, New York

Joseph B. Schwartz

Philadelphia College of Pharmacy and Science
Philadelphia, Pennsylvania

MARCEL DEKKER, INC.   New York and Basel

Library of Congress Cataloging-in-Publication Data
(Revised for vol. 2)

Pharmaceutical dosage forms--tablets.

"In three volumes."
Includes bibliographical references.
1. Tablets (Medicine) 2. Drugs--Dosage forms.
I. Lieberman, Herbert A.   II. Lachman, Leon
          III. Schwartz, Joseph B.
[DNLM: 1. Dosage forms. 2. Drugs--administration &
dosage. QV 785 P535]
RS 201.T2P46 1989   615'.191   89-1629
ISBN 0-8247-8044-2 (v. 1 : alk. paper)

This book is printed on acid-free paper.

MARCEL DEKKER, INC.
270 Madison Avenue, New York, New York 10016

Current printing (last digit):
10 9 8 7 6 5 4 3 2 1

PRINTED IN THE UNITED STATES OF AMERICA

Preface

Several years have passed since the first editions of *Pharmaceutical Dosage Forms: Tablets*, Volumes 1–3 were published. Advances in the science and technology of tablet formulation, processing, and testing are reflected in the updated, revised, and expanded second edition of the volumes.

Tablets are still the most widely used drug delivery system in the pharmaceutical industry. This fact as well as their employment in medical conditions ranging from the most simple to the most serious are factors that make the pharmaceutical scientist a most important part of the health care team. Because of both the importance of tablets in medical practice and their many different types, the formulation, scale-up, production, and quality-control aspects are continually changing and improving. As a consequence, the second edition of this three-volume treatise on tablets is now timely.

Volume 1 covers the many different types of tablet products, their formulations, and methods of manufacture, i.e., wet and dry granulation and direct compression. Volume 2 addresses the various pharmaceutical unit processes involved in tablet manufacture as well as tablet characteristics, test methods, and bioavailability. Volume 3 is concerned with special tablet processes such as coating, particular functions such as controlled release, and manufacturing concerns such as pilot plant, validation, production operation procedures, and also kinetics and quality assurance.

When the first edition was published, its purpose was to assemble the information on tablets that had appeared piecemeal throughout the pharmaceutical literature so that the subject matter would be comprehensive and useful to both novice and experienced tablet technician. The objectives of this second edition are to update the comprehensive collection that made up the first edition, and to expand it to include the most recent technology and references. Although technology and equipment change rapidly, the basic scientific principles do not, and these topics have been largely retained.

Each tablet type requires special formulation techniques; each of the unit operations is involved with specific scientific principles; each subject related to tablet production requires a specific expertise and experience; therefore, a treatise of this magnitude requires highly knowledgeable authors for the many areas covered. A multiauthored text was thus chosen as the preferred way to impart the knowledge necessary to accomplish the desired goals of the editors. To do this we sought the help of experts for each of the various subjects that appear. The authors were selected based on their scientific training, years of particular subject matter experience, and recognized accomplishments in their fields. A goal set for the authors was to combine basic scientific fact with their own practical and current experiences, so that the reader might learn how to do what the authors do.

Volume 2 deals primarily with the various pharmaceutical unit operations involved in the development and production of tablets. Mixing, drying, size reduction, compression and compaction, granulation, bioavailability, and tooling are all aspects that must be understood in order to make effective and cost-efficient tablets.

In this second edition, the mixing chapter has been expanded in the discussion of solid—solid and liquid—solid blending and, in addition, new equipment has been included. The sections on sampling and on scale-up have been expanded and scientific experiences of the authors have been incorporated. The chapter on drying includes a more detailed section on moisture flow, granule drying times, efficiencies, and updated equipment. An extended discussion of fluid bed drying and new sections on both microwave and microwave-vacuum drying represent current trends. The chapter on size reduction or milling contains additional material on equipment and new sections covering the control of raw materials. In the chapter on compression and compaction, the discussion on instrumentation is updated. The discussion of bonding concepts has been expanded, and the "capping" phenomenon is discussed with particular reference to axial and radial tensile strengths. The influence of applied pressure on the extent of solid-state interactions is added.

The chapter on granulation and tablet characteristics is again divided into two parts. The first represents the effect of this operation on granule characteristics; the second addresses tablet properties and behavior. The discussion on the fundamentals of granulation has been significantly expanded. Discussions on granule shapes and sizes and their effects in tableting are included. There is an enlarged section on fluid bed granulation, and a new section on high-shear granulation is added. There are extensive revisions to the chapter on drug bioavailability from tablets. Special descriptions are given to the factors affecting the bioavailability of drugs from conventional and controlled-release tablets. In addition, the new FDA requirements for the bioequivalence of tablets are covered. Statistical and protcol design considerations have been included. The section on dissolution methodology has been updated to include almost all of the technology that has been developed to date for the evaluation of conventional and controlled-release tablets. New approaches to in vitro/in vivo correlations are discussed. Finally, the chapter concerning compression tooling has been revised to contain updated information.

The editors are grateful to the authors for their contributions, the manner in which their subjects are covered and, particularly, with the editors' comments. The subject matter, format, and choice of authors are the responsibility of the editors. Our hope is that the efforts of the contributors and the judgments of the editors have resulted in a text on tablets that will enable the many people who refer to it to practice the technology of tablet production so that industrial pharmacy and medications in tablet form may be further improved.

Herbert A. Lieberman
Leon Lachman
Joseph B. Schwartz

Contents

Contributors

Neil R. Anderson   Head, Pharmacy Research Department, Merrell—Dow Research Institute, Indianapolis, Indiana

Gilbert S. Banker   Professor and Dean, College of Pharmacy, University of Minnesota, Minneapolis, Minnesota

Jens T. Carstensen   Professor, School of Pharmacy, University of Wisconsin, Madison, Wisconsin

Glen C. Ebey   Senior Product Engineer, Engineering Department, Thomas Engineering, Inc., Hoffman Estates, Illinois

Dale E. Fonner   Executive Director, Pharmaceutical Manufacturing Technology, The Upjohn Company, Kalamazoo, Michigan

Roger E. Gordon   Director, Drug Delivery Research and Development — Dry Products, The Upjohn Company, Kalamazoo, Michigan

Russell J. Lantz, Jr.   President, Lantz Consultants, Salem, North Carolina

George F. Loeffler   Director of Engineering, Thomas Engineering, Inc., Hoffman Estates, Illinois

James W. McGinity   Professor, Pharmaceutics Division, College of Pharmacy, University of Texas at Austin, Austin, Texas

Eugene L. Parrott   Professor of Industrial Pharmacy, College of Pharmacy, University of Iowa, Iowa City, Iowa

Thomas W. Rosanske*   Senior Research Scientist, Pharmaceutical Research and Development, The Upjohn Company, Kalamazoo, Michigan

Joseph B. Schwartz   Linwood F. Tice Professor of Pharmaceutics and Director of Industrial Pharmacy Research, Philadelphia College of Pharmacy and Science, Philadelphia, Pennsylvania

Salomon A. Stavchansky   Professor, Department of Pharmaceutics, College of Pharmacy, University of Texas at Austin, Austin, Texas

Kurt G. Van Scoik   Senior Research Scientist, Solid Products Development, Abbott Laboratories, North Chicago, Illinois

Michael A. Zoglio   Associate Scientist, Pharmacy Research, Merrell–Dow Research Institute, Cincinnati, Ohio

Current affiliation: Manager, Technical Development, Marion Laboratories, Inc., Kansas City, Missouri.

Contents of Pharmaceutical Dosage Forms: Tablets, Second Edition, Revised and Expanded, Volumes 1 and 3

edited by Herbert A. Lieberman, Leon Lachman, and Joseph B. Schwartz

VOLUME 3

Contents of Pharmaceutical Dosage Forms: Parenteral Medications, Volumes 1 and 2

edited by Kenneth E. Avis, Leon Lachman, and Herbert A. Lieberman

VOLUME 2

Contents of Pharmaceutical Dosage Forms: Disperse Systems, Volumes 1 and 2

edited by Herbert A. Lieberman, Martin M. Rieger, and Gilbert S. Banker

VOLUME 2

PHARMACEUTICAL DOSAGE FORMS

1

Mixing

Russell J. Lantz, Jr.

Lantz Consultants, Salem, South Carolina

Joseph B. Schwartz

Philadelphia College of Pharmacy and Science, Philadelphia, Pennsylvania

I. INTRODUCTION

Almost every industry depends in some way on a blending or mixing operation at some stage of manufacture. Figure 1 is a tabulation of some typical dry blending operations [1]. Mixing is a process that affects us in almost all walks of life. Many people who may utilize mixing on a daily basis are totally unaware of the principles and theory of this unit operation, e.g., the cook who blends the dry salt, flour, baking powder, etc., for a cake; the mason's helper who learns the importance of pre-blending the sand, gravel, and cement before adding the water; and the gardener who mixes the loams with peat moss and fertilizer to obtain a uniform potting soil. Although each of these examples does not have stringent specifications for completeness (uniformity) of mix, there is some point of mixing below which the outcome of the final product is affected adversely. In pharmacy, however, the mixing objective is clear: one is attempting to obtain dosage units each of which will contain the same quantity of medicament. The most elementary approach to the mixing subject can be illustrated by the hand mixing methods used not too long ago in pharmaceutical dispensing [2].

Spatulation—mixing of small quantities of powders on paper or on a
pill tile using a spatula.

Trituration—mixing powders using a mortar and pestle.

Sifting—passing ingredients through a sieve not only yields mixing,
but also aids the dispersion of agglomerated particles.

Tumbling—mixing ingredients by tumbling in a partially filled, closed
container. This method yields a minimum of mixture particle size
reduction.

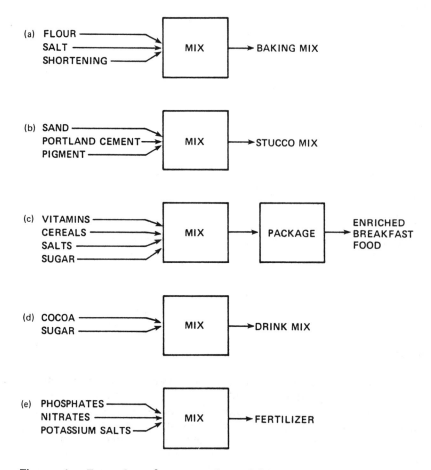

Figure 1   Examples of common dry mixing.

Geometric dilution—in which each of the previous methods may incorporate to aid in the more thorough mixing of potent smaller quantities of active ingredients into the larger bulk of the mix. This
is achieved by first mixing the active ingredient with an equal
amount of diluent; mixing, then adding an amount of diluent equal
to this mix; mixing, etc., until the desired dilution and mixing
has been obtained.

For large-scale industrial pharmaceutical mixing, only the size of the batch
has changed. The same objectives are present.

Assuming that a tablet formula has been developed that performs its
function in the desired manner (i.e., flowability, compressibility, disintegration, dissolution, etc.), the ultimate objective of pharmaceutical
processing is to produce each batch of this product (from hundreds to
thousands of kg/batch) uniformly: not a small task.

A considerable amount of literature has been published on tablet manufacturing, formulation, stability and in vitro—in vivo correlations with formulas, granulating, etc. The authors acknowledge this information. However, the purpose of this chapter is to discuss, from a practical point of view, the unit operation of mixing or blending as it relates to the production of tablets. Although, some basic theory (used to validate the principles involved) and many of the problems encountered during mixing will be discussed, the information for the most part will be based on the authors' experiences and not a literature review of the subject. The basic objectives in mixing are to obtain dosage units each of which contain the same ratio of ingredients, and to replicate this procedure with each batch.

II. THE MIXING PROCESS

A. Definition of Mixing

The American College Dictionary [3] differentiates between the words "mix" and "blend" in that blending is a way of mixing. The definitions are as follows:

> *Mix* (verb): to put together (substances or things, or one substance or thing with another) in one mass or assemblage with more or less thorough diffusion of the constituent elements among one another.
> *Blend* (verb): to mix smoothly and inseparably together.

The terms are very close in definition and are commonly used interchangeably in the industry. However, an attempt will be made to use these two terms properly as they apply to the mixing unit operation in this chapter.

Therefore, from the definition above, mixing is the thorough putting together of ingredients. The mixing of solid particles is accomplished through three principle mechanisms [4-6].

1. Diffusion—the redistribution of particles by the random movement of particles relative one to the other.
2. Convection—the movement of groups of adjacent particles from one place to another within the mixture.
3. Shear —the change in the configuration of ingredients through the formation of slip planes in the mixture.

Diffusion is sometimes referred to in the literature as "micromixing" [7], whereas convection is referred to as "macromixing" [7,8]. These three principal mechanisms are illustrated in Figure 2.

B. Solid—Solid Mixing

The unit operation of solid—solid mixing can be separated into four principal steps [9]:

1. The bed of solid particles expands.
2. Three dimensional shear forces become active in the power bed.

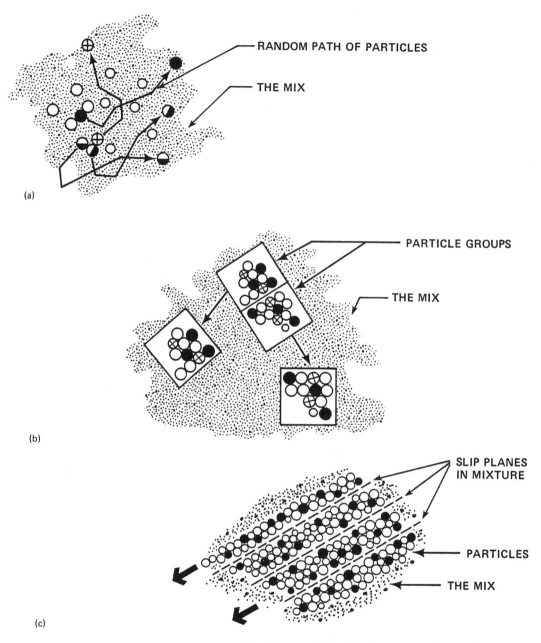

Figure 2   Principal mechanisms of mixing. (a) Diffusion — random action of individual particles in the mix, (b) convection — transfer of adjacent particles groups in the mix, and (c) shear — configuration change through slip planes.

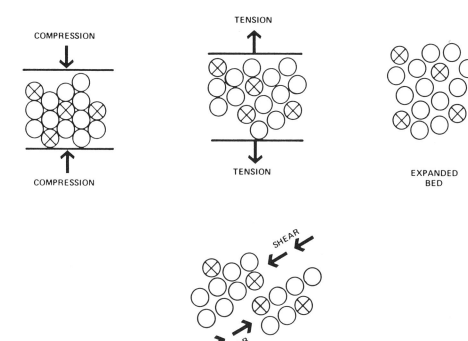

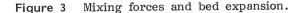

Figure 3   Mixing forces and bed expansion.

3. The powder bed is mixed long enough to permit true randomization of particles.
4. Randomization (no segregation), of the particles is maintained after mixing has stopped.

Initially, when dry materials or particles are loaded into a mixer, they form a static bed. Before mixing or interparticulate movement can take place, this static bed must expand as shown in Figure 3 [9], as a result of mixing forces. It must be noted that before a particle bed can expand for mixing, there must be room for it to expand, i.e., there must be enough additional void space remaining in the mixer for expansion after it has been charged with the ingredients to be blended.

Once particle movement is made possible with the expansion of the powder bed, shear forces are necessary to produce movement between particles. Tension and compression forces merely change the bed volume (Fig. 3).

Induction of movement in all three directions requires adequate three-dimensional stress resulting in the essential random and sometimes turbulent particle movement. Should these forces be inadequate, i.e., high enough to overcome particle surface energies, dead spaces in the form of particle agglomerates in the powder bed move together without being dispersed throughout the powder bed resulting in a poor mix.

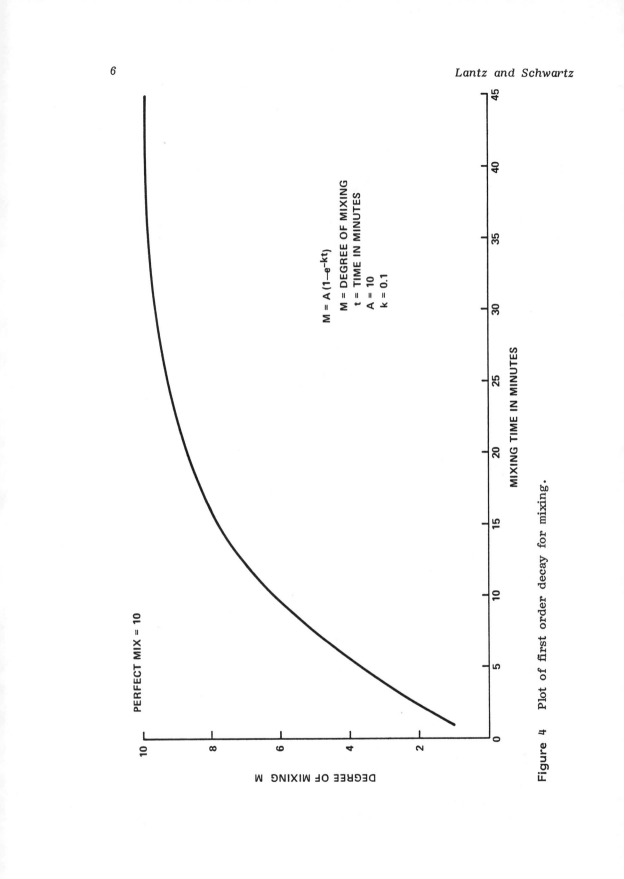

PERFECT MIX = 10

$M = A\,(1-e^{-kt})$

M = DEGREE OF MIXING
t = TIME IN MINUTES
A = 10
k = 0.1

DEGREE OF MIXING M

MIXING TIME IN MINUTES

Figure 4   Plot of first order decay for mixing.

Mixing is an energy-consuming process which produces a random distribution of particles. It is dependent on the probability that an event happens in a given time. The law of mixing appears to follow a first order decay [9]:

$$M = A (1 - e^{-kt})$$
(1)

where

M = resistance to mixing

t = time

A = initial resistance of the dry powder or granules

k = rate at which fine powder components disperse throughout entire system

Therefore, in addition to minimal energy levels required to overcome interparticle forces, mixing results are a function of time. The initial rate of mixing is usually very rapid, while the end point or perfect mixture approaches infinity and in time is not attainable because of the asymptotic characteristic of equation (1) and its relation to the economics of the process.

If we assign 10 to the constant A (fairly high resistance to movement) and 0.1 (an average for this constant depicting dispersion rate) to the constant k, and select specific time intervals, the plot in Figure 4 is obtained. For this particular set of values for the A and k constants, it appears from the curve that the best mixing time, from a practical point of view, would fall between 30 and 35 min. This is valid, because the most rapid change in rate of the slope (mixing rate) has been passed, and the asymptotic portion of the curve has been reached within the 30 to 35 min time period. This will be discussed in more detail later in problems of scale-up.

Once the desired mixing has been attained, it is essential that the particles in the mix cease movement such that the system may exist in a state of static equilibrium without segregation taking place [9]. This is an important point since each subsequent handling of the mixture jeopardizes the static equilibrium. This is particularly true if the mixture is allowed to free-fall during a transfer from one container to another, or the powder mix has been aerated excessively during mixing, while the air escapes rapidly when mixing ceases.

Although unusual characteristics peculiar to specific particulate systems may create complications now and then, poor mixtures usually result from violating one or any combinations of the four principle steps that take place during mixing [9].

C. Liquid–Solid Mixing

In addition to solids–solids blending, the mechanics of liquid–solids blending must also be considered in the "Mixing Process" because it is also a very important process for obtaining tablet products. This process is known as wet granulation. The term liquid–solids blending is used because the liquid which, in most instances, constitutes a minor ingredient

1. AGGLOMERATION

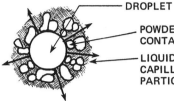

a. INITIAL LIQUID PARTICLE CONTACT

— DROPLET

— POWDER PARTICLES CONTACTING LIQUID SURFACE

— LIQUID MIGRATION BY CAPILLARY ACTION THOUGH PARTICLE INTERSTICES

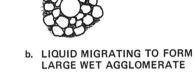

b. **LIQUID MIGRATING TO FORM LARGE WET AGGLOMERATE**

2. AGGLOMERATION BREAKDOWN

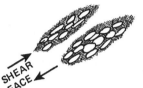

SHEAR FACE

a. **LARGE AGGLOMERATES SHEAR APART BY MIXER FORCE**

b. **MORE DRY PARTICLES CONTACTING AGGLOMERATES**

c. **LESS LIQUID AT PARTICLE SURFACE AS AGGLOMERATES BREAKDOWN**

3. REAGGLOMERATION

PARTICLE POINT CONTACT BRIDGED BY BINDER SOLUTION AND/OR SOLUBILIZED INGREDIENT

4. PASTE FORMATION

WET MASS WITH MUCH LOSS OF DISCRETE PARTICLE UNITS

Figure 5   Stages of liquid solids mixing.

as compared to the percentage of solids, is added to the solids or powder bed.

Granulation may be considered the opposite of size reduction, i.e., particle growth. According to the current technology, granulation may be defined as particle agglomeration. The four general powder properties necessary to yield a satisfactory tablet product include:

1. Compressibility
2. Flow
3. Wetability
4. Lubricity

Compressibility and flow are dictated by the manufacturing method, while wettability and lubricity are usually the result of selected additives incorporated into a formula.

When one is unable to produce a tablet via direct compression, or dry granulation (slugging or compacting) it is necessary to use the wet granulation process. Wet granulation is a complicated process requiring the following steps:

1. Preblending the dry ingredients
2. Addition of the granulating liquid
3. Kneading and/or mixing
4. Wet or coarse milling of the wet granulation
5. Drying the granules
6. Milling the dried granules
7. Mixing the milled granules alone or with additives for lubrication and disintegration, etc.

In steps 2 and 3 above, a number of stages occur during the addition of a liquid to a powder bed being mixed as shown in Figure 5 (a high-shear mixer is necessary for liquid–solid mixing)

1. *Agglomeration*. Droplets of solvent such as water or alcohol or binding solution, e.g., polyvinyl pyrrolidone dissolved in water, contact the moving powder particles that adhere to, and build up around the periphery of each droplet. As more powder particles are wetted by the liquid, the liquid migrates in part by capillary action (pendular and/or funicular) [11] into the particle–particle interstices, and forms large power–liquid agglomerates. It is assumed that the interfacial tension between the liquid and solids in the mixture is low enough to permit at least fair wetting. If this is not the case, the addition of a surface active agent may be necessary. In any case particles adhere to particles, building the agglomerate to a size of 1–5 cm in diameter or greater.

2. *Agglomeration Breakdown*. After the initial large agglomerate formation phase, mixing shear and tensional forces begin to break the large agglomerates down. In this phase, the liquid is carried throughout the mixture via smaller agglomerates which continue to diminish in size as the liquid is more uniformly distributed over the powder particles' surfaces (capillary state) [11]. At this point, no hard agglomerates are detectable, and the wet mass easily crumbles to a powder if compacted by the grip of a hand. It must be noted that liquid bridging is probably the most prevalent force in holding these small agglomerates of small particles together.

3. *Reagglomeration*. As mixing proceeds and the liquid becomes completely distributed throughout the mixture, the powder bed assumes the properties of a wet mass acting very similar to a highly viscous slurry. This slurry resists shear forces and begins to generate heat as particle to particle contact increases requiring more mixer shear force for continued mixing. Increased particle to particle contact is a result of air displacement by liquid at the particle surface. Other resistant shear forces include liquid viscosity and/or partial solubilization of some of the more soluble ingredients that may be present in the formula. This solubilization creates resistance to the high-shear mixing, because it usually contributes to the increased viscosity of the liquid phase of the mixture. A wide size–range of agglomerates can be seen forming in the mixture as mixing

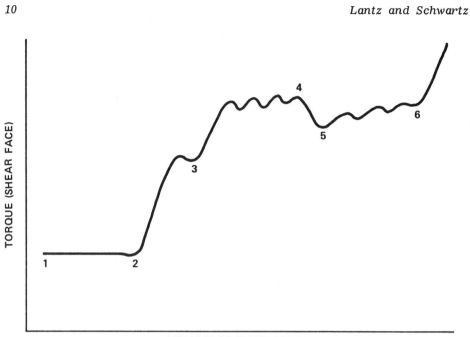

Figure 6   Shear force required during wet-down in wet granulating.

proceeds. The wet granulation mixing end point has heretofore normally
been gauged by how easily a wet compaction (which would not reduce
back to a powder) could be formed in the grip of a hand (near the capillary state and possibly into the droplet state) [11]. More recently,
there have been more scientific approaches to determining this end point.
Measurements of mixer shear force, as seen in Figure 6, show that earlier
scientific approaches were based on mixer power draw measurements.
This was accomplished by a special torque sensing setup on the mixer
blade, since ampere meters were not that accurate nor reproducible [10]
for indicating a granulation end point. A properly granulated formula
may not require a wet milling if it dries easily and forms granules that
are easily dry milled to the desired size, and yields satisfactory flow and
compaction characteristics in the tablet machine.

4. *Paste Formation (the droplet stage).* If mixing is continued beyond the normal granulating end point (which is different for each formula),
a thick wet mass resembling a paste begins to form as a result of solubilization, solvation, etc. This paste, unlike the granulation at its end point,
may be difficult to break up for drying, may dry to extremely hard granules which may be difficult to mill and in many cases forms a poor compaction in the tablet machine.

As one can see, the wetting and kneading steps bring into play very
complex internal forces during wet granulation. Scientifically sorting out
the complexities of these steps is the key to determining an accurate, reproducible wet-granulation-mixing end point. Work conducted by Schwartz
et al. [12] shows the affect of water addition on the viscosity of a

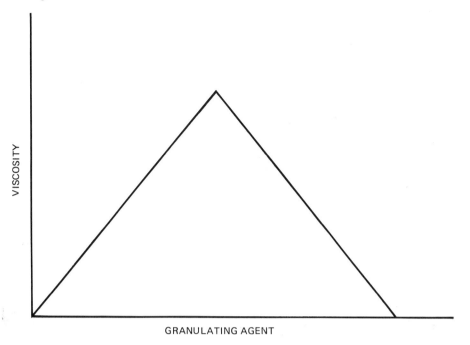

VISCOSITY

GRANULATING AGENT

Figure 7   Hypothetical "viscosity" profile of a powder wetting procedure.

granulation, and is shown diagrammatically in Figure 7.   Experimental work shown in Figure 8, using microcrystalline cellulose, illustrates a "good" and "overwetted" granulation along with a slurry.   Figure 9 shows the difference in wetting profiles for microcrystalline cellulose, calcium phosphate and lactose USP, hydrous.   It is not surprising that different materials yield different profiles.

Schwartz et al. note that granulation viscosity is a function of mixing times, as shown in Figure 10.   These studies extended to further analysis, paralleling the work in Ref. 11, also demonstrate a relation between mixing time and the dried granulation particle (Fig. 11).

D.   Perfect Mixture

As previously illustrated with Eq. (1) (Fig. 4), the mixing process will never yield an ideal or perfect mixture defined as: "that state in which any sample removed from the mixture will have exactly the same composition as all other samples taken from the mix."   The perfect mixture is illustrated in Figure 12a by a chess board with the black and white squares representing two separate components [13].   If one samples two adjacent squares at each sampling, the composition will be identical throughout the lot (also, see Sec. IV, on the sampling and statistics of mixing).

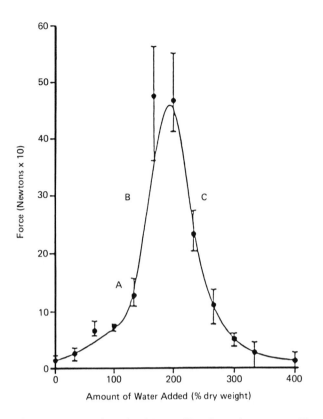

Figure 8 Solid−liquid profile for microcrystalline cellulose PH-101. A = 'good' granulation, B = overwet granulation, C = slurry.

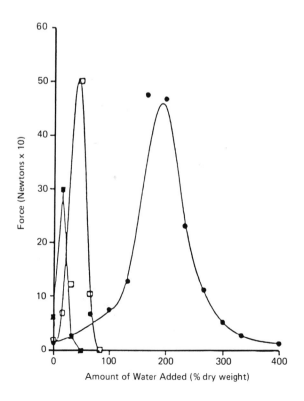

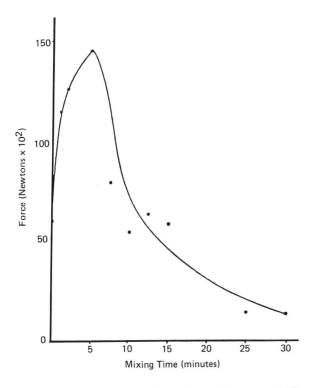

Figure 10 Force readings from the granulation rheology apparatus as a function of mixing time for microcrystalline cellulose PH-101. (From Ref. 12.)

E. Alternatives to the Perfect Mixture

Since the perfect (Fig. 12a) mix cannot be achieved, consideration must be given to other alternatives for obtaining an acceptable mix of a particular formula. First, there is randomization or random mixing which is that state in which the probability of finding a particle of a given component is the same at all points in the mixture [13], and is in the same ratio of components in the entire mixture. A chess board randomization is shown in Figure 12b for two components.

For illustration purposes Lacey [4] takes a binary system of composition "a" and "b" and expresses the theoretical standard deviation (see Sec. IV) of the unmixed components as:

$$\sigma_o = ab \tag{2}$$

Figure 9 Solid—liquid profiles for three common tablet excipients. Key: (●) microcrystalline cellulose PH-101, (○) calcium phosphate, (■) lactose USP, hydrous. (From Ref. 12.)

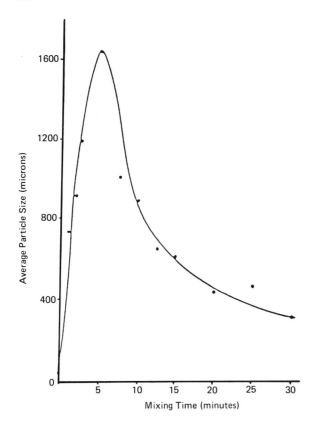

Figure 11 Particle size of the dried granulation as a function of increased mixing time for microcrystalline cellulose PH-101. (From Ref. 12.)

where "a" and "b" are proportions of the two ingredients. Lacey then shows the theoretical standard deviation for the totally randomized mixture to be:

$$\sigma_t = \sqrt{\frac{ab}{n}} \qquad\qquad (3)$$

where n represents the total number of particles in the blend.

Therefore, if one has a particulate system with 20,000 total particles with a fraction of the lower concentration ingredient "a" at 2%, the totally randomized mix at the best attainable level is calculated to be:

$$\sigma_t = \sqrt{\frac{98 \times 2}{20,000}} = 0.099\% \qquad\qquad (4)$$

There is a constraint on this mixing study in that the particle size and densities of both components "a" and "b" were identical. Empirically, degree of randomness is determined by taking a series of samples.

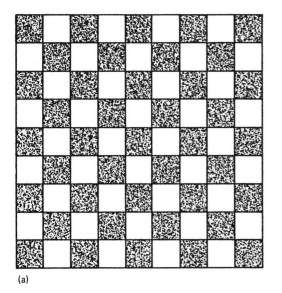 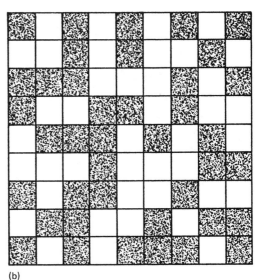

(a)   (b)

Figure 12 Illustrations of perfect and randomized binary mixtures.
(a) Perfect mix and (b) randomized mix.

Referring again to the chess board in Figure 12b, it can be seen that if
two adjacent squares are sampled in the random mix, as they were in the
perfect mix (Fig. 12a), the composition of this sample will not always be
the same, i.e., there is a probability that two black squares or two
squares or two white squares will be sampled instead of a black and white
square. This is the reason that accurately evaluating the quality of a
random mix is dependent on the number and size of samples rather than a
single sample.

For purposes of economics, the extent of the degree of randomization
must also be considered. Referring to the first order of decay plot in
Figure 4, one determines at which point in time a particular mixture has
been mixed long enough to yield an acceptable randomization of the ingredients without using excessive time and energy.

A second alternative to the perfect mixture is ordered mixing. The
theory of ordered mixing was developed by Hersey [14]. Ordered mixing
is described as the use of mechanical, adhesional, or coating forces or
methods to prepare ordered units in the mix such that the ordered unit
will be the smallest possible sample of the mix, and will be of near
identical composition to all other ordered units in the mix [15], e.g., a
dry granule made by wet granulation or a coated particle such as we see
in fluid bed granulating.

Ordered mixing probably comes the closest to yielding the perfect
mix and may be obtained in a number of ways [15]:

1. Mechanical means. Dividing and recombining the powder bed any
   number of times until the desired subdivision unit is obtained as
   illustrated in Figure 13. The smaller the units, the more uniform

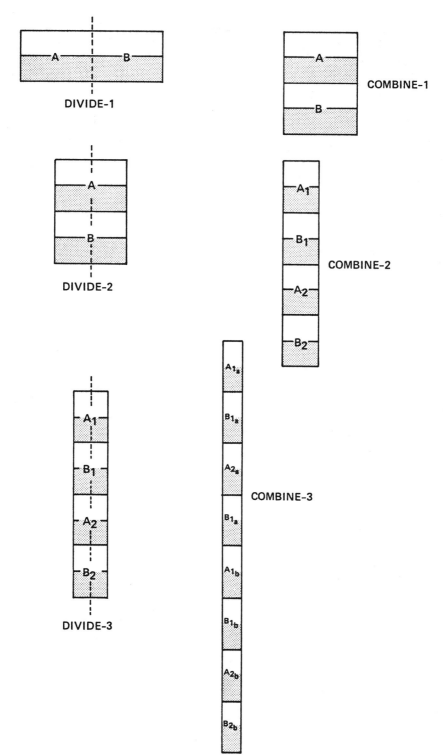

Figure 13 Ordered mixing — mechanically.

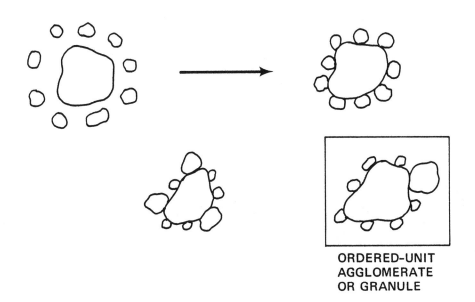

ADHESIONAL OR BINDING FORCES

ORDERED–UNIT
AGGLOMERATE
OR GRANULE

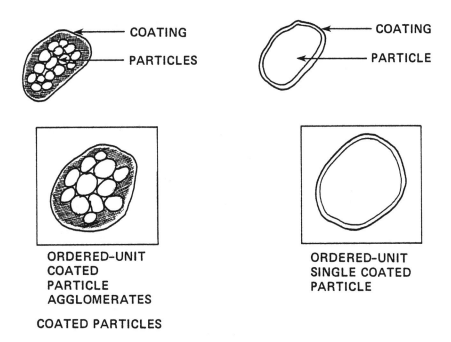

COATING

PARTICLES

COATING

PARTICLE

ORDERED–UNIT
COATED
PARTICLE
AGGLOMERATES

COATED PARTICLES

ORDERED–UNIT
SINGLE COATED
PARTICLE

Figure 14   Ordered mixing by adhesion.

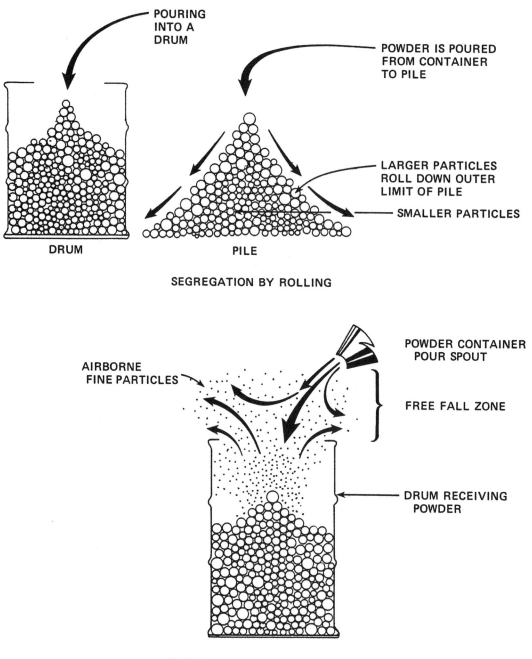

POURING
INTO A
DRUM

POWDER IS POURED
FROM CONTAINER
TO PILE

LARGER PARTICLES
ROLL DOWN OUTER
LIMIT OF PILE

SMALLER PARTICLES

DRUM   PILE

SEGREGATION BY ROLLING

POWDER CONTAINER
POUR SPOUT

AIRBORNE
FINE PARTICLES

FREE FALL ZONE

DRUM RECEIVING
POWDER

SEGREGATION BY DUSTING

Figure 15   Segregation by pouring.

the mix. However, if no particulate adhesion is present, segregation of the mix easily takes place on further handling.

2. Adhesion. Adhesional forces of particles may create ordered units of near identical composition depending on the process. Partial solubilization or the use of a binding agent during wet granulating approximates the same effect as shown in Fig. 14a.

3. Coating. Figure 14b shows that particles in an assemblage may also be coated with other ingredients to give an ordered mix either as individual or coated particle agglomerates.

The major difference between the mechanical and the adhesional and coated ordered mixing is the degree of force holding the ingredients in each type of the ordered units together.

Ordered mixing is not only beneficial in approaching a perfect mixture, but it minimizes the possibility of segregation of a mixture by holding the ingredient ratio constant via the intact ordered units. Segregation occurs primarily as a result of wide differences in particle size in a dry mixture. Segregation may be produced by pouring a powder from one container to the next as is done by emptying the contents of a blender into another hopper or into drums. This is illustrated in Figure 15a. Note that the

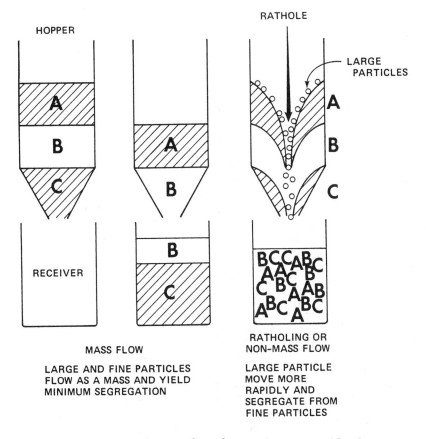

Figure 16   Segregation by flow from a hopper or blender.

larger particles, because of their mass, have a tendency to roll down the outside of the powder pile segregating the coarse and fine particles. A second means of segregation, dusting, may also take place during pouring of a powder, particularly if there is considerable free fall of the particles as shown in Figure 15b. In this case the fine particles become airborne and separate from the bulk of the powder. Segregation may also take place inside the blender when the powder bed does not exhibit mass flow characteristics, i.e., the powder does not flow from a hopper or mixer in the order in which it is situated in the container. This is illustrated in Figure 16, which shows the difference between mass flow and "ratholing." In this case, the large particles move as the power structure breaks down because of their larger mass, leaving the smaller structured particles behind.

III. HOMOGENEITY

It is necessary that one be able to describe the degree of mixing obtained in a given mixing operation. Much of the available mixing literature is devoted to discussions and proposals to measure and compare homogeneity or "degree of mixedness" by some mixing index. These mixing indices are then used to follow a mixing process with time, to compare mixers, to compare the mixing operation as it is scaled up, and to investigate the mechanism of mixing in a given piece of equipment. For the most part, these mixing indices are derived or empirically modified from binary systems which contain monosized particles having the same density. In the opinion of the authors, these are of little, if any utility in solving pharmaceutical mixing problems, from the practical approach. However, they are necessary for developing and illustrating some basic mixing theory. For practical purposes, the authors suggest that the guidelines set forth in the section on "Sampling and Statistics of Mixing" are adequate. The investigator must keep his particular objective in mind when selecting the parameter he or she intends to use.

The majority of mixing indices involve some comparison of the measured standard deviation [5] of the samples of the mixture under study with the estimated standard deviation of a completely random mixture (σ_r). The standard deviation of a completely unmixed system (σ_0) is included by some authors [16]. For this reason, these mixing indices are mentioned here for the sake of information completeness. The use of the associated equations will not be demonstrated. The interested reader is referred to to the following references for further study: Lacey [17], Stange [18], Poole et al. [19], Ashton et al. [20], Williams [21], Buslik [22], and Harnby [23].

The various mixing indices, over thirty in all, were reviewed and tabulated by Fan et al. [24]. In a separate report [25], Fan and Wang selected the nine most frequently used mixing indices and related them, one to another. Several of these are listed in Table 1. Several other parameters have been suggested as methods of determining degree of mixedness including Hersey's "Mixing Margin" and Buslik's "Homogeneity Index" [26]. In addition Lai and Wang and Fan have suggested the use of nonparametric statistics to sampling in solid mixing [27].

Unless one is investigating the mechanism of mixing, the authors recommend that the method used to determine homogeneity in a mixture be

Table 1 Mixing Indices

Mixing index	Comment	Ref.
$M = \dfrac{\sigma_R}{\sigma}$	This ratio is less than one	24
$M = \dfrac{\sigma_0 - \sigma}{\sigma_0 - \sigma_R}$	This ratio is less than one	4
$M = \dfrac{\sigma_0^2 - \sigma^2}{\sigma_0^2 - \sigma_R^2}$	This ratio is less than one	4
$M = \dfrac{\sigma}{\sigma_R}$	Ratio greater than one. Better differentiation between mixtures	19
$M^2 = \dfrac{\log \sigma_0^2 - \log \sigma^2}{\log \sigma_R^2 - \log \sigma_0^2}$		20

M = degree of mixedness, σ_0 = standard deviation of unmixed system, and σ_R = standard deviation of completely randomized mixture.

suited to the objective at hand. Other primary configurations include: the effort (including analytical support available), and the accuracy required.

IV. SAMPLING AND STATISTICS OF MIXING

Sampling is an integral part of the statistics of mixing. This is particularly true during the evaluation and qualification of new or existing mixing equipment, and is absolutely necessary for the mixing operation of a product validation. From many years of experience, the authors have found that in a majority of cases, people do not often have mixing problems, but actually have sampling problems.

To begin with, random samples are used to generate the data necessary to estimate the true mean and standard deviation of the mixture. This is accomplished in two stages (28):

1. The estimation of the true arithmetic mean and the true standard deviation of a mixture
2. An accuracy and precision assessment of these estimates

Precision is normally expressed in terms of confidence in which these estimates will fall within specified limits [28]. These limits are derived from the assays of the samples which, with few exceptions, follow a Gaussian distribution yielding a normal or bell type curve.

The data for the statistics are developed by assaying, or in some manner identifying the active ingredient(s) in a number of random samples taken from the blend at a specified time. The mean assay value of a group of random samples taken from a mixture is a measure of the central tendency of the batch population (active ingredient content). The arithmetic mean value is given by

$$\overline{y} = \sum_{i}^{n} y_i/n \qquad\qquad (5)$$

where

y_i = the value of a given sample

n = the number of samples

Since it is impractical to sample and assay the entire batch to obtain a true mean $\underline{u}$, a limited number of samples are taken and an estimate of the true mean $\overline{y}$ is calculated from these samples. In addition to the estimated mean $\overline{y}$ of the true mean $\underline{u}$, an additional statistic is calculated to describe or characterize the spread or dispersion of individual samples about the mean $\overline{y}$. This is the standard deviation S for n number of random samples, which is given by

$$S = \sqrt{\frac{\sum_{i}^{n} (y_i - \overline{y})^2}{n - 1}} \qquad\qquad (6)$$

Based on the numbers of samples used to obtain the $\overline{y}$ estimate of the true mean $\underline{u}$, so the standard deviation S is an estimate of the true population standard deviation σ of the total mixture.

For computational purposes the standard deviation may also be expressed as

$$S = \sqrt{\frac{\sum_{i}^{n} \overline{y}^2 - \frac{1}{n}\left(\sum_{i}^{n} \overline{y}\right)^2}{n - 1}} \qquad\qquad (7)$$

The square of the stand deviation S^2 is called the variance which is also used to characterize a mixture because of its additive properties.

$$S^2 = \frac{\sum_{i}^{n} (y_i - \overline{y})^2}{n - 1} \qquad\qquad (8)$$

Again, this value is an estimate of the true variance σ^2 of the mixture.

Table 2 Five- and 10-Min Mix-Time Assay
Data

Sample No.	5-min mix time	10-min mix time
1	4.90	5.20
2	5.10	5.00
3	5.10	5.00
4	5.10	5.10
5	4.80	5.00
6	4.90	4.90
7	5.30	5.10
8	5.00	5.00
9	5.20	5.00
10	4.90	5.00
11	4.90	4.90
12	4.70	4.90
13	5.10	4.80
14	5.00	5.00
15	4.80	5.20
16	5.00	5.10
17	5.00	4.80
18	5.00	5.10
19	5.20	4.90
20	5.00	5.00

It is logical that the simple course is to take random samples from different parts of the mixer and analyze them for the component of interest.
An example of tabulated assay data from a mixture mixed for 5 and 10
min is shown in Table 2. These data are put into frequency distribution
curves in Figure 17. Each sample has a mean assay $\bar{y}$ of 5.00. However, note that the scatter about the mean or standard deviation S is
greater at the shorter mixing time.

The higher standard deviation indicates less uniformity of the mixture
assuming minimal variation in the assay method.

One may also follow the mixing operation in a given process by plotting
the standard deviation as a function of time as shown in Figure 18.

If one wishes to compare the efficiency of two or more mixing operations and has different sample sizes or different compositions, the relative
standard deviation (RSD) should replace the standard deviation as a
measure of sample uniformity. The relative standard deviation is the
standard deviation divided by the mean, i.e.

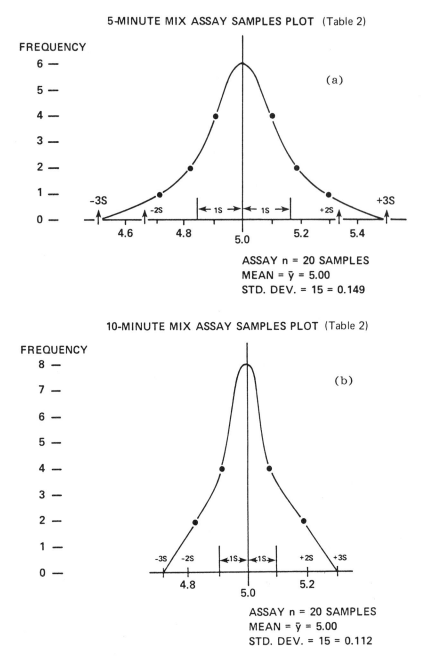

Figure 17 Frequency distribution curves. (a) Five-min mix assay samples plot (Table 2) and (b) 10-min mix assay samples (Table 2).

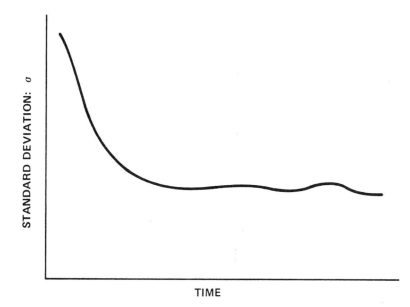

Figure 18   Standard deviation of a mixture as a function of time.

$$\mathrm{RSD} = \frac{\sigma}{\bar{y}} \qquad\qquad (9)$$

This value is usually expressed as a percent, by multiplying the values by 100.

It is important to note at this point that differences in the assay mean from the assay theory may not only indicate homogeneity problems, but may also be the result of poor or inadequate sampling, improper handling of the powder for assay in the lab, or may point up an assay method problem. The same is true when considering the standard deviation of a mixture. Therefore, it is essential that each of these variables, which may contribute to differences in the mean and standard deviation of a mixture, be investigated thoroughly. In this manner, one may determine the extent to which these variables contribute to the overall mean and standard deviation of the mixture.

A mixture begins with the unmixed dry ingredients represented in Figure 19a, as a binary mixture. After mixing an adequate length of time, a randomized mixture results as seen in Figure 19b. For comparison, refer back to the perfect mixture as represented in Figure 12a. The problem is how to differentiate between the three mixtures, i.e., how to determine the quality of each mixture. To illustrate the problems one may encounter, both the unmixed and randomized mixture have several possible sample sizes shown (sample through X for 1/2 the mix; sample through Y for 1/8 the mix; and sample through Z for 1/32 of the mix). Each sample when assayed will show 50% white and 50% black squares. This indicates a perfect mix for each example. It is obvious these are erroneous results

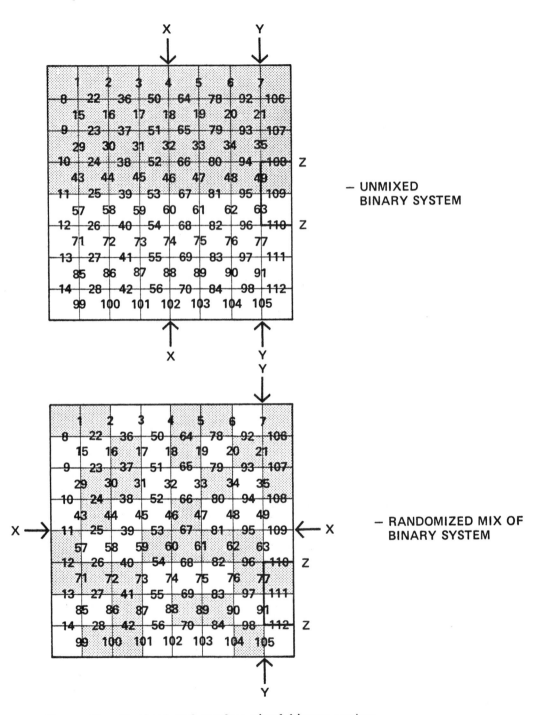

Figure 19   Unmixed and random mixed binary system.

because the two samples have not been distinguished from the perfect mix, or from each other, and all three examples are different mixtures.

The solution to the problem lies within certain statistical guidelines including:

1. The proper number of samples required should be no less than 20, preferably 30, and more ideally 100. The larger the number of samples obtained and assayed per granulation sampling time, the greater the confidence in estimating the true mean and standard deviation of the mixture at that time. Since economics plays a major role in limiting the number of samples assays in a production atmosphere, many of the examples shown in this chapter will be composed of 20 samples. From a more realistic point of view, uniformity of a mix is determined on 10 individual sample assays for validation of the mixing process. This is based on the 10 individual tablet uniformity tests cited in the (USP) [29]. It is advisable to take at least 20 unit dose samples and use them only if necessary. In this way validation batches will not have to be rerun perchance one or more of the original samples have been handled improperly, spilled, or lost.

2. Random sampling is the method of choice for the statistic.

3. The sampling size for determining content uniformity should approximate the unit dose size of the final product. This is an absolute necessity to show process control at the mixing stage of the product manufacture.

4. Comparison between the mean value of the sample analysis and the target value gives the first estimate of the degree of mixing.

5. If the mean value of the sample analysis is on or near the target value, then calculation of the standard deviation (and/or variance) will give an indication of the uniformity of the samples. The acceptance criteria for uniformity is the USP test [29] for tablet uniformity.

Applying these guidelines to the examples in Figures 19a and b, the unit sample or smallest unit dose is two adjacent squares, since the example is a binary mixture.

To illustrate the random sampling of each of these examples, the units of all two adjacent square possibilities in Figures 19 a and b have been numbered on each chess board. Both examples have been randomly sampled for 20 samples using a table of random numbers. This sampling has been repeated three times as shown in Tables 3 and 4. Note the differences in assays of each table. There is one overlap at 55%, but the unmixed system shows a much wider spread from the theoretical mean in the three assay groups than does the random mixed sample. Note that the random mixed sample shows some variation as it should when compared to the perfect mixture which will show no spread in the assay if samples in the same manner.

Statistically, one may sample using one or two approaches: (a) by not returning the sample to the mixture after evaluating it, or (b) by returning the sample to the mixture after its evaluation. Destructive testing

Table 3   Random Sampling of Unmixed Binary System

Sample no.	Assay group 1			Assay group 2			Assay group 3		
	*	B	W	*	B	W	*	B	W
1	42	0	1	9	1	0	39	½	½
2	6	1	0	102	0	1	37	1	0
3	56	0	1	83	0	1	112	0	1
4	101	0	1	32	1	0	110	0	1
5	51	1	0	77	0	1	45	1	0
6	74	0	1	80	1	0	54	0	1
7	42	0	1	38	1	0	75	0	1
8	77	0	1	47	1	0	7	1	0
9	86	0	1	64	1	0	94	1	0
10	64	1	0	41	0	1	108	1	0
11	7	1	0	54	0	1	107	1	0
12	29	1	0	98	0	1	102	0	1
13	110	0	1	88	0	1	73	0	1
14	4	1	0	34	1	0	74	0	1
15	46	1	0	72	0	1	53	½	½
16	70	0	1	37	1	0	47	1	0
17	87	0	1	19	1	0	35	1	0
18	55	0	1	108	1	0	52	1	0
19	83	0	1	55	0	1	5	1	0
20	76	0	1	43	1	0	18	1	0
		7	13		11	9		12	8

Percent of active (B):   7/20 = 35%   11/20 = 55%   12/20 = 60%

Theoretical mean = 50%

*Random number selection.

Table 4   Random Sampling of Random Mixture of Binary System

Sample no.	Assay group 1			Assay group 2			Assay group 3		
	*	B	W	*	B	W	*	B	W
1	100	1	0	55	0	1	91	0	1
2	84	$\frac{1}{2}$	$\frac{1}{2}$	53	$\frac{1}{2}$	$\frac{1}{2}$	83	$\frac{1}{2}$	$\frac{1}{2}$
3	98	$\frac{1}{2}$	$\frac{1}{2}$	22	$\frac{1}{2}$	$\frac{1}{2}$	76	$\frac{1}{2}$	$\frac{1}{2}$
4	44	$\frac{1}{2}$	$\frac{1}{2}$	74	0	1	108	$\frac{1}{2}$	$\frac{1}{2}$
5	5	1	0	102	0	1	69	$\frac{1}{2}$	$\frac{1}{2}$
6	10	0	1	24	1	0	104	$\frac{1}{2}$	$\frac{1}{2}$
7	17	$\frac{1}{2}$	$\frac{1}{2}$	17	$\frac{1}{2}$	$\frac{1}{2}$	86	$\frac{1}{2}$	$\frac{1}{2}$
8	99	$\frac{1}{2}$	$\frac{1}{2}$	30	1	0	102	0	1
9	73	$\frac{1}{2}$	$\frac{1}{2}$	15	0	1	62	1	0
10	93	$\frac{1}{2}$	$\frac{1}{2}$	54	$\frac{1}{2}$	$\frac{1}{2}$	98	$\frac{1}{2}$	$\frac{1}{2}$
11	20	$\frac{1}{2}$	$\frac{1}{2}$	99	$\frac{1}{2}$	$\frac{1}{2}$	6	$\frac{1}{2}$	$\frac{1}{2}$
12	53	$\frac{1}{2}$	$\frac{1}{2}$	105	$\frac{1}{2}$	$\frac{1}{2}$	12	1	0
13	35	$\frac{1}{2}$	$\frac{1}{2}$	93	$\frac{1}{2}$	$\frac{1}{2}$	18	$\frac{1}{2}$	$\frac{1}{2}$
14	62	1	0	89	1	0	3	0	1
15	111	$\frac{1}{2}$	$\frac{1}{2}$	33	$\frac{1}{2}$	$\frac{1}{2}$	13	$\frac{1}{2}$	$\frac{1}{2}$
16	13	$\frac{1}{2}$	$\frac{1}{2}$	40	$\frac{1}{2}$	$\frac{1}{2}$	30	1	0
17	17	$\frac{1}{2}$	$\frac{1}{2}$	42	1	0	79	$\frac{1}{2}$	$\frac{1}{2}$
18	36	$\frac{1}{2}$	$\frac{1}{2}$	83	$\frac{1}{2}$	$\frac{1}{2}$	75	0	1
19	2	$\frac{1}{2}$	$\frac{1}{2}$	35	$\frac{1}{2}$	$\frac{1}{2}$	33	$\frac{1}{2}$	$\frac{1}{2}$
20	79	$\frac{1}{2}$	$\frac{1}{2}$	8	$\frac{1}{2}$	$\frac{1}{2}$	37	1	0
		11	9		10	10		10	10

Percent of active (B)	11/20 = 55%	10/20 = 50%	10/20 = 50%

Theoretical mean = 50%.

*Random number selection.

such as putting the sample into solution for assay will not permit the
latter sampling approach (b). Therefore, it is necessary to use destructive sampling when checking for distribution of ingredients in a mixed
formula. On the other hand, when working in production quantities
(hundreds of kg), the unit dose sampling of 20−100 samples is infinitely
small when compared to the entire population and may be tested as in
(b) above (returning the samples to the mix before the next sampling).
There are two golden rules of sampling [30]:

1. "a powder should be sampled when it is in motion."
2. "the whole of the stream of powder should be taken for many
   short increments of time, in preference to part of the stream
   being taken for the whole time"

Although these rules are the ultimate in sampling, from a practical point
of view one must be satisfied with less than the ultimate. This is usually
not the choice of the experimenter, but rather limitations of the system.
For example: a number of ingredients are placed in a blender for mixing.
The mixer is activated for various lengths of mixing time. After each
time interval, a number of samples are removed to determine homogeneity
of the mixture. The object: to determine the optimum blending time.
How is each sample removed from a mixer to follow "the golden rule of
sampling"? The powder mixture usually cannot be sampled from a moving
stream because of (a) the configuration of the mixer (i.e., bowl shape
does not lend itself to dumping), (b) the size of the batch (large volumes
are not conducive to routine transfer from the blender to drums or into
large hopper type collectors), and (c) the possibility of mixture segregation biasing the sample. Therefore, one is left with several less than
desirable options including:

1. scoop sampling of the bulk mixture
2. thief probing of the bulk mixture

Each of the sampling options above has limitations and, although they
are discussed at length in the chapter on Size Reduction, comment must
also be made here.
Scoop sampling has two basic drawbacks:

1. Scooping from the top of a container of powder may produce a
   sample which has segregated on standing, i.e., smaller particles
   have sifted down through the interstices of the larger particles
   biasing the sample to the larger particles; or entrapped air
   escaping to the top of the mixture causing locally high concentrations of smaller particles near the surface of the powder bed.
2. Scooping cannot remove a sample from the middle or bottom of a
   blender or container without considerable disturbance of the
   mixture.

The thief probe also has several drawbacks:

1. As the thief is inserted into the powder bed, some compaction
   takes place around the thief and flow into the thief opening may
   be poor.

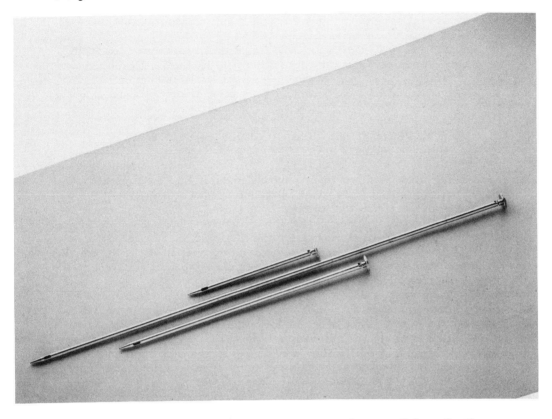

Figure 20   Unit dose thief samplers. (Courtesy Sampco, Salem, South
Carolina.)

   2. As the thief is inserted in the powder bed it may carry material
       from the surface of the mixture down into the mixture depending
       on the diameter of the thief. This may place a portion of "top
       sample" down at the lower portion of the thief, and if a compart-
       mentalized thief is used, the lower samples are biased or contamin-
       ated with top sample.

However, from a practical point of view, the thief probe sample is preferred over the scoop because samples can be taken from deep within the
powder bed, and a reasonable degree of random sampling is achieved. To
further minimize the drawbacks using a thief probe, a small diameter thief
probe is available (see Fig. 20) which allows sampling of mixers, hoppers,
and drums with a minimal of carry-down of top material. The sample
sizes that are removed approximate a tablet unit dose. This allows assay
of the entire sample after it has been removed, which eliminates inad-
vertent excessive handling of a large sample in the lab to obtain a small
enough sample to assay. This eliminates possible segregation before the
sample has been assayed. Excessively handled, large samples usually do
not represent the population removed from the sampled enclosure, or the

population being samples in the enclosure (drum, mixer, storage hopper, etc.).

Probably the most significant measure of quality of a mixture is how the blend actually performs, and the uniformity of the final product. However, Current Good Manufacturing Practice (CGMP) Regulations require documentation of a controlled process at each step of manufacturing.

V. MATERIAL PROPERTIES: BASIC CONCEPTS OF DRY BLENDING—THE UNIT PARTICLE

Since mixing plays such an important role in tableting, an understanding of the characteristics of the materials being mixed is paramount. Many of the studies presented in the literature, and used previously in examples, deal with binary mixtures of physically and chemically similar materials which can easily be differentiated for the study by color, size, or assay. However, pharmaceutical, binary, particulate systems in tableting are the exception, and results dealing with binary systems have limited applicability in industrial practice.

Each component in a mixture has distinct physical characteristics which contribute to, or detract from, the completeness (uniformity) of a mixture. Therefore, it is important to define and characterize the unit particles that make up the mixture, whether it is a premix of a wet granulation, a direct compression formula, or the addition of lubricants, etc., to a granulation. Figure 21 is an illustration of several different types of particles handled in tablet granulation mixing.

The unit particles in a system may range from the less-than-1 μm-size pure substance raw material particle to the 8 to 12 mesh multicomponent granule held together by a binder. Since dry mixing is a dynamic state of an assemblage of particles, the properties of the unit particle must be discussed in terms affecting these dynamics.

There are three properties intrinsic to each component in the mixture: "composition (physicochemical structure), size (and size distribution), and shape" [31].

Composition of each particle is "its qualitative and quantitative makeup" [32]. Each unit of pure substance has its own molecular composition and arrangement that distinguishes it from all other materials, and dictates its behavior in part as a powder per se, or in combination with other tablet mixture ingredients. Chemical composition is important, because chemical reactivity limits a material's use with other tableting components, e.g., acids and bases such as aspirin and phenylpropanolamine would not be blended together because of their potential to react. The same applies to components that may affect the stability of a mixture such as the potential Schiff Base reaction between certain sugars and amines when in contact even in the dry state.

Physically, the molecular makeup determines crystallinity manifested as color, hardness, tackiness, general appearance, etc.

Particle size and size distribution of the unit particles have considerable impact on the flow properties of powders and therefore, the dynamics of mixing. Table 5 shows, in general, the effect of particle size on the flow properties of powders. Table 6 is a list of some common substances used in the pharmaceutical industry, and their flow characteristics. A very complete and detailed list of materials and their characteristics

PURE
SUBSTANCES
DIFFERENT SHAPE
CONFIGURATIONS
INDIVIDUAL
PARTICLES

PURE SUB-
STANCES
AGGLOMERATED
BY FREE SURFACE
ENERGY, ELECTRO-
STATIC FORCES,
ETC.

PURE SUB-
STANCES
AGGREGATED
WITH A
BINDER

PURE SUBSTANCE
COMPACTED AND
MILLED

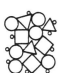

BINARY MIXTURE
AGGLOMERATED BY
FREE SURFACE
ENERGY, ELECTRO-
STATIC FORCES, ETC.

BINARY MIXTURE
AGGREGATED WITH
A BINDER

MULTICOMPONENT
MIXTURE

WET GRANULATED
MULTICOMPONENT
MIXTURE-MILLED

Figure 21   Several different types of particles encountered in tablet granulation dry blending.

may be found in the reference text: *Handbook of Pharmaceutical Excipients* [33].

Large (sieve size range >60 mesh) dry particles have a tendency to flow better than the smaller dry particles, because they have greater mass. Smaller particles (<100 mesh) may create mixing problems because surface areas are very great, and may give rise to strong electrostatic forces as a result of processing and/or inter-particle friction from movement. These forces may prevent the desired distribution of these smaller particles throughout a mixture because of fine particle agglomeration.

As the particle size approaches 10 μm and below, weak polarizing electrical forces called van der Waals forces or cohesive forces also begin to affect the flow of the powder. Both van der Waals and electrostatic forces usually inhibit powder flow through particle agglomeration as mentioned above. However, in some instances improved flow results because

Table 5   Effect of Particle Size on Powder Flow

Particle size	Type of flow[a]	Reason
200–250 μm (10–60[b] mesh)	Flow is usually good if shape is not interfering	Mass of individual particles is relatively large
250–75 μm (60 mesh–200 μm)	Flow properties may be a problem with many pure substances and mixtures	Mass of individual particles is small and increased surface area amplifies effects of surface forces
<100–75 μm	Flow becomes a problem with most substances	Cohesive forces or free surface energy forces are large as well as static electrical forces relative to particle size

[a]Assume particle shape is constant and does not interfere with flow.

[b]U.S. standard mesh size.

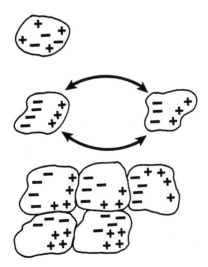

NEUTRAL PARTICLE (electrical charge evenly distributed over particle)

PROCESSING AND/OR DRY PARTICLE MOVEMENT CAUSES POLARIZATION OF FINE PARTICLES (static electric forces)

POLARIZATION CAUSES AGGLOMERATION OF FINE PARTICLES (electrical charges inducted by one particle on another van der Waals forces)

Figure 22   Effect of electrical forces on fine particles.

the agglomerated particles behave as a single large mass particle (Fig. 22). Flow may be better in this case, but the dynamics of distributing these small particles during mixing is very poor.

Increased surface exposure of fine particles to the atmosphere may present oxidation and/or moisture adsorption/absorption problems which should be avoided if possible. Fine powder particles also create potential dust conditions which may require operators to wear respirators for safe handling, and may also create potentially dangerous dust explosion hazards.

Particle size distribution of unit particles as suggested in the above discussion may also have an effect on the flow of a powder, i.e., too large a percentage of fine particles with cohesive forces, or free surface energy may inhibit flow. Although it has been stated that cohesive forces are strong in powders composed of particles 10 μm or less in size, each powder has a "critical size" where cohesive forces begin to affect the powder flow properties. An example of this is shown in Table 7.

The "angle of repose" (α) or the "angle of slip" is a relative measure of the friction between powder particles but also is a measure, for the most part, of the cohesiveness of fine particles. The angle of repose may be measured in several ways as shown in Figure 23. Methods 1 and 2 are both dynamic angle of repose measurements: the powder in Method 1 flows from a filled powder funnel onto a smooth surface where the angle is measured as illustrated, and in Method 2 the powder is moving in a rotating drum while the angle is measured as shown. Method 3 gives the static angle of repose, because the powder container is removed and the powder does not, or is not flowing before the measurement.

Since many factors enter into the angle of repose such as particle size, shape, moisture content, etc., there is some question as to its value in characterizing a powder. However, certain generalizations can be made regarding the angle of repose:

1. α is >60° for cohesive powders.
2. α is <25° for non-cohesive particles.
3. High (α) usually means poor powder flow and the particles are usually less than 75 to 100 μm in size.
4. Low (α) usually mean good powder flow and the particles are usually greater than 60 mesh or 250 μm in size.

The tangent of the angle repose (tan α) is termed the "coefficient of friction" of a powder and is preferred by some in referring to the flow properties of a powder. For example, a powder with an angle of repose of 65° will have a coefficient of friction of

tan 65° = 2.14

Whereas, a powder with an angle of repose of 35° will have a coefficient of friction of

tan 35° = 0.700

Table 6   Flow Characteristics of Some Common Substances

Material	Working bulk density (gm/cm3)	Type of powder	General comments on flow
Acrawax C	0.46	Very fluid powder	Dusty, slippery material
Ammonium chloride	0.75	Nonuniform powdered granules	May form hard lumps, as a result of hygroscopicity
Calcium carbonate	0.92	Fluid cohesive powder	Flow becomes very poor if powder is packed
	0.36	Cohesive powder	
di-Calcium phosphate	0.99	Uniform granules	Powder form is very dusty. Material is hygroscopic which reduces flowability
	1.31	Very fluid granules and powder	
Cellulose	0.09	Fibrous not free flowing and crystalline free flowing	Flow depends on size of fibers or crystals
Kaolin	0.48	Fluid powder	Dusty material which has poor flow when powder is packed excessively

Magnesium hydroxide	0.56	Fluid powder	Dusty material which is hygroscopic. Flowability is reduced considerably when powder is packed excessively
Sodium chloride	1.10	Uniform granule or fluid granules and powder	Material is very hygroscopic and cakes at relative humidity: 40–50% at room temperature
Sodium bicarbonate	0.96 / 1.08	Fluid cohesive powder / Uniform powdered granules	Very little dustiness. Material is hygroscopic which decreases flowability
Corn starch	0.56	Very fluid powder	Very dusty. Material is hygroscopic which decreases flowability
Talc	0.67 / 0.19	Fluid powder / Fluid cohesive powder	The two density powders are slippery and very dusty. Material is hygroscopic which decreases flowability
Titanium dioxide	0.56	Cohesive powder	Flow becomes extremely poor if packed
Zinc oxide	0.45 / 0.74	Fluid cohesive powder / Cohesive powder	Dusty, tends to lump. Flow becomes poor when packed. Some dustiness tends to lump. Flow becomes poorer when packed

Source: Carr, R. L., Jr., *Chem. Eng.*, Feb., 1:69–72 (1965).

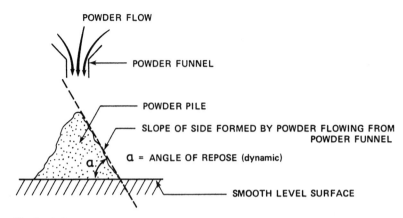

Method 1

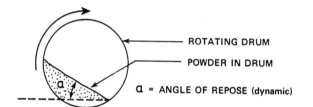

Method 2

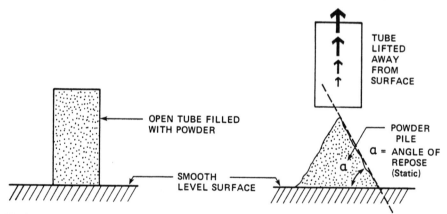

Method 3

Figure 23   Angle of repose.

Table 7   Critical Particle Size of Raw
Materials

Raw material	Critical particle[a]
Wheat starch	$20-25$ μm
Boric acid	$150-170$ μm

[a]Cohesive forces diminish at this particle size range and have little affect on raw material flow properties as the particle size increases above this range.

Size distribution of a powder also has an effect on the packing characteristics, and therefore the bulk density of the powder. This is illustrated in Figure 24, which shows how the smaller particles of a size distribution occupies interstices between the larger particles creating a more densely packed powder. Densely packed powders usually have flow difficulties.

    Particle shape affects powder inter-particle friction, and consequently the flow properties of the powder. Figure 25 shows general particle shapes and their effects on powder flow. Materials composed of particles with rounded edges such as (a) and (b) in Figure 25, will flow more readily than those with sharper edges (c), or two dimensional flat, flake-like particles (e). Poor flow is usually encountered with particles having

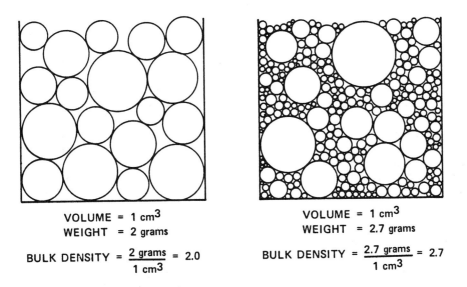

VOLUME = 1 cm³
WEIGHT = 2 grams

BULK DENSITY = $\dfrac{2 \text{ grams}}{1 \text{ cm}^3}$ = 2.0

VOLUME = 1 cm³
WEIGHT = 2.7 grams

BULK DENSITY = $\dfrac{2.7 \text{ grams}}{1 \text{ cm}^3}$ = 2.7

Figure 24   Effects of particle size distribution on the bulk density of a powder.

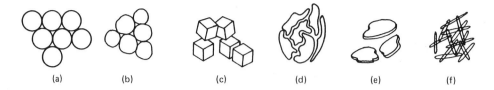

Figure 25   General particle shapes and their effect on power flow. (a) Spherical particles — normally flows easily, (b) oblong shapes with smooth edges — normally flows easily, (c) equidimensionally shaped sharp edges such as cubes — does not flow as readily as (a) or (b), (d) irregularly shaped interlocking particles — normally shows poor flow and easily bridges, (e) irregularly shaped two-dimensional particles such as flakes — normally shows fair flow and may cause bridges, (f) fibrous particles — very poor flow, and bridges easily. Bridging refers to the stoppage of powder flow as a result of particles which have formed a semirigid or rigid structure within the powder bulk.

an interlocking shape or of a fibrous configuration illustrated in Figure 25 (d) and (f), respectively.

It is apparent that particle shape affects the angle of repose of a powder, particularly powders with low magnitude surface forces as found with particles greater than 100 μm, and some low free-surface energy-fine powders such as talc (hydrous magnesium silicate) and cornstarch [34]. It must be remembered that all of the properties discussed above are intimately interrelated, and, although each one must be considered individually, they must also be considered as an entire group of variables when evaluating powder flow properties.

VI. MIXING EQUIPMENT

A general classification of mixers is shown in Table 8. Types of mixers can be divided first into two broad categories: (a) batch type, and (b) continuous. By far and large, the most prevalent type used in the pharmaceutical industry today is the batch type that mixes a sub-lot or total lot of a formula at one time, i.e., all ingredients are placed in the mixer, the materials are mixed and removed as one unit lot or sub-lot. The continuous mixer, on the other hand, is usually dedicated to a single high-volume product. Ingredients are continuously proportioned into the mixer and collected from the continuous discharge. The lot size is usually determined by a specified length of mixing time which may range from 8 to 24 hr, depending on the process.

A. Batch-Type Mixers

The first general class of mixers are those that create particle movement by rotation of the entire mixer shell or body. A schematic of four types listed in Table 8 is seen in Figure 26, while a slant, double-cone mixer (a modification of the double cone) is shown in Figure 29. Both the

Table 8 Mixer Classification

A. Batch Type

    1. Rotation of the entire mixer shell or body with no agitator or mixing blade

        a. Barrel
        b. Cube
        c. V-shaped
        d. Double cone
        e. Slant double cone

    2. Rotation of the entire mixer shell or body with a rotating high-shear agitator blade

        a. V-shaped processor
        b. Double cone formulator
        c. Slant double cone formulator

    3. Stationary shell or body with a rotating mixing blade

        a. Ribbon
        b. Sigma blade
        c. Planetary
        d. Conical screw

    4. High-speed granulations (stationary shell or body with a rotating mixing blade and high-speed agitator blade)

        a. Barrel
        b. Bowl

    5. Air mixer — stationary shell or body using moving air as agitator

        a. Fluid bed granulator
        b. Fluid bed drier

B. Continuous type

    "Zig Zag"

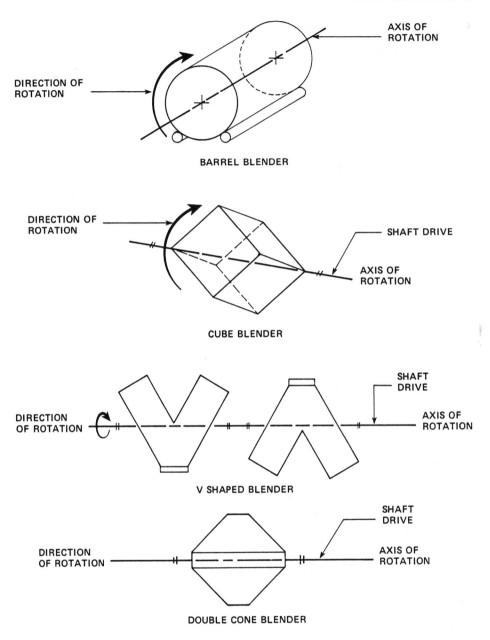

BARREL BLENDER

CUBE BLENDER

V SHAPED BLENDER

DOUBLE CONE BLENDER

Figure 26   Schematic of rotating shell blenders.

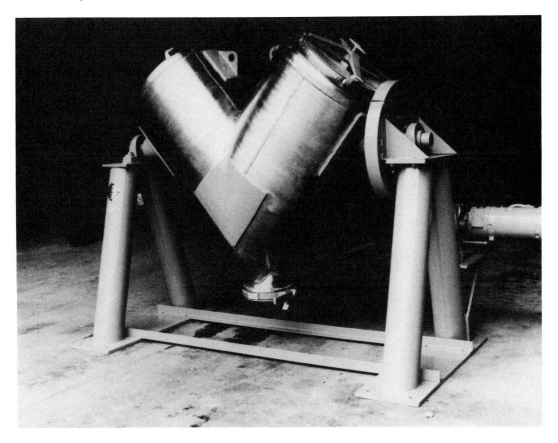

Figure 27   The twin shell V-blender. (Courtesy of Patterson-Kelley Company, Division of HARSCO Corporation, East Stroudsburg, Pennsylvania.)

barrel and cube mixers are not used to any great extent in the industry today. However, the V-shaped blender (Fig. 27), the double-cone (Fig. 28), and slant double-cone (Fig. 29) blenders, each ranging in size from 3 to 150 ft^3 or larger, are used extensively for blending. The term blending is used in relation to these pieces of equipment because they mix the dry powders with a minimum of energy imparted to the powder bed as a result of tumbling the powders. The rotating shell blenders with no high speed agitator bar are used only for dry mixes and have no packing glands (seals) around shafts entering the chamber to cause potential problems. Modifications, such as the addition of baffles, to increase mixing shear have been made to these types of blenders. The slant, double cone design is unique in that it eliminates the dead spot that may occur in the double cone mixer (Fig. 29) at the trunnions (area where drive shaft connects to the shell). The advantage of using the V-shaped, double-cone, and slant double-cone blenders include:

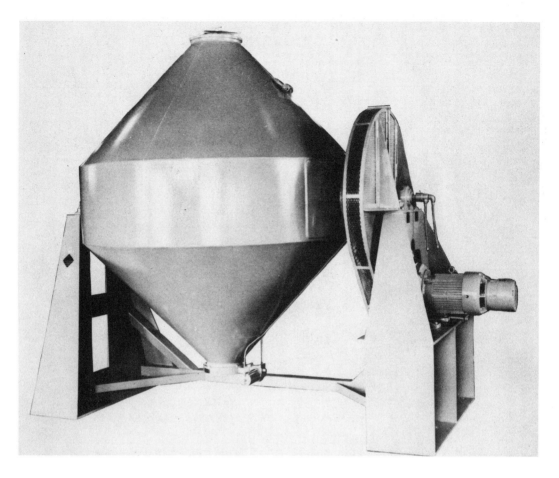

Figure 28 Double-cone blender. (Courtesy of Patterson-Kelley Company, Division of HARSCO Corporation, East Stroudsburg, Pennsylvania.)

1. Minimal attrition when blending fragile granules
2. Large capacity equipment available
3. Easy to load and unload
4. Easy to clean
5. Minimal maintenance

The primary disadvantages are:

1. High head space needed for installation (particularly with V-shaped mixers)
2. Segregation problems with mixtures having wide particle size distribution and large differences in particle densities
3. Tumbling-type blenders not suitable for fine particulate systems because there may not be enough shear to reduce particle agglomeration
4. Serial dilution required for the addition of low dose active ingredients if powders are free flowing

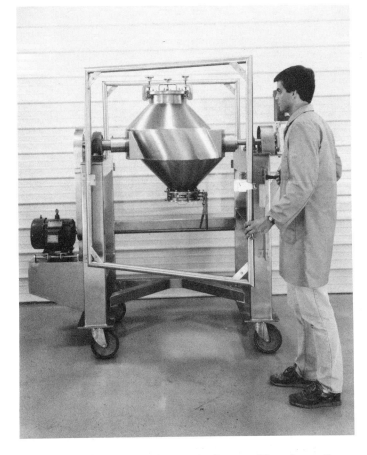

Figure 29   Slant double-cone mixer. (Courtesy Gemco, Middlesex, New Jersey.)

These blenders are operated by adding material to be blended to a volume of approximately 50 to 60% of the blender's total volume. Blending efficiency is affected by the load volume factor as shown in Table 9.

Blender speed may also be a key to mixing efficiency in that the slower the blender, the lower the shear forces. Although higher blending speeds provide more shear, more dusting may be prevalent causing segregation of fines, i.e., as the mixture is tumbling, the fines become airborne and settle on top of the powder bed after blending has ceased. There is also a critical speed which, if approached, will diminish blending efficiency of the mixer considerably. As the revolutions per minute (rpm) increase, the centifugal forces at the extreme points of the mixing chamber will exceed the gravitation forces required for blending, and the powder will gravitate to the outer walls of the blender shell. It should be noted that bench scale blenders turn at much higher rpm than the large blenders, usually in proportion to the peripheral velocity of blender extremes.

Table 9   Effect of Powder Fill on Blending Time of Double-Cone
Blenders[a]

Volume percent of blender filled with powder charge	Approximate blend time (minutes) in production-size blenders
50	10
65	14
70	18
75	24
80[b]	40[b]

[a]Blending done in double-cone blenders and times measured to obtain comparable blends.

[b]Uniform blend not attainable with this fill level.

Source: Sweitzer, G. R., Blending and Drying Efficiency Double Cone vs. V-Shape, GEMCO, Newark, New Jersey.

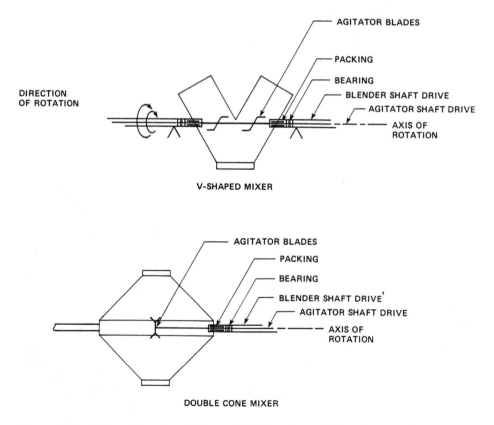

Figure 30   Schematic of rotating shell blenders with agitator mixers.

Both the V-shaped and the double-cone blenders may have a variable speed drive for adjusting the mixing speed of the shell. The double-cone blender is usually charged and discharged through the same port, whereas the V-shaped blender may be loaded through either of the shell hatches or the apex port. Emptying the V-shaped blender is normally done through the apex port.

The second general class of mixers is a modification of the tumbling blenders shown schematically in Figure 30 with the addition of a high-speed (1200 – 3000 rpm) agitator mixing blade. This agitator blade is situated as shown in Figure 31, and gives added versatility to the tumbling blenders by virtue of the high shear attainable. The advantages with the addition of the agitator bar to the tumbling blender include:

1. Good versatility in that both wet and dry mixing can be accomplished in the blender.

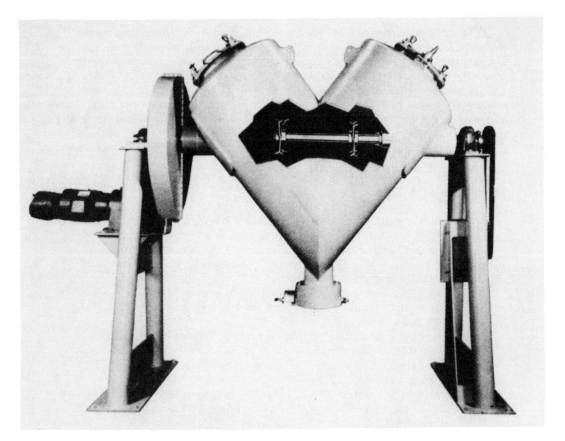

Figure 31 V-shaped blender with agitator mixing assembly. (Courtesy of Gemco, Middlesex, New Jersey.)

2. A wide range of shearing force may be obtained with the agitator bar design permitting the intimate mixing of very fine as well as coarse powder compositions.
3. Serial dilution more than likely may not be needed when incorporating low dose active ingredients into the mixture.

The disadvantages include:

1. Possible attrition of large more friable particles or granules in a mixture as a result of the high-speed agitator mixer.
2. Scale-up can prove to be a problem in that direct scale-up based on geometry, size, and peripheral velocity in many cases does not work. Experimental work is advised on the size mixer planned for the process if possible.
3. Cleaning may be a problem depending on design, since the agitator assembly must be removed and packings changed for a product changeover.
4. Potential packing (seal) problems (packings are used to prevent leakage through the shaft entrance into the mixing chamber and to prevent the blender contents from contaminating the bearings).

The mixers with agitator bars, in most cases, are also available with a separate liquid dispensing system (Fig. 32), or incorporated into the agitator bar so that a solids−liquid blend can be easily prepared without stopping the mixer for the addition of the granulating liquid. These units, known as "processors" or "formulators" may also have a steam jacket around the shell of the blender for heating the wet powder or granulation, and a vacuum system to remove the granulating liquid vapors during drying. In essence, the entire granulating and drying step may be accomplished in one piece of equipment. A schematic of this operation is shown in Figure 33.

A typical sequence of operating steps for the processor or formulator would read as follows:

1. Prepare granulating solution and adjust feed rate through pump.
2. Charge the blender with ingredients to be granulated.
3. Turn on vacuum to 15 in. of mercury and start condenser unit.
4. Premix the dry solids at normal processor shell rpm and run agitator mixer during blending.
5. Pump granulating solution into processor or formulator (with agitator bar running) and turn on full vacuum (27−29 in. of mercury).
6. Mix until granulation is properly wet up (stop processor or formulator, relieve vacuum, and open to examine granulation).
7. Shut off agitator mixer and reduce the blender shell speed to minimum rpm for drying.
8. Dry until solvent collector contains the specified quantity of solvent to be removed from the granulation (do a material balance of solvent "in" and solvent "out." The difference equals solvent remaining in chamber).
9. Check the loss of drying (LOD) after drying is completed. Empty granulation into a hopper or drums for further processing.

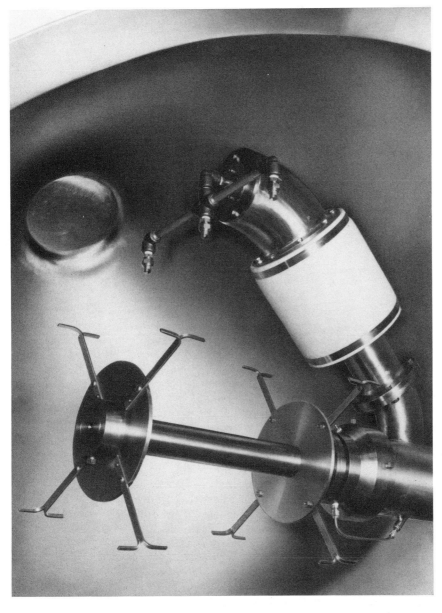

Figure 32 Separate liquid dispensing system. (Courtesy of Gemco, Middlesex, New Jersey.)

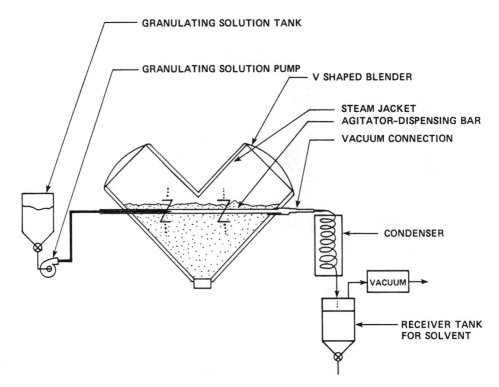

Figure 33   Schematic of V-shaped blender, processor.

The problems encountered with the operation include packing gland (seal) leakage under vacuum, and the granulation sticking to the sides of the blender shell. These problems can be often overcome by careful packing of the agitator mixer packing gland(s), optimizing the shell temperature and granulation composition and optimizing the granulating solution addition rate, and developing the proper sequence of steps during granulating. The processors and formulators are loaded and unloaded the same way as the V-shaped and double-cone blenders.

The third category of mixers is mechanically different from the tumbling shell-type blenders, i.e., the mixing forces are transferred to the powder bed by moving blades moving in a fixed (nonmovable) shell that confines the ingredients. The blades naturally have different configurations for each of the specific designs, and move the solid−solid or liquid−solid mixtures by the force exerted through a motor driven drive shaft. Schematics of the more commonly used designs are seen in Figure 34.

The ribbon mixer derives its name from the ribbon shaped blades which transverse the entire length of the U-trough and are attached to the drive shaft by struts not shown in the side view of the Figure 34a schematic. The ribbon mixer (Fig. 35) can be used for either solids−solids or liquid−solids mixing and gives somewhat less shearing action than the sigma or planetary mixer. The top of the mixer is covered during mixing because considerable dust may be created during dry blending, and granulating solution may evaporate during wet granulating. The normal procedure is to open the discharge spout several times during

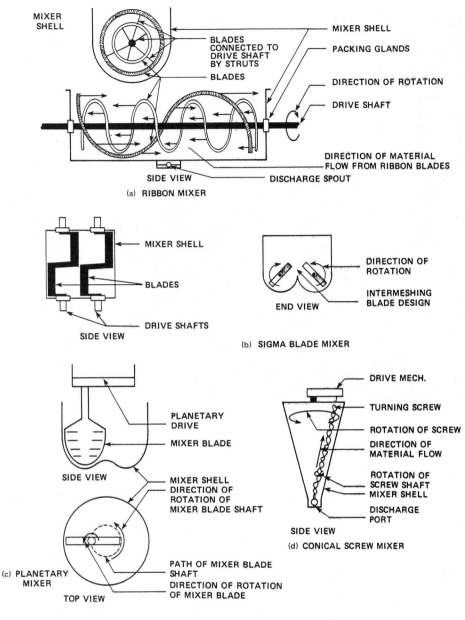

Figure 34   Schematic of fixed-shell, moving-blade mixers.

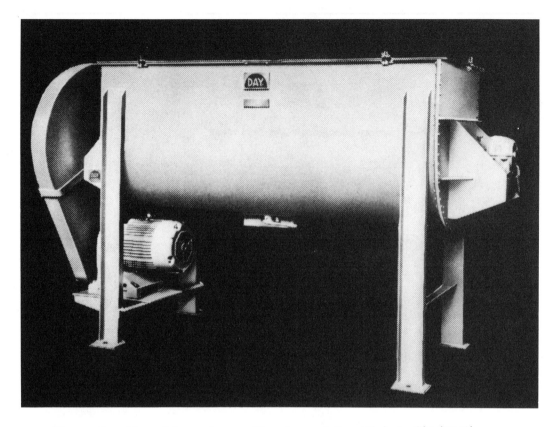

Figure 35   The ribbon mixer. (Courtesy of Day Mixing, Cincinnati, Ohio.)

mixing, returning the discharged material to the mixer. This eliminates unmixed material from becoming trapped in this spout. This is a good all-purpose mixer, but has one main disadvantage which is the possibility of dead spots (areas that remain unmixed) at the ends and in the corners of the mixer. For the same mixer volume, head room requirements are less for the ribbon mixer. The ribbon mixer is top loading with a bottom discharge port.

The sigma blade mixer (Fig. 34b) is commonly used for dough mixing in the baking industry because of tis high shear and kneading action created by the intermeshing blades. The mixer is therefore an excellent choice for wet granulating where heavy wetted powders require kneading for good liquid—solid distribution. The mixer is probably the most heavily constructed of the mixers and has close tolerances between the side walls and bottom of the mixer shell. This creates a minimum of dead space during mixing. The sigma blade mixer is used primarily for liquid—solids blending, although it can be used for solids—solids blending. The mixer is top loading, and is emptied by tilting the entire shell, via a rack and pinion drive.

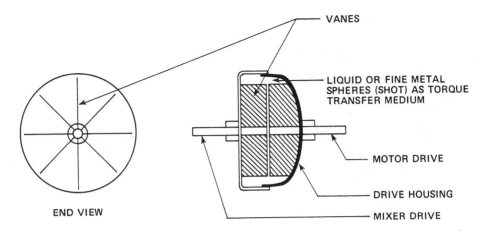

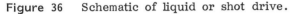

Figure 36   Schematic of liquid or shot drive.

Both the ribbon and sigma blade mixers are a fixed speed drive, and on large units that motor drive is usually connected to the blade shaft through either a fluid drive or a shot drive (Fig. 36). This prevents the high torque developed by the drive motor from breaking gears or twisting drive shafts if the mixer is turned on while loaded with a wet granulation. Each of these drives absorbs the initial torque while the blades begin to move against the granulation.

The planetary mixer (Fig. 34c) is so named because the mixing shaft is driven by a planetary gear train shown in Figure 37. As the small planetary gear, attached to the mixing blade, is driven in the indicated direction around the ring gear, it rotates the mixer blade. Therefore, the mixer blade shaft position is rotational as well as the mixer blade itself. This mixer is also a high-shear mixer and is normally built with a variable speed drive. This allows slow blade speed for pre-mixing dry powder (minimizes dusting) and faster speeds for the required kneading action in wet granulating. The mixer shell is a mixing bowl which is removed from the mixer by either lowering it beneath the blade, or raising the blade above the bowl, or both, as is the case with the larger size (340 quart) planetary mixers. There are literally no dead spaces in the mixing bowl, and extra bowls permit the mixing of one sub-lot after another if so desired. The big disadvantage with this equipment is the limited size batch which can be made at one time. The common practice is to mix several sub-lots and then make a final blend of the sub-lots in a large tumbling mixer. For small batch work this may fit the need very well, but the granulation of large lots may be done more easily in large-volume granulating equipment such as found with the processor or formulator, the ribbon and sigma blade mixers. It must be noted that since the mixer blade is mounted from above the mixer bowl, there are no packing glands in contact with the product, eliminating the need for repacking between lots and product changes. Emptying the bowls may be done by hand scooping or by obtaining a dumping mechanism which lifts and dumps.

The last of the more commonly used stationary shell mixers is the conical screw type (Fig. 38). Again, as with the planetary mixer, the

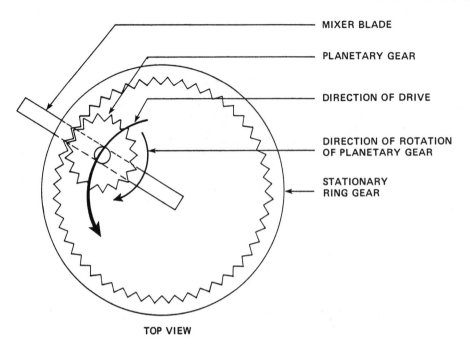

MIXER BLADE

PLANETARY GEAR

DIRECTION OF DRIVE

DIRECTION OF ROTATION
OF PLANETARY GEAR

STATIONARY
RING GEAR

TOP VIEW

Figure 37   Schematic of planetary gear.

screw shaft rotates around the periphery of the cone and the screw turns
such that the pitch transfers the material from the bottom of the mixer to
the top as illustrated in Figure 34d. This mixer provides a very mild
shearing action and was, at one time, used only for solids–solids blending.
However, with several modifications, the mixer may also be used for liquid–
solids blending in wet granulating. Probably the biggest drawback to the
conical screw mixer is the high head space required for installation of commercial size ($30-100$ ft^3) units. The big advantage with the unit is that
when filled to any height, the same mixing action is obtained. For example, if a 10 ft^3 lot of material is to be scaled up to 50 ft^3, the 10 ft^3 lot
may be blended in the 50 ft^3 blender, and the same mixing action that a
50 ft^3 lot receives will be obtained. The conical screw mixer is top loading
with a bottom discharge port.
     The fourth category of mixers is the high-speed granulators. These
are stationary shell mixers with a large mixer–scraper blade that mixes the
ingredients, eliminates dead spots in the mixer container, and presents
the mixer contents to a high-speed chopper blade which intimately mixes
the ingredients. The high-speed chopper is driven by a motor separate
from that driving the larger more slowly rotating mixer–scraper blade, and
is located at the side of the mixing bowl or chamber. Schematics of the
barrel type and bowl type are illustrated in Figure 39. The advantage of
this equipment is extremely rapid, intimate solids–solids mixing or liquid–
solids mixing. Granulating times may be only $6-10$ min long, which includes dry blending and wet granulating. The product is usually a fairly

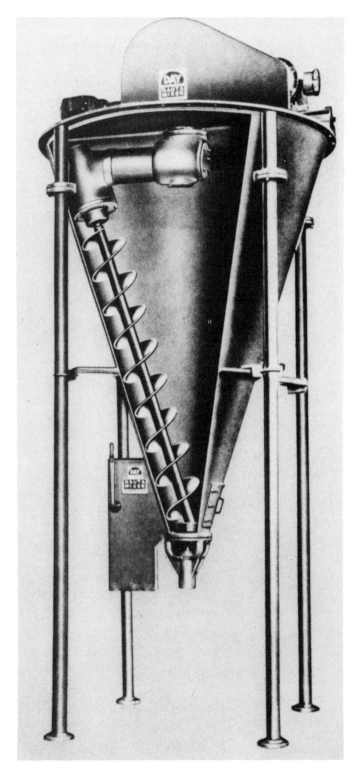

Figure 38 The conical screw mixer. (Courtesy of Day Mixing, Cincinnati, Ohio.)

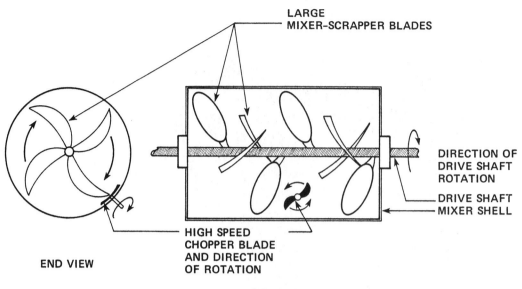

a. BARREL TYPE

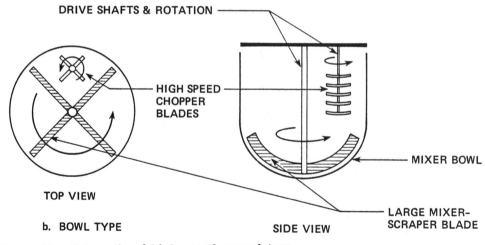

b. BOWL TYPE

Figure 39   Schematic of high-speed granulators.

uniform wet granule size of 14−8 mesh (1400−2400 μm) that needs no further wet milling or screening. The granules are usually emptied directly into a fluid bed drier.

Disadvantages may include product contamination from the packing gland where the shaft passes through the mixer shell. This has been remedied somewhat by the use of mechanical seals or the air flushed packing glands; a positive low pressure air is continually flushed through the glands into the mixer to prevent contamination of the bearings with the product and contamination of the product from bearing grease, etc. A second disadvantage may be the batch size limitation since there is some expense limit in purchasing larger models of the equipment. As with bowl mixers, this may mean the use of a second, larger tumbling blender when sub-lots made in the high-speed granulator are to be blended.

The barrel-type mixers are top loading and have bottom discharge doors while the bowl types are top loaded and may also have a special rapid discharge port located at the bottom of the mixer shell. The high-speed granulators are made from small (2 ft^3) to production sizes (1000 Kg+, about a volume of 35 ft^3) depending on production needs. Because mixing is so rapid, it is almost standard procedure to time the mixing accurately or put an ampere meter or watt meter on the high-speed chopper motor to determine the end point of wet mixing. Care must be taken during dry mixing because too long a mixing time may cause unwanted particle-size reduction which could change the characteristics of the final granulation.

The last general category of mixer is the air mixer which has a stationary shell or body using moving air as the agitator. Figure 40 shows a general schematic of the fluid bed granulator, which mixes very intimately and efficiently. By fluidizing the powder bed, enough shear is developed to mix some of the smallest size particle beds with very gentle action. The action is so gentle that even soft granules mix with little or no attrition. The equipment is used in its mixing capacity usually in the case where a wet granulation is made in the granulator. A material that must be mixed and not granulated in the fluid bed granulator normally is not mixed in the granulator. The same mixing action may be obtained with fluid bed driers, but this equipment is also usually reserved for the drying of pre-made wet granules.

It must be noted that, although the fluid bed granulator and/or drier is an excellent mixer, it also may segregate the very fine powder particles from the remainder of the mix. These fine particles collect on the discharge air filter bags and drop only at the end of fluidizing when a final shake of the filter bags is completed, i.e., the fine particles always settle on top of the powder batch mass, and usually the entire mix must be made uniform by tumble mixing. This is of little concern when possibly three lots or more of fluid bed granulated material is mixed together to increase the batch size in a large tumbling mixer. This combining of smaller lots into a larger batch is termed "sublotting," which is a common practice in the industry.

B. Continuous Mixers

Continuous mixing in the pharmaceutical industry is reserved for the large volume product which requires between 8 and 24 hr a day mixing all year

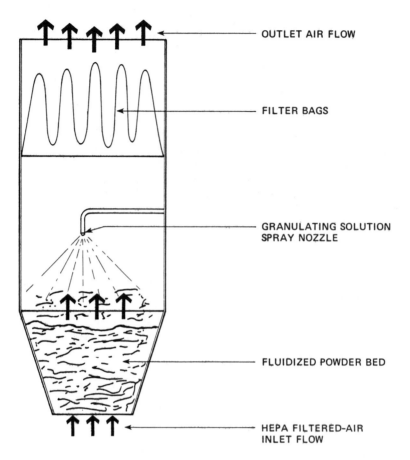

OUTLET AIR FLOW

FILTER BAGS

GRANULATING SOLUTION
SPRAY NOZZLE

FLUIDIZED POWDER BED

HEPA FILTERED-AIR
INLET FLOW

Figure 40   Schematic of fluid bed granulator – mixer.

round to meet marketing demands.   In all cases of continuous mixing, the
ingredients to be mixed are carefully and accurately metered into the
mixer at one end and are discharged as a homogenous mix at the other end
ready for further processing.   The batch size is determined by a specific
period of time, so that lot numbers of raw materials and weighing records
can be traced to reflect the composition of the final product from day to
day.

The primary problems associated with continuous mixing are associated
with material handling technology and raw material properties.   Material
handling technology problems are merely planning and selecting the
auxiliary equipment to be used with a particular continuous mixing process.
Such equipment as storage hoppers, automatic weighting units, conveying
methods and metering equipment must be selected to handle the formula
ingredients and scheduled volumes.   There must also be enough flexibility
to be able to increase or reduce the process throughput to meet the market
demands.   The materials handling system must be continuously monitored
for accuracy of blend composition, and accurate operating records maintained.

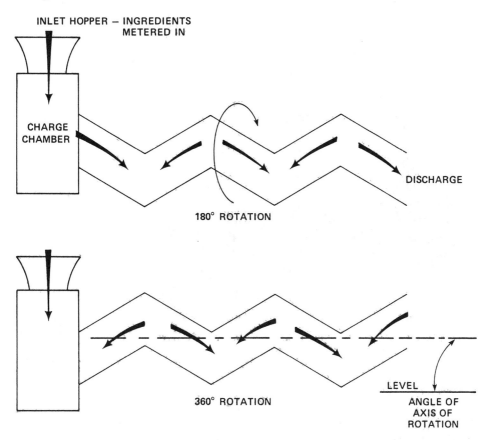

INLET HOPPER — INGREDIENTS METERED IN

CHARGE CHAMBER

180° ROTATION

DISCHARGE

360° ROTATION

LEVEL

ANGLE OF AXIS OF ROTATION

Figure 41   Schematic of "Zig Zag" continuous blender. (Courtesy of Patterson-Kelley Company, Division of HARSCO Corporation, East Stroudsburg, Pennsylvania.)

All of this work in designing and planning may be of little use if an effective raw material control is not put into play. As discussed in Sec. V, there are many variables that may cause problems with powder flow, density, etc., that must be tested for and controlled as closely as possible to make and keep a continuous mixing operation working.

There may be only one continuous mixer that should be mentioned that is in current use in the pharmaceutical industry. This mixer is a rotating shell type, except that the shell takes the shape of several V-shaped blenders in series, with lower cone angles shown schematically in Figure 41. Figure 42 is a photograph of the mixer. As the material is metered into the rotating mixer, the throughput rate is determined in part by the angle of the axis of rotation which can be varied, i.e., as the angle increases, the throughput increases. The blender works on the principle that a single pre-weighed charge can be dumped into a charge chamber, portions of which gravitate into the V-shaped tubular sections as the shell rotates. With each rotation, one-half of the blend in each downward V recycles back to the preceding chamber and one-half moves

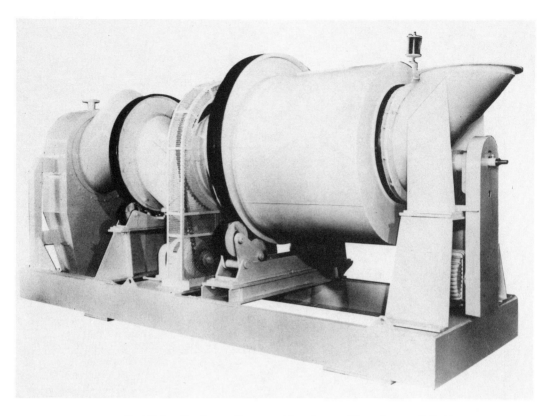

Figure 42   The "Zig Zag" continuous blender. (Courtesy of Patterson-Kelley Company, Division of HARSCO Corporation, East Stroudsburg, Pennsylvania.)

forward to the next leg of the blender. Because of the inclined axis of rotation toward the discharge, material movement is always forward, or out of the mixer discharge end. As the first charge clears the mixer, which may take only several minutes, the next charge is added. The mixer may also be operated using a continuous accurate metering of feed materials, uniformty of blend depending on flow properties of the ingredients. Although initially this equipment was intended for only solids – solids blending, a high intensity chopper and liquid dispenser permits liquid – solid mixing on a continuous basis.

Depending on the size of the continuous blender, very large quantities (500 tons/hr) of materials may be blended if required.

VII. MIXING PROBLEMS

From a practical point of view, it is necessary to learn how to use production equipment to achieve the same results obtained with a formula on both the development and pilot scale level. The scale-up to large mixers can be a very discouraging and frustrating step in putting a tablet formula into commercial production. This is primarily so because there are no hard, fast rules or equations to direct one to the use of a particular size and type of mixer during scale-up. Results are usually empirical and the starting point is dependent heavily on the experience of the people responsible for the project. The frustration and problems in scale-up are further amplified by the fact that the tablet and/or granulation production department already has specific sizes and certain type of mixers on hand. As a result, the mixing unit operation for a new formula must be adapted to this equipment. Unless the product has a large potential market and/or is a large volume product where facilities must be expanded to accommodate this volume, one normally does not have the luxury of selecting and purchasing a new blender suited for a specific new product. In addition to the above aspects of the commercial mixing unit operation, product scheduling often times prefers, or requires, that a product have the potential of being mixed using several different types of mixers.

All of these constraints are difficult to adhere to and yet obtain the desired end product. However, there are several general approaches that are used in the industry today for dealing with some potentially difficult mixing problems. Several of these potential mixing problems are listed in Table 10 with suggested approaches commonly used to overcome the difficulties. Note that the problems and suggested approaches in Table 10 are of a general nature and cannot be expected to cover all possibilities.

The first problem (A) encountered is usually one of uniformity dispersing a low-dose high-potency active ingredient in a diluent used to make a tablet large enough to compress and monitor tablet weights with ease. Dilution of the active ingredient on a small scale may be done by several dilution by hand. However, large-scale work can only approach the serial dilution method. In the dry state where a direct-comparison tablet is desired, and can be successfully compressed with the proper combination and ratio of diluents, the active ingredient must be of a small enough particle size to allow relatively large numbers of particles to be distributed in each dosage unit. When this occurs, one often runs into surface electrical charge problems as described in Sec. V. Assuming a minimum of surface, etc., problems, 10 kg of the active ingredient to be blended into 200 kg of the final granulation, for example, is usually milled or passed through a small screen (20 – 40 mesh or smaller) with an equivalent amount, or enough diluent to obtain an amount of triturate which is easily handled (20 – 40 kg in this case). The mill may have knives or hammers at medium to high mill speeds, depending on the degree of dispersion required.

After the active ingredient has been passed through the mill, the mill is cleared of active ingredient by passing another portion of diluent through the mill, adding to the triturate. The triturate and "mill cleaning" diluent is added to the mixer with about one-half of the remaining diluent and mixed for 10 to 15 min in any of the mixers without high-speed agitation, such as the tumbling mixers, the sigma blade, ribbon and conical screw type mixers. The remainder of the diluent and additives, such as the disintegrating and lubricating agents, are then added to the mixer for the final mixing.

A second alternative may be used if high-speed agitation equipment is available such as the V-shaped or double-cone blenders with agitator blades, or the high-speed granulating equipment with the chopper blade. This type of equipment permits the addition of all the ingredients at once to the

Table 10 Summary of Mixing Problems and Suggested Approaches

Problem	Suggested approaches	Suggested equipment
A. Uniformly disperse high-potency low-dose active ingredient in a diluent for direct compression	1. Mill or pass active ingredient and equal amount of diluent through a small screen. Rinse screen with more diluent. Place in mixer with 1/2 of remaining diluent and mix. Add remaining diluent and additives (starch, microcrystalline cellulose, etc.) and mix to a final mixture.	1. Cutting or hammer mill with small screen or moisturized sifter. Use tumbling mixer: V-shaped or double cone. May use sigma, ribbon, or conical screw-type mixers. Should create minimum dust.
	2. Place active ingredient, all of diluent and additives in mixer with high speed for mixing bar or chopper. Mix to a final blend.	2. V-shaped or double-cone blender with high-speed agitator bar, horizontal or vertical high-speed granulator (may have batch size restriction in these type mixers).
B. If uniform dispersion of active ingredient cannot be achieved above	1. Dissolve active ingredient in a granulating solution solvent and wet granulate in preblended diluent and additives to uniformly disperse	1. Sigma blade, ribbon, planetary, conical screw, or high-speed mixer. The mixer must have high enough shear to distribute granulating-active ingredient solution in preblended diluent, and additives. May also use a fluid bed granulator for this. Fluid bed drying is recommended to minimize active ingredient migration during drying. A mill may also be necessary to bring to final granule size.

C. Uniformly disperse small quantities of dye lakes throughout diluent with low-dose high-potency active ingredient for direct compression

1. Use same approach as in A1 above, milling active ingredient and dye lake together with diluent.

   1. Same as A1 above.

2. Use same approach as in A1 above, milling active ingredient and dye lake separately with diluent. No. 1 above is preferred above this approach because material handling is minimized.

   2. Same as A1 above.

3. Use of high-speed mixer bar or chopper with all diluent and additives.

   3. Same as A2 above.

D. Uniform dispersion of small quantities of dye lake throughout high-dose, large-volume product for direct compression

1. Mill or pass dye lake and small quantity of additives through a small screen. Rinse screen with more additive. Place in mixer with 1/2 of remainder of ingredients and mix. Add remainder of ingredients and mix to final blend.

   1. Same as A1 above.

E. Uniform dispersion of dyes in high- or low-dose products

1. Use same wet granulation technique as B1 above.

   1. Same as B1 above.

F. Poor flowing cohesive powders in general

1. Use high-shear equipment.

   1. Sigma, ribbon, and planetary mixers. V-shaped and double-cone blenders with agitator bars or high-speed granulators.

2. Fluidized bed.

   2. Fluid bed granulators.

Table 10   (Continued)

Problem	Suggested approaches	Suggested equipment
G. Over mixing of lubricants yielding granulation or formula dry mixture with poor lubricating properties	1. Cut blending time if it does not interfere with homogenicity of final blend.	1. High shear mixing equipment, e.g., ribbon, sigma, high-speed granulators and tumbling mixers with agitator blades.
	2. Use lower shear mixer if it does not interfere with homogenicity of final blend.	2. Tumbling mixers.
	3. Leave lubricant out of final final blend until last 5–10 min of mixing.	3. Both G1 and G2 above.

mixer. No pre-mixing is required because the mixing action is so intense. Mixing times are relatively short and must be watched carefully so that unwanted size reduction does not take place with the more friable materials, if present. Perchance the active ingredient cannot be successfully dispersed in a dry state (problem B, Table 10), it may be dissolved in the granulating solution solvent and wet granulated in the pre-mix diluents and internal additives (additives which are granulated are internal additives, and additives which are added to the dried granulation are called external additives). This is usually determined in the development stages of the product.

Wet granulating mixing equipment is used as listed in Table 10. It should be pointed out that slow drying of the wet granules may cause migration of the solubilized materials in the granulating solution including the active ingredient. This could present uniformity problems in the dry granulation. This may show up in the final dosage unit if the granulation is not milled to a small enough particle size. This problem may be prevented by rapid drying in a fluid bed drier or by granulating in a fluid bed granulator.

The uniform dispersion of small quantities of dye lakes throughout the granulation as in problems C and D in Table 10, follows very closely to the problem A suggested approaches. It should be noted that the mixing process must be optimized by reducing materials handling to a minimum. This includes pre-milling, pre-mixing, and mixing times.

The uniform dispersion of dyes in high or low dose active ingredient wet granulations follows closely the suggestions in problem B1 discussed above, as well as the equipment suggestions.

In general, poor flowing cohesive powders can be mixed as suggested in problem F, Table 10, by using high-shear equipment such as the high-speed granulators, or even the fluid bed granulator. The use of this equipment for mixing poor flowing ingredients will require some experimentation to determine the amount and type of shear required and the mixing time to yield a uniform mixture.

In some instances where new mixers are brought on stream (put into production use) for established products and/or the efficiency of mixing is not anticipated for both established and new products, more mixing may take place than is needed. This is the case in point in problem G, Table 10, where very thorough mixing affects the lubricity of a granulation. Experience has shown that in many cases where poor lubrication is noted, it is a result of too intimate a mixing of the lubricant, i.e., the lubricant is dispersed too well throughout the mixture. Usually, working directions call for the lubricant to be added initially in a direct-compression mixture. They may also be added with the remaining external ingredients during the final blend of a dried, milled, wet granulation. If poor lubrication during compression of the granulation is noted, a number of steps may be taken other than increasing the concentration of the lubricant (New Drug Application permitting). First, the mixing time may be decreased if it does not affect the homogeneity of the overall mixture. This is particularly useful if high-shear mixing equipment is used and the mixing time has not been optimized (blend time may be too long initially). It may even be necessary to change mixers before the lubricant is added as noted in the second suggestion, using a lower shear mixer. The third suggestion, which also works well, consists of adding the lubricant for the last 5−10 min of mixing. The higher the mixing shear, the shorter the mixing time required to obtain satisfactory lubrication dispersion.

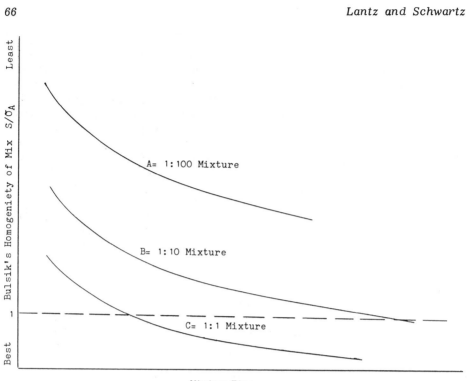

Figure 43   Effect of active ingredient concentration on homogeneity of mixture. (Adapted from J. A. Hersey, Industrial Awareness Seminar, Powder and Bulk Solids Conference/Exhibit, Philadelphia, May 1979.)

It is also noteworthy while discussing mixing problems to address and bring to the readers' attention the work done by Hersey [35] showing the effect of mixing different proportions of ingredients in the same size tumble mixer at the same tumble speed. Figure 43 shows digramatically that plotting Buslik's Index of Homogeneity [36] against mixing time gives significantly different results. This plot indicates that the 1:100 mixture could never be mixed to meet an allowable variation around the mean of the mixture. On the other hand, a 1:1 ratio of ingredients easily dispersed within acceptable limits in a reasonable time. This has important meaning when scaling up a low concentration active ingredient in a tumble mixer. The same is true when decreasing particle size to obtain maximum uniformity [35]. One may substitute small particles for line A in Figure 43 and coarse particles for line C in Figure 43. The least homogeneity is seen with the smaller particles size mixture. This is not what one would expect. However, considering the increased surface energy of smaller particles because of their much greater surface area, one can see why this situation may exist. To obtain the required particle dispersion and desired content uniformity, more energy than just tumbling must be imparted to the mixture. In order to make large volume batches (50 to 250 ft^3 in volume, approximating 500 to 4000 kg lots), it is suggested that these large tumble mixers should have high-speed agitator bars in them when they are purchased. This will minimize the previous potential problems. This will also be pointed out in the scale-up section to follow.

VIII. SCALE-UP AND MIXER SELECTION

Once a tablet formula has been carefully developed, the next biggest problem is scale-up from development to pilot to commercial production. As mentioned before, there are no set formulas for scaling up because each particulate system, dry or wet, has its own particle–particle interactions. In addition, there has been very little mixing data accumulated to provide a solid data base for a mathematical scale-up model. Several recent references may give the reader more insight into both the practical and theoretical aspects of scale-up to date [5,37,38]. The authors' own experiences in mixing, again relating to dry powder mixes in the 500 to 4000 kg or more batch sizes (50 to 250 ft^3 working capacity), show that purchasing large tumble-type mixers as described above, without a high-speed agitator bar, may make a production size mixing step a very labor intensive operation. This is particularly true if milling (to obtain adequate dispersion of fine particles in a mixture) and serial dilution is necessary. During the evaluation of mixers for a process upgrade or an increase in mixer capacity, work usually begins with the smaller bench type mixer models or even units that may hold 2 to 5 ft^3 of material. Initially, one attempts to minimize the amount of a high-potency, low-dose active ingredient during these tests, because the costs may become prohibitive since the material usually has limited availability, and is usually discarded after testing. Many times, it is felt that if a satisfactory content uniformity is obtained in a 3 ft^3 tumbling blender, that scale-up to a 50 or 100 ft^3 unit will present few if any problems. This is a poor assumption. Figure 44 illustrates this.

Figure 44 is a comparison of the same formula (8:100 ratio of active ingredient to toal granulation weight) made up from the same lots of dry ingredients, and mixed in double cone blenders of three different sizes (no high-speed agitator bars in the blenders). Each blender size was charged with material to the recommended working capacity. A superimposed line has been drawn in Figure 44 representing a 3 RSD as the maximum allowable scatter about the mean of the assays. Note that the 3 ft^3 mixer yields a more than satisfactory mixture in a relatively short mixing time. The shell tumble speed on the 3 ft^3 mixer was 20 rpm. Line B represents a 50 ft^3 mixer that also yields a satisfactory mixture in about 3 times the mix time of the 3 ft^3 unit. The 50 ft^3 mixer-shell tumble-speed was 12 rpm. The data creating line A indicates that, regardless of the mixing time, the mixture may never comply with the 3 RSD limits. The 100 ft^3 mixer shell tumble speed was 8 rpm. When one looks at the horsepower of each mixer and develops a mass/horsepower ratio, the 100 ft^3 mixer shows the highest mass-per-unit horsepower. Since mixing is an energy operation it becomes apparent that the large mixers do not impart enough energy to the powder mixture mass to overcome the adhesional and cohesional forces resisting particle movement within the powder mass. This is particularly applicable to ratios of active ingredient to total granulation weight of 1:10 or less. One's comment might be to increase the rpm of the large tumbling mixer. This is a valid suggestion. However, equipment this size is not built for high speeds. High speeds

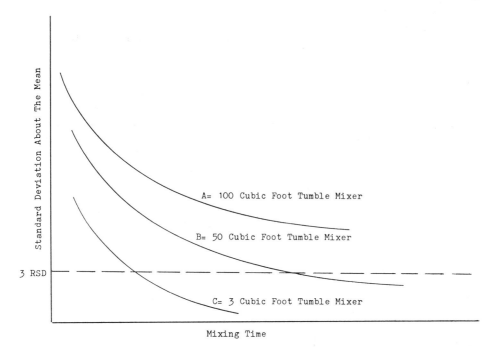

Figure 44   Effect of tumble mixer on mixture content uniformity.

would exceed design stress safety factors, and might even approach that
critical velocity, mentioned earlier, where powder particles would centrifu-
gate to the extremities of the rapidly tumbling chamber. This would cease
all mixing motion. The major point here is, again, the use of the high
speed agitator bar to impart the required energy to effect the desired
particle dispersion. It is a must with small cohesive powder mixes. This
is quite apparent from results obtained with the high-shear bowl-type
mixers with high-speed chopper blades.

The best advise is to use common sense and optimize mixing in the
size mixer intended for use in pilot or production where possible. This
may sound like an expensive approach but, in actuality, it means working
with mixers that a company's staff already has considerable experience
with and knows with some certainty the results that may be obtained.

On the other hand, if a mixing process is to be upgraded by changing
the mixer, or a new product requires a mixer other than those already
available in the research, pilot or commercial production facility, a logical
plan for mixer selection is flow charted by Hersey in Figure 45. The
chart is clear, self-explanatory, and covers most mixing pitfalls.

Do your homework. If a mixer is going to be changed to upgrade
product quality and/or improve the economics of a process, begin collecting data on all products intended to be processed via the new mixer, i.e.,
if the products are being mixed satisfactorily now on existing equipment,
establish the characteristics of what makes the powder mix satisfactory
with this equipment. Determine bulk densities, screen analysis, content
uniformities, moisture content, flow characteristics, angle of repose, etc.,

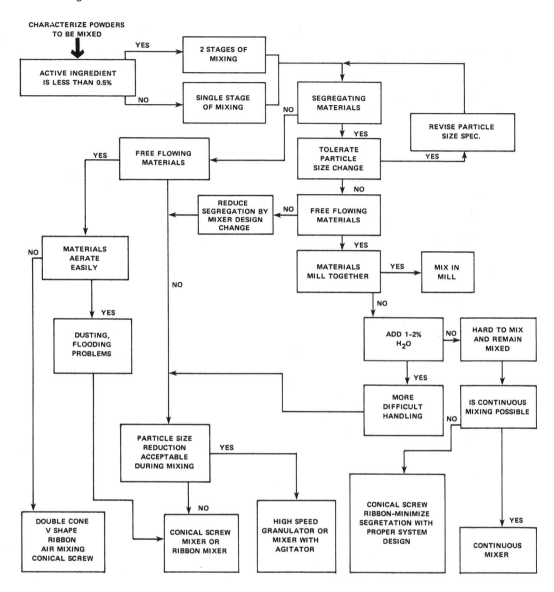

Figure 45 Flow chart for mixer selection. (From J. A. Hersey, "Powder Mixing," presented at An Industrial Awareness Seminar—Powder and Bulk Solids Conference Exhibition, May 1979.)

on all of these products per their current mode of mixing. Collect data on at least 10 lots if not 20 on high-volume products to establish an idea of what type of variance is tolerable with each product. By spending this time and effort, one will have a basis of comparison or an acceptance criteria to use for the existing products being mixed with ε new type or size mixer. If this data is not available, it may be impossible to trace down problems that might arise as a result of changing a mixer type or volume.

REFERENCES

1. Fischer, J. J., Solid–solid blending, a report from *Chemical Engineering*, August:107–128 (1962).
2. Martin, E. W., ed., *Husa's Pharmaceutical Dispensing*, Sixth ed., Mack Publishing Company, Easton, Pennsylvania, 1966, pp. 63–84.
3. Barnhart, C. L., ed., *The American College Dictionary*, Random House, New York, 1967.
4. Lacey, P. M. C., *J. Appl. Chem.*, 4:257 (1954).
5. Wang, R. H. and Fan, L. T., *Chemical Engineering*, May 17, 1974, pp. 88–94.
6. Lee, D. A., *Powder/Bulk Solids*. Sept. 1984.
7. Cahn, D. S. and Fuerstenau, D. W., *Powder Tech.*, 2:215–222 (1968/1969).
8. Cahn, D. S. and Fuerstenau, D. W., *Powder Tech.*, 1:174–182 (1967).
9. Train, D. J., *Am. Pharm. Assoc.*, 49:265–271 (1960).
10. Travers, D. N., Rogerson, A. G., and Jones, T. M., *J. Pharm. and Pharmacol.*, 27(Suppl.):3P (1975).
11. Newett, D. M. et al., *Trans. Inst. Chem. Eng.*, 36:422 (1958).
12. Schwartz, J. B. et al., *Drug Dev. and Ind. Pharm.*, 14(14):2071–2090 (1988).
13. Williams, J. C., *Powder Tech.*, 2:13–20 (1968/1969).
14. Hersey, J. A., *Powder Tech.*, 11:41–44 (1975).
15. Hersey, J. A., *Seminar on Bulk Solids Handling: Powder Mixing*, presented May 1979, Philadelphia, Pennsylvania.
16. Hersey, J. A., *J. Soc. Cosm. Chemists*, 21:259 (1970).
17. Lacey, P. M. C., *J. Appl. Chem.*, 4:257 (1954).
18. Stange, K., *Chem. Ingr. Tech.*, 26:331 (1954).
19. Poole, K. R., Taylor, R. F., and Wall, G. P., *Trans. Inst. Chem. Eng.*, 42:T305 (1964).
20. Ashton, M. D. and Valentin, F. H. H., *Trans. Inst. Chem. Eng.*, 44:T166 (1966).
21. Williams, J. C., *Powder Tech.*, 3:189 (1969/1970).
22. Buslik, D., *Bul. Am. Soc. Test. Mats.*, 165:66 (1950).
23. Harnby, N., *Trans. Inst. Chem. Eng.*, 45:CE270 (1967).
24. Fan, L. T., Chen, S. J., and Watson, C. A., *Ind. and Eng. Chem.*, 62:53 (1970).
25. Fan, L. T. and Wang, R. H., *Powder Tech.*, 7:111 (1975).
26. Buslik, D., *Powder Tech.*, 7:111 (1973).
27. Lai, F. S., Wang, R. H., and Fan, L. T., *Powder Tech.*, 10:13–21 (1974).
28. Harnby, N., *Powder Tech.*, 5:81–86 (1971/1972).
29. U.S.P. XXX-NF XI, *United States Pharmacopeial Convention, Inc.*, Rockville, Md., 1985.

30. Allen, T., *Particle Size Measurement*, Second Ed., Chapman and Hall Ltd., London, England, 1975.
31. Lopper, C. E. J., *Stanford Res. Inst.*, 3rd Quarter, 5:95 (1961).
32. *Webster's New Collegiate Dictionary*, G&C Merriam Company, Springfield, Massachusetts, 1976.
33. Boylan, J. C., Cooper, J., Chowan, Z. T., Lund, W., Wade, A., Weir, R. F., and Yates, B. J., *Handbook of Pharmaceutical Excipients*, American Pharmaceutical Association, Washington, D.C., 1986.
34. Carr, R. L., Classifying flow properties of solids, *Chem. Eng.*, 69–72, Feb. 1 (1965).
35. Hersey, J. A., Statistics of solids mixing, an industrial awareness seminar, Pwd and Blk Solids Conf./Exhibition, Philadelphia, Pennsylvania, May 1979.
36. Buslik, D., *Powder Tech.*, 7:111 (1973).
37. Schofield, C., *Chem. Ind.*, 3:105 (1977).
38. Yip, C. W. and Hersey, J. A., *Drug Dev. and Ind. Pharm.*, 3:429 (1977).

2

Drying

Kurt G. Van Scoik

Abbott Laboratories, North Chicago, Illinois

Michael A. Zoglio

Merrell–Dow Research Institute, Cincinnati, Ohio

Jens T. Carstensen

University of Wisconsin, Madison, Wisconsin

I. INTRODUCTION

In the manufacture of tablets it is often necessary to include a wet
granulation step. Wet granulation serves several purposes, including increasing particle size, supplying a binder to the formulation, improving
flow and compression characteristics, and improving content uniformity
[1–6]. In the context of drying of wet granulations, drying is usually
understood to mean the removal of water (or other liquid) from a solid or
semisolid mass by *evaporative* processes.

The moisture content of a dried substance varies from product to
product. It must be kept in mind that drying is a relative term, and
means simply that the moisture content has been reduced from some initial
value to some "acceptable" final value. This final value depends on the
material being dried. For example, a stable hydrate may be considered
"dry" after all free, or chemically unbound water has been removed.

In describing equipment that may be used for drying pharmaceutical
granulations, there are several classifications that may be used. One
such classification is whether or not the process is a batch process or a
continuous process. Batch equipment is usually favored when production
rates are low (as they are in the production of pharmaceuticals, compared
to bulk chemicals), when residence time in the unit is long, or when
many different products are to be dried in the same unit. This is not
meant to imply that continuous processes are inferior to batch processes; indeed, the converse may be true. A continuous process, if
designed properly, is a steady state process. This can lead to greater
product uniformity, control improvements due to reduced transients in
process conditions, higher throughput, and possibly reduced labor costs.

However, due to the relatively low batch size of most pharmaceuticals, there are relatively few continuous drying operations in the pharmaceutical industry [7]. It is more common to see pseudo-continuous processes, such as granulation followed by drying in fluidized bed equipment.

Another useful classification is whether or not a dryer is a direct or indirect contact drier. A direct contact drier is one in which the material is dried by exposure to a hot gas, whereas in an indirect contact drier the heat required for evaporation is transferred from a heating medium through a metal wall to the material. Generally, direct heat driers are more efficient. Drier efficiency is the fraction of energy supplied to the drying equipment which actually causes the evaporation of the liquid. As we shall see later in the chapter, heating is not always necessary to achieve drying.

One further classification is the dynamic state of the granulation bed in the dryer. A *static* bed is achieved when the particles are positioned one on top of another and experience no relative motion among each other. This is also sometimes referred to as a *stagnant* bed. An example of this would be traditional tray drying. A *moving* bed is one in which the particles flow one over another, but where the volume of the bed is only slightly expanded. Solids motion is induced by either gravity or mechanical agitation. A *fluidized* bed is obtained when the particles are supported in an expanded state by gases moving up through the bed. The velocity of the gas must be less than the entrainment velocity, or conveyence will occur. The solids and gases are mixed together more or less uniformly, and when considered as a whole the system behaves like a boiling fluid.

The nature of the product also influences the choice of the dryer. It must be kept in mind that drying of granulations requires the handling of solids or semisolids. It is important to consider the capability of the equipment in this regard. Obviously, fragile crystals or friable granulations must not be subjected to severe mechanical stress while being loaded, dried, or unloaded from a dryer.

Another consideration in choosing equipment is cost. Drying costs are determined by factors such as labor, energy, and equipment cost; construction of facilities to house the equipment, and other plant overhead. Each individual process should be thought of in terms of how it fits into the "big picture" of the entire production scheme. Examples of cost analyses of drying processes may be found in the engineering literature [8,9].

There is no single theory of drying that covers all materials and dryer designs. Differences in the method of supplying the heat required for vaporization, the mechanism of flow of moisture through the solid, and moisture equilibria make it impossible to present a single unified treatment. Therefore, some of the more important components of drying will be discussed individually, while some may be presented together.

Solids drying involves two fundamental processes. Heat is transferred to the granule to evaporate liquid, and mass is transferred as a liquid or vapor within the solid and as a vapor from the surface into the surrounding gas phase. The factors that influence the rates of these processes determine the drying rates. Since drying involves both mass and heat transfer, it must be kept in mind that these two phenomena may impact on one another. For example, the vaporization of solvent will cool the granulation. Therefore, provision must be made for the addition of heat energy to provide for the enthalpy of evaporation in addition to heating bulk solid and liquid in the material being dried.

II. MODES OF HEAT TRANSFER

There are three means of heat transfer that apply to drying processes. These are convection, conduction, and radiation. Conduction is the transfer of heat from one body to another part of the same body, or from one body to another body in direct physical contact with it. This transfer of heat must occur *without* significant displacement of particles of the body other than atomic or molecular vibrations. Some examples of conduction would include heating of metal pipes by a hot liquid inside of them, or heat supplied to a solids bed via a metal shelf in the case of vacuum drying.

Convection is the transfer of heat from one point to another within a fluid (gas, liquid, or solid) by the mixing of one portion of the fluid with another. In natural convection, the motion of the fluid is caused by gradients in density caused by temperature and gravity. In forced convection, the motion is caused by mechanical means. An example of convection drying would include the use of hot air in tray dryers and fluid bed dryers.

Radiation is the transfer of heat energy (or any other kind of radiant energy) between two separate bodies not in contact with each other by means of electromagnetic waves moving through space. Examples of this are infrared and microwave drying. It should be pointed out that microwave, or dielectric heating, has been considered by some authors to be a fourth method of heat transport [10]. In this case the energy source is an alternating electromagnetic field which generates heat by causing friction between molecules. This is probably the only mode of drying in which the temperature inside the material may exceed the temperature at the surface. Whether or not microwave drying should be considered as a fourth mode of heat transfer is debatable. Material which does not contain polar molecules will not be significantly heated by microwave radiation.

All three (or four) types of heat transfer may occur at the same time, or in various combinations. For example, in convection drying, there is a flow of hot gas past the wet surface of a granule. However, at the immediate surface of the granule, there is a relatively quiet layer of gas known as the film, or stagnant layer. Heat is transferred from the bulk gas through the film to the granule via molecular conduction. The resistance of this stagnant layer or film to heat flow depends primarily on its thickness. This is one of the reasons why increasing the velocity of the drying air will increase the heat transfer coefficient. As the velocity of the drying air increases, the stagnant layer becomes thinner. However, under the conditions used in the convective drying of granulations, there will always be a thin film of stagnant air surrounding each granule.

In summary, when discussing modes of drying, one predominant mode is usually associated with a particular dryer design for the sake of simplicity.

In discussing drying processes, it may be helpful to define a number of terms used in chemical engineering and drying technology. Useful compilations of drying terminology may be found in many reference books [11,12].

Bound moisture is water (or other solvent in nonaqueous systems) held by a material in such a manner that it exerts a lower vapor pressure than that of the pure liquid at the same temperature. Water may be chemically or physically bound. *Unbound moisture* is therefore moisture in association with a solid which exerts the same vapor pressure as the pure liquid. In a discussion of bound versus unbound water, it should be pointed out that not only are different equilibria to be considered, but that the binding energies and kinetics are also different. These topics have been addressed in both the pharmaceutical and the food sciences literature.

The *free moisture content* of a substance is the amount of moisture which can be removed from the material by drying at a specified temperature and humidity. The amount of moisture which remains associated with the material under the drying conditions specified is called the *equilibrium moisture content*, or EMC.

Any study of how a solid dries may be based on either the internal mechanism of liquid or vapor flow, or on the effect of external conditions such as temperature, humidity, air flow, particle size, and surface area.

III.   INTERNAL MECHANISM OF MOISTURE FLOW

There are three kinds of transport of moisture in a granular solid: capillary flow, liquid diffusion, and vapor diffusion. Capillary flow occurs when moisture held in interstices, as liquid on the surface, or as free moisture held in capillaries moves by gravity and capillary forces. A requirement for this kind of transport is that passageways for continuous flow are present, either through the material or around the individual particles. Liquid flow resulting from capillarity applies to liquid which is not held in solution, and to all moisture in a granule above the equilibrium moisture content at the specified atmospheric conditions. An example of this kind of flow might be water through a bed of sand as it is dried.

The next kind of moisture flow to be considered is vapor diffusion. Moisture may move through a granule via vapor diffusion provided that a vapor pressure gradient is established, either by heating or by subjecting the material to an atmosphere in which the partial pressure of the solvent is lower than the vapor pressure of that solvent within the granule. This kind of flow may occur in any solid where heating takes place at one surface and evaporation from another surface, or when the material is heated from the inside, such as in microwave drying.

Liquid diffusion is restricted to a granule in which the equilibrium moisture content is below the point of atmospheric saturation, or to a system in which the moisture and the solid are mutually soluble, such as in a water soluble paste.

External conditions which affect drying rates are usually much easier to quantitate. These include such parameters as temperature, relative humidity, airflow, particle size, degree of agitation of the granule bed, the method of supporting the granules, and the degree of contact between the drying phase and the wet granules.

One of the most important external conditions in drying operations is the capacity of the drying medium to transfer heat to the granulation and carry moisture away. This leads to the subject of *psychrometry*.

IV. PSYCHROMETRY

Psychrometry can be defined as the study of the relationships between the material and energy balances of water vapor/air mixtures. If a system other than air and water is involved, then psychrometry is concerned with the mass and energy balances for the particular solvent(s) and gas(es) at hand. The air/water vapor system is the most common system encountered in the drying of pharmaceutical granulations, but the air/ethanol or air/ethanol−water systems are also frequently encountered.

Before going any further, it is important to emphasize the fact that drying is largely a mass transfer problem; mass transfer considerations are usually more important than heat or other energy transfer phenomena in drying processes. The evaporation of water or other solvents is dominated by the concentration gradient which must exist between the moist granule and the surrounding atmosphere. For drying to occur, there must be a difference between the vapor pressure of the particular solvent(s) at the evaporating surface of the granule and the vapor pressure of the solvent(s) in the drying gas (or vacuum). In other words, before drying can begin, the moist solid must be heated to a temperature at which the vapor pressure of the liquid to be evaporated exceeds the partial pressure of the liquid (in vapor form) in the surrounding gas. Obviously, under vacuum conditions the vapor pressure may be exceeded at room temperature.

The reader must be aware that in a general discussion of vapor pressures, concentration gradients, and the effects that changing temperatures can have on these phenomena, the individual components of the system must be kept in mind. For example, if one is drying a granulation made with a hydroalcoholic solution, a change in the humidity may have a dramatic effect on how fast the water dries, but will have little to no effect on how fast the alcohol dries. In other words, increasing the temperature of an air stream will change the relative humidity and the drying rate of the water (because of changes in the concentration driving force, not the temperature). However, because the original concentration of organic solvent in the air was probably zero and remains zero, there will be less of an effect on the drying rate of the alcohol. The practical significance of this is that the manner in which the solvents come off of the granulation can change the structure of the resultant particle.

The concentration of water vapor in air is called the *humidity* of the air. However, humidity may be expressed in several different ways. To understand the interrelationships between temperature, vapor pressure, heat energy, and humidity, one may consult *psychrometric charts*, which may be found in most chemical engineering handbooks [11−13]. A particularly lucid discussion of the use of the psychrometric chart may be found in Ref. 14.

Since there are several different definitions of humidity that may be considered in a discussion on drying, it will be helpful to define some of them. The term "dry air" is used frequently (but loosely). Very rarely would an air sample contain 0% moisture, particularly on the scale required for an industrial drying process. Therefore, there must be some means of specifying the actual amount of water vapor (or other vapor) in a given quantity of air. The *absolute humidity* is defined as the mass of water vapor per unit mass of air. Since the driving force for the transfer of water from the wet surface of the granulation to the surrounding air is dominated by the vapor pressure gradient, it follows that the lower the vapor pressure (partial pressure) of water in the air, the greater the rate and extent of evaporation, all other things being equal.

The *saturation humidity* is the absolute humidity at which the partial pressure of water vapor in the air is equal to the vapor pressure of pure bulk water at a particular temperature. Since there would be no difference in vapor pressure, there would be no concentration gradient and hence no evaporation at the saturation humidity.

The *dew point* is the temperature to which a particular mixture of air and water vapor must be cooled to become saturated with respect to the water vapor. If the mixture is cooled below the dew point, then the system becomes supersaturated and it will separate into a two-phase system of saturated air and liquid water. Many of the best humidity meters are actually dew point detectors.

The *relative humidity* may be expressed as the ratio of the actual concentration of water vapor in the air to the saturation concentration of water vapor in the air under the same conditions of temperature and atmospheric pressure. Relative humidity may be defined as

$$100 \times \frac{\text{measured vapor pressure of water in air}}{\text{saturation vapor pressure of water in air}} \qquad (1)$$

Relative humidity is probably the most familiar expression of moisture content in the air.

Two other quantities of interest are the *wet-bulb* temperature and the *dry-bulb* temperature of a thermometer. The dry-bulb temperature is simply the temperature measured by an ordinary thermometer. The wet-bulb temperature is read from a thermometer whose tip containing the temperature indicating medium (e.g., mercury) is wrapped in a material which may be soaked in water. If there is a difference between the vapor pressure of the water surrounding the tip of the thermometer and the vapor pressure of water in the surrounding atmosphere, some of the water will evaporate. This (to an extent governed by the latent heat of evaporation) will cool the evaporating surface to a point below that of the air. As the tip of the thermometer cools, heat will flow from the surrounding air into the cooler region. Eventually, the rate of heat transfer to the surface will equal the rate of heat loss by evaporation. Once this equilibrium is established, one may determine the relative humidity by recording the temperatures on the two thermometers and consulting a psychrometric chart. This principle is utilized in the *sling psychrometer*, which is a simple device used to obtain the relative humidity.

The psychrometric chart can be used for a number of other purposes, since it is really just a graphical means of presenting the relationships between the material and energy balances in air/water vapor systems. It may be pointed out that psychrometric charts exist for systems other than air/water vapor. The charts may be drawn in different ways, but they usually include a basic temperature (dry-bulb) and humidity (absolute

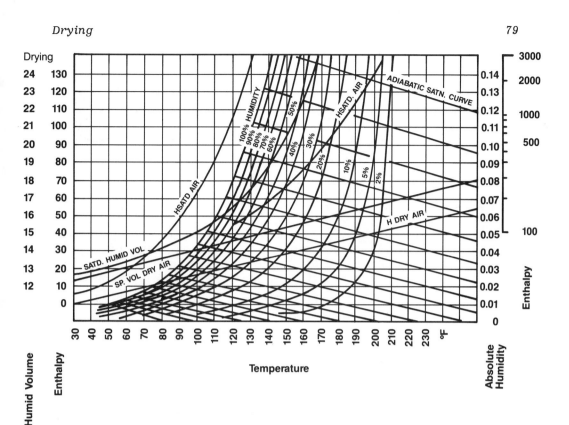

Figure 1 Psychrometric chart. The units given are °F, Btu, ft^3, and lb. These can be converted to new units (°C, joules, m^3, and kg) by the following conversion factors: to convert from °F to °C, subtract 32 from °F and divide by 1.8; to convert from ft^3 to m^3, multiply ft^3 by 0.027; to convert from Btu lb^{-1} to J kg^{-1}, multiply Btu lb^{-1} by 2324; to convert from lb to kg, divide lb by 2.2. (From Ref. 29.)

humidity) set of coordinates (Fig. 1). Additional lines or parameters that are usually included are:

1. Constant relative humidity lines
2. Constant moist volume (humid volume) lines
3. Adiabatic cooling lines which are the same as wet-bulb lines for water, but not for other solvents
4. The 100% relative humidity, or saturated air curve
5. Enthalpy values

With any two values known, the chart can be used to determine any other value of interest.

In an air sample, the partial pressures of the various gases and water vapor add up to some total pressure, which is usually one atmosphere. The amount of water and of air can be estimated by employing a form of the Ideal Gas Law; PV = nRT:

$$n_{water} = \frac{P_{water} \, V}{R \, T} \tag{2}$$

where n denotes the number of moles, V the volume (in liters), R is the universal gas constant (0.083 liter-atmospheres moles^{-1} degree K^{-1}), and T is temperature in degrees Kelvin. It follows that if the total pressure is one atmosphere, then $P_{air} = 1 - P_{water}$, so that

$$n_{air} = \frac{(1 - P_{water}) V}{R \, T} \tag{3}$$

It is therefore possible to calculate the amount of each component in a particular volume (e.g., one cubic meter) of moist air, simply by knowing the water vapor pressure. For instance, in saturated air at 50°C, given that P_{water} is 0.1217 atm, it follows that P_{air} is $1 - P_{water}$, or 0.8783 atm. The molecular weight of water is 0.018 kg/mol, and that of air is 0.029 kg/mol. The masses M of water and of air in a 1 m^3 (10^3 liters) sample of saturated air at 50°C are, therefore:

$$M_{water} = \frac{0.1217 \times 10^3 \times 0.018}{0.083 \times 323.15} = 0.0817 \text{ kg}$$

$$M_{air} = \frac{0.8783 \times 10^3 \times 0.029}{0.083 \times 323.15} = 0.9496 \text{ kg}$$

The absolute humidity is therefore 0.0817 ÷ 0.9496 = 0.086 kg water per kg of dry air.

One would like to assume that for 50% relative humidity that the absolute humidity would be one-half of that found above. This is not quite correct, as a quick calculation would show:

$$P_{water} = \frac{1}{2} \times 0.1217 = 0.06085 \text{ atm, so } P_{air} = 1 - 0.06085 = 0.93915 \text{ atm}$$

$$M_{water} = \frac{0.06085 \times 10^3 \times 0.018}{0.083 \times 323.15} = 0.0408 \text{ kg}$$

$$M_{air} = \frac{0.93915 \times 10^3 \times 0.029}{0.083 \times 323.15} = 1.0154 \text{ kg}$$

The absolute humidity is therefore $\frac{0.0408}{1.0154} = 0.0402$ kg H_2O/kg dry air. As we can see, 0.0402 is close to 0.5 × 0.86 = 0.043, but it is not the same.

One can approximate the results of these calculations by using a psychrometric chart (Figure 1). Actually, a psychrometric chart is created from these kinds of calculations. To use the chart to obtain the same results as above, first locate the dry bulb temperature on the abcissa (50°C or 120°F). Follow the vertical line up until it intersects with the curve labeled "50% humidity." At the intersection, follow the horizontal line to the right, which ends at the absolute humidity of 0.04 kg of water per kg of dry air.

Drying of a granulation is actually evaporation of water (or other solvent) which is accomplished by providing heat energy, Q (in joules or Btu's) to the granulation. If the heat of vaporization of water is L^* joules per kilogram, then the amount of water that can be evaporated is Q/L^* kg. If one knows the heat content (the enthalpy H in joules/kg of the incoming dry air, it is possible to calculate the heat Q given off to the granulation as the difference in the enthalpy between the incoming (H_i) and the outgoing (H_0) air. The heat content of air samples can be determined by the use of the psychrometric chart.

The psychrometric chart can also be used to determine relative humidities using the sling psychrometer. Although modern instruments allow the direct determination of the moisture content of the air, it may be of interest to explain how the sling psychrometer can be used for this purpose. For example, after twirling the sling psychrometer, suppose the wet bulb temperature is 100°F and the dry bulb temperature is 120°F. Draw a vertical line upwards from 100° on the abscissa of the psychrometric chart until it intersects the 100% humidity curve. From that point, draw a line parallel to the adiabatic saturation curve until it intersects with a vertical line drawn upwards from 120° on the abscissa. The intersection is on the 50% relative humidity curve. For a deeper understanding of the many uses of psychrometric charts, the reader is urged to consult chemical engineering handbooks and textbooks [11–13].

In the actual drying operation there is a certain rate of air going into the dryer, W kilograms of dry air per minute, for example. On a dry basis, the same amount of air leaves the dryer as entered it. However, on a moist basis a larger amount of air leaves the dryer than entered it, because the outgoing air contains the mass of water it evaporated during its residence time in the dryer. By means of the psychrometric chart and by measuring the flow rate of air and the drying time, it is possible to calculate the theoretical mass of water M_1 which can be evaporated. This should equal the amount of moisture (M_2) lost by the granulation as determined by moisture assay or weight loss before and after drying. In reality, M_2 will never equal M_1, and the ratio of M_2 to M_1 is a measure of the efficiency of the dryer.

V. DRYING MECHANISMS — PERIODS OF DRYING

Since it may be difficult to study liquid and vapor movement within a granulation, drying time and drying rate data are easier to collect and model. Time and rate data are also generally of more use in practical drying applications.

A. Drying Profiles

Drying behavior of a granulation may be conveniently studied by starting with experimental drying time profiles. In this case, the moisture content of the solid is expressed on a dry basis; that is, as mass of liquid per

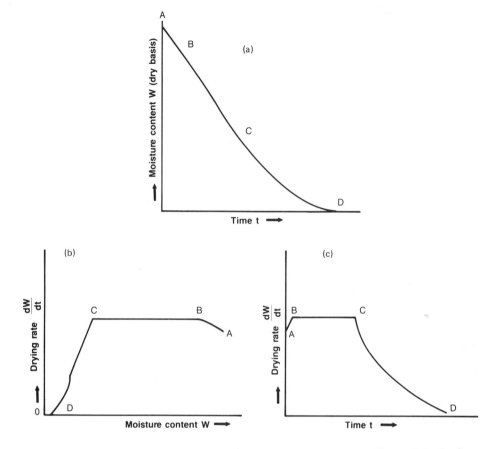

Figure 2 Drying profiles. (a) Moisture content versus time, (b) drying rate versus moisture control, and (c) drying rate versus time. (Adapted from Ref. 11.)

mass of dry solid. Moisture content W (kg water/kg dry solid) determinations may be made on samples of the granulation at preselected time points. If W is then plotted versus time t, then a graph such as shown in Figure 2a may be obtained. The slope of the curve dW/dt at any particular time is denoted the drying rate at that time.

Since the drying rate may be subject to variation with respect to time and moisture content, it may be more informative to plot dW/dt versus W, or dW/dt versus t. dW/dt may be determined graphically or by numerical differentiation of the curve in the W versus t graph. Figures 2b and 2c show the respective plots of the data in Figure 2a after determination of dW/dt values. As can be seen in these graphs, there are a number of portions of the curves which may be identified as different drying periods. One particular feature of Figure 2c is that a plot of this sort shows how long each drying period lasts.

Segment A−B on each curve is a warming-up or initial *induction period* in which the wet material is heated to the drying temperature. Segment B−C represents the *constant rate (or steady state) period* during which the drying rate per unit surface area is constant. At point C, the granulation reaches the point which is commonly called the *critical moisture content*. The portion C−D of the curve is termed the *falling rate period* (of which there may be more than one if different moisture transport mechanisms apply). Each of these drying periods will be discussed in more detail in the next few paragraphs. It should be pointed out now that in drying profiles, some of the periods may not be observed. For example, if the initial moisture content of a granulation is below the critical moisture content, then a constant rate drying period will not be observed.

B. Constant Rate (Steady State) Period

In the constant drying rate period, the granulation behaves as if there is a free liquid surface of constant composition and vapor pressure. Moisture movement to the surface is rapid enough to provide sufficient bulk liquid to ensure that the evaporation is essentially independent of the granule's structure. The rate of drying is governed by the rate of heat transfer to the evaporating surface. Water (or other solvent) diffuses from the saturated surface, through the stagnant diffusion layer, and into the surrounding atmosphere. This atmosphere may be the drying gas (convection) or a vacuum (conduction or radiation). The rate of mass transfer balances the rate of heat transfer and while the steady state period is maintained, the temperature of the saturated surface remains constant.

If heat is transferred solely by convection from a hot gas, the surface temperature of the granulation will approach or reach the wet-bulb temperature. If conduction and/or radiation contribute to heat transfer, the surface temperature of the material will reach a temperature between the wet-bulb temperature and the boiling point of the liquid. Thus, combining convection with conduction and/or radiation may allow an increase in the rate of heat transfer (with a resultant higher drying rate) provided that the vapor pressure gradients can be maintained.

If conduction or radiation is the predominant mode of heat transfer, the surface (and possibly the interior) moisture may literally boil regardless of the temperature or the humidity of the environment. This may be readily demonstrated by microwave drying. Thus, if control of granulation temperature is important, direct heat (convection) dryers usually offer greater control and product safety since the material's surface does not exceed the wet-bulb temperature during the steady state period. However, it will be shown later in this chapter that properly controlled dielectric drying may also be used to dry heat sensitive materials.

The simultaneous heat and mass transfer balances occurring during constant rate drying may be expressed in the steady state equation

$$-\frac{dW}{dt} = \frac{h_t A (T - T'_s)}{L_s} = k_a A (p'_s - p) \tag{4}$$

where

$\frac{dW}{dt}$ = drying rate, $\frac{kg\ H_2O}{second}$

h_t = the sum Σ of all convection, conduction, and radiation components of heat transfer, in units of $\frac{kilowatts}{meter \cdot degrees\ K}$

A = surface area for heat transfer and vaporization, $meters^2$

L_s = latent heat of vaporization at T'_s, $\dfrac{k \text{ joule}}{kg \text{ } H_2O}$

k_a = mass transfer coefficient $\dfrac{kg}{hour \cdot meter^2 \cdot kPa}$

T = average source temperature for all components of heat transfer, °K

T'_s = liquid surface temperature, °K

p'_s = liquid vapor pressure at T'_s, kPa

p = partial pressure of vapor in the gas environment, kPa

The magnitude of the constant drying rate depends on five factors:

1. The heat transfer coefficient
2. The mass transfer coefficient
3. The surface area exposed to the drying medium.
4. The temperature gradient between the wet surface of the solid and the gas stream
5. The vapor pressure gradient between the wet surface of the solid and the gas stream

It should be noted that all of these factors are *external* variables.

For convenience, Eq. (4) may be rewritten in terms of the decrease in moisture content rather than the mass of solvent evaporated. If we consider the case of evaporation from a stationary bed of granulation spread on trays:

$$- \frac{dW}{dt} = \frac{h_t a}{\rho_m d_m L_s} (T - T'_s) \tag{5}$$

where

$\dfrac{dW}{dt}$ now has units of $\dfrac{kg \text{ } H_2O}{kg \text{ dry material} \cdot second}$

ρ_m is the dry material bulk density, $\dfrac{kg}{m^3}$

d_m is the thickness of the bed of granulation in meters

a is the heat transfer area per unit bed of volume, $\dfrac{1}{m}$

ρ_m can be measured, but the quantity h_t is usually calculated by inserting experimentally obtained data in Eq. (5)

C. Critical Moisture Content

When discussing drying processes, the critical moisture content may be defined as the moisture content of the granulation at the end of the constant drying rate period. This moisture content is a function of the chemical nature of the material being dried (as well as porosity and other physical properties), the constant drying rate, and the particle size. It must be pointed out that critical moisture content may be of little use for standardization of drying operations unless the drying method and conditions are carefully specified. For example, particle size distribution determines surface area to mass ratios. The smaller the particles, the shorter the distance the internal moisture must travel to reach the surface. Therefore, large particles usually have higher critical moisture contents than small particles.

Another phenomenon which may effect the critical moisture content is known as case-hardening. In this case, the surface of the material is dried so rapidly that a layer of dry, nonporous material forms. This overdried surface acts as a barrier to moisture diffusion, since diffusivity decreases with moisture concentration. This may occur in vacuum drying, which will be discussed later in the chapter. To reduce the risk of case-hardening, the relative humidity of the drying gas may be increased to assist in maintaining a higher surface equilibrium moisture content until the internal moisture has diffused to the surface.

D. The Falling Rate Period

After the constant rate period ends, the falling rate period begins. This period may be seen as one or more of the terminal segments of the drying profile. The falling rate period begins when the rates of heat and mass transfer are no longer balanced, usually because internal moisture cannot move to the surface quickly enough to maintain the saturated character encountered in the steady state period. The internal mass transfer mechanisms which control falling rate drying include: Capillarity in porous and fine granular materials; liquid diffusion in continuous materials, in which the liquid is soluble (e.g., gelatin/water systems); and pressure-induced flow of liquid and vapor when material is heated on one side (or in the interior by dielectric heating) and vapor escapes from the opposite surface.

Even though one mass transfer mechanism can usually be invoked to approximate the drying kinetics at any particular time, in reality several mechanisms may occur simultaneously. For this reason it may be difficult or impossible to accurately model drying kinetics in the falling rate period.

In many, if not most of all pharmaceutical drying operations, the drying profiles *are* or may *appear* to be in the falling rate period, i.e., corresponding to segment C–D in Figure 2a. In this case, the slope (Fig. 2b) is linear in W, so that the drying equation will be of the type $\ln W = \ln W'_0 - kt$, where W'_0 is the moisture content at the critical point.

VI. PHARMACEUTICAL GRANULATION DRYING METHODS

The three most common drying methods for pharmaceutical granulations are tray drying, fluid bed drying, and vacuum drying (not necessarily in that order). Other less common methods include dielectric (microwave) drying, tunnel drying, rotary current drying, and various combinations such as dielectric-vacuum drying. Some of the more modern methods such as microwave-vacuum drying are beginning to be appreciated for their unique capabilities and the advantages they offer.

A. Tray Drying

Although tray drying is slow and relatively inefficient, it is still a commonly used method of drying and has been widely reported in the literature
[15-17]. In tray drying, wet granulation or wet product is placed on
trays which are then placed into a drying oven (Fig. 3). The trays are
usually made of metal and more often than not are lined with paper. The
trays themselves may be placed onto racks in the oven, or may be placed
on a large rack with wheels called a truck. This "truck" is then wheeled
into a large oven or room for drying. This particular arrangement is
known as truck drying.

Tray drying and truck drying are obviously batch procedures, and
are labor intensive. Most tray dryers are direct dryers, in that hot gas
or air is circulated over (or through) the granulation bed. Most tray drying operations do not employ trays with fine wire mesh on the bottom, so
that drying can take place only from the upper surface of the bed. Tray
dryers can be used to dry most materials. Drying by circulation of air
over the stationary top layers of granulation is slow, and drying cycles
may be as long as 48 hr a batch. Drying in a through-circulation unit, in
which the drying air is forced through the solids bed in a perpendicular
direction, is much more rapid than in a conventional cross-circulation unit.
However, through circulation is usually neither economical nor necessary in
a batch dryer, because shortening the drying cycles does not reduce the
amount of labor required for each batch.

Tray and truck dryers are not limited to the drying of granulations.
One application in which this mode is particularly useful is in the drying of soft shell capsules. A typical processing temperature might be
37°C with a relative humidity of 10%. The air can be dried by either
passing it over silica gel or through a column with a saturated solution
of lithium chloride. In the former case the unit that dries the air

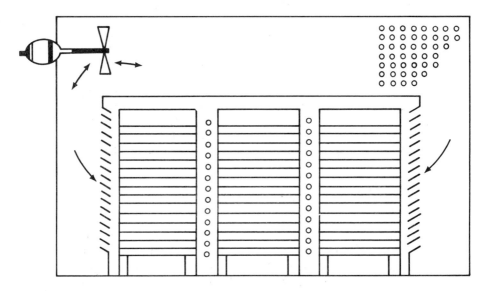

Figure 3   Tray/truck drying oven. (From Ref. 29.)

consists of two or more drying towers. One tower contains dry dessicant and the air to be dried passes through this unit. The other tower contains spent dessicant which is regenerated by passing hot gases through it. This way, when the dessicant in one tower becomes exhausted, the air stream can be switched to the other tower with dry dessicant, while the exhausted dessicant is regenerated. The drying of soft shell capsules is a diffusion process, in which a model of diffusion out of a cylinder can be used (x1). In this case, the drying equation is

$$\ln(c - c_\infty) = \frac{-t}{\alpha} + \ln(c_0 - c_\infty) \tag{6}$$

where

$$\alpha = \frac{h^2}{5.8D} \tag{7}$$

In these equations, c is the moisture content at time t, c_0 is the initial moisture concentration, and c_∞ the equilibrium moisture content of the capsule. h is the thickness of the gelatin film, and D the diffusion coefficient of the gelatin film. One must make the simplifying assumption that D is independent of the moisture content of the gelatin. α is defined in Eq. (7). Drying of soft shell capsules generally does adhere well to a drying equation such as Eq. (6). The drying endpoint is critical, because overdrying causes the capsules to become brittle, and insufficient drying imparts an excessive plasticity to the capsules so that they will adhere to each other and deform on storage.

The above equations can be used to calculate capsule drying time. Suppose a soft shell capsule reaches the required moisture level after 24 hr of drying. If the capsule shell wall thickness is increased 20%, how long will it take to dry the new capsules to the same moisture content c*? *Solution*: Using Eqs. (6) and (7), it is seen that if h is increased by 20% to 1.2 h, then α increases by a factor of $(1.2)^2 = 1.44$. For $(c^* - c_\infty)/(C_0 = C_\infty)$ to have the same value as for the thinner capsule shell, t must also be increased by a factor of 1.44 (i.e., increased so that t/α remains the same). The drying time for the thicker shell, therefore, is 1.44 × 24 hr = 35 hr.

It has been shown [15,16] that the mechanism of drying in a stationary bed appears to be evaporation from the surface of the bed, with the movement of liquid water up through the bed to maintain a water concentration gradient. This was supported by the fact that calculated diffusion coefficients were on the order of those expected for liquid water diffusion rather than water vapor diffusion. The temperature dependence of the calculated difficent coefficients were also in agreement with what would be expected for liquid water diffusion. This leads to the following drying equation:

$$\ln(M - M') = -kt + \ln(M_0 - M') \tag{8}$$

where M is the mass of the wet granulation at time t, M' is the mass of the dry granulation, and M_0 is the mass of the wet granulation at time zero. In casual interpretation, Eq. (8) corresponds to the falling rate period.

These findings are also supported by the fact that a water soluble material (dyes, for example) may migrate in a stationary bed as heat energy is supplied [17]. In the case of tray drying by convection from air passed over the surface, the solute tended to concentrate in the surface layer of the bed. In the same study, infrared radiation, microwave radiation, and vacuum drying were also used to study migration in a stationary granulation bed. The greatest migration occurred when infrared radiation was used, with solute concentrating near the middle of the bed. The granules dried in a vacuum and by microwave radiation experienced very little migration of solute.

To illustrate the processes occurring in tray drying in a more quantitative fashion, we will assume that a tray is filled with a wet granulation to a depth of a meters and that the rate limiting step in drying is the transfer of moisture from the bed into the airstream. The rate of moisture loss will follow the equation:

$$-D \left(\frac{\partial C}{\partial x} \right) = \alpha (C_o - C_s) \tag{9}$$

where

D = diffusion coefficient (m^2/sec) of water vapor

C = concentration of water vapor in the void space of the bed (kg/m^3)

$\partial C / \partial x$ = moisture vapor gradient over the interface between the bed and the airstream (kg/m^4)

α = proportionality constant

Subscripts o and s = bed and airstream, respectively

The airstream is assumed to be perfectly dry, so that $C_s = 0$; therefore C_o may be denoted simply as C in the following treatment. Initially, when the granules contain surface moisture, the vapor in the void space is at saturation pressure P_{sat} (N/m^2):

$$C = \frac{P_{sat}}{RT} \, 0.018 \text{ kg m}^{-3} \tag{10}$$

where R = the gas constant in units of 8.3143 Nm mol^{-1} deg^{-1}. At this point C is constant, and application of Fick's law gives the drying rate, dM/dt (kg per sec), as

$$-\frac{1}{\varepsilon A} \frac{dM}{dt} = -D \left(\frac{\partial C}{\partial x} \right) = \alpha C \tag{11}$$

where A is the surface of the tray and ε is the bed porosity (i.e., $A\varepsilon$ is the cross section through which diffusion occurs). Combining Eqs. (9) – (11) then gives the zero-order rate of evaporation as

$$-\frac{dM}{dt} = A\alpha\varepsilon \frac{P_{sat}}{RT} \, 0.018 \tag{12}$$

It is possible to calculate α from the slope of the initial drying curve if the granules contain surface moisture.

As drying proceeds, the surface moisture of the granules will eventually be exhausted and the vapor pressure in the void space of the granulation will drop below P_{sat}. Now, if in this period both evaporation from the granules *and* the internal equilibration of water vapor in the bed are rapid compared to the transfer of moisture over the bed-stream interface, then the diffusion equation can be solved [19]. Using the dimensionless parameter

$$J = \frac{a\xi}{D} \tag{13}$$

the first-order approximation of the solution can be written as

$$\ln\left[1 - \left(\frac{c_t}{c_\infty}\right)\right] = -\left(\frac{\beta^2 D}{a^2}\right)t + \ln\left[\frac{2J^2}{\beta^2(\beta^2 + J^2 + J)}\right] = -Gt + \ln K \tag{14}$$

Here, $-G$ and $\ln K$ represent slope and intercept, respectively, β is the smallest possible root of

$$J = \beta\tan\beta \tag{15}$$

c_t denotes the mass (kg) of water in the granulation at any particular time, and c_∞ is the equilibrium amount of moisture in the granulation, usually that obtained by proper drying of the product.

Equation (4) shows that the amount of moisture left in the granulation, less the equilibrium moisture c_∞, is log linear in time. Also, β^2 can be calculated from the negative slope $(-G)$:

$$\beta^2 = \frac{Ga^2}{D} \tag{16}$$

Figure 4 shows a typical example of tray drying data, with a bed depth of $a = 2.5$ cm, treated according to Eq. (14) [20]. The least squares fitting slope is -0.102 hr^{-1} and the intercept is -0.021.

B. Countercurrent Drying

Countercurrent drying is carried out in rotary dryers. These are long cylinders with internal baffles (sometimes helical) which direct the product in the direction opposite to that of the air flow. Because of the rotation, the granules continuously cascade down through the airstream. Because of the countercurrent nature of the product flow, the drier the product, the drier the air it counters. Countercurrent drying is usually applied only to large volume products, and only in automated or semiautomated processes. Pitkin and Carstensen [21] have shown that in countercurrent drying the rate-limiting step is the moisture movement within the granule. They showed this in the case

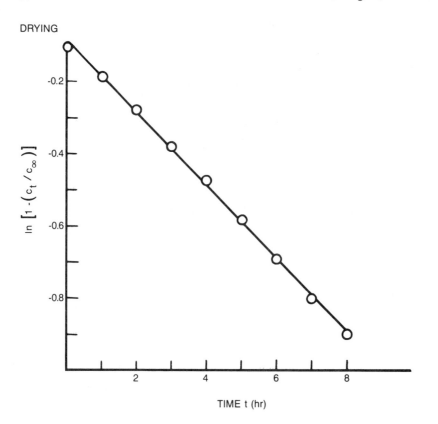

Figure 4 Tray drying data. Treated according to Eq. (12). (From Ref. 29.)

$$\frac{c - c_\infty}{c_o - c_\infty} = \frac{6}{\pi^2} \sum_{j=1}^{\infty} \frac{1}{j^2} \exp\left(-\frac{j^2 t}{K}\right) \tag{17}$$

where

$$K = \frac{a^2}{4\pi^2 D} \tag{18}$$

where j is a running index, a is the diameter of the granule, t is time, and D is the diffusion coefficient of water in the granule. D is temperature dependent by the relation

$$D = D_o \exp\left(\frac{-E'}{RT}\right) \tag{19}$$

where E' is an activation energy for diffusion, T the absolute temperature, and R the gas constant. Where a range of different particle sizes emerge from the drier, keep in mind that the moisture content will depend on the particle diameter, since from Eq. (17) the drying time t is the same for all particles. When t is of a realistic magnitude, the terms in Eq. (17) with j larger than 1 become negligible, and we may write

$$\ln \frac{c - c_\infty}{c_0 - c_\infty} = - \frac{t' 4\pi^2 D}{a^2} \ln \frac{6}{\pi^2} \tag{20}$$

that is, $\ln(c - c_\infty)/(c_0 - c_\infty)$ should be linear in $1/a^2$, with an intercept of $\ln(6/\pi^2) = -0.5$.

Since the rate of diffusion of liquid water within a granule is influenced by the porosity (ε) of the granule, we can use the above equations to show how drying times can change with changes in granule porosity brought about by changes in kneading times. For example, if it is assumed that D is proportional to ε, what effect will long kneading have on the drying rate for a wet granulated product? If a granulation is kneaded for 5 min and has a porosity of 0.3 after drying, and if after 10 min of kneading it would have a porosity of 0.2 after drying, what is the difference in drying time of the two granulations? *Solution*: Increased kneading time causes a decrease in porosity, and hence an increase in drying time because of the decrease in the diffusion coefficient. *In the following, subscripts denote kneading time.* Refer to Eqs. (17) and (19). For $(c - c_\infty)/(c_0 - c_\infty)$ to be the same, t/K must be the same (i.e., t_{10}/t_5 must equal K_{10}/K_5). Since $D_5 = (0.3/0.2)D_{10}$, it follows that $K = (0.2/0.3)K_{10}$ [Eq. (18)]. Hence, $t_{10}/t_5 = K_{10}/K_5 = 1.5$, so that the drying time increases by 50%.

Since prolonged kneading is a squeezing process, suppose that a decrease in ε from 0.3 to 0.2 is a result of a decrease by 10% in the diameter of the granules. What is the new drying time? *Solution*: Using Eq. (18),

$$K_{10} = \frac{a_{10}^2}{4\pi^2 D_{10}}, \quad K_5 = \frac{a_5^2}{4\pi^2 D_5} = \frac{1.11^2 a_{10}^2}{4\pi^2 1.5 D_{10}} = 0.82$$

so the drying time increases by a factor of $1/0.82 = 1.22$, or by 22%.

C. Fluid Bed Drying

Fluid bed drying is a process in which a drying gas is forced through a solids bed at a velocity sufficient to partially suspend the granules. The velocity must be less than that required to entrain and convey the particles, but must be great enough to overcome gravity (at least temporarily). The bed of particles is expanded relative to its stationary volume. The particles are continuously being lifted by drag forces from the gas and falling back down under the influence of gravity. Together, the gas phase and the solids phase may be described as behaving like a boiling fluid.

As the drying air passes through the bed of particles, it will undergo a pressure drop which can be expressed by the Kozeny-Carman equation under conditions of low air velocities:

$$\Delta P = \frac{q \, (\varepsilon_b)^3}{d^2 \, (1 - \varepsilon_b)^2} \qquad\qquad (21)$$

Where P is air pressure, ε_b is the porosity of the granulation bed, and d is diameter. This pressure drop remains fairly constant at low air velocities.

As the air velocity v increases, the incipient fluidization velocity, v' (m sec^{-1}) will be reached and the bed will expand and fluidize. Increasing the velocity further will expand the bed further (i.e., increase the bed porosity). At a higher particular velocity v_e (the entrainment velocity), air entrainment (conveyance) will occur. Fluid bed drying should be conducted at air velocities well below the entrainment velocity.

A plot of ε versus v should be linear, with v_e obtained by extrapolation. ε can be calculated from the bed thickness a (meters), which can be observed directly through viewing ports which are present on many commercial fluid-bed dryers. The drying chamber can be assumed to be cylindrical with cross section A meters^2. Let a equal the bed thickness, where a_0 is the smallest bed thickness at $\varepsilon = 0$. If ζ is the density of particles (kg m^{-3}), then S kg of granulation can be given by the expression $S = Aa_0\zeta$. Thus, bed porosity ε can be calculated via

$$\varepsilon = 1 - \frac{S}{A\zeta a} \qquad \text{or} \qquad a = \frac{S}{A\zeta(1 - \varepsilon)} \qquad\qquad (22)$$

As an example of how these relationships can be used, consider the following: Suppose the expansion chamber in a fluid-bed dryer is cylindrical with a cross scetional area of 1 m^2. The product change is 300 kg of material with a particle density of 1.5 g cm^{-3}. At an air flow rate of 4.5 m^3 sec^{-1}, the height of the bed was measured to be 0.5 m. When the air flow rate is 5.4 m^3 sec^{-1}, the porosity of the bed is $\varepsilon = 0.78$. What is the entrainment velocity in m sec^{-1}?

Solution: The flow rates are equal to linear velocity in m sec^{-1} because the cross sectional area is 1 m^2. The porosity of the bed at a flow rate of 4.5 m^3 sec^{-1} can be calculated as follows. The weight of the bed is equal to the (particle) powder density times the solids volume fraction $(1 - \varepsilon)$ times the volume. The particle density is 1.5×10^3 kg m^{-3}, so $1500 \, (1 - \varepsilon)(0.5 \times 1) = 300$, from which $1 - \varepsilon = 300/(1500 \times 0.5) = 0.4$ (i.e., $\varepsilon = 0.6$). At $v = 4.5$, $\varepsilon = 0.6$; and at $v = 54$, $\varepsilon = 0.78$. The slope of the ε versus v line with ε as the ordinate and v as the abscissa using this data is $(0.78 - 0.6)/5.4 - 4.5 = 0.2$. Thus, we can write the equation of the line in the form $y = mx + b$ as $\varepsilon - 0.6 = 0.2 \, (v = 4.5)$, or $\varepsilon = 0.2 \, v - 0.3$. Entrainment occurs when $\varepsilon = 1$, and $\varepsilon = 1$ when $0.2 \, v = 1 + 0.3$. Solving for v, we obtain $v_e = 6.5$ m sec^{-1} or 6.5 m^3 sec^{-1} due to the dimensions of our dryer.

Fluidized drying techniques are efficient for the drying of solids because of their effiency in promoting heat and mass transfer. Drying times may be reduced from hours or days to minutes [22]. Each granule is surrounded by a layer of drying gas which is constantly being exchanged. This creates a high surface area for evaporation, and helps to maintain the concentration gradient necessary for evaporation to take place. In the ideal situation, the dimensions of the heat and vapor paths are no larger than the diameter of the individual granules. This layer of gas may also act as a cushion between impinging particles and container surfaces. Furthermore, the boiling action of the bed promotes efficient mixing between the gas and solid phases, which helps to maintain a more uniform temperature throughout the fluid bed.

Zoglio et al. have shown that the rate limiting step in fluid bed drying is the diffusion of water vapor through the stagnant air film surrounding the granule and into the surrounding fluidizing air [23]. It has also been shown that the drying rate is a function of particle diameter, as shown in Figure 5. It should be noted that although the movement of granules in a fluid bed dryer may seem violent, the relative velocities of the individual granules are small. Therefore, the degree of attrition in a properly fluidized bed is usually moderate to small. Thus, particle size distributions do not change much upon fluid bed drying.

When aqueous-based granulations are dried in fluid bed driers, the process parameter which has the greatest impact on drying rate is the humidity of the drying air. Once again, this is because the driving force in aqueous drying operations is the vapor pressure difference between the moist solid and the drying air. As long as the surface of the granules are moist, the surface of the granules will not exceed the wet bulb temperature of the drying gas. However, towards the end of the drying

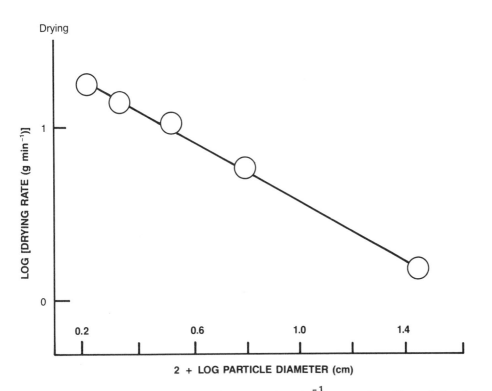

Figure 5 Logarithm of the drying rate (g min^{-1}) as a function of the log of particle diameter (cm) in a fluidized bed drying experiment. (From Ref. 29.)

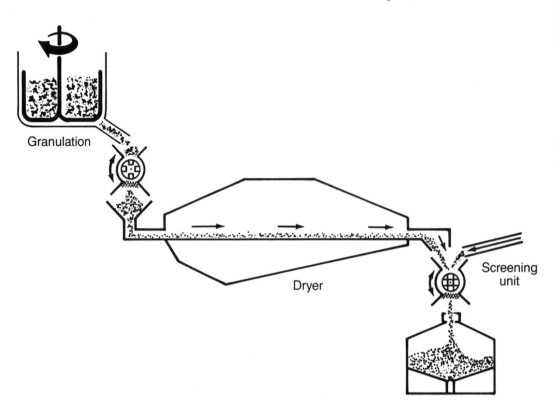

Figure 6   The sequence of continuous granulation and drying. (From
Ref. 63.)

cycle some of the particles will approach the dry bulb temperature of the
gas. For this reason, heat sensitive materials must be dried at an appropriate temperature to prevent degradation.

    Fluid bed drying may be conducted in a batch or continuous manner
[7]. For continuous processes, a horizontal fluid bed design is usually
employed, such as that shown in Figure 6. For batch processes, the
more familiar vertical design shown in Figure 7 is employed. Most fluid
bed systems incorporate similar features regardless of their design.
There must be a source of fluidizing air, and a means of heating (and
dehumidifying, if necessary) the air. There must be a screen or plate to
distribute the incoming air as it enters the dryer, and to prevent the
granulation from falling out of the dryer when the air is not flowing.
There is usually some kind of dust collection system to prevent fines from
escaping into the atmosphere or collecting on the blades of the fan which
pulls the air through the drier (since such particulates could cause mechanical damage). Finally, if organic solvents are used in coating, the
device should be explosion-proof, with a means of dealing with the rapid
pressure buildup that would be seen in an explosion.

    Modern fluid bed systems are often extensively instrumented and com-
puterized for validation and process control reasons. One advantage of

Fluid Bed Processing Installation

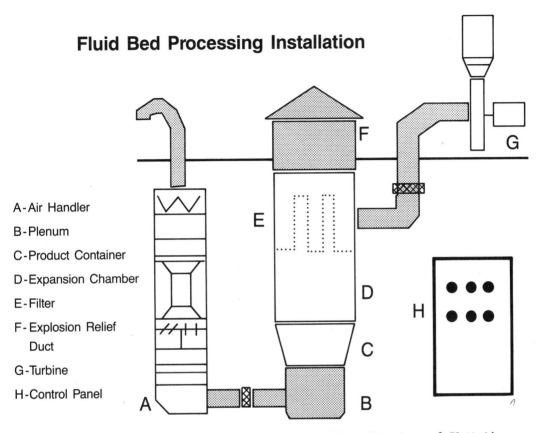

A - Air Handler

B - Plenum

C - Product Container

D - Expansion Chamber

E - Filter

F - Explosion Relief
    Duct

G - Turbine

H - Control Panel

Figure 7 Typical fluid bed processing schematic. (Courtesy of Glatt Air Techniques, Inc., Ramsey, New Jersey.)

this instrumentation is that it allows materials to be dried with a temperature profile which is either programmed or controlled automatically by the process itself. This profile may make use of the different drying rate periods. Moisture evaporating from the granules will cool the drying air. As long as the material is in the constant rate period, the energy consumed by evaporating moisture will be reflected in the constant temperature difference between the incoming warm, dry air and the cooler, more humid exhaust air. As drying proceeds, and the granulation enters the falling rate period, the abrupt increase in temperature of the exhaust air can be rapidly detected and the temperature of the drying air can be reduced to prevent overheating and overdrying.

One additional means of assuring a well-defined drying cycle is to monitor the power used by the fan that moves the air through the system. At the beginning of the drying cycle the air being pulled past the fan will be cool and damp. As the process continues, the air will become warmer and dryer, requiring less work from the fan motor. If the power to the fan is not cut back (or the pressure change the fan "sees" is not increased), air flow through the unit will increase, which could lead to

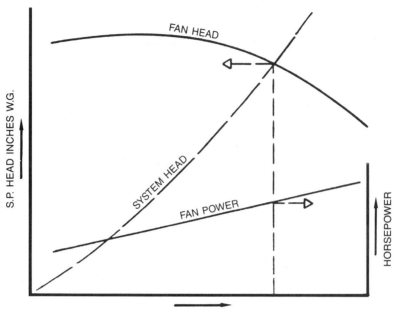

Figure 2.8 Typical fan performance curve. (Courtesy of Fluid Air, Inc., Naperville, Illinois.)

overdrying or increased attrition of the granules being dried. The relationship between pressure change (or "head") and air flow is shown in Figure 8. By programming a damper to respond to changes in the load on the fan motor (a quantity which can be measured quickly and accurately), the relationship between motor load and damper opening can be established which allows air flow to remain constant throughout the drying cycle, or varied in a desired and well-controlled manner.

It is important to point out that fluid bed dryers, as well as other dryers, present safety hazards when flammable organic solvents are used. Considerable static electricity may be generated in a fluid bed operation, and steps should be taken to safely drain off any static buildup [24,25]. All fluid bed dryers used for granulation or drying with organic solvents should be equipped with explosion relief vents which will allow any rapid increase in pressure to be safely vented to the outside of the building in which the dryer is housed. Another safety measure which may be taken is to use noncombustable gases such as nitrogen or carbon dioxide, although this approach is likely to be prohibitively expensive in open systems. A better strategy would be to operate at air flow rates which allow the air vapor mixture to remain below the lower explosion limit of the particular solvent in question.

D. Vacuum Drying

In the evaporation of solvent from any moist solid (which is what thermal drying is), the drying potential is the difference between the vapor pressure of the solvent in or at the surface of the wet granule, and the vapor pressure of the solvent in the surrounding gas. The drying (at least in the constant rate period) is also a function of A, the liquid surface area (or the surface area of the granules), and is inversely proportional to the heat of evaporation of the liquid, L* (J/kg). Thus, the drying rate may be written:

$$\text{Rate} = N \frac{A}{L*} (P_0 - P_1) \qquad (23)$$

where P_0 is the solvent vapor pressure at the wet granule surface and P_1 is the solvent vapor pressure in the surrounding gas. The proportionality constant N is a transfer coefficient which is dependent on both heat and mass transfer. It depends, for example, on the interfacial energy between the liquid and the gas.

Pure water at 25°C has a vapor pressure of 25 torr. If the pressure of the atmosphere surrounding a wet granule is reduced to less than 25 torr, the water will boil. If the water contains dissolved material, then its vapor pressure will of course be less than 25 torr. When the solvent boils, the bubbles which form greatly increase the surface area A. Therefore, it stands to reason that subjecting a wet granulation to a sufficiently low pressure should result in rapid drying at a low temperature [26].

The chief advantage of vacuum drying is, in fact, its capability of drying substances at a low temperature. Theoretically, vacuum drying should be more rapid than tray, truck, or countercurrent drying, but not as rapid as fluid bed drying. However, a high vacuum can cause fast surface drying, leading to case-hardening. Therefore, some empirical manipulation of vacuum drying conditions may be necessary. Other advantages of vacuum drying also exist, such as the ability to reduce oxidation, contain dust, and reduced energy costs.

Vacuum dryers may be equipped with a means of providing heat to their load. This is advantageous, since the evaporation of the liquid will lower the temperature of the solid. This heat may be supplied by jacketing the drier (Fig. 9), by providing heated shelves similar to those in a freeze-dryer, or by installing microwave or infrared heat sources.

E. Dielectric or Microwave Drying

Dielectric or microwave drying is a method of drying in which electromagnetic radiation (radio frequency from 3–150 MHz or microwave frequency at 915 or 2450 MHz) is applied to the material to be dried. If polar solvent molecules such as water or alcohols are present, the electromagnetic field will tend to induce orientation of the dipoles in the molecules. As the field oscillates, the polar solvent molecules will attempt to oscillate with the field, resulting in increased kinetic energy from the dipolar molecules and their collisions with other molecules. This increase in kinetic energy is manifested as thermal, or heat energy. Since electromagnetic radiation is able to penetrate the entire granule or bed of granules (depending on field strength and dielectric properties of the solid being dried), heating and vaporization of solvent can occur evenly throughout the mass (Fig. 10). Rapid heat generation within the granule or the bed with subsequent solvent vaporization results in the vapor pressure gradient which is required for drying. Drying rates are proportional to the rate of vapor diffusion rather than liquid diffusion.

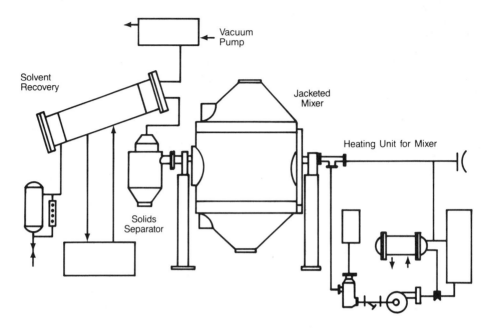

Figure 9   Schematic setup of vacuum drying. (Courtesy Patterson Kelly Co., East Stroudsburg, Pennsylvania.)

Microwave or dielectric drying has been reported in the pharmaceutical literature as being comparable or superior in terms of efficiency, energy consumption, and cost compared to conventional batch or continuous fluid-bed drying methods [27]. Energy saving of as much as 70% in industrial settings have been reported [14]. Microwave drying may be conducted in a vatch or continuous manner, with or without fluidization. It has been shown [27] that a dielectric, vibrating, fluidized bed produced drying rates at low temperatures that were superior to tray drying at 105°C and fluid bed drying with an inlet air temperature of 105°C (Fig. 11). It was found that by using dielectric radiation with the proper combinations of bed thickness and airflow, even thermally unstable materials could be dried safely and rapidly.

In dielectric drying, the rate of heating is proportional to the dielectric constant of the materials placed in the energy field. If there are large differences between the dielectric constants of the materials in the granules, then rapid and fairly selective drying is possible. For example, since water has a dielectric constant of 70, if the dielectric constant of the granule itself is around 10, then water will be heated much more rapidly than the other components of the granule. This may be shown in Eq. (24):

$$P = Z f E^2 \epsilon' \tan \delta \tag{24}$$

where

    P = power absorbed (watts per unit volume)

    Z = geometric constant times the dielectric constant of a vacuum

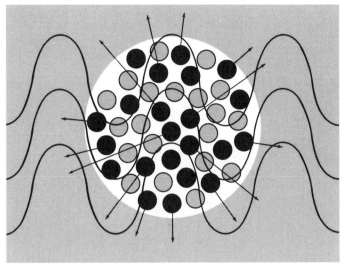

(a)

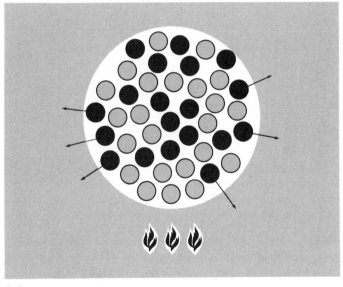

(b)

Figure 2.10 Microwave penetration of granules during drying compared (a) with convection drying (b). (Courtesy of the Fitzpatrick Co., Elmhurst, Illinois.)

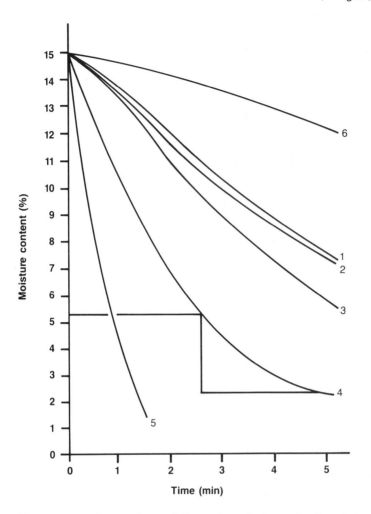

Figure 11   Comparison of the rates of six methods of drying granulate A,
which had an initial moisture content of 16%.   1 = drying cabinet, 10 mm
layer, 105°C air temperature; 2 = high frequency field, static bed, 25 mm
layer; 3 = high frequency field, fluidized bed, 23 mm layer, 43°C air
temperature; 4 = high frequency field, vibrating fluidized bed, 23 mm
layer, 65°C air temperature, two passes of material through dryer; 5 =
high frequency field, vibrating fluidized bed, 12 mm layer, 22°C air temperature; 6 = batch fluidized bed, 15 kg batch, 105°C air temperature.
(From Ref. 22.)

> f = the frequency of the applied field
>
> E = the field strength (volts per unit distance)
>
> ε' = the relative dielectric constant of the material being heated
>
> tan δ = the loss tangent or dissipation factor of the material

It can readily be seen that the higher the dielectric constant of the material being heated, the more power it will absorb and therefore the faster it will be heated.

F. Microwave-Vacuum Drying

Although drying methods based on convection, such as fluid bed drying and tray drying, are more widely used than vacuum and microwave drying at this time, the use of the latter techniques should increase as the capabilities of these methods become better known. Several manufacturers of pharmaceutical equipment have brought commercial- and laboratory-scale microwave vacuum dryers to the market in the very recent past. These units offer many advantages in the drying of solids. With the production of very low vapor pressures combined with the molecule-selective energy-coupling of microwaves, polar solvents may be evaporated at low temperatures. For example, at a typical process pressure of 45 millibar (about 35 mm mercury), water based granulations can be dried at 31°C [28]. Another advantage of combining vacuum and microwaves is that the process is practically independent of ambient atmospheric conditions such as relative humidity and temperature, which can have such dramatic effects on conventional drying techniques. Installation of the equipment is fairly straightforward, since elaborate air ducts and explosion relief vents are not necessary. These units are very efficient at their containment of product, which is important in the processing of hazardous or highly potent drugs. A further advantage is the recovery of solvents when organic solvents have been used in the granulation step. One particular design is shown in Figures 12 and 13.

While it may be difficult to utilize microwave and vacuum technology in continuous processes, an alternate strategy is to combine the unit operations of mixing a dry powder blend, wet granulating, drying, and lubricating of the granulation in the same unit. This approach has been taken by at least one manufacturer. These units have capacities varying from 15 kg (dry weight) to 400 kg, depending on the size of the unit and properties of the bulk powder.

Several methods can be used to monitor the drying process in microwave-vacuum drying [28]. Generally, watching temperature and/or electric field changes will afford adequate control. One can also make a priori predictions of the length of drying times required by knowing the latent heat of evaporation of the solvent involved, the mass of solvent to evaporate, and the energy output of the magnetrons in the dryer. When drying begins, there is usually free solvent present, which will couple with the microwave energy. Thus, a low electric field strength will be measured in the drying chamber. This low field strength will continue to be measured as the bulk of free solvent is evaporated. This portion of the drying cycle will amount to a "steady state" phase. It should be pointed out that water of crystallization does not couple with microwave

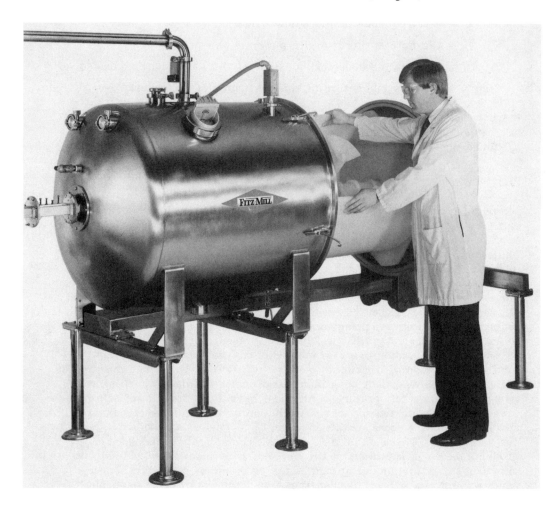

Figure 2.12   Microwave–vacuum dryer.   (Courtesy of Fitzpatrick Company, Elmhurst, Illinois.)

energy in the same manner as free or unbound water due to the presence of the crystal lattice.

The measured electric field will rise sharply as the free solvent becomes exhausted and the microwaves attempt to couple with the ever-decreasing solvent load (or the product load). At this time, the temperature may also sharply rise. Therefore, it is imperative to cut back on the amount of microwave energy going into the chamber when the end of the steady state phase is reached. By proper instrumentation of the dryer, careful monitoring of the drying process should allow the operator to prevent overheating of the product. The relationship between the electric field and temperature can be determined experimentally on small batches.

It must be noted that the stringent guidelines associated with the manufacture of pharmaceutical products put constraints on the kinds of

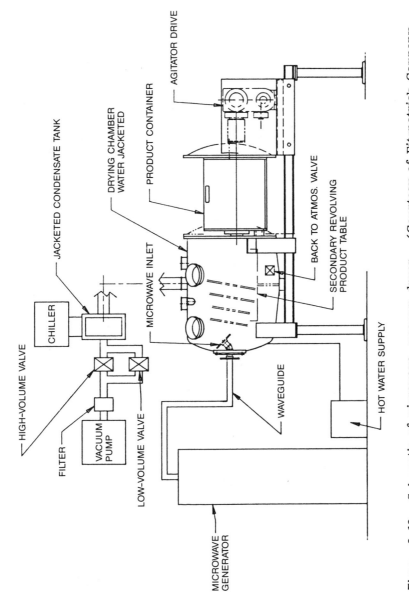

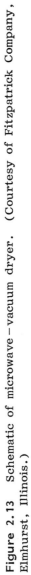

Figure 2.13 Schematic of microwave–vacuum dryer. (Courtesy of Fitzpatrick Company, Elmhurst, Illinois.)

drying equipment that can be used. Since few pharmaceuticals are produced in such quantity that drying equipment is dedicated to only one product, the equipment must allow thorough cleaning and validation of the cleaning process. Surfaces that contact the product are usually polished stainless steel, which increases cost. Not only is the stock 316 stainless steel more expensive as a starting material, it requires special expertise to fabricate and weld. The welds should be polished to increase cleaning efficiency and decrease pores and crevices in which chemical contaminants or microorganisms may reside.

The relatively small volumes of pharmaceutical products make the use of some kinds of continuous process equipment inefficient or prohibitively expensive. However, innovations in engineering and technology have created production scale equipment in which several steps such as mixing, granulating, and drying may be combined. These kinds of multifunction units, when appropriate, should be considered for their potential time and energy-saving qualities. In any event, when the purchase of equipment for use in the drying of granulations is being considered, the basic principles of drying and the specific limitations of the equipment must be kept in mind. The pharmaceutical scientist may seel the advice of a competant chemical engineer in order to develop the best process possible.

REFERENCES

1. Carstensen, J. T., in *Pharmaceutics of Solids and Solid Dosage Forms*, Wiley, New York, 1977, pp. 210–213.
2. Jones, T. M. and Pilpel, N., *J. Pharm. Pharmacol.*, *17*:440 (1965).
3. Jones, T. M. and Pilpel, N., *J. Pharm. Pharmacol.*, *18*:81 (1966).
4. Jones, T. M. and Pilpel, N., *J. Pharm. Pharmacol.*, *18*:182S (1966).
5. Jones, T. M. and Pilpel, N., *J. Pharm. Pharmacol.*, *18*:429 (1966).
6. Ridgway, K. and Rupp, R., *J. Pharm. Pharmacol.*, *21*:30S (1969).
7. Koblitz, T. and Erhardt, L., *Pharm. Tech.*, *9*(4):62 (1985).
8. Sapakie, S. F., Mihalik, D. R., and Hallstrom, D. H., *Chem. Eng. Progr.*, *75*(4):44 (1979).
9. Peters, M. S. and Timmerhaus, K. D., *Plant Design and Economics for Chemical Engineers*, 2nd Ed., McGraw-Hill, New Yorl, 1968.
10. McCormick, P. Y., Drying, in *Kirk-Othmer Encyclopedia of Chemical Technology*, Vol. 8 (M. Grayson and D. Eckroth, eds.), 3rd Ed., Wiley, New York, 1979, pp. 75–113.
11. Porter, H. F., Schurr, G. A., Wells, D. F., and Semrau, K. T., Solids drying and gas–solids systems, in *Perry's Chemical Engineer's Handbook* (R. H. Perry and D. Green, eds.), 6th Ed., McGraw-Hill, New York, 1984, Chap. 20.
12. McCabe, W. L. and Smith, J. C., in *Unit Operations of Chemical Engineering*, McGraw-Hill, New York, 1956.
13 Himmelblau, D. M., *Basic Principles and Calculations of Chemical Engineering*, 3rd Ed., Prentice-Hall, Englewood Cliffs, New Jersey, 1974.
14. Rankell, R. S., Lieberman, H. A., and Schiffman, R. F., Drying, in *The Theory and Practice of Industrial Pharmacy* (L. Lachman, H. A. Lieberman, and J. L. Kanig, eds.), 3rd Ed., Lea & Feabiger, Philadelphia, 1986.
15. Carstensen, J. T. and Zoglio, M. A., *J. Pharm. Sci.*, *71*:35 (1982).

16. Samaha, M. W., El Gindy, N. A., and El Maradny, *Pharm. Ind.*, *48*: 193 (1986)
17. Travers, D. N., *J. Pharm. Pharmacol.*, *27*:516 (1975).
18. Jost, W., in *Diffusion*, Academic Press, New York, 1960, p. 46.
19. Crank, J., in *The Mathematics of Diffusion*, 4th Ed., Oxford (Clarendon) Press, Oxford, England, 1970, p. 56.
20. Carstensen, J. T. and Zoglio, M. A., "Drying," American Pharmaceutical Society Meeting, Kansas City, Missouri, Nov. 1979, abstracts, p. 10.
21. Pitkin, C. and Carstensen, J. T., *J. Pharm. Sci.*, *62*:1215 (1973).
22. Kulling, W. and Simon, E. J., *Pharm. Tech.*, *4*:79 (1980).
23. Zoglio, M. A., Streng, W. H., and Carstensen, J. T., *J. Pharm. Sci.*, *64*:1869 (1975).
24. Simon, E., *Manuf. Chem. Aerosol News*, *49*:23 (1978).
25. Roschin, N. I. and Avakyan, V. A., *Pharm. Chem. J. (U.S.S.R.)*, *13*:649 (1980).
26. Cooper, M., Schwartz, C. J., and Suydam, W., Jr., *J. Pharm. Sci.*, *50*:67 (1961).
27. Koblitz, T., Korblein, G., and Erhardt, L., *Pharm. Tech.*, *10*:32 (1986).
28. Waldron, M. S., *Pharm. Eng.*, *8*:9 (1988).
29. Zoglio, M. A. and Carstensen, J. T., Drying, in *Pharmaceutical Dosage Forms: Tablets* (H. A. Lieberman and L. Lachman, eds.), Vol. 2, 1st Ed., Marcel Dekker, New York, 1981.

3

Size Reduction

Russell J. Lantz, Jr.

Lantz Consultants, Salem, South Carolina

I. INTRODUCTION

Size reduction is the process of reducing larger size solid unit masses to smaller size unit masses by mechanical means. The complexity of the process has resulted in few if any theories of general applicability. For the most part, the subject is primarily a conglomeration of ideas and theories of limited scope describing the size reduction of specific cases of single- and multicomponent particulate systems. A considerable amount of literature, past [1,2] and present [3], has accumulated over the last 25 years on the subject of size reduction, and because of its scope is impossible to summarize within the space limitations of a chapter in a text of this type.

In the past, there has been a continuing quest by researchers in the field to express or define size reduction in terms of a general mathematical model. This was not too successful prior to 1975, because of:

1. The lack of a generally accepted theory of comminution
2. The individuality of each size reduction case, i.e., each milling operation requires its own analysis
3. The lack of a practical mathematical term to better represent the characteristics of a particle or an assemblage of particles in terms of size, shape, density, fracturability, etc. [4]

However, this status may be changing as a result of a relatively new branch of mathematics developed over 20 years of work by Dr. Benoit Mandelbrat. The mathematics is called fractal geometry because it is composed of fractional portions of specific geometric shapes. It is best demonstrated by computer imaging, since repetition of a "family of irregular

shapes" [12,13] may be randomized to any number of degrees to yield irregularly shaped objects such as one might find in an assemblage of powder
particles. The degree of randomness yielding the degree of particle shape
irregularity.

Size reduction is a rate process [5] depending on the starting size of
the feedstock (material being fed into the mill), its orientation and residence time in the mill. The process may or may not follow a first order
equation depending on the deviations that take place during milling, e.g.,
(a) residual stresses within powder particles due to plastic deformation
and/or changes in internal particle stresses from uneven thermal changes
during size reduction [6]; (b) distribution of particle strengths [7]; and
(c) caking or reagglomeration of smaller particles to each other and/or to
larger particles. Reagglomeration and agglomeration occur simultaneously
to the size reduction process [8].

The principal means of accomplishing size reduction is by cutting or
shearing, compressing, impacting, and attrition. The majority of size reduction equipment design is based on these four principles [9].

Because of the complexity, there are a number of differences of opinion as to exactly what takes place during size reduction of powder particles or granules. However, the literature appears to agree, for the most
part, on the following sequence of events.

Assume an assemblage of particles of uniform composition, which may
or may not be irregular in shape and which are to be reduced in size.
These particles may be subjected to one or a combination of four forces:
shear, compression, impaction, or tension (i.e., shear = the cutting
force; compression = the crushing force; impaction = the direct, high-
velocity collision force; and tension = the force that works to elongate or
pull a particle apart).

Each of the particles in the assumed assemblage will have initial flaws
or differing degrees as well as possible internal stress as a result or
prior manufacturing operations [6]. A flaw in a unit particle, be it
crystalline or amorphous, is a discontinuity or imperfection in the structure. This flaw constitutes a weakness in the particle structure that may
result in failure at the point when external milling forces applied to the
particle exceed the cohesive forces of the particle flaw. This failure man-
ifests itself as a crack or cracks that eventually may lead to particle
cleavage at the crack with additional force and/or repeated force applications. Cleavage yields two or more particles; hence, additional surface
area is created. During milling, the shear, the compression, the impaction, and the tension initially produce a flexing or bending of the particle
or granule. The particle or granule attempts to return to its more
stable, original shape when energy application is removed and the particle
or granule is not fractured. This results in the release of energy (which
caused the flexing or bending) in the form of heat, and is known as the
heat of "plastic deformation." If the milling forces are great enough to
overcome the inner- or intra-particle cohesive forces, flaws or cracks are
generated. Particles may cleave (Fig. 1) at various locations such as
through the mass of the particle itself as a result of shear; or compression, impact and/or tension and at the outermost edges as a result of attrition. Attrition usually creates a distribution of smaller size particles.

Essentially the same holds true for an assemblage of dried granules
that are being reduced in size for proper flow and bulk density in tableting. Again, cleavage occurs at the weakest point or points in the granule:

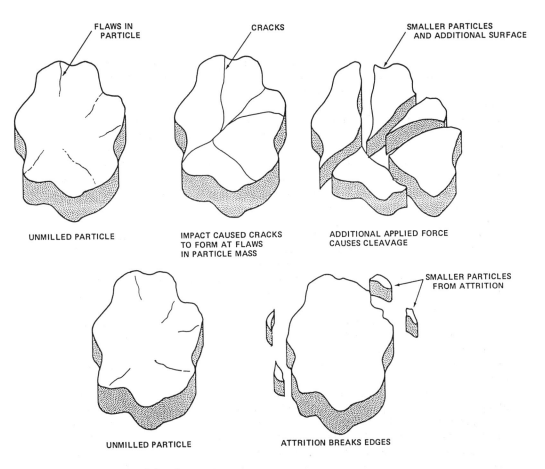

Figure 1   Particle cleavage.

1.   The binder – particle interface
2.   The bridge of binder between the individual ingredient particles being granulated
3.   Flaws in the individual ingredient particles within the granule
4.   A combination of any of the above

Granules held together with lower strength binding agents such as polyvinyl pyrrolidone will require less severe grinding conditions because the fractures take place primarily at the binder bridge and/or the binder – particle interfaces.

Comminution or milling is an extremely inefficient unit operation with only 0.05 to 2% of the applied energy [10,11] being utilized in the actual reduction of the particle size. Milling efficiency is dependent upon the type of mill and the characteristics of the material being milled (feedstock). A large portion (10–50%) of the expended energy ends up as heat generated from:

1.   Plastic deformation of particles that are not fractured
2.   Friction of the particles contacting the mill

3. Friction of the particles colliding with each other
4. Friction of the mechanical parts of the mill

A considerable research expenditure has been made in developing
theoretical and practical approaches to improve efficiency [14] and to solve
the problems of scale-up milling from the laboratory to production. This
expenditure was being carried primarily by "heavy industry," namely the
coal, coke, ore (steel included), cement, and paint industries. Because of
the enormous volume of materials handled in these industries (tons to
thousands of tons per hour), the scale-up, purchase, fabrication, and installation of equipment that handle these material volumes — and withstand
the loads and wear encountered — constitute major investments for the cor-
porations involved. With the exception of a number of continuous pharmaceutical manufacturing processes now in operation, pharmaceutical production does not approach the production scale encountered in "heavy industry." This is the primary reason why the pharmaceutical industry is
not oriented toward designing and testing new size reduction equipment.
A number of smaller equipment companies appear to be meeting the pharmaceutical industries' needs by getting into the size reduction of biological
products, and have merely extended their line to include the size reduction of solids. Size reduction and scale-up problems in the pharmaceutical
industry are very similar to those found in "heavy industry," and are
more often solved empirically rather than through the theoretical route.
There is some application of mathematics developed for specific size reduction equipment, and this will be discussed in Sec. II, Size Reduction
Equipment.

Size reduction is nothing new to pharmacy, as evidenced by the array
of age-old metal, wooden, and ceramic mortars and pestles that have been
preserved from antiquity and which were used in the early apothecaries in
the preparation of powder mixes, pills, and plant and animal extracts.

Size reduction, as it applies to tablet production, falls into three basic
categories, namely: (a) the reduction in size of oversized and/or agglomerated raw materials, (b) the reduction in size of wet and dry granular
materials usually of multi-ingredient compositions, and (c) the reduction in
size of tablets or compactions which must be milled for dry granulating or
reworking.

Size reduction and the use of size reduction equipment creates certain
advantages in tablet formula development and their subsequent production,
including:

1. Increase in surface area, which may enhance an active ingredient's
   dissolution rate and hence, its bioavailability. This is particularly
   important with compounds that are slightly soluble, such as
   phenacetin. The affect in phenacetin dissolution rate and bioavailability as a result of small particle size differences is illustrated in Figure 2. Improved bioavailability with improved dissolution rate has been demonstrated by Ullah et al. [16]. Effects
   on pharmaceuticals has been well documented by E. L. Parrott
   [17]. It must be noted, however, that active ingredients reduced
   in particle size to gain the advantage of increased surface area,
   may not retain all of this advantage after being incorporated into
   a wet or dry granulation mix, and compressed into tablets.
2. Improved tablet to tablet content uniformity by virtue of the increased number of particles per unit weight. The more particles

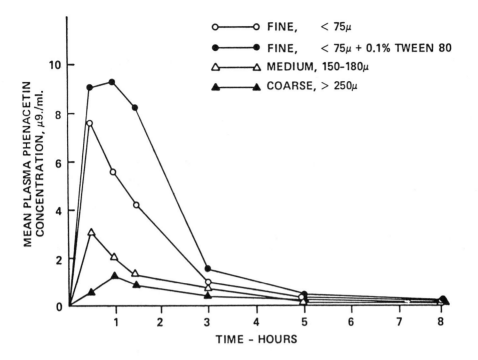

Figure 2 Mean plasma phenacetin concentration in 6 adult volunteers following administration of 1.5-Gm doses of penacetin in different ranges of particle size. (From Ref. 15.)

of active ingredient available, statistically diminishes the probability that any single tablet will contain too few or too many drug particles to place it below or above the allowable assay limits. This is very important in formulas containing highly potent low dose medicaments, and is of concern in the manufacture of tablets containing 10% by weight or less of an active ingredient.

3. Improved flow properties of some raw materials that are needle-shaped or extremely irregular in shape and tend to form a structure that resists flow. This type of flow-resistant structure, when encountered in a hopper, storage bin, or silo is called "bridging." Flow is improved by virtue of minimizing shape irregularity by attrition, and eliminating oblong needle-like particles.

4. Improved color and/or active ingredient dispersion in the tablet excipient diluents by proper use of the size reduction equipment to effect a more complete or intimate serial dilution of the ingredients. Small particle size active ingredients and pigment particles have a tendency to agglomerate. Milling may reduce this tendency.

5. Uniformly sized wet granules promote uniform drying. This will tend to lend uniformity to granules during drying because color and active ingredient migration to the surface of the granules is also more uniform when it occurs. Nonuniform color migration usually results in mottling while nonuniform active ingredient

migration may yield content uniformity problems in the final compressed tablet.

6. Controlled particle size distribution of a dry granulation or mix to promote better flow of the mixture in tablet machine feed hoppers and tablet dies. This assures one of tablet weight uniformity when compressing on high-speed gravity or force-feed rotary tablet machines.
7. Controlled particle size distribution of a dry granulation or dry mix to minimize segregation of fines and/or active ingredients while handling and tableting.
8. Surface area reproducibility for excipients as well as active ingredients is now paramount in high speed automated granulating equipment for obtaining lot to lot granulation physical characteristic uniformity.

There are also disadvantages to size reduction that may play an important part in the desicion as to whether a powder component(s) should be milled, and to what extent. These disadvantages include:

1. A possible change in polymorphic form of the active ingredient, rendering it less (or totally) inactive or unstable because of the possible heat generated during milling.
2. Possible degradation of the drug as a result of oxidation or adsorption of unwanted moisture due to the increased surface area created.
3. A decrease in bulk density of the active compounds and/or excipients that may cause flow problems and segregation in the mix. Many times a wet or dry granulation (compaction) is used in lieu of a direct compression formula because of the bulk density differences between formula components.
4. A decrease in raw material particle size usually creates increased particle surface energies. These static charge problems cause the small drug particles to agglomerate, thereby effectively decreasing its surface area. This may diminish the solid—liquid interface, which may in turn decrease the dissolution rate.
5. An increase in surface area from size reduction may promote adsorption of air, which may inhibit wettability of the drug to the extent that it becomes the limiting factor in the dissolution rate.

The milling process is not an easily contained unit operation from the Current Good Manufacturing Practices (CGMP) viewpoint because of the high possibility of cross contamination. It is said that if you can have a supplier do the milling to your specifications, do it. It could save considerable time and money. However, of first importance is the need for in-process control, which is best accomplished under a pharmaceutical manufacturer's own roof.

Whether used to reduce size or distribute coloring or active ingredients, the milling process is an important [18,19], integral part of the successful development and mass production of a formula of particulates which, when compressed, yield tablets that are uniform and reproducible and are physically and chemically stable.

II. SIZE REDUCTION EQUIPMENT

All milling or comminution equipment have three basic components (Fig. 3):

1. A structure for feeding material to the mill
2. The milling chamber and its working parts
3. A take-off to a receiver or collector in which the milled product is deposited.

One exception to this is the small-batch ball mills, which do not have a means for continuous feed or milled product removal.

Many mills now are also fitted with cyclones, centrifugation, etc., for classifying the particles by size, so that the larger and unmilled particles may be separated from the smaller milled material and recycled through the system for remilling [20]. Each of these basic components will be discussed in detail with each particular mill type.

Table 1 is a general characterization of milling equipment commonly used in tableting. The mills are listed roughly in the order of the milled product they may yield, starting from the smallest to the largest particle

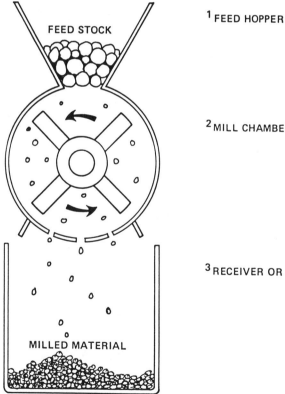

FEED STOCK

MILLED MATERIAL

[1] FEED HOPPER

[2] MILL CHAMBER

[3] RECEIVER OR COLLECTOR

Figure 3   Three basic mill components.

Table 1 General Characteristics of Milling Equipment Used Commonly in Tablet Production and Powder Raw Material Processing

Mill action and setup	Use	Type and size of feedstock	Expected results	Materials not recommended for mill
1. *Fluid energy mill*				
Attrition and impact: (Compressed gases 80–150 psig)	Ultra fine grinding	20–200 mesh moderately hard materials	30–5 μm or less with narrow size range	Soft, tacky, fibrous
2. *Ball mill or rod mill* Attrition and impact:				
a. Wet:	Fine grinding closed system	4–100 mesh moderately hard abrasive materials	100–5 μm or less	Soft, tacky, fibrous
b. Dry:	Fine grinding closed system	4–100 mesh moderately hard abrasive materials	200–10 μm or less	Soft, tacky, fibrous
3. *Hammer mill* Impact, some attrition				
a. High speed—peripheral speed at 20,000 ft/min (1) Small screen (2) Large screen (3) No screen	Fine grinding depending on screen size	2–20 mesh, non-abrasive to moderately abrasive, brittle dry material	100–325 mesh depending on material—narrow size distribution	Sticky, fibrous material, low melting point

Equipment / Speed	Application	Product / feed	Particle size	Materials not recommended
b. Low speed—peripheral speed at 1500–300 ft/min	Moderate grinding	2–20 mesh, nonabrasive soft dry materials	40–100 mesh depending on material—wide size distribution	Sticky, fibrous materials, low melting point. Hard abrasive material
(1) Small screen	Dispersion of dry powder blends and some size reduction of soft granules	Coarsely blended powders less than screen size used—10–40 mesh	Dispersion of powders 80–100 mesh granules	Sticky, fibrous materials and hard abrasive materials
(2) Large screen	Coarse dispersion of powder blends and size reduction of wet granulations	Coarsely blended powders 100 mesh and wet granulations	Dispersion of powders 10 to 40 mesh—wet granules	Sticky, fibrous materials and hard
(3) No screen				
4. Cutting mill — Cutting or shear and some attrition				
a. High speed—peripheral speed at 20,000 ft/min	Usually do not use these milling conditions	Dry powders, fibrous materials wet granulation regarding compressed tablets	Dispersion of dry powders chopping of fibrous materials and reduced wet granule size	Hard abrasive materials
(1) Small screen	Coarse dispersion of powders and wet granulation size reduction			
(2) Large screen				
(3) No screen				
b. Low speed—peripheral speed at 1500–3000 ft/min	Usually do not use these milling conditions	Wet and dry granulation tablet reworks, slugged of chilsonated granulations and wet granulation	4–80 mesh	Hard abrasive materials
(1) Small screen	Size reduction of large dry and wet granulations			
(2) Large screen				
(3) No screen				

Table 1 (Continued)

Mill action and setup	Use	Type and size of feedstock	Expected results	Materials not recommended for mill
5. *Oscillating granulator* Attrition and shear				
a. Small screen (20 mesh)	Dry granulation size reduction, rework of tablets	Tablet reworks and dried granulation	20–60 mesh	Wet granulation
b. Large screen (4 mesh)	Stepwise size reduction	Tablet reworks, dry and wet granulation	10–40 mesh	
6. *Extruder* Shear—large and small openings in head	Primarily for continuous preparation of wet granulations	Wet granulations formulated for continuous extrusion. Batch work may also be done	Granular and spaghetti-like wet granules	Dry material
7. *Hand screen* Shear and attrition	Dispersion and delumping of powders—small scale size reduction of wet and dry granulations	Raw materials, small batch wet and dry granulations	Powder dispersion, delumped, narrow size distribution with both wet and dry granulation	Hard, abrasive materials

Table 2 Examples of Pharmaceutical Raw Materials of Different Hardness

Material	General hardness classification
Talc	Soft — abrasiveness varies
Chalk	Soft to brittle
Boric acid	Soft
Cellulose	Soft but plastic (resiliency)
Aspirin	Moderately hard — brittle
Lactose	Moderately hard — brittle
Ammonium chloride	Moderately hard — brittle
Sucrose	Moderately hard — brittle
Dextrin	Hard — brittle
Sorbitol	Hard
Kaolin	Hard
Magnesium oxide	Hard — abrasive
Calcium lactate	Hard — abrasive
Amobarbital	Very hard — abrasive

sizes. The speeds of the mills listed in this table are approximations as are the screen sizes. Each milling process (operation) is usually an individualized case and must be treated according to the individually defined parameters. These parameters will be discussed later in the text. Table 2 has been included to give examples of hard, abrasive, moderately hard, etc., raw materials mentioned in Table 1. An excellent reference text for tableting excipients is the recently published *Handbook of Pharmaceutical Excipients* [21].

A. Fluid Energy Mill

The fluid energy mill, which is reviewed extensively by Albus [22], has no moving parts and is a rapid and relatively efficient method of reducing powders to 30 microns (μm) and below in size, with a relatively narrow particle size distribution [23]. Figure 4 is a schematic of one type of this mill. The mill operates on the principle of impact and attrition in that a velocity air stream introduces the powder to the milling chamber usually by way of a venturi tube (high-velocity air stream passing an opening containing the powder produces a vacuum in the opening and draws the powder into the air stream). Larger feedstock sizes must be reduced in size before they can be fed to, and milled by fluid energy (pre-reduction in size is usually accomplished via a hammer mill operation). Milling takes place immediately because of the high velocity collisions

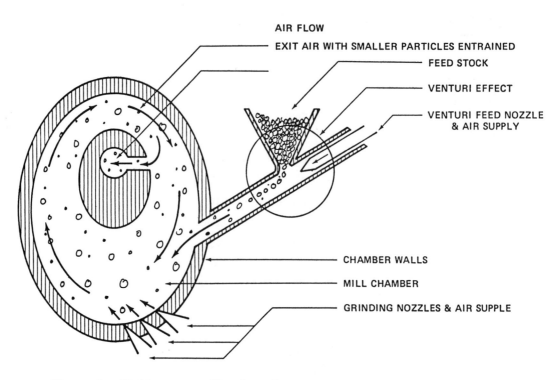

AIR FLOW
EXIT AIR WITH SMALLER PARTICLES ENTRAINED
FEED STOCK
VENTURI EFFECT
VENTURI FEED NOZZLE
& AIR SUPPLY

CHAMBER WALLS
MILL CHAMBER
GRINDING NOZZLES & AIR SUPPLE

Figure 4   Fluid energy mill schematic.

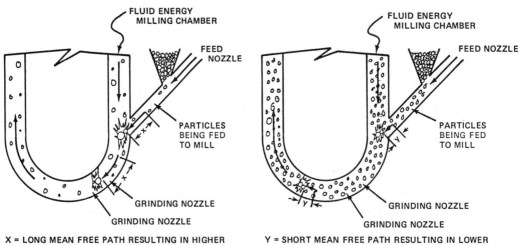

FLUID ENERGY
MILLING CHAMBER

FEED
NOZZLE

PARTICLES
BEING FED
TO MILL

GRINDING NOZZLE
GRINDING NOZZLE

FLUID ENERGY
MILLING CHAMBER

FEED NOZZLE

PARTICLES
BEING FED
TO MILL

GRINDING NOZZLE
GRINDING NOZZLE

X = LONG MEAN FREE PATH RESULTING IN HIGHER
PARTICLE IMPACT VELOCITY – SMALLER PARTICLES
(LOW FEED RATE OF POWDER PARTICLES)

Y = SHORT MEAN FREE PATH RESULTING IN LOWER
PARTICLE IMPACT VELOCITY – LARGER PARTICLES
(HIGH FEED RATES OF POWDER PARTICLES)

Figure 5   Effect of mean free path of particles on the impact in fluid
energy milling.

between particles suspended within the air stream (see Fig. 5). A limitation of this mill, as with other mills, is the rate at which a material is fed to the mill. Effective grinding depends to a large part on the particle mean free path (the distance a particle travels before colliding with another particle) and the energy gained for collision in a longer mean free path (illustrated by dimension "X" in Fig. 5). Therefore, higher feed rates diminish the length of the mean free path (illustrated by dimension "Y" in Fig. 5) and may teduce milling effectiveness and efficiency.

A number of grinding nozzles (usually from 2 to 6, depending on the size of the mill), which may be placed tangentially or opposite to the initial powder flow path (Fig. 6), increases particle velocity, resulting in higher impact energy. Grinding appears to depend on the number of particle collisions, the probability of breakage on collision, and whether attrition or impact is the principal mechanism [24]. The air from the grinding nozzles acts to transport the powder in the elliptical or circular track of the mill to the classifier that removes the smaller particles by entrainment. The entrained particles are removed by cyclone and bag filters (Figs. 7 and 8). Because of the mass of the larger particles and the opposing drag and centrifugal forces, they recirculate, colliding again with each other and the new incoming feedstock particles. The particles remain in the mill until they are reduced sufficiently in size to exit via the classifier; hence, the narrow particle size distribution. The mean particle size and distribution appears to be dependent not only on the size, distribution, hardness, and elastic properties of the feedstock but also on the configuration of the mill, the placement of the nozzles, the design of the classifier, and the energy input to the mill.

Effects of feed rate on particle size distribution during milling of Calcite E or $CaCO_3$ (99.4%) may be seen in Figures 9 and 10. Figure 9 is a set of conventional cumulative distribution curves, while Figure 10 is a three-dimensional set of frequency distribution curves of the same data. The frequency distribution curves depict more clearly how the size distribution is affected by feed rate [25], i.e., as feed rate decreases, particle size also decreases. Figures 11 and 12, with the same type graphics representation, indicate that, at constant feed rate, product particle size decreases with increased grinding pressure, provided the mill is operated within its feed rate design limits.

Figure 13 shows several frequency distributions of amobarbital, an extremely hard substance, before and after several passes through a fluid energy mill. Each succeeding pass was made at a higher nozzle pressure at the same feed rate using the material obtained from the previous pass through the mill. Two things become obvious from this figure, namely, the narrow size distribution, and the near absence of change in size distribution between product from passes 2 and 3 (from author's experience).

The mill surfaces that contact the product may be made from a variety of materials ranging from the softer stainless steels to the tough ceramics, which are used for exceptionally abrasive materials such as barium sulfate and amobarbital (data shown in Fig. 13). Usually the mills are constructed such that the contact surfaces are merely linings which can be removed and replaced if excessively eroded after use.

Size reduction using the fluid energy mill has the advantage that heat labile substances can be milled with little danger of thermal degradation.

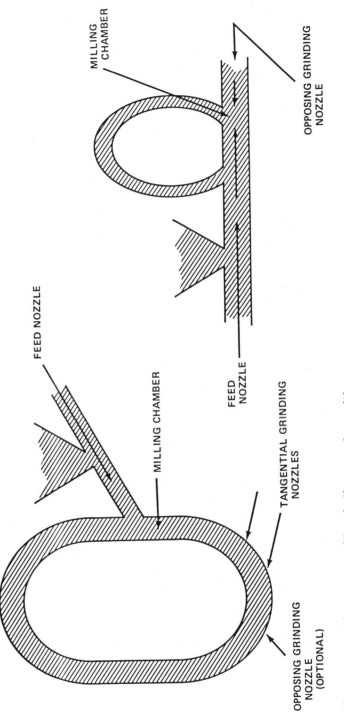

Figure 6   Fluid energy mill grinding nozzle positions.

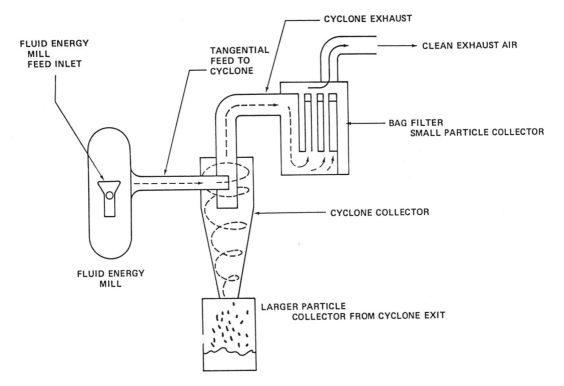

FLUID ENERGY
MILL
FEED INLET

TANGENTIAL
FEED TO
CYCLONE

CYCLONE EXHAUST

CLEAN EXHAUST AIR

BAG FILTER
SMALL PARTICLE COLLECTOR

CYCLONE COLLECTOR

FLUID ENERGY
MILL

LARGER PARTICLE
COLLECTOR FROM CYCLONE EXIT

Figure 7   Schematic of fluid energy mill and particle collection system.

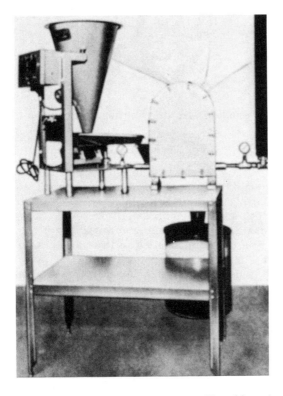

Figure 8   Trost fluid energy mill. (Courtesy Plastomer Products, Newton, Pennsylvania.)

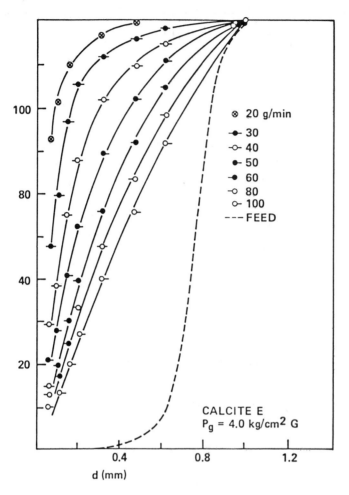

Figure 9 Effect of feed rate on product size distribution. (From Ref. 11.)

This is a result of the cooling effect of the expanding gases (with the exception of steam as a gas) and the rapid heat exchange between particle and milling gases. It must be noted that gases used for milling must contain little if any moisture. If any appreciable moisture were present, the expanding gases could decrease temperatures in the milling chamber below the gas dew point. This would cause moisture condensation in the mill and on the particles. Gases used for fluid energy milling should have dewpoints below 5–10°C. Inert gases may also be used to minimize or eliminate oxidation of susceptible compounds that may occur with compressed air. Soft materials such as waxes may be milled by pre-chilling in liquid nitrogen to make them brittle (Cryogenic milling is reviewed by Chinnis in Ref. 25). Again, protection against moisture condensation is extremely important.

Fluid energy milling is usually used (a) to reduce the particle size of active ingredients that require a very small particle size to assure both

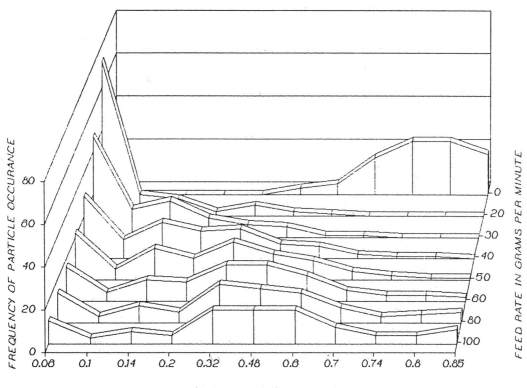

PARTICLE SIZE FREQUENCY DISTRIBUTION

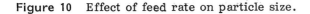

Figure 10   Effect of feed rate on particle size.

maximum surface area for solubilization and bioavailability and (b) for tablet
content uniformity, particularly in dry granulations. Although it is not
used in tablet granulating per se, fluid energy milling may be used as a
means of intimately dispersing a coarse mixture of powders, drying, or even
intimate mixing of small amounts of liquid with a fine powder [22]. However, one must be careful that classification does not segregate the different
admixture ingredients by virtue of their differences in particle size, hardness, and absolute density and/or moisture content.

B. Ball Mill

Ball milling is also used to obtain extremely small particles, but not used
in tablet granulating per se. Considerable study has been directed to ball
milling [26] in attempting to predict the action of this type of mill as well
as to express the "dynamic characteristics" in mathematical terms. Potentially these terms may then be used to more closely control this process by
computer. Scale-up and mill design are also areas that can be realized as

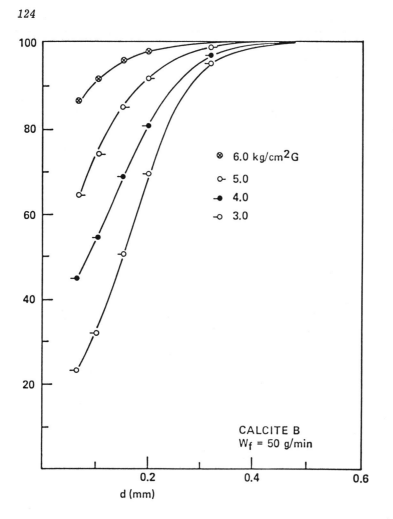

CALCITE B
W_f = 50 g/min

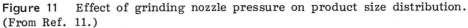

Figure 11   Effect of grinding nozzle pressure on product size distribution.
(From Ref. 11.)

a result of the work that has been accomplished to date with the ball mill.
Since the theory cannot be dealt with adequately within the space of this
text, the reader is referred to the available wealth of literature [27,28]
dealing with various theoretical aspects of ball milling. The discussion to
follow takes a more practical point of view for those who will be, or who
are, involved in the milling of raw materials in tablet making.

The ball mill (Figs. 14 and 15) is a cylindrical or conical shell usually
filled to about half its volume with grinding media that can be varied in
both size (1/4 in. or smaller to 3 in. diameter), size distribution, shape
(balls, cylinders, cubes, etc.) and composition (Fig. 16). The shell rotates on its central axis by means of motor-driven rollers on which it
rests. The drive may also be through a "bull gear" that follows the cir-
cumference of the outer shell. The ball mill designed for batch milling

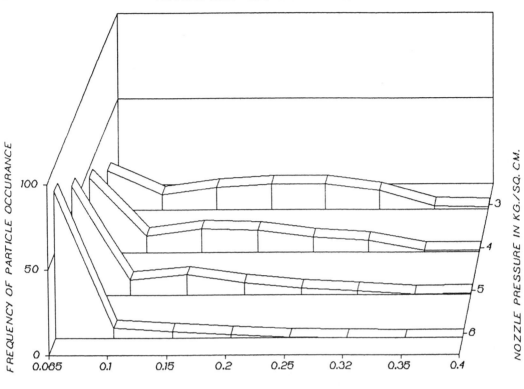

Figure 12   Effect of grinding pressure on particle size frequency distributions.

usually has a removable end plate or side entrance hatch cover, depending on the size of the installation, where the grinding media and unmilled material can be loaded, and then unloaded when milling is complete.

The continuous milling design (Fig. 17) is usually a conical shell with grinding media of equal or varied sizes. The feedstock enters through the hollow trunion at one end of the mill, and milled material exits through a grating or small ports at the opposite end of the chamber. Continuous closed circuit milling (Fig. 18) is arranged using the continuous mill with a gas or liquid classifying system. In this arrangement, the air swept dry milling introduces the gas (in most cases air) and feed through the hollow trunion at one end of the mill. The large feedstock drops into the milling zone while the smaller particles become entrained in the air stream flowing through the opposite end to a particle classifier. The classifier removes the smallest of the particles, or the fraction of particles it is designed to remove, while the larger particles are recycled to the mill inlet for further size reduction. Wet milling with a liquid can also be carried

PARTICLE FREQUENCY DISTRIBUTION

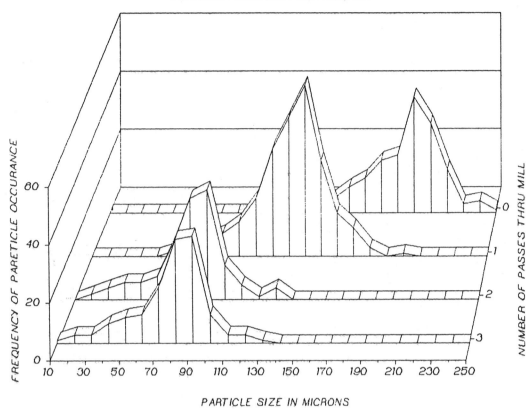

Figure 13   Fluid energy milling.

out in a very similar manner with certain mill and classifier modifications.

In general terms, milling takes place as the charged cylindrical or conical chamber rotates. The grinding media (balls, cubes, etc.) are made to climb the chamber walls (Fig. 19) as a result of the chamber rotation, and drop from the elevated position to the bed of media below resulting in the primary means of particle fracture by impact. The higher the grinding media are carried up the chamber wall, the greater the capacity of the mill, and the more effective the impact grinding.

However, it must be noted that a critical mill speed may be reached where the centrifugal force on the grinding media becomes greater than the gravitational force, and the media no longer drop to the bottom of the mill, but is held at the rotating chamber wall. This critical speed may be calculated using the following equation:

$$Nc = \frac{76.6}{\sqrt{D}}$$

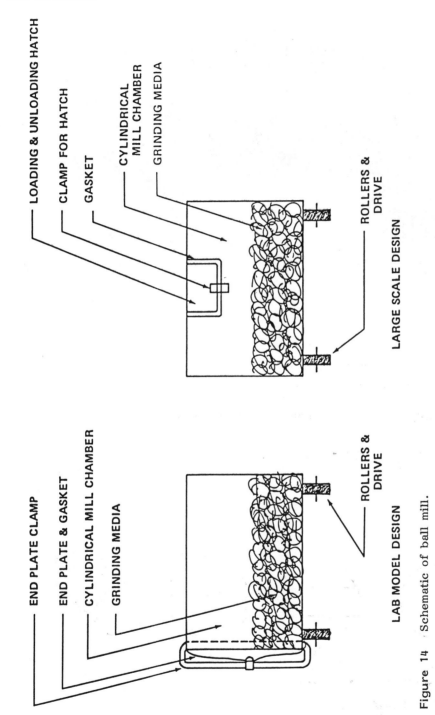

Figure 14   Schematic of ball mill.

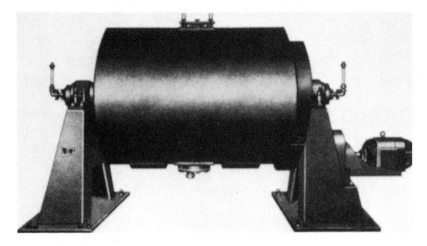

Figure 15   Ball or pebble mill.   (Courtesy of Paul O. Abbe, Inc., Little Falls, New Jersey.)

where

    Nc = the critical speed in revolutions/min

    D = the inside mill diameter in ft

For example, the critical speed of a 6-in. diameter mill would be:

$$Nc = \frac{76.6}{\sqrt{0.5}} = 108 \text{ rpm}$$

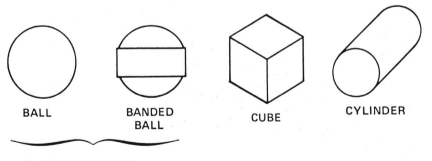

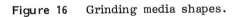

Figure 16   Grinding media shapes.

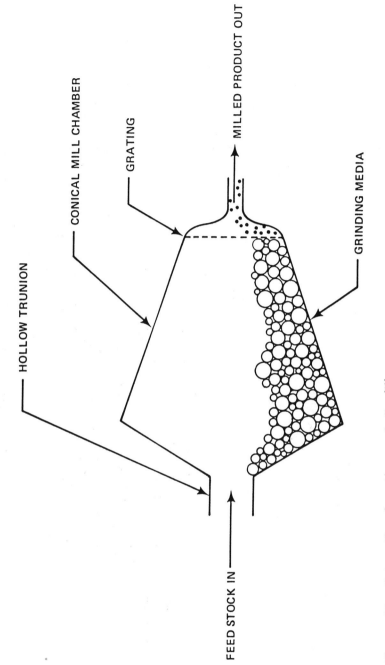

Figure 17 Schematic of continuous ball milling.

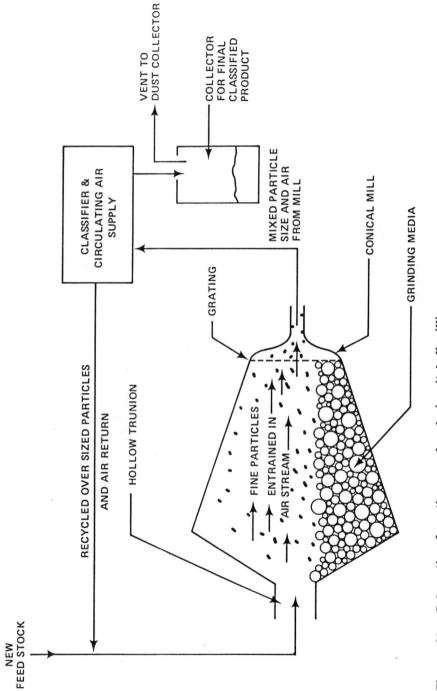

NEW FEED STOCK

RECYCLED OVER SIZED PARTICLES AND AIR RETURN

CLASSIFIER & CIRCULATING AIR SUPPLY

VENT TO DUST COLLECTOR

COLLECTOR FOR FINAL CLASSIFIED PRODUCT

MIXED PARTICLE SIZE AND AIR FROM MILL

GRATING

HOLLOW TRUNION

FINE PARTICLES ENTRAINED IN AIR STREAM

CONICAL MILL

GRINDING MEDIA

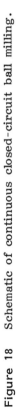

Figure 18   Schematic of continuous closed-circuit ball milling.

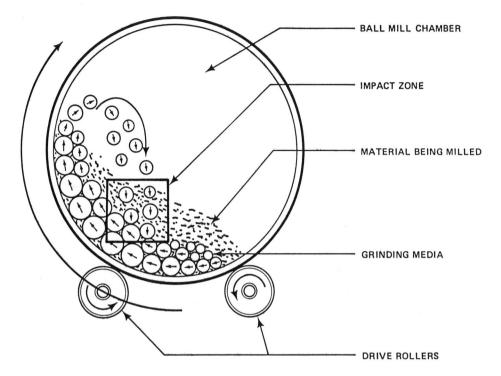

BALL MILL CHAMBER

IMPACT ZONE

MATERIAL BEING MILLED

GRINDING MEDIA

DRIVE ROLLERS

Figure 19 Schematic of ball mill and grinding media action.

In comparison, the critical speed of a 24-in. diameter mill would be

$$Nc = \frac{76.6}{\sqrt{2.0}} = 54 \text{ rpm}$$

At the critical speed and above, the mill is said to be "centrifuging" and milling all but ceases. Therefore, milling must be carried out below the critical speed of the mill at some optimum speed where the grinding media are carried to the highest point in the chamber without "centrifuging." This speed is dependent on chamber size, grinding media size, material size distribution, shape, density, and the amount used in the mill. The optimum speed may range between 60 to 85% of the critical speed, and may be calculated from the empirically derived equation:

$$N_o = (57) - 40 \ (\log D)$$

where

N_o = the optimum speed in revolutions per min

D = the inside diameter of the mill in feet

Calculating the optimum speeds for the previous examples, the percentages of the critical speeds are:

6-in. diameter mill:

$$N_o = (57) - 40 \text{ (log } 0.5) = 69 \text{ rpm} = 64\% \text{ of the critical speed}$$

24 in. diameter mill:

$$N_o = (57) - 40 \text{ (log 2)} = 45 \text{ rpm} = 83\% \text{ of the critical speed}$$

Grinding also takes place by attrition as the media move against one another and against the walls of the mill. Slower-than-optimum speeds may be used such that attrition is the primary type of milling taking place. Milling at slower speeds yields finer grinding but requires considerably longer milling times. Finer grinding may also be achieved, in most cases, by using smaller size grinding media and/or by wet milling.

Wet milling utilizes a liquid in which the material to be ground is insoluble. This liquid may also contain additives such as surfactants, if necessary, to prevent particle flocculation. Wet milling is usually attempted when it is found that dry milling causes caking of the material to the grinding media and the chamber wall which in turn acts to cushion both the impact and attrition action in the mill. This diminishes milling efficiency, and creates problems in recovery of caked material from the mill.

The amount of grinding media and powder charge may vary in the mill but are very important factors affecting milling efficiency and fineness of grind. The grinding media usually occupies from 30% to no greater than 50% of the mill chamber volume. The powder charge is usually gauged to fill the volume of the grinding media interstices with enough excess to just cover the top of the grinding media bed. This is not a hard fast rule, but should act as the upper limit, since large powder charges tend to cushion and absorb impact energy of the grinding media.

The disadvantages in using the ball mill is the difficulty in cleaning it, long milling times, and the high power requirements (considerable energy is expended in moving and lifting the griding media for grinding). However, the mill is very well suited for milling highly abrasive materials. Typical materials of mill construction include: chrome manganese alloy and porcelain, both a standard and a high density grade. Recently, another concept in ball milling is being marketed (by Brinckman Instruments, Inc., Westbury, New York) where the mill container is held upright, and the balls accomplish milling by virtue of centrifugal force.

Figure 20 shows the difference in particle size distribution between the ball and pebble mill, and the fluid energy mill after milling the same starting material. Again, a narrower size distribution is seen using the fluid energy mill.

C. Hammer Mill

The hammer mill, which can be either the horizontal or vertical shaft type (Fig. 21), is one of the most versatile and widely used mills in the pharmaceutical industry. Intermediate (10 to 100 mesh) to fine (100 to <325

PARTICLE SIZE FREQUENCY DISTRIBUTION

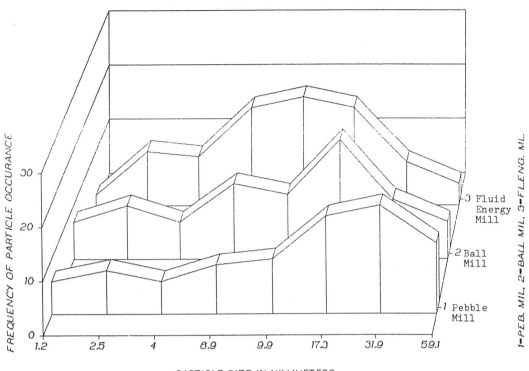

Figure 20   Effect of milling equipment.   (From Ref. 22.)

mesh) milling can be obtained with this mill as well as coarse to thorough
dispersion of powder mixes by simply changing hammer speeds, and/or
screen sizes and feed rates.   Evaluation of this type of mill in the pharmaceutical industry is very limited because the information is usually of a
proprietary nature.   Some data are available from mill manufacturers as to
what type of material has been milled, the milling conditions, and the results in terms of screen analysis and throughput rates.   Examples are
shown in Tables 3 and 4.   These materials are usually pure compounds
and do not include various types of tablet granulations.

   The principle of the operation of the hammer mill is one of impact between rapidly moving hammers mounted on a rotor (Fig. 22) and the
powder particles.   The problem in design of the hammer mill is in presenting the particles to the hammers such that enough force is imparted
to the particles to shatter them.   This can be difficult, because the air
currents created by the rotating hammers cause the powder particles to
travel in the same direction as the hammers.   Because of their low mass
and the fluid drag forces, the particles seldom reach the velocity of the
hammers, so some impact is achieved.   One mill (Fig. 23) is equipped with

Table 3 Commercial Milling Data

Material	Character	Remarks	Mill model	Hammers
Aspirin	Brittle, light	None	#1SH	LFS
			#1S1	Rigid, sharpened
Alginic acid	Fibrous, light, slightly hygroscopic	Runs hot	Bantam	FT
Ascorbic acid	Brittle, light	None	#1SH	LFS − SS
Benzoic acid	Brittle, heavy	None	#1SH	1/8 × 1"
Caffeine	Fibrous, light, soft	None	#1SH	L. lined
Sugar cane	Brittle, heavy, free flowing	None	#2TH	1/8 × 1"

Source: Courtesy of Pulverizing Machinery Division, Milropul Corporation, United States Filter Corporation, Summit, New Jersey.

specially designed deflectors around the mill inner periphery that alter the path of the traveling particles by deflecting them back into the path of the hammers.

A much greater velocity differential between powder particles and hammers is achieved with the deflectors. This results in increased milling effectiveness. For the deflectors to work properly, there is apparently a critical clearance between the hammers and deflectors, i.e., if the clearance is too great, the particles will not deflect, and if the clearance is too small, considerable heat may be developed during milling.

Another device used with the hammer mill is the screen that is placed over the milling chamber outlet (the bottom of the horizontal shaft mills and 360° around the vertical shaft mills). These screens serve to retain the larger particles in the milling chamber for further size reduction and also act in part as a classifier in allowing only certain size particles and smaller to pass out of the milling zone into the collector. The screens do not act as sieves, i.e., one cannot expect the largest particle leaving the

Speed (rpm)	Screen	Grind	Output (lb/hr)	Horsepower
9,600	020HB	98.2% < 150 mesh 96.0% < 200 mesh	200	3
986	1/8Rd.	53.4% < 110 mesh 22.0% < 60 mesh	2140	Idle
14,000	020Rd.	94.8% < 100 mesh	30	1/2
8,000	035HB SS	2.4% < 100 mesh 16.2% < 200 mesh 81.4% < 325 mesh	667	3
8,000	3/64HB	99.7% < 30 mesh 82.5% < 100 mesh	860	—
3,000	1/4Rd.	99.3% < 40 mesh	425	Idle
1,750	020HB	88.7% < 40 51.2% < 60 35.5% < 100 19.8% < 200	2400	3

mill to be 20 mesh if the mill is fitted with the equivalent to a 20-mesh screen. This is due to the particle velocity and the angle at which it approaches and exits through the screen as seen in Figure 24.

Screen thickness is also a factor in the exiting particle size. If one assumes the same particle velocity for different screen thicknesses, Figure 25 illustrates screen thickness effect on the particle size.

The screen is usually an integral part of the hammer mill in the pharmaceutical industry, and because of the large forces they are subjected to, they usually are not of the woven wire type seen in hand screens and the oscillating granulator. The screen strength required for much of the hammer milling is obtained by using sheet metal of various thicknesses with perforated holes or slots as shown in Figure 26. The holes may range in size and open area as seen in Table 5. The slots may also vary in size and pattern. Slot patterns often used are the herring-bone or the cross slot configuration also shown in Figure 26. Table 6 shows typical applications of the different screen configurations.

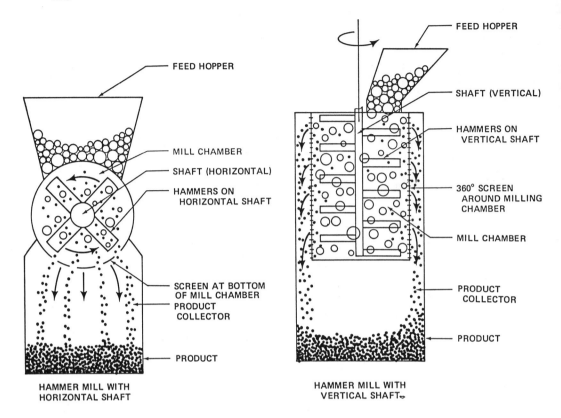

Figure 21   Schematic of two types of hammer mills.

Hammers may take several shapes as shown in Figure 27.   However, the two basic shapes are the stirrup and the bar; the bar-shaped hammers being used extensively in tablet granulating.   The hammers are usually made of hardened steel, stainless steel, or a mild steel with impact surfaces made of an extremely abrasive resistant material such as haystellite (imbedded carbaloy particles) or carbaloy.   Most of the work in pharmaceuticals does not require the hardest of alloy hammers, and in most cases stainless steel may suffice.

Hammers (Fig. 28) may also be free swinging.   The free swinging hammer has the advantage or disadvantage of increasing hammer to screen clearance if excessive buildup occurs within the mill.   This will minimize mill damage if the milled raw material fuses from heat, or it may decrease output rate if the material is extremely difficult to mill.

As mentioned previously, the hammers may be mounted on either a horizontal or vertical shaft.   Vertical shaft mills such as the Stokes Tornado (Sharples-Stokes, Division Pennwalt Corporation, Clark, New Jersey) mill have feed inlets at the top where powder enters the milling chamber perpendicular to the swing of the hammers.   There is some tendency to segregate the powder or powder mix by size, because the

Table 4 Commercial Milling Data[a]

Milling variables	Run 1	Run 2	Run 3	Run 4
Rpm	5000	7200	7200	7200
Screen hole size (in.)	0.020	0.020	0.010	0.012
Blade type	125	125	125	125
Forward	Impact	Impact	Impact	Impact
Feeds size and type	S-throat	4 × 4	4 × 4	4 × 4
Feed setting no.	Gravity	3.0	3.0	1.0
Rotor amperes	–	12.0	16.0	11.0
Equipment model no.	DAS06[b]	VFS-DAS06	VFS-DAS06	VFS-DAS06

Sieve analysis (%)[c]	Original	Run 1	Run 2	Run 3	Run 4
>20	0.18	0	0	0	0
20–50	67.1	0	0	0	0
50–60	12.1	0	0	0	0
60–100	14.4	0	0	0	0
100–140	4.6	31.0	17.7	21.4	0
140–200	0.4	13.7	17.7	25.0	5.0
200–325	0.9	31.0	28.6	28.5	45.0
<325	0.09	24.1	36.8	25.0	50.0

[a]Material: medium grade sucrose.
[b]Fitzpatrick mill model number.
[c]Mesh (U.S. standard).
Source: Fitzpatrick Company, South Plainfield, New Jersey.

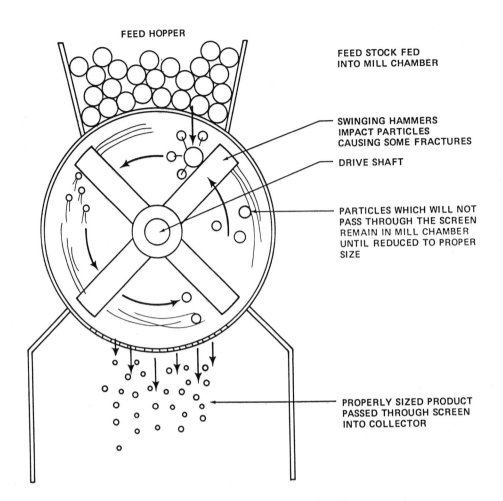

FEED HOPPER

FEED STOCK FED
INTO MILL CHAMBER

SWINGING HAMMERS
IMPACT PARTICLES
CAUSING SOME FRACTURES

DRIVE SHAFT

PARTICLES WHICH WILL NOT
PASS THROUGH THE SCREEN
REMAIN IN MILL CHAMBER
UNTIL REDUCED TO PROPER
SIZE

PROPERLY SIZED PRODUCT
PASSED THROUGH SCREEN
INTO COLLECTOR

Figure 22   Hammer mill and particle impact and sizing.

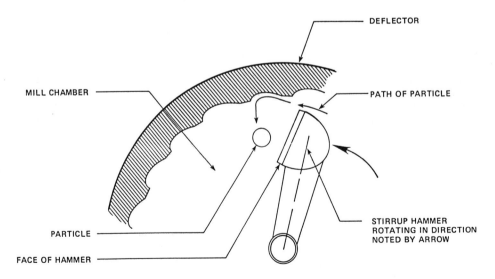

DEFLECTOR

MILL CHAMBER

PATH OF PARTICLE

STIRRUP HAMMER
ROTATING IN DIRECTION
NOTED BY ARROW

PARTICLE

FACE OF HAMMER

Figure 23   Hammer mill with deflector. (Courtesy Pulverizing Machinery
Mikropul Corp., Subsidiary of United States Filter Corporation, Summit,
New Jersey.)

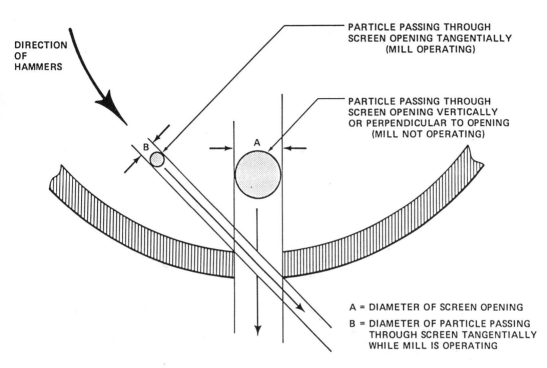

Figure 24 Effect of exiting particle angle through mill screen on exiting particle size. (Courtesy Fitzpatrick Company, Elmhurst, Illinois.)

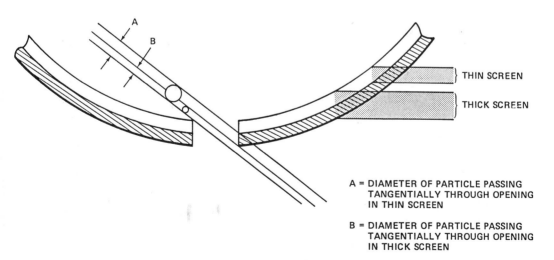

Figure 25 Effect of mill screen thickness on exiting particle size. (Courtesy Fitzpatrick Company, Elmhurst, Illinois.)

Table 5   Model D6 Screens

	Round hole screens			
Number	Hole size (in.)	Open area	Gage	Old number
1532-0020	0.020	24%	28	000
1532-0024	0.024	24%	26	00
1532-0027	0.027	23%	24	0
1532-0033	0.033	29%	24	1
1532-0040	0.040	30%	22	1A
1532-0050	0.050	33%	22	1B

Note: Above mounted on 18-gage 18-hole backing frames.

Number	Hole size (in.)	Open area	Gage	Old number
1531-0065	0.065	26%	18	2
1531-0079	0.079	41%	18	2AA
1531-0093	0.093	33%	18	2A
1531-0109	0.109	45%	18	2B
1531-0125	0.125	40%	18	3
1531-0156	0.156	46%	18	3AA
1531-0187	0.187	51%	18	3A
1531-0218	0.218	45%	18	3B
1531-0250	0.250	48%	18	4
1531-0312	0.312	47%	18	4A
1531-0375	0.375	51%	18	4B
1531-0500	0.500	47%	18	5
1531-0625	0.625	47%	18	5A
1531-0750	0.750	51%	18	6
1531-1000	1.000	58%	18	7

	Square hole screens			
Number	Hole size (in.)	Open area	Gage	Old number
1533-0200	0.200	64%	18	15S
1533-0250	0.250	45%	18	14S
1533-0312	0.312	51%	18	516S
1533-0375	0.375	56%	18	38S
1533-0437	0.437	64%	18	716S
1533-0500	0.500	53%	18	12S
1533-0625	0.625	59%	18	58S
1533-0687	0.687	54%	18	1116S
1533-0750	0.750	57%	18	34S
1533-0875	0.875	68%	18	78S
1533-1000	1.000	64%	18	100S
1533-1125	1.125	53%	18	1-18S
1533-1500	1.500	64%	18	1-12S

Table 5 (Continued)

Mesh screens	
Number	Mesh size
1536-0004	4
1536-0006	6
1536-0008	8
1536-0010	10
1536-0012	12
1536-0014	14
1536-0016	16
1536-0020	20
1536-0024	24
1536-0030	30
1536-0040	40
1536-0050	50
1536-0060	60
1536-0080	80
1536-0100	100
1536-0120	120
1536-0150	150
1536-0200	200
1536-0250	250
1536-0325	325

Note: All mesh screens reinforced with suitable backing frames.

Special screens					
Number	Type of hole	Hole size	Open area	Gage	Old number
1532-5001*	Round	0.020	30%	26 (18 BF)	N-000
1539-0018	Square	0.625	59%	14	58S
1539-0019	Square	0.687	54%	14	1116S
1539-0032	Square	0.875	68%	14	78S
1539-0020	Square	1.000	64%	14	100S
1539-0021	Square	1.125	53%	14	118S
1539-0022	Square	1.500	64%	14	112S
1539-0024	Square	1.000	64%	12	100S
1539-0025	Square	1.125	53%	12	1-18S
1539-0026	Square	1.500	64%	12	1-12S

Note: All screens listed above are of 18−8 stainless steel except nickel material on item indicated by an asterisk.

Source: Courtesy of The Fitzpatrick Company, Elmhurst, Illinois.

Table 6   Applications of Different Mill Screen Configurations

Perforation shape	Recommended use	Comments
Round holes	Fibrous materials	Clogs more quickly; lower hole size limited because of structural strength
Herringbone slot	Amorphous and crystalline material	Slightly coarser grind than equal diameter round perforation
Cross slot	Amorphous and crystalline material	Some grind size as equal size round perforation; finer slot size attainable than round perforations

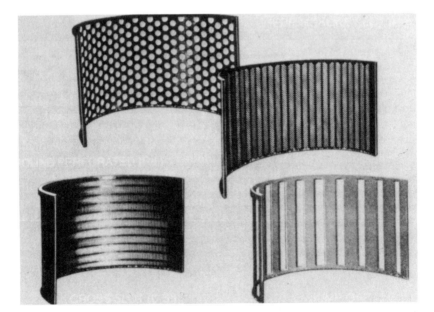

Figure 26   Different screen configurations. (Courtesy of Pulverizing Machinery, Division of Mikropul, Subsidiary of United States Filter Corporation, Summit, New Jersey.)

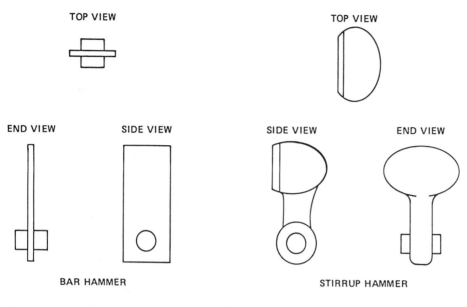

Figure 27 Two popular hammer mill hammer shapes.

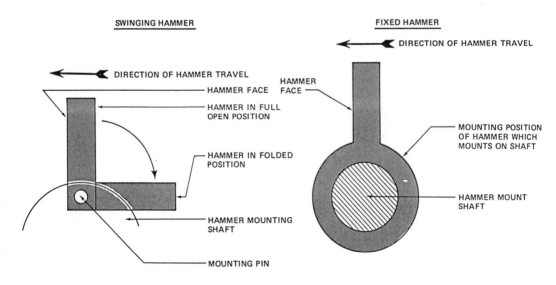

Figure 28 Swinging and fixed hammers.

smallest particles exit through the screen near the top while the larger particles with more mass have a tendency to fall to the bottom of the mill before complete dispersion through the screen. This is contrasted to the power feed tangential to the hammer swing as found in the horizontal shaft Micropulverizer (Mikropul Corporation, Summit, New Jersey) and Fitzpatrick (Fitzpatrick Company, Elmhurst, Illinois) mills. The vertical shaft mills, by virtue of the 360° surrounding screen, normally have higher through-put potential than the horizontal shaft equipment where the screen is mounted at the mill chamber bottom outlet.

There is also an air swept hammer mill very similar to the ball mill depicted in Figure 18, where the air is forced through the milling chamber entraining and carrying the smaller particles out of the milling chamber. This air suspension of particles passes through a classifier where the larger particles are further separated and recirculated back to the mill, and the small particles are collected. This type of mill is particularly useful where a small uniform particle size is required with heat sensitive materials, i.e., the circulating air cools the particles and the mill. This type of mill is normally used for the milling of non-heat sensitive raw materials but is not commonly used in the preparation of tablets.

Maximum mill versatility is obtained by utilizing a hammer with a cutting blade on the trailing edge of the bar. With a simple mechanical manipulation, the cutting edge is available for use in the mill. In the case of the Fitzpatrick mill, the milling head is so designed that a 180° rotation of the drive shaft and attached hammers exposes the trailing edge of hammers, which is the cutting edge.

The particle size of a milled material is inversely proportional to the hammer speed which may vary from 1000 to 20,000 ft/min, depending on hammer length and rpm. Changes in speed are accomplished by variable speed drive or by manually changing the hammer drive and motor pulley ratio. Mill speeds should be recorded as part of the operating conditions during size reduction of a material.

The advantages of the hammer mill include:

1. Ease of setup, teardown, and cleanup
2. Minimum scale-up problems provided the same type mill is used
3. Ease of installation
4. Wide range in size and type of feedstock that can be handled
5. Small space requirements (under normal circumstances where special or elaborate equipment for recycling of coarser material is not needed)

The disadvantages include:

1. Potential clogging of screens
2. Heat buildup during milling with possible product degradation
3. Mill and screen wear with abrasive materials

D. Cutting Mill

The use of cutting mills in tablet making are primarily for intimate dispersion of powder mixes such as a premix of two or more powders, milling wet and dry granulations, and size reduction of tablet batches requiring rework for one reason or another. This equipment is akin to the hammer mill, because the cutters are usually on the trailing edge of the bar hammers as mentioned previously. In some cases, hammers can easily be replaced with cutters using the same shaft and milling chamber. The cutters are used with both woven and perforated hole screens. In some cases, as with soft, dry, or wet granulations, size reduction or powder dispersion may not require a screen.

Although size reduction in the cutting mill may be primarily the result of shearing action, one must not forget the increase in force per unit area created at the leading edge of a cutting blade. An example is given in the following paragraph.

A hammer mill is running at some constant peripheral velocity (x) ft/min, and the impact surface area of the hammer is 9/16 in.^{2} (hammer blade is 3 in. long by 3/16 in. wide). If one were to substitute a cutting edge of 3/64 in.^{2} area for the hammer surface area (blade is 3 in. long and the cutting edge is 1/64 in. wide) using the same peripheral velocity, the increase in potential pressure (force per unit area) of the cutting edges would be 9/16 in.^{2} divided by 3/64 in.^{2}, or 12 times that of the faces. Although potential impact force (pressure) of the mill hammer has been increased by 12 times, the probability of particle contact has been reduced by just as much, because of the reduced potential surface contact area. Although over-simplified, this illustrates why the knife edges are not as effective in size reduction as the larger surface area hammers.

The same variables encountered with the hammer mill must be considered when using the cutting mill, i.e., size and size distribution of the feedstock, cutter speed, screen size, and feed rate.

The conical screen mill (Quadro Comil, Quadro, Inc., Park Ridge, New Jersey) is also very effective for the dry and wet milling of soft to medium-hard materials. The material is fed through an opening in the top of the milling chamber where it falls via gravity into a conical screen area with a rotating impellor. The impellor-screen clearance is maintained such that minimal heat is generated and optimum size reduction efficiency is obtained with fairly high material throughputs. Variables include screen sizes, impellor designs, and speed.

E. Oscillating Granulator

The oscillating granulator (Fig. 29) is used in the pharmaceutical industry almost exclusively for size reduction of wet and dry granulations, and to some extent reducing tablets and compactions that must be recompressed. This equipment consists of an oscillating bar contacting a woven wire screen. A hopper above the oscillator and screen provides a receptacle for the feedstock that is forced through the screen by the oscillating motion of the bar(s). Size reduction is primarily by shear with some attrition. Collection of the product may be directly onto trays in the case of wet granulations, or into drums via a sleeve from a specially fitted collector funnel which minimizes dust during the processing of a dry granulation. The oscillator speed is constant, and the screens, which are readily interchangeable, range in size from 4 to 20 mesh.

The outstanding characteristic about the oscillating granulator is the narrow size range and minimum amount of fines obtained during size reduction of a dry granulation, and the very uniform wet granulation size,

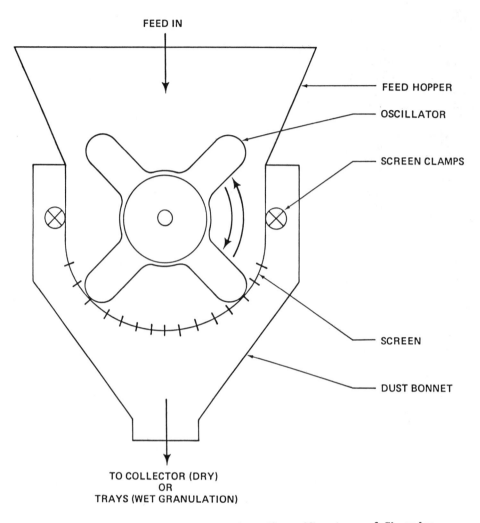

Figure 29   Oscillating granulator schematic.   (Courtesy of Sharples-Stokes, Division of Pennwalt Corporation, Clark, New Jersey.)

which promotes uniform drying. The disadvantages with this equipment are the low throughput rates, wear on the screens, the possibility of product contamination by metal particles abraded away from the screen by oscillator, and the fact that size reduction of large particles or granules (4 mesh or larger) must be done stepwise, i.e., passed through successively smaller screens until the desired granule size is obtained.

   To illustrate the effect of different milling conditions, using a hammer and cutting mill and an oscillating granulator, an acetaminophen wet granulation was prepared using the following formula:

   Acetaminophen   88%
   Microcrystalline cellulose   10%
   Polyvinyl pyrrolidone (PVP)   2%
   Deionized water (q.s. to make a 7.5% PVP solution)

The wet granulation was not milled but spread on trays and dried to 1% moisture at 45°C.

Equal proportions of the dry granulation were put through a Model D Fitzpatrick Mill at the same feed rate under the following operating conditions:

1. Low speed ⎫
2. High speed ⎬ large screen ⎫
3. Low speed ⎫ ⎬ Hammers forward
4. High speed ⎬ small screen ⎭

5. Low speed ⎫
6. High speed ⎬ large screen ⎫
7. Low speed ⎫ ⎬ Knives forward
8. High speed ⎬ small screen ⎭

The same granulation was passed through a Stokes Oscillating Granulator using a large screen (10 mesh woven wire) and then a small screen (14 mesh woven wire). A screen analysis was performed on each milled granulation and the unmilled granulation using 10, 20, 30, 40, 70, and 140 U.S. Standard mesh screens. The screens were nested from the largest mesh opening (10 mesh) to the smallest with a collector pan nested below the smallest screen (140 mesh). One hundred grams of sample were coned and quartered out of each mill sample and placed at the top of the nest of screens and the collector pan was mounted in the Rotap (W. S. Tyler, Inc., Mentor, Ohio) screen shaker and allowed to shake for 15 min. The screens and collector pan were removed at the end of the time interval and weighed individually. The differences in weight were calculated and expressed as a percent of the total collected on each screen, i.e., amount collected less than 10 mesh but greater than 20 mesh, and plotted as shown in Figures 30−36.

In Figures 30 and 31, note that a low speed using the large screen, very little change in size distribution takes place when compared to the unmilled granulation (compare 0 and 1).

However, a change to a smaller screen reduces the granule size considerably (compare 0 and 3). At high speed the screen size does not yield as big a change as seen at low speed (compare 2 and 4). Mill speed changes using the large screen (compare 1 and 2) does not show as great an effect on the granule size distribution as seen with the small screen (compare 3 and 4).

Figure 32 shows that the basic changes in granulation size distribution using knives with the large screen size are very similar to those seen with the hammer mill in that there is almost no change from the unmilled granulation. However, at high speeds, both the large and small screens show significant size distribution changes. These changes are not as great as those seen with the hammer mill.

Using both large and small screens, Figures 33 and 34 illustrate that the the hammer mill yields a smaller particle size than the cutting mill at high speeds. Note that, except for the distribution obtained using knives forward with a small screen (No. 8), the size distributions are all very similar (near parallel lines and frequency distributions) but different in average particle size at high mill speed.

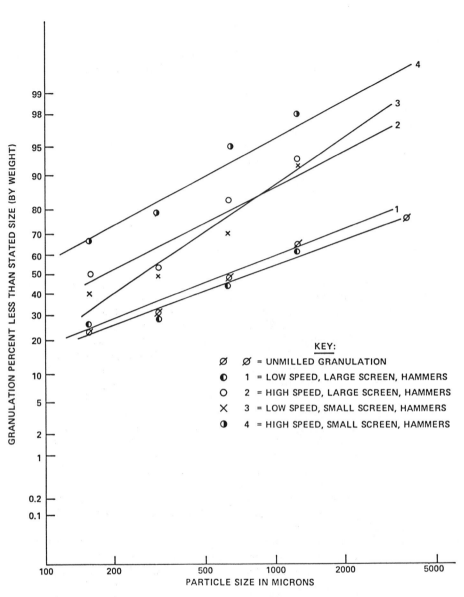

Figure 30   Effect of screen size and speed on acetominophen granulation size distribution using a hammer mill.

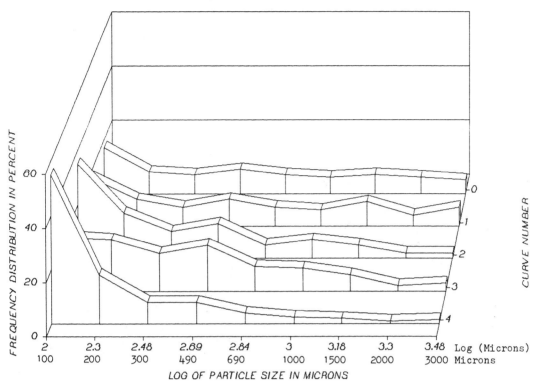

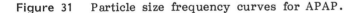

Figure 31   Particle size frequency curves for APAP.

Screen size or mill type makes very little difference in granulation size distribution at low speeds, as shown in Figure 35.

Although reduced in size, Figure 36 shows that the screen sizes used did not make much difference in the size distribution of the acetominophen granulation passed through the oscillating granulator.

Only the most general conclusions may be drawn from work of this type since granulations with different characteristics will give differing results on the same equipment using the same milling conditions.

F. Granulation Cracker

A slightly different design and unique piece of equipment has been tested and found to be very effective in reducing the size of compactions. These compactions may originate from a compactor, a slugging machine, or compressed tablets which do not meet compression specifications, e.g., weight,

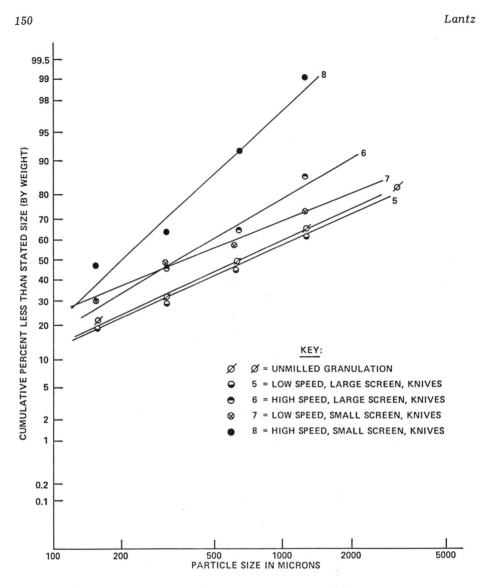

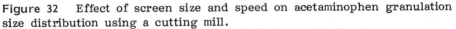

Figure 32   Effect of screen size and speed on acetaminophen granulation size distribution using a cutting mill.

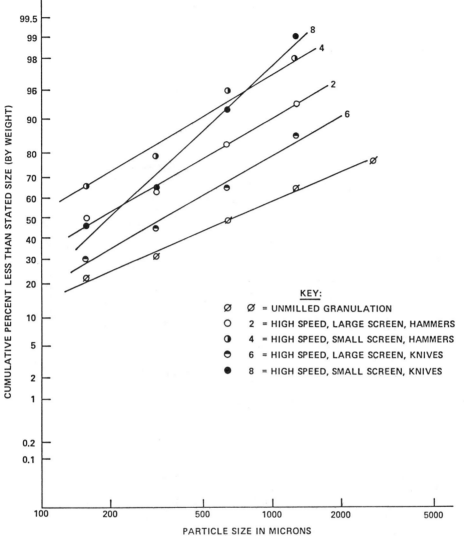

Figure 33   Effect of mill type and screen size on acetaminophen size distribution at high mill speed.

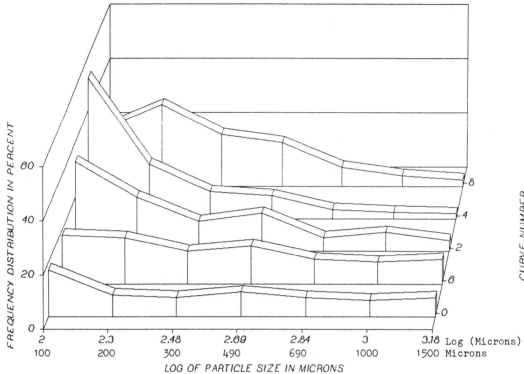

Figure 34   Particle frequency curves for APAP.

hardness, and thickness. The Crack-U-Lator is comprised of several sets
of horizontally positioned, parallel rolls. The top set of rolls have the
largest mating corrugations on each roll. The space between the rolls can
be set to accommodate the largest slug or tablet size. As the slug or
compaction pieces pass between the turning corrugated rollers, they are
literally cracked to a size small enough to pass through these rolls.
Below these rolls are up to six additional sets of rolls, with successively
smaller corrugations, and each of which has a reproducible means of
setting the spaces or gaps between the rolls. Fewer than six sets of
rolls may be selected to do the size reduction if desired, since each set of
rolls is a module that can be added or left out as desired. As the compaction is fed from the top hopper and passes each set of rolls with sequen-
tially smaller corrugations and gaps between the rolls, one may literally
size a compaction to a desired granule size distribution.

    Table 7 shows a tablet granulation made by the wet method and milled
to size for tablet compression. For some reason, the tablets were unsatisfactory, and had to be reprocessed. The reprocessing was done using
the Crack-U-Lator, and yielded the granule size distribution shown in the
last column of Table 7. With no added lubricant, the tablets were

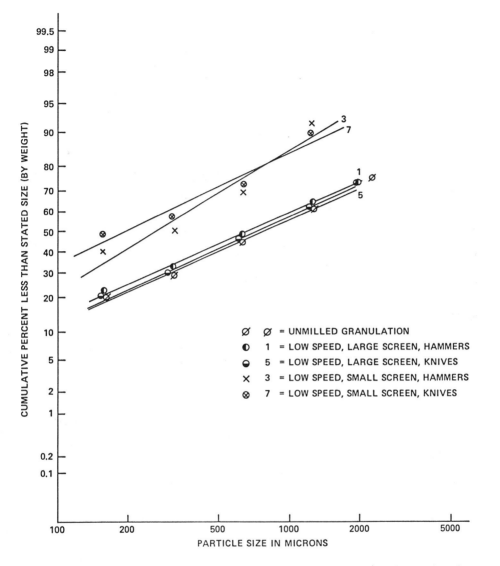

Figure 35 Effect of mill type and screen size on acetaminophen granulation size distribution at low mill speed.

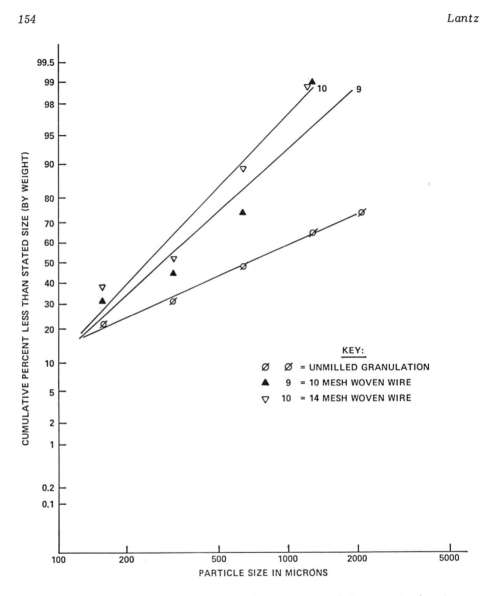

Figure 36   Effect of oscillating granulator screen size on acetaminophen granulation size distribution.

Table 7   Analysis of an Original Tablet Granulation Before
and After One Pass Through the Crack-U-Lator

U.S. standard sieve size	Percent retained on the stated screen size	
	Original	Crack-U-Lator
>16 mesh	0.4	–
<16>20 mesh	5.0	–
<20>40 mesh	13.7	0.9
<40>60 mesh	10.7	37.8
<60>80 mesh	11.4	6.2
>100 mesh	46.2	33.6

recompressed to fall within the product's physical and chemical specifications. This has been demonstrated with a number of products. However, there have been occasional products which have shown softer tablets when compressed after being passed through the Crack-U-Lator. The equipment is noteworthy.

G. Extruder

The extruder (Fig. 37) is considered here only from the view that it is a means of uniformly sizing a wet granulation. The extruder is used primarily for continuous wet granulating, i.e., the dry pre-mixed powder and granulating solution is metered into the equipment where mixing of the two components take place. The resulting mass is forced out of a series of small orifices. This yields a spaghetti-shaped mass that is easily broken up and may be dried on trays, in fluid bed driers, in a continuous belt drier, or a drum-type drier.

H. Hand Screens

These are the forerunners to the oscillating granulator and are used primarily in tablet making for screen analysis of powder raw materials or granulations. They are also used in product development for size reduction of wet and dry granules on a small scale, and in the mixing of small amounts of powder ingredients. It may be noted that those screens that are used in the manufacture of a granulation should not be used for screen analysis work since forcing materials through a screen alters the spacing of the woven wires. This leads to nonuniformity in size opening over the screen surface which would lead to inaccurate screen analysis results.

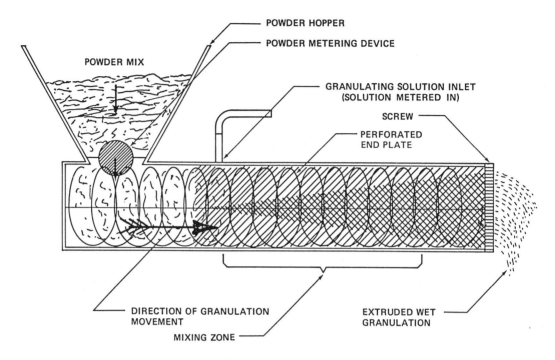

Figure 37   Extruder schematic.

Hand screens are made of brass or, preferably, stainless steel. They consist of a woven wire cloth stretched in a circular or rectangular frame (Fig. 38), the upper portion of the frame being constructed high enough above the wire cloth to contain a dry or wet powder mass which is to be screened. Table 8 is a list of mesh sizes available and their corresponding openings in microns (μm). A detailed discussion on wire mesh screens is found in Ref. 29.

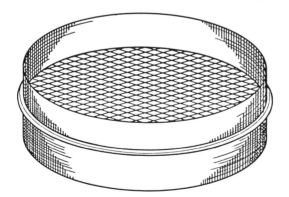

Figure 38   Hand screen.

Table 8 U.S. Standard Screen Sizes

U.S. Std.	Equivalent		Mesh openings	
	British Std.	Tyler	in.	μm
325		(325)	0.0017	44
270	(300)	(270)	0.0021	53
230		(250)	0.0024	62
200		200	0.0029	74
170	170	170	0.0035	88
140	150	150	0.0041	105
120	120	115	0.0049	125
100			0.0059	149
80	85		0.0070	177
70	72		0.0083	210
60			0.0098	250
50			0.0117	297
45		42	0.0138	350
40			0.0165	420
35	30		0.0197	500
30		28	0.0232	590
25			0.0280	710
20			0.0331	840
18			0.0394	1000
16			0.0469	1190
14			0.0555	1410
12			0.0661	1680
10			0.0787	2000
8			0.0937	2380
7			0.1110	2830
6			0.1310	3360
5			0.1570	4000
4			0.1870	4760

III. POWDER CHARACTERIZATION

The evaluation of the effect of milling is made by comparing the characteristics of a powder before and after milling. At the present level of mathematics and computer sophistication, the basic properties of particles escape
expression in a single precise mathematical term. As mentioned previously,
fractal geometry (geometry of irregular shapes) holds some promise to
filling this need. Until this void is filled it is necessary to treat these
characterizing properties as separate and sometimes overlapping entities.
In order to discuss the characterization of powders and their constituent
particles, the term *particle* is defined in the scope of this text as having:

1. Single- or multiple-ingredient composition within the unit
2. Homogeneous or heterogeneous mixtures within the unit
3. Nonporous or porous structures within the unit
4. An approximate unit particle size range between 2000 μm (10 mesh)
   and 0.5 μm.

Powder composed of spherical or irregularly shaped particles of a single
size or distribution of sizes are characterized by a number of parameters
including density, porosity, surface area, shape, and particle size and
distribution.

A. Sampling

Characterizing a powdered or granular material whether it is milled or unmilled is heavily dependent upon the method of obtaining a sample from the
bulk since it must be representative of the entire lot or batch of material.
   Sampling small lots of material is fairly uncomplicated because the
sample may simply be coned and quartered or riffled. Coning and quartering involves a thorough premixing of the entire sample, and then a careful pouring of the sample into a pile, which usually forms a cone with a
base angle referred to as the "angle of repose" of the powder. The cone
is then divided into approximately four equal parts (Fig. 39).
   Two opposite quarters are combined and mixed well while the remaining two quarters are returned to the original container. This procedure
is repeated no less than four times until the desired sample is obtained.
If four repeats cannot be made because of a small sample size, repeat the
procedure using the material returned to the original container. Because
of the propensity for segregation of admixtures, coning and quartering is
not the sampling method of choice.
   The second method is via the riffler which is a mechanical splitting
device shown schematically in Figure 40. After each pass through the
splitter, one or several portion(s) is(are) retained depending on the number of portions developed by one pass through the riffler (this may vary
from two to eight). The number of passes through the riffler will depend
on the desired sample size. Again, the possibility of segregation of powder
admixtures as a result of free fall into the riffler receptacles must be
considered.
   The above two sampling methods may or may not be satisfactory for
batch sizes of powders or granules that can be manipulated on a bench
top depending on their compaction. However, batches of hundreds or
even thousands of kilograms require a different approach. Usually

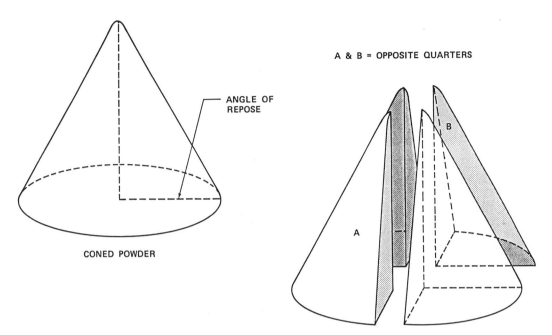

ANGLE OF
REPOSE

CONED POWDER

A & B = OPPOSITE QUARTERS

A

B

QUARTERED CONE OF POWDER

Figure 39   Coning and quatering.

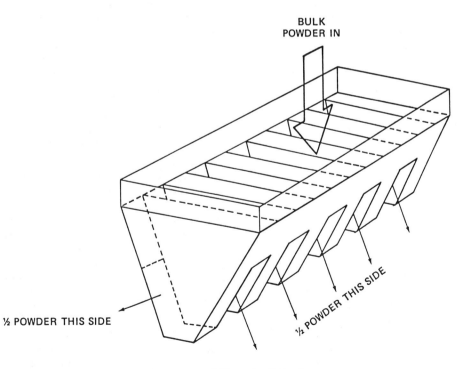

BULK
POWDER IN

½ POWDER THIS SIDE

½ POWDER THIS SIDE

Figure 40   Schematic of powder riffler (splitter).

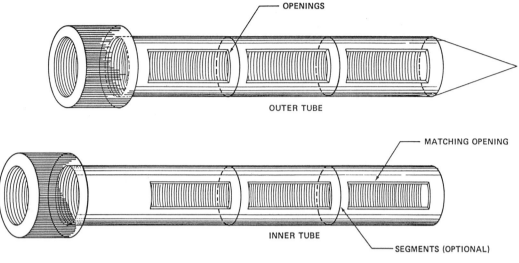

OPENINGS

OUTER TUBE

MATCHING OPENING

INNER TUBE

SEGMENTS (OPTIONAL)

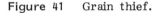

INNER TUBE IS INSERTED INTO OUTER TUBE

Figure 41   Grain thief.

unmilled, homogeneous raw material as received from the source is not
blended before sampling for identification and purity. On the other hand,
if physical characteristics such as bulk density and particle size distribution are a part of the initial testing or the powder is a heterogeneous
mixture, representative sampling is essential.

One of the more common sampling instruments for sampling large
powder bulks has been the grain thief. The grain thief (Fig. 41) is made
up of an inner and outer tube with matching openings along its length that
can be closed off by rotating the inner and outer tubes to a point where
the openings to the inner tube are covered.

The closed shaft is inserted vertically to the bottom of the drum and
the inner tube is rotated to open the sampling chamber. The powder
theoretically fills the thief chamber, the inner tube is rotated to close the
sampling chamber and the thief, with its sample, is withdrawn from the
drum of powder. Although the procedure appears quite simple, a number
of possibilities exist that may prevent a representative sampling:

1. The contents of the drum may have segregated on handling (small
   particles have sifted through the larger particles to the bottom of
   the drum). The contents of the lower sections of the drum may
   be packed material, which will not flow freely, while the contents
   of the upper section may be less packed, more free flowing larger
   particles. As the thief is opened for sampling, the larger free
   flowing particles enter from the top opening and flow down to the
   bottom of the thief. This prevents adequate sampling of the lower
   portion of the drum biasing the particle size distribution.
2. The thief, when inserted into the powder, may carry a portion of
   the upper contents to the middle or lower sections of the drum
   biasing the sample particle size distribution.

3. The thief may have to be moved or rotated within a 2 to 4 cm radius distance to obtain a sample of packed powder (this is usually very difficult with a packed powder bed). During movement, crystals or granules may be reduced in size biasing the sample particles size distribution.

4. As the powder sample is emptied via the upper end of the thief by tipping it vertically, the smaller particles may become airborne because of the rapid powder flow and/or impact on the collecting surfaces. This dust or some fraction of fine particle segment of the particle size distribution is lost, and the analysis again becomes biased.

The author has found that by using a specially designed thief shown in Figure 42, that individual small-volume (1 to 2 cm^3) samples may be taken from random locations in the drum (bin, hopper, mixer, etc.), analyzed separately, or combined to give larger sample volumes for screen analysis or particle counter use. The shaft is small enough in diameter to minimize or eliminate the "carry-down" of sample. This equipment eliminates "free fall" segregation and permits analysis of the entire sample(s) without prior manipulation.

It is essential that duplicate and triplicate sampling be carried out to provide enough material for duplicate particle size analysis. Usually agreement of two or more analyses indicates satisfactory sampling. There is no substitute for care during the sampling procedure and the handling of the sample(s).

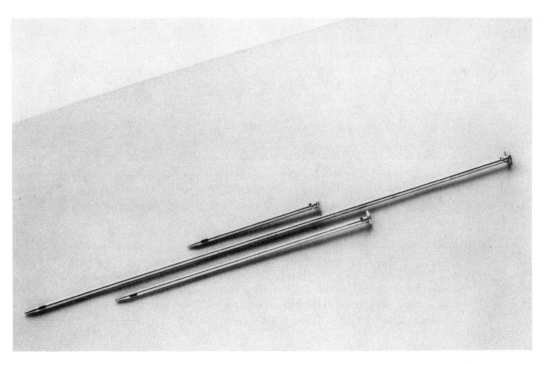

Figure 42   Unit dose thief samplers. (Courtesy Sampco, Salem, South Carolina.)

Another sampling method in common use today is done by removing the cover from each container and taking a scoop of powder from the top of the contents. This is totally unacceptable when sampling for physical characterization and content uniformity. The pitfalls of this method are obvious and should be avoided. For continuous processes such as a conveyor carrying granulation from a drying oven or the exit from a continuous blender where granulation must be sampled, timed mechanical devices are used to sample at one convenient point in the process.

A fact: particle size analysis data is only as representative as the sample(s) from whence it came.

For sampling large bulk batches, the following methods may be used, but are listed in order from the best to the least probability of obtaining a representative sample. Experience dictates that one can never be certain of the container to container or overall uniformity of size distribution of a powder material received from a vendor; or as a powder is collected in containers from a mill and/or handled in transit from one place to another:

1. Blend the entire batch and random thief sample in the blender using a small single-chamber thief. Analyze individually or mix samples thoroughly. Analyze the entire sample mix.
2. If the batch is too large to blend as one unit, select $\sqrt{n} + 1$ (where n = total number of containers in the lot being tested as suggested in the Military Standards [30]) number of containers at random and blend them. Random thief sample from the blender and proceed as in #1 above.
3. One may also proceed as in #1 and #2 above, but return the blend to the containers and thief sample these containers.
4. Random thief sample (using a small single-chamber thief per #1 above) all containers with no blending.
5. Select $\sqrt{n} + 1$ number of containers at random, and random thief sample them with no blending.
6. It is important to note that in the above, all the sample(s) be tested individually or combined after one random sampling.

B. Density and Porosity

Density is the weight to volume ratio of a substance, expressed in g/cm^3 or lb/ft^3. Powders that the pharmacist deals with are several different densities that can be manipulated to give useful information about a powder and its constituent particles.

First, the true or absolute density is the weight to volume ratio of only the solid portion of the powder particles. True density is determined by degassing (vacuum) an accurately weiged sample of the powder in a known volume container and emitting a fluid which wets but does not dissolve the powder. In this way, the void spaces around the powder particles, particularly irregularly shaped particles, can be measured. The volume determination of the powder particles is shown schematically in Figure 43.

The calculation is straightforward:

$$D_t = \frac{W}{(V_c - V_{cs})}$$

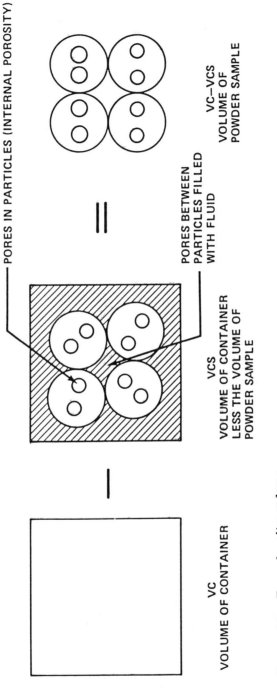

Figure 43 True density volume.

where

$$D_t = \text{true density}$$
$$W = \text{weight of the powder sample}$$
$$V_c = \text{volume of container}$$
$$V_{cs} = \text{volume of container less the volume of the powder sample}$$
$$(V_c - V_{cs}) = \text{volume of powder particles}$$

Since very few substances are completely devoid of all void spaces, the pharmacist usually deals with powder particles and granules that have varying degrees of internal porosity that cannot be easily measured. Internal porosity may or may not be used in characterizing powder particles or granules in quality control.

The most common method of accurately determining the volume of the solids in the true density determinations is by weighing the fluid occupying the void space around the powder particles at a specific temperature and calculating its volume via the density formula:

$$\text{Volume of fluid} = \frac{\text{Weight of fluid}}{\text{Density of fluid}}$$

For example: (modified ASTM density procedure) [31].

A container known as a pycnometer (Fig. 44) with a known-volume is accurately weighed:

(a) Weight of pycnometer = 22.000 g

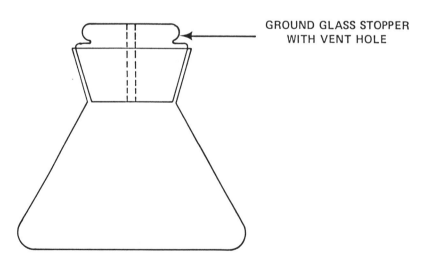

GROUND GLASS STOPPER
WITH VENT HOLE

Figure 44 Powder pycometer.

The pycnometer is filled with water at 25°C and accurately weighed (assume water will not solubilize the powder sample):

(b) Weight of pycnometer + water = 42.000 g

The pycnometer is emptied and dried and a water insoluble powder sample is added and an accurate weight is taken:

(c) Weight of pycnometer + sample = 26.000 g

Water is added to the pycnometer containing the powder sample, and another accurate weight is taken:

(d) Weight of pycnometer + sample + water at 25°C = 48.000 g

The density calculation is as follows:

(e) Weight of water at 25°C = (b) − (a) = 42.000 g − 22.000 g

   = 20.000 g

(f) Weight of sample at 25°C = (c) − (a) = 25.000 g − 22.000 g

   = 3.000 g

(g) Weight of sample + water at 25°C = (d) − (a)

   = 47.000 g − 22.000 g = 25.000 g

(h) Weight of water displaced by sample = (g) − (e) − (f)

   = 25.000 − 20.000 − 3.000 = 2.000 g

(i) Volume of sample

$$= \frac{\text{wt water displaced}}{\text{density of water at 25°C}} = \frac{2.000 \text{ g}}{0.99707 \text{ g/cm}^3} = 2.006 \text{ cm}^3$$

(j) "True" density $= \dfrac{3.000 \text{ g}}{2.006 \text{ cm}^3} = 1.496 \text{ g/cm}^3$

The second density term is the bulk density, or the ratio of the weight of a powder to the volume it occupies expressed in the same terms as the true density. This density term accounts not only for the volume of the solid portion of the particles (true density), and the voids within each particle (internal porosity), but also for the voids between the particles. Because of its dependence on particle packing, the bulk density should be reported at a particular packing condition. For example, the "poured" bulk density of a powder sample is determined by taking 50 g of the powder and gently pouring it into a 100 ml-graduated cylinder and recording the volume. The "packed" bulk density may be determined by dropping the graduated cylinder containing the "poured" 50 g sample 3 times at 1 sec intervals through a distance of 1.90 cm [32]. The packing may be extended by tapping any number of times until the volume ceases to change. This is shown schematically in Figure 45.

$$\text{BULK DENSITY} = \frac{\text{SAMPLE WEIGHT}}{\text{SAMPLE VOLUME}} = \rho_B = \frac{W}{V}$$

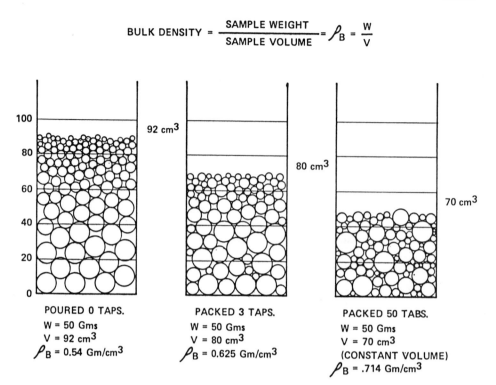

POURED 0 TAPS.
W = 50 Gms
V = 92 cm^3
ρ_B = 0.54 Gm/cm^3

PACKED 3 TAPS.
W = 50 Gms
V = 80 cm^3
ρ_B = 0.625 Gm/cm^3

PACKED 50 TABS.
W = 50 Gms
V = 70 cm^3
(CONSTANT VOLUME)
ρ_B = .714 Gm/cm^3

Figure 45   Bulk density volume.

Bulk density is very important in determining the size containers needed for handling, shipping, and storage of raw material and granulation. It is also important in sizing hoppers and receivers for milling equipment and for sizing blending equipment in the scale-up to pilot and to commercial production.

Porosity is the measure of void spaces within a powder and can be calculated by manipulating the "true" and bulk densities. For example, using the densities determined previously, porosities may be calculated by subtracting the reciprocal of the true density from that of the bulk density.

Reciprocal (1/D):

$$D_B = \text{Bulk density} = 0.498 \text{ g/cm}^3 = 2.008 \text{ cm}^3/\text{g}$$

$$D_t = \text{True density} = 0.722 \text{ g/cm}^3 = 1.385 \text{ cm}^3/\text{g}$$

$$\text{Volume difference or porosity} = 0.623 \text{ cm}^3/\text{g}$$

The porosity may also be expressed in percent void space:

$$\% \text{ Voids} = \frac{0.623}{2.008} \times 100 = 31.0\%$$

Reciprocals 1/D (from Fig. 45):

	Poured	3 taps	50 taps constant volume
$\left(\dfrac{1}{D_B}\right) =$	1.852 cm^3/g	1.600 cm^3/g	1.400 cm^3/g
$\left(\dfrac{1}{D_t}\right) =$	1.385 cm^3/g	1.385 cm^3/g	1.385 cm^3/g
Porosity $(1/D_B) - (1/D_t) =$	0.467 cm^3/g	0.215 cm^3/g	0.015 cm^3/g

% Void space

$$\frac{(1/D_B) - (1/D_t)}{(1/D_B)} \times 100 \quad = \quad 25.2 \qquad\qquad 13.4 \qquad\qquad 1.1$$

The porosity of a powder indicates the type of packing a powder undergoes when subjected to vibration, when stored, and when being fed into tablet machine feed hoppers or feed frames, emptying it from drums, tote bins, or hoppers. A powder or granulation with more void spaces will have a greater chance of flowing freely than a densely packed, low-porosity powder.

Milling may affect the density of a powder in several ways:

Bulk density decrease: Powder particle size has been reduced and more air is absorbed onto the surface of each particle yielding a high porosity (loose packing). Very small particle size powders by virtue of their size may not flow even though their porosity is high because of adsorbed moisture and/or Van der Waals forces which may act to agglomerate the powder particles.

Bulk density increase: Powder particle size distribution has been changed such that smaller particles filter into the interstices created by the orientation of the large particles.

True density increase: This may occur when the internal porosity has been minimized as a result of reducing the powder particle size.

True density — no change: Powder particles essentially lack internal porosity and size reduction has no effect on true density.

C. Surface Area

The effectiveness and efficiency of a size reduction unit operation is measured by the change in a powder's particle size distribution and/or the corresponding change in its surface area. As the particle size distribution shifts to the smaller size range, the surface area increases as a result of the new surface created.

Surface area may be calculated from particle size distribution data making the assumption that the particles are spherical. In this manner, calculations can be made using one dimension, namely, the diameter of the particle. Example: Assume a powder is composed of spheres of three different diameters havin a certain number of particles at each diameter:

Given: Surface area for a sphere = $4\pi r^2$

Number of particles at each stated size

The surface area for each size and for the total number of particles of each size is as follows:

Diameter:		Surface area/ particle (cm^2)	Number of Particles at stated diam. in 1 g powder	Total surface area for all particles (cm^2)
(μm)	(cm)			
20	2×10^{-3}	1.26×10^{-5}	100	1.26×10^{-3}
40	4×10^{-3}	5.03×10^{-5}	200	10.05×10^{-3}
60	6×10^{-3}	1.13×10^{-4}	300	33.93×10^{-3}
		Total powder particles/g of powder =	600	45.24×10^{-3} cm^2

The sum of the surface areas = the total calculated surface area for 1 g of powder = 45.24×10^{-3} cm^2.

Problems arise when the particles are irregular in shape rather than spherical, because the calculation now becomes an estimate, the accuracy of which depends on how closely the particle shape approaches that of a sphere. Unfortunately, spherical particles are "the exception rather than the rule."

Surface area may be measured by a number of methods. Probably the most popular technique is the Brünarer-Emmett-Teller, or B.E.T., method which measures specific surface area by the volume of nitrogen adsorbed as a monomolecular layer on the surface of unit mass of powder [33-36].

Referring to Figure 46, the basic steps in determining surface area by the B.E.T. method include:

1. Determining the volume of each section of the apparatus by filling it with known volume of gas at a known pressure.
2. Pretreating the sample by degassing it. More rapid degassing may be accomplished if thermal stability of the sample permits heating to above 100° C.
3. The sample in its container (L) of known volume [to value (A)] is attached to the apparatus, immersed in a liquid nitrogen bath, and degassed (temperature dependence of the method dictates that the system be maintained at liquid nitrogen temperature in the Dewar flask "Φ").
4. The adsorption isotherm (constant temperature conditions) is determined by introducing clean, dry nitrogen in small increments

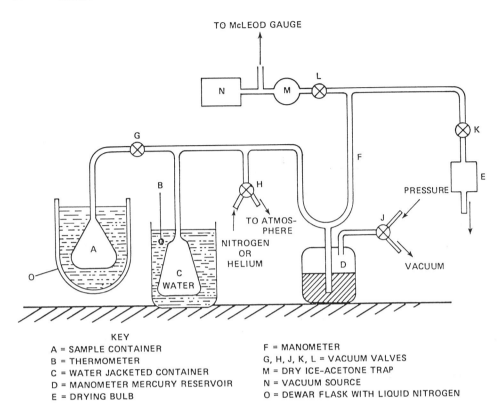

Figure 46   Schematic of Emmett type setup for B.E.T. surface area determination. (From G. Herdan, *Small Particle Statistics*, Academic Press, New York, New York.)

and recording the pressure as each equilibrium point is reached. Since the volume of the sample and the container are known, any difference in pressure is a measure of the number of molecules adsorbed on the sample surface per the ideal gas law:

$$\text{No. of molecules} = \frac{(\text{volume})\ (\text{change in pressure})\ (\text{Avogadro's No.})}{(\text{gas constant})\ (\text{absolute temperature})}$$

or

$$n = \frac{V \times \Delta P \times 6.23 \times 10^{23}}{0.082 \times T}$$

where

V is in liters

ΔP is in atmospheres

gas constant (0.82) is in liter-Atm/degree-mole

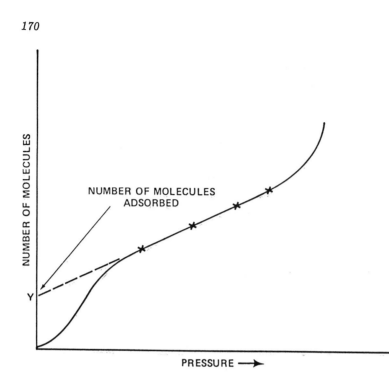

Figure 47   Example of B.E.T. absorption isotherm. (From J. T. Cartensen, *Pharmaceutics of Solids and Solid Dosage Forms*, Wiley, New York, 1977.)

5. Each of these points are plotted as shown in Figure 47, and the linear portion of the line is extrapolated to the y axis, which is a measure of the number of molecules adsorbed as a monolayer on the sample surface.

The cross-sectional area of the nitrogen molecule is 16×10^{-16} cm^2. This constant multiplied by the number of molecules in the monolayer is a measure of the surface area of the sample; and divided by the number of grams in the sample yields the specific surface area or surface area/g.

For example, if the line in Figure 47 is extrapolated to point y $(25 \times 10^{20}$ molecules) for a 2.2 g sample, the surface area would be:

$$\frac{(25 \times 10^{20}) \ (16 \times 10^{-16} \ cm^2)}{(2.2 \ g)}$$

or

1.82×10^{6} cm^2/g (specific surface area)

The advantage of using surface area measurement is the exactness with which milling effectiveness can be measured, particularly in the milling of small particle size raw materials. Surface area measurement normally is not used to evaluate the milling of tablet granulations, although it can be done. There are several companies that determine surface area of

Table 9 Average Griseofulvin Blood Levels[a] in Humans as a
Function of Specific Surface Area

Specific surface area (m²/g)	Dose (g)	Fourth hour blood levels (μg/ml) (suspension dosage form)
0.41	0.5	0.70
1.56	0.5	1.60

[a]Average of 6 to 12 subjects per group.
Source: Ref. 37.

a granulation admixture before wet-up of the granulation. Surface area
measurements indicate very closely how much binder solution is needed to
obtain uniform consistency from batch to batch. With the advent of automation and high speed granulating, it is strongly suggested that some
measure of particle size or surface area be a part of the quality control
acceptance criteria of raw material intended for use in these operations.
Without control of the surface area parameter, high-speed mixing and/or
automation may be of no consequence.

Surface area data is also very useful, since surface area may be the
cause of dissolution rate differences in milled lots of raw materials and
subsequently have a significant effect on the adsorption rate of an active
ingredient, as shown in Table 9.

The big disadvantage in evaluating milled raw materials and granulations by surface area measurement is the care and lengthy time involved in
evaluating each sample. Although, current day technology has reduced
testing time, testing equipment is expensive, and this should be considered
when anticipating the upgrading of a granulating operation.

D. Particle Shape and Dimension

The first step in characterizing a powder by shape and size is the examination of the units which make up the powder. In the case of granules
and powder particles greater than 40 − 60 mesh, a macroscopic observation
reveals the shape of the particle. Below 60 mesh (250 μm) it is necessary
to observe particle shape through a microscope. This is done by dispensing a small amount of powder sample in mineral oil or other liquid medium
in which the particles are easily wetted and not solubilized. A drop of
this slurry is placed on a slide with a cover slip. The slide is mounted
on the microscope stage and the field is scanned with a magnification between 20× and 200×, depending on the size range of the particles in the
sample.

Figure 48 illustrates several general particle shapes and how they contribute to power flow in general. The generalizations in Figure 48 pertain
to powder particles greater than 200 mesh (74 μm) since surface characteristics such as static charge and adsorbed moisture usually overshadow the
particle shape effect on powder flow characteristics below this size.

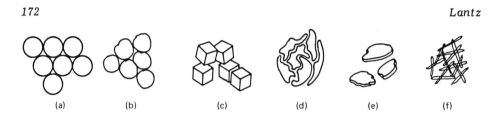

(a)   (b)   (c)   (d)   (e)   (f)

Figure 48   General particle shapes and their effect on powder flow.
(a) Spherical particles —normally flows easily, (b) oblong shapes with
smooth edges —normally flows easily, (c) equidimensionally shaped sharp
edges such as cubes —does not flow as readily as (a) or (b), (d) irregularly shaped interlocking particles —normally shows poor flow, and easily
bridges*, (e) irregularly shaped two-dimensional particles such as flakes —
normally shows fair flow and may cause bridges, (f) fibrous particles —
very poor flow and bridges easily.

   Particle shape also plays an important role in particle size analysis.
Spherical particles are the ideal in treating not only surface area calculations, but particle size and size distribution.   However, since irregular
particle shape is the rule, the single diameter dimension which amply
describes a sphere's size becomes a term which must be defined when
sizing particles in a single plane, e.g., observation of particles through a
microscope or by microprojection.   For example, there are a number of possible particle diameters which may be used to size the particle in Figure 49.

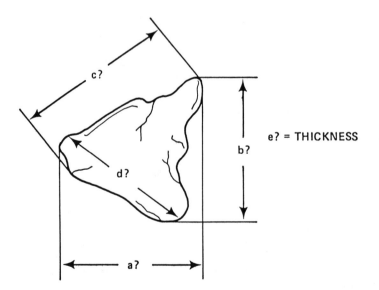

Figure 49   Particle dimension possibilities.

---

*Bridging refers to the stoppage of powder flow as a result of particles
which have formed a semirigid or rigid structure within the powder bulk.

A number of approaches have been used to solve this dilemma and they include:

1. Volume of the equivalent sphere. The volume of the particle is determined by displacement of a liquid and the diameter of an equivalent sphere is calculated:

$$d = \sqrt[3]{\frac{6V}{\pi}}$$

   This method cannot be used per se but is the principle on which the stream scanning electrical resistant particle counter is based which will be discussed in Sec. III.E.
2. Projected area of an equivalent circle. Particles of a powder sample are projected down onto a white working surface or are photographed and enlarged. The area is measured with a plainimeter and the equivalent circle diameter is calculated:

$$d = \sqrt[2]{\frac{4A}{\pi}}$$

   This method is time consuming when measuring hundreds of particles, but is the principle on which the stream scanning, light obstruction, electronic particle counting equipment is based, and will be discussed in Sec. III.E.
3. Statistical particle diameters. For counting particles by microscope observation, by microprojection, or from microphotographs, two statistical approaches to dimensioning irregularly shaped particles known as Feret's and Martin's diameter are used.

The use of Feret's and Martin's diameters fixes the direction in which the particle is measured regardless of its orientation [35] in the microscopic field, as shown in Figure 50. The significance of measuring particle diameter by this method will be discussed later in the chapter.

E. Particle Size Analysis

From a practical point of view, particle size distribution change is more easily visualized, and is the physical measurement of choice in characterizing unmilled and milled raw materials, powder mixtures, and granulations in tablet making. Particle size analysis is the means by which change in size distribution of powder particles is determined as a result of milling, and for purposes of tablet making, can be divided into two ranges (the exact cut-off points are arbitrary):

1. Subsieve size range — 100 μm (140 mesh) or smaller
2. Sieve size range — 44 μm (200 mesh) or larger

Although there is an area of overlap, each particle size range requires different methods of analysis, but both ranges use essentially the same mathematics for characterizing the size distribution. The basic steps in performing a particle size analysis include:

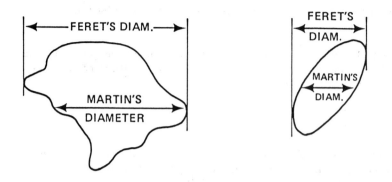

Martin's diameter = mean length of line paralleling the direction of measure-
    ment bisecting the particle, and terminating at the particle boundaries

Faret's diameter = mean length of line paralleling the direction of measure-
    ment and terminating at two tangents to the outer-most boundaries of
    the particle

Figure 50   Statistical diameters.

1. Sampling the material to be analyzed (discussed earlier in this
   chapter
2. Preparing the sample for analysis (see Sec. IV)
3. Generating the data
4. Treatment and presentation of the data

F. Particle Size Statistics

In generating the data, individual or groups of particles from each sample
are sized and counted. The sizing and counting follow a particular pattern
in order to put this data into an orderly, meaningful form which can be
statistically analyzed for interpretive and comparative purposes. For example, it will be assumed that initial microscopic observation of a sample
reveals a size range between 0.5 to 60 μm. To begin the statistics, this
range is divided into convenient equal parts known as class intervals and
the mean of each class interval is determined. For convenience of calculation, the lower limit of the first class interval is assumed to be zero. The
particles are sized, counted, and tallied under their proper class interval
as shown in Table 10.

For the statistical calculation all the particles counted in each class
interval are assumed to be equal to the mean of their respective class
interval. This data can now be put into bar graph or histogram form as
shown in Figure 51. If the means of each class interval are connected by
a smooth line, a distribution curve results as shown in Figure 52. This
frequency curve is bell-shaped and is known as a Gaussian curve if sym-
metrical. The sample represented by the curve is said to have a
Gaussian distribution. To normalize the data, the percentage of particles
can be calculated in each class interval (Table 11), added cumulatively,
and plotted to give the number distribution curve seen in Figure 53.

Table 10   Microscopic Count Data

Class interval (μm)	Mean of the class interval (μm)	Number of particles counted in each class interval
0 – 5	2.5	96
5 – 10	7.5	105
10 – 15	12.5	116
15 – 20	17.5	129
20 – 25	22.5	150
25 – 30	27.5	212
30 – 35	32.5	148
35 – 40	37.5	127
40 – 45	42.5	114
45 – 50	47.5	101
50 – 55	52.5	93
55 – 60	57.5	88

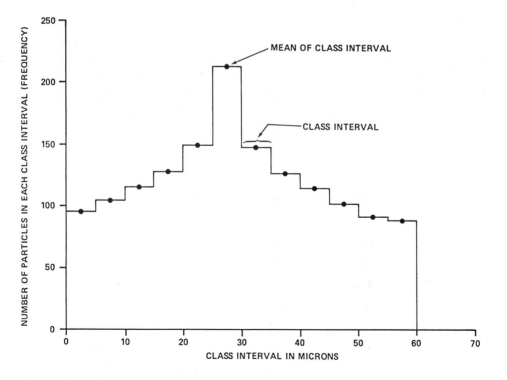

Figure 51   Histogram.

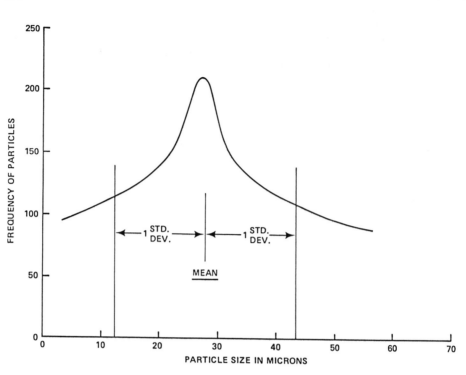

Figure 52 Frequency curve.

Table 11 Calculations of Cumulative Percent

Class interval (μm)	Means (μm)	No. of particles	% of particles	Cumulative %
0 − 5	2.5	96	6.5	6.5
5 − 10	7.5	105	7.1	13.6
10 − 15	12.5	116	7.8	21.4
15 − 20	17.5	129	8.7	30.1
20 − 25	22.5	150	10.1	40.2
25 − 30	27.5	212	14.3	54.5
30 − 35	32.5	148	10.0	64.5
35 − 40	37.5	127	8.6	73.1
40 − 45	42.5	114	7.7	80.8
45 − 50	47.5	101	6.8	87.6
50 − 55	52.5	92	6.2	93.8
55 − 60	57.5	88	5.6	99.4

Total = N = 1478

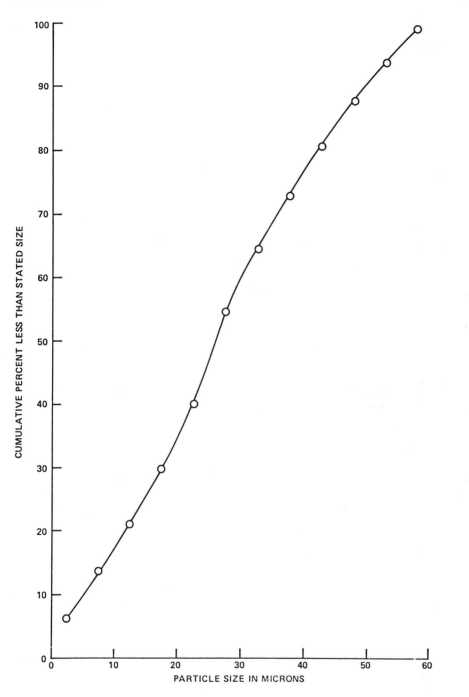

Figure 53   Cumulative distribution curve.

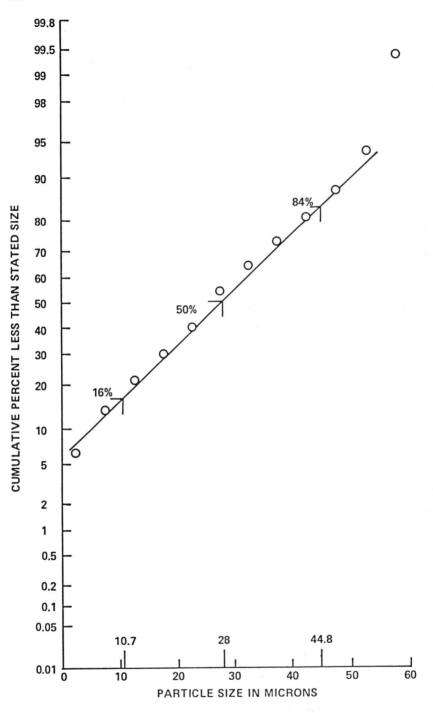

Figure 54   Normal-probability plot.

The cumulative percent as plotted in this graph is interpreted as percent of the number of particles which are less than the stated size, e.g., 99.4% of all particles are less than 57.5 µm, and 50% of the particles are less than 28 µm in diameter (assume the particles to be spherical). Note that this curve is typically "S" shaped. If this same data is plotted on probability paper as shown in Figure 54, a straight line can usually be drawn if the distribution has a relatively narrow size range. This would be characteristic of the milling of soft granules and more friable raw materials. These materials are said to have a "normal" distribution.

The 50% point on this normal probability plot approximates the arithmetic mean or average particle size of the sample. A second very important term is used in combination with the mean to describe the scatter or dispersion around the mean. This term is the "standard deviation" which can be approximated graphically by taking the 16% and 84% points on the line, which come out to be 10.7 and 44.8 µm, respectively [35]. By subtracting the size at 50% from the size at 84% (28 − 10.7 = 17.3 µm), or subtracting the size at 16% from the size at 50% (44.8 − 28 = 16.8 µm), the standard deviation is approximated. The standard deviation is also illustrated on the frequency curve in Figure 52 to better show the range covered by this term. The standard deviation and the mean can also be determined more accurately by calculation using the following equations:

$$\overline{X}_a = \frac{\Sigma n_i X_i}{N}$$

where

$\overline{X}_a$ = arithmetic mean or average particle size

n_i = frequency or number of particles in each class interval in series
$n_1 + n_2 + {}'n_3 + n_4 + {}' \ldots n_i$

X_i = mean of each class interval in the series $X_1 + X_2 + {}'X_3 + {}'$
$X_4 + {}' \ldots X_i$

N = total number of particles in the distribution

Σ = summation of

$$S_a = \sqrt{\frac{\Sigma n_i X_i^2 - (\Sigma n_i X_i)^2/N}{N - 1}}$$

where

S_a = arithmetic standard deviation

The following is an example of the calculation of the mean and standard deviation of the data plotted in Figure 54 (from Table 12):

Table 12 Calculation of the Arithmetic Mean

Class interval (μm)	Mean of class interval X_i (μm)	Frequency		
		n_i	$n_i X_i$	$n_i X_i^2$
0 – 5	2.5	96	240	600
5 – 10	7.5	105	788	5910
10 – 15	12.5	116	1450	18125
15 – 20	17.5	129	2258	39515
20 – 25	22.5	150	3375	75938
25 – 30	27.5	212	5830	160325
30 – 35	32.5	148	4810	156325
35 – 40	37.5	127	4762	178575
40 – 45	42.5	114	4845	205912
45 – 50	47.5	101	4798	227905
50 – 55	52.5	92	4830	253575
55 – 60	57.5	88	5060	290950

$$\Sigma n_i = N = 1478$$

$$\Sigma n_i X_i = 43046$$

$$\Sigma n_i X_i^2 = 1613655$$

$$\overline{X}_a = \frac{43046}{1478} = 29.1 \; \mu m$$

$$S_a = \sqrt{\frac{1613655 - (43046)^2/1478}{1478 - 1}} = 15.6 \; \mu m$$

If the distribution has a wide range in size, then the data should be plotted on log probability paper which will usually straighten out the "S" curve obtained on arithmetic paper (a wide distribution range is more convenient to plot on log probability paper because of the range attainable with the log scale). This is known as a "log normal" distribution and is typical of results seen from the milling of hard granules and less friable raw materials.

Empirical data from numerous milling studies show that milled materials fit a log-normal distribution as a ruler rather than a normal distribution. Therefore, the calculations that describe the log-normal distribution are important in particle size analysis. The difference in the normal and log-normal size distribution means is shown in Table 13 with the data obtained from a material which was ball milled.

The equation for the geometric mean $\overline{X}_g$ is:

$$\log \overline{X}_g = \frac{\Sigma n_i \log X_i}{N}$$

and,

$$\log \overline{X}_g = \frac{10712}{15656} = 0.6842$$

$$\overline{X}_g = \text{antilog } 0.6842 = 4.83 \ \mu m$$

The arithmetic mean $\overline{X}_a$ for this same data is calculated:

$$\overline{X}_a = \frac{\Sigma n_i X_i}{N} = \frac{80906}{15656} = 5.17 \ \mu m$$

The geometric mean is always smaller than the arithmetic mean. The geometric standard deviation "S_g" may be calculated from the plot of Table 13 data in Figure 55, using the equation:

$$S_g = \frac{50\% \text{ point}}{16\% \text{ point}} = \frac{84\% \text{ point}}{50\% \text{ point}} = \frac{5.9}{3.8} = 1.55 \ \mu m$$

Except for the ball milled data above, the examples depicting the basic statistics have been based on the count or numbers of particles in each class interval. It is more convenient and meaningful if this data is converted to a distribution based on the particle surface area or the volume or weight of the particle.

Particle size distribution by number may be converted to a distribution by surface or by volume by assuming all the particles are spherical and calculating the total surface or volume in each class interval. Cumulative surface or volume percentages are calculated and plotted against the mean of the corresponding class interval. The plots of these three distributions in Figure 56 show the differences between the means. It must be noted, however, that the conversion from number to surface or volume distribution is an approximation if the particles are not spherical. This estimate should be used for comparisons of the same milled material only, since it is particle shape dependent.

Table 14 is a tabulation of the different means or average particle sizes which can be calculated from their corresponding mathematical equations.

A comparison of the means calculated from the data in Table 11 is shown in Tables 15 and 16.

The deviations of these various particle size means are not presented in this chapter but the reader may review them in texts by Herdan [35] and Cadle [38].

Table 13 Particle Size Data From Ball Milled Material

Class interval (μm)	Mean of class interval X_i (μm)	Log X_i	Frequency			% by weight	Cumulative %
			n_i	$n_i X_i$	$n_i \log X_i$		
1–3	2	0.301	1097	2194	330	7.00	7.00
3–5	4	0.602	7365	29460	4434	47.00	54.00
5–7	6	0.778	5014	30084	3901	32.00	86.00
7–9	8	0.903	1567	12536	1415	10.00	96.00
9–11	10	1.000	423	4230	423	2.70	98.70
11–13	12	1.079	141	1692	152	0.90	99.60
13–15	14	1.146	39	546	45	0.25	99.85
15–17	16	1.204	8	128	10	0.05	99.90
17–19	18	1.255	2	36	2	0.01	99.99

$$\Sigma n_i = N = 15656 \qquad \Sigma n_i K_i = 80906 \qquad \Sigma n_i \log X_i = 10712$$

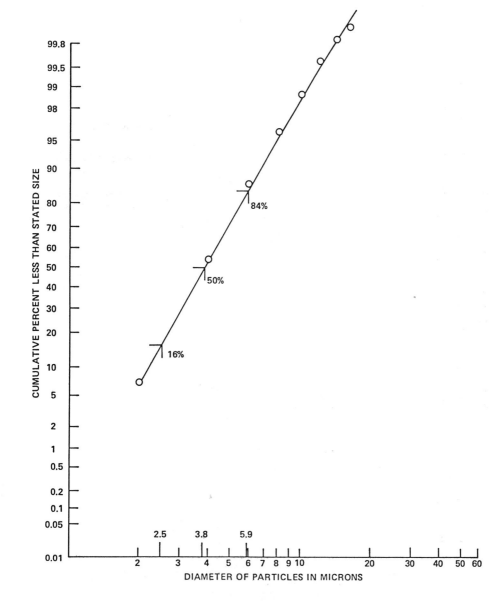

Figure 55   Log-probability plot of ball milled material.

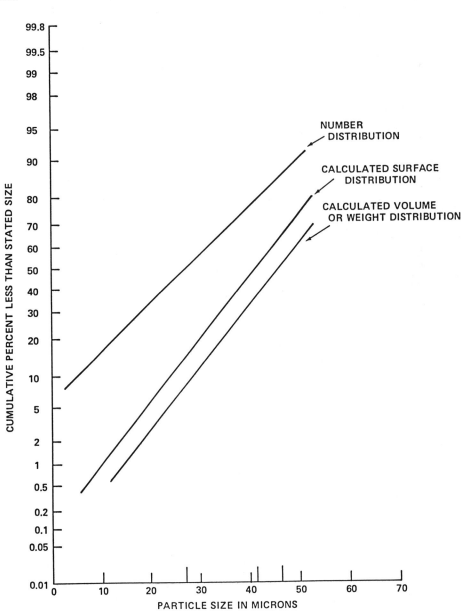

Figure 56   Three distributions from the same number frequency data.

Table 14 Equations for Calculating Different Particle Size Means

Mean diameter	Equations
Arithmetic mean $\overline{X}_a$	$\dfrac{\Sigma n_i X_i}{N}$
Surface mean $\overline{X}_s$	$\sqrt{\dfrac{\Sigma n_i X_i^2}{N}}$
Volume mean $\overline{X}_v$	$\sqrt[3]{\dfrac{\Sigma n_i X_i^3}{N}}$
Volume-surface mean $\overline{X}_{vs}$ (Sauter mean)	$\dfrac{\Sigma n_i X_i^3}{\Sigma n_i X_i^2}$
Weight mean $\overline{X}_w$	$\dfrac{\Sigma n_i X_i^4}{\Sigma n_i X_i^3}$

Table 15 Calculations for Comparison of Means

Class interval (μm)	Class interval mean X_i (μm)	n_i	$n_i X_i$	$n_i X_i^2$	$n_i X_i^3$	$n_i X_i^4$
0 – 5	2.5	96	240	600	1500	3750
5 – 10	7.5	105	788	5910	44325	332438
10 – 15	12.5	116	1450	18125	226562	2832031
15 – 20	17.5	129	2258	39515	691512	12101469
20 – 25	22.5	150	3375	75938	1708605	38443612
25 – 30	27.5	212	5830	160325	4408938	121245781
30 – 35	32.5	148	4810	156325	5080562	165118281
35 – 40	37.5	127	4762	178575	6696562	251121094
40 – 45	42.5	114	4845	205912	8751260	371928550
45 – 50	47.5	101	4798	227905	10825988	514210656
50 – 55	52.5	92	4830	253575	13312688	698916094
55 – 60	57.5	88	5060	290950	16729625	961953438

$\Sigma n_i = N = 1478$

$\Sigma n_i X_i = 43046$

$\Sigma n_i X_i^2 = 1613655$

$\Sigma n_i X_i^3 = 68477628$

$\Sigma n_i X_i^4 = 3138207194$

Table 16   Calculated Mean Particle Sizes

Mean diameter	Equation	Calculation	Calculated mean in μm
Arithmetic mean $\overline{X}_a$	$\dfrac{\Sigma n_i X_i}{N}$	$\dfrac{43046}{1478}$	29.1
Surface mean $\overline{X}_s$	$\sqrt{\dfrac{\Sigma n_i X_i^2}{N}}$	$\sqrt{\dfrac{1613655}{1478}}$	33.0
Volume mean $\overline{X}_{vs}$	$\sqrt[3]{\dfrac{\Sigma n_i X_i^3}{N}}$	$\sqrt[3]{\dfrac{68477628}{1478}}$	35.9
Volume surface mean $\overline{X}_s$	$\dfrac{\Sigma n_i X_i^3}{\Sigma n_i X_i^2}$	$\dfrac{684477628}{1613655}$	42.4
Weight mean $\overline{X}_w$	$\dfrac{\Sigma n_i X_i^4}{\Sigma n_i X_i^3}$	$\dfrac{3138207194}{68477628}$	45.8

Source: Data from Table 14.

As discussed previously, different average particle sizes based on number, weight, etc., can be obtained from a single powder sample. Table 16 lists the more common methods of counting particles and the average particle size obtained from the listed data.

IV. METHODS OF PARTICLE SIZE ANALYSIS

There are many methods of analyzing particle size distribution and mean particle size. However, the discussion in this text is limited to the most common and practical methods (items 1−7, Table 17) used in tablet production and raw material processing.

A. Sieve Analysis

This is the most widely used method of determining the size distribution of a granulation. The method is described previously for the comparison of the effect of milling conditions on an acetaminophen granulation (page 137).

The data collected from the difference in the tare weight of each screen and the total weight of the tare and the powder is entered in table form, and the cumulative percentages calculated. The class intervals are restricted to the selection of sieve sizes available as shown in Table 18.

Table 17 Common Particle Counting Method and Resulting Average Particle Size

Method of counting	Size range covered (approx.)	Resulting average particle size[a]
1. Sieve	44 and greater (325 mesh)	Average by weight X_w
2. Light scattering	1–200 μm (70 mesh)	Average by volume or weight X_v or X_w
3. Electronic sensing zone	1–300 μm (50 mesh)	Average by volume; X_V volume of equivalent sphere
4. Light obstruction	2–300 μm (50 mesh)	Average by volume; X_V as calculated from cross sectional area of an equivalent sphere
5. Air permeation	0.05–150 μm (100 mesh)	Average by surface and volume; X_{vs}
6. Sedimentation in gas or liquid	2–200 μm (70 mesh)	Average by weight; X_w
7. Optical microscope	0.5–100 μm (140 mesh)	Average by number; X_a Average by surface; X_s Average by volume; X_V

[a]Data from Table 16.

For the screen analysis shown in Figures 30, 32, 33, 35, and 36, screens were selected such that each smaller size screen was one-half the size opening of the screen preceeding it.

The mean of the class interval was obtained by taking the average of each pair of adjacent screens in the nest, e.g., 12 mesh = 1680 μm and 20 mesh = 840 μm: the mean of the class interval would calculate to be

$$\frac{1680 + 840}{2} = 1260 \ \mu m$$

A sample calculation for the unmilled acetaminophen granulation is shown in Table 19.

B. Stream Scanning

There were essentially four stream scanning methods in wide use today, which are based on electrical resistance, light obstruction, and light scattering. The methods are electronic and count large numbers of

Table 18 Sedimentation Data

Time of sample in seconds (t)	Mean of class interval of corresponding equivalent spherical diameter (μm)	Weight of sample collected (mg)	Weight % of sample	Cumulative weight (%)
25	80	—	0	0
29	75	1	0.5	100.0
33	70	2	1.3	99.5
39	65	4	2.7	98.2
45	60	8	6.5	95.5
54	55	14	9.0	89.0
65	50	21	14.0	80.0
81	45	30	17.0	66.0
102	40	90	16.7	49.0
133	35	37	14.7	32.3
182	30	20	8.0	17.6
262	25	13	5.2	9.6
410	20	7	2.8	4.4
728	15	3	1.2	1.6
1638	10	1	0.4	0.4
6553	5	—	0	0

Total weight = 251 mg

$\rho = 2.2$ g/cm^2, $h = 0.005$ poise, $G = 981$ cm/sec^2. $\rho = 0.8$ g/cm^3, $H = 25$ cm.

Where ρ = density, h = viscosity, H = sedimentation distance, G = acceleration of gravity.

Table 19 Sample Screen Analysis Data of Unmilled Acetaminophen Granulation

U.S. Std. sieve size	Sieve opening (μm)	Mean of class interval (μm)	Granulation weight on the smaller screen (g)	%	Cumulative %
> 12	1680	–	32.7	33	98
12–20	1680–840	1260	16.7	17	65
20–40	840–420	630	17.4	17	48
40–70	420–210	315	8.9	9	31
70–140	210–105	157	21.0	21	22
<140	<108	–	0.9	1	–
		Totals	98.6	98	

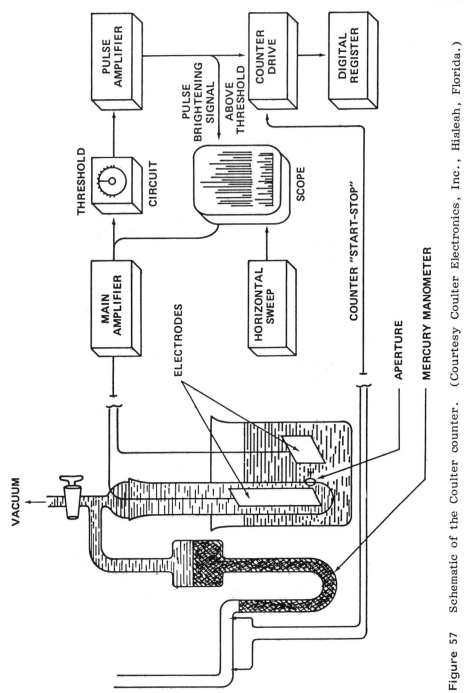

Figure 57   Schematic of the Coulter counter.   (Courtesy Coulter Electronics, Inc., Hialeah, Florida.)

particles (10,000 to 100,000+) very rapidly, and yield highly reproducible results.

Because of the large numbers of particles, the statistics yield a high level of confidence in the distribution of a sample.

A schematic of the electrical conductivity method is shown in Figure 57 [39], which labels the basic parts. The counter determines the number and size of particles suspended in an electrically conductive liquid in which the sample is not soluble. This is accomplished by forcing a thoroughly dispersed suspension of particles through a small orifice on either side of which is an electrode. As each particle passes through the aperture it changes the resistance between the electrodes because the volume of the particle displaces an equivalent volume of electrolyte. This in turn produces a short duration voltage pulse of a magnitude proportional to the volume of the particle.

These pulses are sized and counted electrically. The data yields volume (or weight) distribution of equivalent spheres. Precautions that should be noted in using this equipment include: cost of equipment, possible sensor blockage, the selection of an electrolyte in which the material to be counted is insoluble, and the possibility of picking up background electrical "noise" which could lead to erroneous results.

The light obstruction method is shown schematically in Figure 58 [40]. A liquid in which the sample disperses easily and is not dissolved, passes

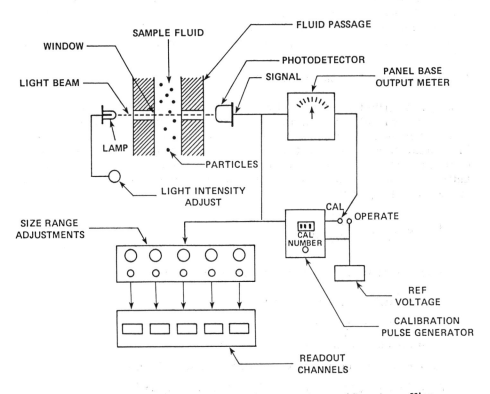

Figure 58   Schematic of the Hiac particle counter. (Courtesy Hiac Instrument Division, Pacific Scientific Company, Montclair, California.)

a window which is transversed by a light source. The light source is detected by a photo detector which senses loss of light transmitted through the suspending medium when a particle interrupts the light beam.

The amount of light blocked from the detector by a particle is proportional to the cross-sectional area of the particle. This creates short duration electrical pulses that are sized and counted electronically. The data yields a distribution based on the cross-sectional area of equivalent spheres which is easily converted to a weight distribution as shown earlier in the discussion under Particle Size Statistics.

The precautions with this equipment include keeping the sensing zone windows clean, adhering to particle concentrations that will prevent coincident counting, and making certain a thorough dispersion of particles is obtained.

The disadvantages with this method are: cost of equipment and, possible sensor blockage.

Light scattering is carried out using either a nonlaser or a laser light beam. The principle is one of light from the beams of known intensity refracting or scattering as the beam is interrupted by the particles in either liquid or air. Photo-sensors detect the intensity of scattered light and the variations in intensities (pulse variations) are electronically classed according to pulse intensity. The refracted light intensity is a measure of the particle size which can be displayed via CRT or hard copy in the form of a histogram, cumulative size distribution curve, or just an average particle size. There are a multitude of manufacturers who sell this type of equipment, and can be found in most of the current equipment advertising trades published today. The advantages to this equipment is the high concentrations of suspended particles that can be sized with certain models.

C. Sedimentation in Gas or Liquid

A weight distribution of a powder sample can be determined by using one of several available sedimentation methods. In each method the weight distribution is obtained by allowing a dispersed powder to settle in air or in a liquid in which it is not soluble, and weighing the particles in each class interval separately or cumulatively on a balance. The relationship between the particle settling time and the size of the particle is expressed in the Stokes equation:

$$d = 10^4 \sqrt{\frac{18\eta h}{(D - D_o)gt}}$$

where all particles are assumed to be spheres and

d = particle diameter in microns

η = viscosity in poise

h = distance of fall in cm

D = absolute density of the powder particles in g/cm^3

D_o = density of the fluid settling medium in g/cm^3

g = gravity acceleration constant: 981 cm/sec^2

t = time in seconds

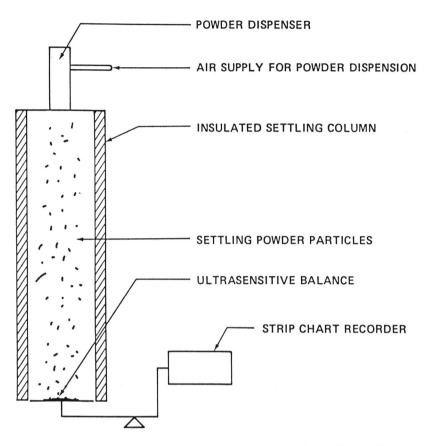

POWDER DISPENSER

AIR SUPPLY FOR POWDER DISPENSION

INSULATED SETTLING COLUMN

SETTLING POWDER PARTICLES

ULTRASENSITIVE BALANCE

STRIP CHART RECORDER

Figure 59   Schematic of the Micromerograph air sedimentation apparatus.
(Courtesy of Sharpless Corporation, Philadelphia.)

Using either the Micromerograph (where the powder particles settle in air),
or the Cahn Sedimentation Balance (where the powder particles settle in a
liquid) shown schematically in Figures 59 and 60, respectively, the sample
is dispersed in its respective settling medium, and the powder particles
settle per the Stokes equation onto an ultrasensitive balance. Weight is
recorded cumulatively against time, the time being the only variable in
the equation related to the particle diameter, i.e., all other components in
the equation remain constant so that particle diameter is proportional to
the settling time.

Each of the pieces of equipment mentioned above record this data electronically, yielding a hard copy size distribution curve. The diameter axis
is adjusted to the constants in the Stokes equation, and the data can be re-
plotted on normal or log-probability paper for final representation.

Another method that is still in use is the Andreasen Pipet. This apparatus is shown in Figure 61, and is also based on the Stokes equation.
This apparatus is designed for a settling liquid medium that will not dissolve the sample and can be easily and completely evaporated by heat
and/or vacuum. With this apparatus, the settling liquid is filled to the

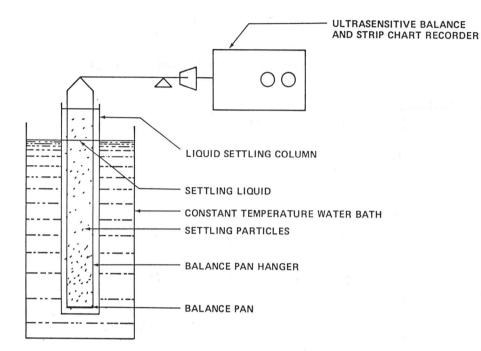

ULTRASENSITIVE BALANCE
AND STRIP CHART RECORDER

LIQUID SETTLING COLUMN

SETTLING LIQUID

CONSTANT TEMPERATURE WATER BATH

SETTLING PARTICLES

BALANCE PAN HANGER

BALANCE PAN

Figure 60   Schematic of a Cahn Sedimentation Balance liquid sedimentation apparatus. (Courtesy of Cahn Division, Ventron Instruments Corp., Paramount, California.)

top line. The sample is weighed and pre-dispersed in a small amount of the settling medium. This dispersion is then added to the top of the settling medium column and time zero is recorded. At specified recorded time intervals which have been predetermined from the Stokes equation and the constants used, 5, 10, or 20 ml samples are withdrawn into clean pre-tared evaporating pans. The settling medium is evaporated and each sample is weighed. Diameters are calculated and cumulative weight percents are plotted against them on normal or log-probability paper for presentation. An example of an Andreasen Pipet sedimentation determination is shown in Table 18, and the plotted data is shown in Figure 62.

Each of the sedimentation methods is accurate and reproducible, but each has a lower particle size limit of about $2-3$ μm because of the inordinately long settling times required with the very fine powder particles. Several precautions must also be observed when using the sedimentation methods including:

1. Temperature control of the settling medium is critical because of possible changes in density with temperature.
2. Microscopic examination of the predispersed sample is essential to determine that dispersion is complete, and the particle size range is within the $2-200$ μm limits.

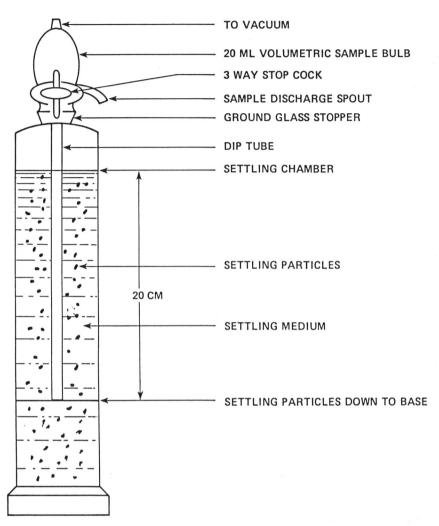

TO VACUUM

20 ML VOLUMETRIC SAMPLE BULB

3 WAY STOP COCK

SAMPLE DISCHARGE SPOUT

GROUND GLASS STOPPER

DIP TUBE

SETTLING CHAMBER

SETTLING PARTICLES

20 CM

SETTLING MEDIUM

SETTLING PARTICLES DOWN TO BASE

Figure 61 Schematic of the Andreasen Pipet.

3. Particle concentration in the settling medium. It has been shown that the higher the particle concentration, the higher the settling velocity of the powder particles. It may be necessary to try several sample concentrations until duplication of distribution is obtained at two different concentrations.

D. Optical Microscope

Probably one of the least popular but very practical methods of sizing and counting particles in the subsieve size range is by optical microscope. The advantage of this method is the relatively low cost for equipment with

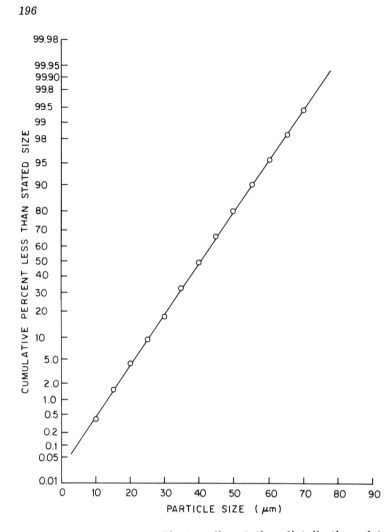

Figure 62   Andreasen Pipet sedimentation distribution plot.

fairly good accuracy. The big disadvantage is the length of time required to size a powder sample. The greatest chance for error is that too few numbers of particles will be counted. This will lessen the level of confidence in the statistics.

Table 20 is a partial list of particle size analysis equipment available for measuring particle size and particle size distribution. Selection is dependent upon the user's applications.

Table 20 Particle Size Analysis Equipment

Equipment name	Manufacturer	Principle of operation	Size range	Suspending media
Horiba	Horiba Instruments, Inc. Irvine, CA	Change in optical observance during gravitational or centrifugal settling	$0.04-300$ μm	Any liquid compatible with system
PCSV-P Particle Size Analyzer	Insitec Pittsburgh, PA	Intensity of light scattering change in laser beam in line measuring	$0.2-200$ μm	Gases compatible with system
Microscan	Quantachrome Syosset, NY	Sedimentation	$0.1-300$ μm	Gas
LUMOSED	PAAR Warminster, PA	Sedimentation	$0.5-500$ μm	Any liquid compatible with system
Sedigraph 5100	Microminetics Norcross, GA	Sedimentation	$0.1-300$ μm	Any liquid compatible with system
Aerodynamic Particle Sizer	TSI, Inc. St. Paul, MN	Light scattering particle detection	$0.5-50$ μm	Any gas compatible with system
Multisizer	Coulter Electronics Hialeah, FL	Change in liquid resistance containing particles	$0.4-1200$ μm	Electrolyte liquids
Omnicon 3600	Artek Systems Farmingdale, NY	Image analyzer	Subsieve	Dry or wet
Model 2010 Direct Particle Size Analyzer	Brinkman Instruments Westbury, NY	Scanning laser and image analyzing	$0.7-1200$ μm	Any media

197

Table 20 (Continued)

Equipment name	Principle of operation	Size range	Suspending media
Microtrac II SRA	Leeds & Northrup North Wales, PA	Light scattering	0.7–700 μm	Gas
Malvern	Malvern Instruments Southborough, MA	Laser defraction	0.5–1800 μm	Gas or liquid
H L Free Swinging Sifter	Great Western Manu-facturing Co., Inc. Levenworth, KA	Screen analysis	0.25–400 mesh	Wet or dry
Hiac/Royco Series 4300	Pacific Scientific Claremont, CA	Light beam interruption or light scattering	0.25–9000 μm	Liquids or gases

REFERENCES

1. Snow, R. H., Bibliography of Size Reduction, 9 Vols., *Natl. Tech. Inform. Service*, Springfield, Virginia, 1974.
2. Schonert, K., *Fortschr Verfahrenstich*, 10(B2):204−222 (1970/1971).
3. Moir, D. N., *Chem. Eng.*, 91(8):54−68 (1984).
4. Melloy, T., Open Forum—"Future Directions for Research in Powder Technology," held at the International Powder and Bulk Solids Handling and Processing Conference/Exhibition 76, Chicago, Illinois (1976).
5. Dustin, L. G., *Powder Technol.*, 5:1−17 (1971/1972).
6. Herschhorn, J. S., *Powder Technol.*, 4:1−8 (1970/1971).
7. Gupta, V. K. and Kapur, P. C., *Powder Technol.*, 12:81−83 (1975).
8. Berg, O. T. G. and Avis, L. E., *Power Technol.*, 4:27−31 (1970/1971).
9. McCabe, W. L. and Smith, J. C., Size reduction, in *Unit Operations of Chemical Engineering*, 2nd Ed., McGraw-Hill, New York, 1967, p. 809.
10. Perry, R. H., ed., Principles of size reduction, *Perry's Chemical Engineer's Handbook*, 4th Ed., McGraw-Hill, New York, 1963, p. 2.
11. Ramanujam, M. and Venkateswarlu, D., *Powder Technol.*, 3:93−101
11. (1969/1971).
12. *Understanding Computers — Computer Images*, Time Life Books (1986); Mandelbrot, B., *The Fractal Geometry of Nature*, San Francisco: W. H. Freeman (1982).
13. Thibert, R., *J. Pharm. Sci.*, 77:724−726 (1988).
14. Stoner, K., *Powder and Bulk Eng.*, 1(6):46 (1987).
15. Prescott, L. F., Steel, R. F., and Ferrier, X, X., *Clin. Pharmacol. and Therap.*, 11:496 (1970).
16. Ullah, I. and Cadwallader, D. E., *J. Pharm. Sci.*, 60:230−233 (1971).
17. Parrot, E. L., *Pharm. Manufac.*, 2(4):31−37 (1985).
18. Brooke, D. J., *Pharm Sci.*, 62:795−798 (1973).
19. Ikekawa, A. and Kaneniwa, N., Parts I through IX, *Chem. Pharm. Bull.*, 1967, 1968, 1969.
20. Klumpar, I. V., *Powder and Bulk Eng.*, 1(8):42−58 (1987).
21. Boylan, J. C., Cooper, J., Chowman, Z. T., Lund, W., Wade, A., Weir, R. F., and Yates, B. J., *Handbook of Pharmaceutical Excipients*, American Pharmaceutical Association, Washington, D.C., 1986.
22. Albus, F. E., *Powder and Bulk Eng.*, 1(6):32−47 (1987).
23. Dobson, B. and Rothwell, E., *Powder Technol.*, 3:213−217 (1969/1970).
24. Rumanujam, M. and Venkateswarlu, D., *Powder Technol.*, 3:92−101 (1969/1970).
25. Chinnis, L. E., *Powder and Bulk Eng.*, 1(10):12−16 (1987).
26. Snow, R. H., *Advances in Particle Science and Technology* (D. Wasan, ed.), Academic Press, New York, 1973.
27. Snow, R. H., *Powder Technol.*, 5:351−364 (1971/1972).
28. Snow, R. H., *Powder Technol.*, 10:129−142 (1974).
29. Nushart, S., *Powder and Bulk Eng.*, 1(8):14−19 (1987).
30. Ref. Military Standard.
31. Standard Method of Test for Specific Gravity of Pigments, ASTM Designation: D153-54, 1954, reapproved (1961).
32. *Drug Standards*, 20:22 (1952).

33. Brunaur, S., Emmett, P. H., and Teller, E., *J. Am. Chem. Soc.*, *60*:309 (1938).

34. Emmett, P. H., deWitt, *Ind. Eng. Chem. (Anal.)*, *13*:28 (1941).

35. Herdan, G., *Small Particle Statistics*, Academic Press, New York, 1960.

36. Carstensen, J. T., *Pharmaceutics of Solids and Solid Dosage Forms*, Wiley, New York, 1977.

37. Atkinson, R. M., Bedford, C., Child, K. J., and Tomich, E. G., *Antibiot. Chemo.*, *12*:232 (1962).

38. Cadle, R. D., *Particle Size Theory and Industrial Applications*, Reinhold Publishing, New York, 1965.

39. Instruction Manual, Coulter Counter Industrial Model B, Coulter Electronics, Inc., Hialeah, Florida.

40. High Accuracy Products, Operation and Service Manual—HIAC S, Montclair, California.

4
Compression

Eugene L. Parrott

University of Iowa, Iowa City, Iowa

I. THE PROCESS OF COMPRESSION

Compression is the process of applying pressure to a material. In pharmaceutical tableting an appropriate volume of granules in a die cavity is compressed between an upper and a lower punch to consolidate the material into a single solid matrix, which is subsequently ejected from the die cavity as an intact tablet. The subsequent events that occur in the process of compression are (a) transitional repacking, (b) deformation at points of contact, (c) fragmentation and/or deformation, (d) bonding, (e) deformation of the solid body, (f) decompression, and (g) ejection.

A. Transitional Repacking or Particle Rearrangement

In the preparation of the granulation to be placed in the hopper of the tablet press, formulation and processing are designed to ensure that the desired volume of the granulation is fed into each die cavity so that at a fast production rate the weight variation of the final tablets is minimal. The particle size distribution of the granulation and the shape of the granules determine the initial packing (bulk density) as the granulation is delivered into the die cavity. In the initial event the punch and particle movement occur at low pressure. The granules flow with respect to each other, with the finer particles entering the void between the larger particles, and the bulk density of the granulation is increased. Spherical particles undergo less particle rearrangement than irregular particles as the spherical particles tend to assume a close packing arrangement initially. To achieve a fast flow rate required for high-speed presses the granulation is generally processed to produce spherical or oval particles;

thus, particle rearrangement and the energy expended in rearrangement are minor considerations in the total process of compression.

B. Deformation at Points of Contact

When a stress (force) is applied to a material, deformation (change of form) occurs. If the deformation disappears completely (returns to the original shape) upon release of the stress, it is an elastic deformation. A deformation that does not completely recover after release of the stress is known as a plastic deformation. The force required to initiate a plastic deformation is known as the yield stress. When the particles of a granulation are so closely packed that no further filling of the void can occur, a further increase of compressional force causes deformation at the points of contact. Both plastic and elastic deformation may occur although one type predominates for a given material. Deformation increases the area of true contact and the formation of potential bonding areas.

C. Fragmentation and Deformation

At higher pressure, fracture occurs when the stresses within the particles become great enough to propagate cracks [1,2]. Fragmentation furthers densification, with the infiltration of the smaller fragments into the void space. Fragmentation increases the number of particles and forms new, clean surfaces that are potential bonding areas. The influence of applied pressure on specific surface area (surface area of 1 g of material) is shown in Figure 1. The specific surface of the starch and sulfathiazole granulation was 0.18 m^2/g; the tablet compressed at a pressure of 1600 kg/cm^2 had a specific surface of 0.9 m^2/g [3].

With some materials fragmentation does not occur because the stresses are relieved by plastic deformation. Plastic deformation may be thought of as a change in particle shape and as the sliding of groups of particles in an attempt to relieve stress (viscoelastic flow). Such deformation produces new, clean surfaces that are potential bonding areas.

D. Bonding

Several mechanisms of bonding in the compression process have been conceived, but they have not been substantiated by experimentation and have not been useful in the prediction of the compressional properties of materials [4]. Three theories are the mechanical theory, the intermolecular theory, and the liquid-surface film theory.

The mechanical theory proposes that under pressure the individual particles undergo elastic, plastic, or brittle deformation and that the edges of the particles intermesh, forming a mechanical bond. If only the mechanical bond exists, the total energy of compression is equal to the sum of the energy of deformation, heat, and energy adsorbed for each constituent. Mechanical interlocking is not a major mechanism of bonding in pharmaceutical tablets.

The molecules (or ions) at the surface of a solid have unsatisfied intermolecular forces (surface free energy), which interacts with other

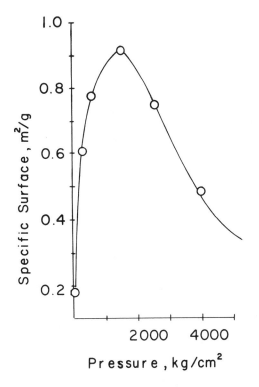

Figure 1 The effect of applied pressure on the specific surface of sul-fathiazole tablets. (From Ref. 3, with permission of the copyright owner, The American Pharmaceutical Association.)

particles in true contact. Absolutely clean surfaces will bond with the strength of the crystalline material, whereas adsorbed materials restrict bonding. According to the intermolecular forces theory, under pressure the molecules at the points of true contact between new, clean surfaces of the granules are close enough so that van der Waals forces interact to consolidate the particles. A microcrystalline cellulose tablet has been described as a cellulose fibril in which the crystals are compressed close enough together so that hydrogen bonding between them occurs [5]. It appears that very little deformation or fusion occurs in the compression of microcrystalline cellulose. Although aspirin crystals undergo slight de-formation and fragmentation at low pressure, it appears that hydrogen bonding has strongly bonded the tablets, because the granules retain their integrity with further increases in pressure [6].

The liquid-surface film theory attributes bonding to the presence of a thin liquid film, which may be the consequence of fusion or solution, at the surface of the particle induced by the energy of compression. During compression an applied force is exerted on the granules; however, locally the force is applied to a small area of true contact so that a very high pressure exists at the true contact surface. The local effect of the high pressure on the melting point and solubility of a material is essential to bonding.

The relation of pressure and melting point is expressed by the Clapeyron equation,

$$\frac{dT}{dP} = \frac{T(V_1 - V_s)}{\Delta H} \tag{1}$$

in which dT/dP is the change in melting point with a change in pressure, T is the absolute temperature, ΔH is the molar latent heat of fusion, and V_1 and V_s are the molar volumes of the liquid melt and the solid, respectively.

As the latent heat of fusion is positive, the Clapeyron equation states that for a solid, which expands on melting ($V_1 > V_s$), the melting point is raised by an increase in pressure. As most solids expand on melting, the Clapeyron equation predicts that during compression it would be unlikely that fusion would occur. The Clapeyron equation is derived for a thermodynamically reversible process in which the system is uniformly exposed to a pressure. In fact, the compression of a pharmaceutical tablet is nonreversible, and the pressure is not uniformly distributed.

Equating the free energy of the liquid and solid phases, Skotnicky [7, 8] derived an equation relating the heat of fusion, volumes of the liquid and solid phases, temperature, and the pressures applied to the liquid and solid phases. For an ideal process in which the material is exposed to a uniform pressure, the relation reduced to the Clapeyron equation. If the pressure at the points of true contact is exerted only on the solid, and the liquid phase is subjected to a constant atmospheric pressure, the relationship simplifies to

$$\frac{dT}{dP_s} = \frac{V_s T}{\Delta H} \tag{2}$$

As dT/dP is positive, regardless of the expansion or contraction of the solid, the pressure acting locally at the points of true contact lowers the melting point.

For surface fusion at the points of true contact, a localized temperature at least equal to the melting point of the material is attained. With some mixtures the melting point may be depressed by other ingredients and fusion will occur at a temperature lower than the melting point of the pure material. For most pharmaceutical solids, the specific heat is low and the thermal conductivity is relatively slow. The heat transfer to the surface can be estimated by dividing the compressional energy by the total time of compression. Using the derivation of Carslaw and Jaeger [9] for heat transfer, Rankell and Higuchi [8] estimated for the compression of 0.4 g of sulfathiazole that if the area of true contact were 0.01 to 0.1% of the total area, the surface termperature would melt medicinal compounds and pharmaceutical excipients. Then upon release of the pressure, solidification of the fused material would form solid bridges between the particles. Gross melting does not occur during the compression of most tablets because the energy expended (2 cal for 0.4 g of sulfathiazole) causes only a small temperature (5 to 10°C), which is not sufficient to melt the material being tableted.

By analogous reasoning, the pressure distribution in compression is such that the solubility is increased with increasing pressure. With an increase in solubility at the points of true contact, solution usually occurs in the film of adsorbed moisture on the surface of the granule. When the applied pressure is released and the solubility is decreased, the solute dissolved in the adsorbed water crystallizes in small crystals between the particles. The strength of the bridge depends on the amount of material deposited and the rate of crystallization. At higher rates of crystallization, a finer crystalline structure and a greater strength are obtained.

The poor compressibility of most water-insoluble materials and the relative ease of compression of water-soluble materials suggest that pressure-induced solubility is important in tableting. The moisture may be present as that retained from the granulating solution after drying or that adsorbed from the atmosphere. Granulations that are absolutely dry have poor compressional characteristics [10]. Water or saturated solutions of the material being compressed may form a film that acts as a lubricant, and if less force is lost to overcome friction, more force is utilized in compression and bonding, and the ejection force is reduced. In formulations using solutions of hydrophilic granulating agents, there may be an optimum moisture content. It has been reported that the optimum moisture content for the starch granulation of lactose is approximately 12% and of phenacetin is approximately 3% [11].

E. Deformation of the Solid Body

As the applied pressure is further increased, the bonded solid is consolidated toward a limiting density by plastic and/or elastic deformation of the tablet within the die as shown in Figure 2. The compressional behavior of solids under uniaxial pressure is discussed in Sec. V, Transmission of Forces.

F. Decompression

The success or failure to produce an intact tablet depends on the stresses induced by elastic rebound and the associated deformation processes during decompression and ejection. Often, if capping or lamination of the ejected tablet has occurred, the individual pieces are dense, hard, and strongly bonded indicating that sufficient areas of true contact existed during compression. In such cases, the mechanism of failure is different from that of a crumbly tablet. As the upper punch is withdrawn from the die cavity, the tablet is confined in the die by a radial pressure. Consequently, any dimensional change during decompression must occur in the axial direction.

Ideally, if only elastic deformation occurred, with the sudden removal of axial pressure the granules would return to their original form breaking any bonds that may have formed under pressure. Also the die wall pressure would be zero as the elastic material recovered axially and contracted radially. Actually under nonisostatic pressure, pharmaceutical materials undergo sufficient plastic deformation to produce a die wall pressure in excess of that that may be relieved by elastic recovery accompanying removal of the upper punch. As the movement of the tablet is restricted by the residual die wall pressure and the friction with the die wall, the stress

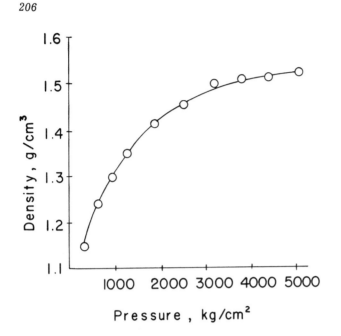

Figure 2   The effect of applied pressure on the apparent density of tablets of sulfathiazole. (From Ref. 3, with permission of the copyright owner, The American Pharmaceutical Association.)

from the axial elastic recovery and the radial contraction causes splitting (capping) of the tablet unless the shear stress is relieved by plastic deformation.

Thus, capping is due to uniaxial relaxation in the die cavity at the point where the upper punch pressure is released [12] and some may also occur at ejection [13]. It has been demonstrated that if decompression occurs simultaneously in all directions capping is reduced or eliminated [14, 15].

Stress relaxation of plastic deformation is time dependent. Materials having slow rates of stress relaxation crack in the die upon decompression. In Figure 3 the ratio of the pressure at time t to the maximum pressure is plotted against the logarithm of the time [12]. The change of the initial slope suggests some prominent mechanism of bonding soon becomes negligible. The initial slope reflects the ability of the materials to relieve stress during decompression. The rate of stress relieve is slow for acetaminophen so cracking occurs while the tablet is within the die. With microcrystalline cellulose the rate of stress relieve is rapid, and intact tablets result. If stress relaxation is slow and cracking is a problem, a slower operational speed provides more time for stress relaxation. A tablet press that provides precompression allows some stress relaxation before the final compression. To optimize stress relaxation, before the final compression, the precompressional pressure should approach the maximum pressure that will not by itself introduce lamination. The time dependent nature of plastic flow may be responsible for the different tablet presses and with various adjustments for a given press.

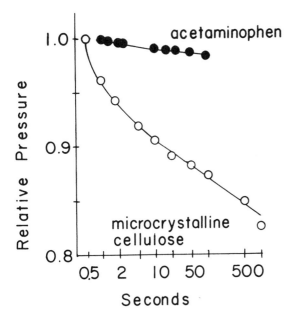

Figure 3   Relative punch pressure against logarithm of time. (From Ref. 12, with permission of the copyright owner, The American Pharmaceutical Association.)

A shape of tablet may be selected to reduce stress gradients within the tablet. With deep oval punches the larger quantity of material in the dome is expanding radially during ejection, and as the main body of the tablet can not expand radially but is constrained by the die wall, larger shear stresses develop. Flat-faced punches would form tablets that avoid this large shear stress.

G. Ejection

As the lower punch rises and pushes the tablet upward there is a continued residual die wall pressure and considerable energy may be expanded due to the die wall friction. As the tablet is removed from the die, the lateral pressure is relieved, and the tablet undergoes elastic recovery with an increase (2 to 10%) in the volume of that portion of the tablet removed from the die. During ejection that portion of the tablet within the die is under strain, and if this strain exceeds the shear strength of the tablet, the tablet caps adjacent to the region in which the strain had just been removed.

H. Descriptions of Process

The process of compression has been described in terms of the relative volume (ratio of volume of the compressed mass to the volume of the mass at zero void) and applied pressure as shown in Figure 4. In transitional

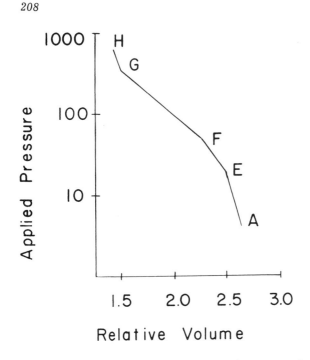

Figure 4   Events of the process of compression in terms of applied pressure and relative volume.

repacking the granules are packed to an arrangement in which the particles are immobile and the number of intergranular points of contact has increased.   The decrease in relative volume during transitional repacking is represented by the segment AE.   With a further increase in pressure, temporary supports between the particles are formed as represented by the segment EF.   Fragmentation and/or plastic deformation is represented by the segment FG.   As some higher pressures bonding and consolidation of the solid occur to some limiting value as indicated by segment GH.

For the compressional process, Heckel [16] proposed the equation

$$\ln \frac{V}{V - V_\infty} = kP + \frac{V_o}{V_o - V_\infty} \qquad (3)$$

in which V is the volume at pressure P, V_o is the original volume of the powder including voids, k is a constant related to the yield value of the powder, and V_∞ is the volume of the solid.

The Heckel relationship may be written in terms of relative density ρ_{rel} rather than volume

$$\log \frac{1}{1 - \rho_{rel}} = \frac{KP}{2.303} + A \qquad (4)$$

in which P is the applied pressure, and K and A are constants.   The Heckel constant K has been related to the reciprocal of the mean yield

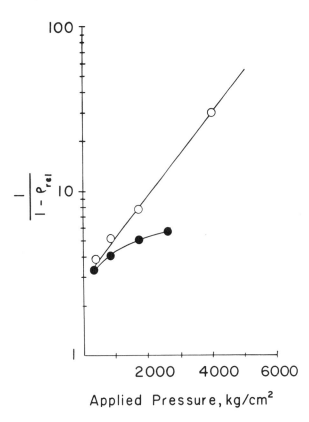

Figure 5 Density-applied pressure relationship according to the Heckel plot. Key: (●), dibasic calcium phosphate dihydrate; and (○), with 4.5% starch. (From Ref. 19, with permission of the copyright owner, The American Pharmaceutical Association.)

pressure, which is the minimum pressure required to cause deformation of the material undergoing compression [17]. The intercept of the curved portion of the curve at low pressure represents a value due to densification by particle rearrangement. The intercept obtained from the slope of the upper portion of the curve is a reflection of the densification after consolidation. A large value of the Heckel constant indicates the onset of plastic deformation at relatively low pressures [18].

A Heckel plot permits an interpretation of the mechanism of bonding. For dibasic calcium phosphate dihydrate, which undergoes fragmentation during compression, the Heckel plot in Figure 5 [19] is nonlinear and has a small value for its slope (a small Heckel constant). As dibasic calcium phosphate dihydrate fragments, the tablet strength is essentially independent of the original particle size. For sodium chloride a Heckel plot is linear indicating that sodium chloride undergoes plastic deformation during compression. With no significant change in particle size during compression, the strength of the compressed tablet depends on the original particle size of the sodium chloride [20].

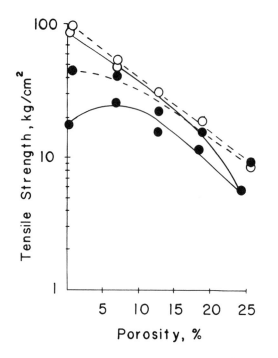

Figure 6   Tensile strengths—porosity relationship of the logarithmic form
of the Ryshkewitch equation for dibasic calcium phosphate dihydrate
granules with 1.2 (———) and 4.5% (– – – –) starch. (●) axial and
(○) radial tensile strength. (From Ref. 19, with permission of the copyright owner, The American Pharmaceutical Association.)

Binders (starch paste) are added to a material to increase bonding.
As shown in Figure 5 the linear relationship and the lower mean yield
pressure (1904 kg/cm^2) with 4.5% starch compared to the nonlinear relationship and the mean yield pressure (4303 kg/cm^2) of dibasic calcium
phosphate dihydrate indicate that the addition of the binder had conferred
plastic characteristics to the material.
  Ryshkewitch [21] observed that

$$\log \sigma_x = \log \sigma_{max} - b\varepsilon \tag{5}$$

in which σ_x is the radial tensile strength, σ_{max} is the theoretical radial
tensile strength at zero void, ε is the porosity, and b is a constant. In
the Ryshkewitch plot in Figure 6 the increase in concentration of starch
from 1.2 to 4.5% increases the radial tensile strength 47% at a porosity of
25%. This increase in starch increases the radial tensile strength only
12% as zero void is approached. Similarly, with lactose granulated with
povidone, an increase in concentration of povidone from 1 to 9% increases
the radial tensile strength 58% at a porosity of 20% and only 34% near zero
void.

It appears that the concentration of binder has a greater influence in more porous tablets than in those approaching zero void. As the applied pressure is increased and the porosity of the tablet is decreased, the interparticular distances through which bonding forces operate are shorter. Thus, the bonding force of the material is stronger at lower porosity, and a lesser quantity of binder is required to produce a tablet of desired strength.

The quotient of the applied force and the area of true contact is the applied deformation pressure at the areas of true contact. Thus, under pressure a desired maximum area of true contact is established merely by applying adequate pressure. However, when the applied force is removed, the area of true contact may change. It has been stated that smaller particles yield larger areas of true contact and thus bond more strongly. However, the compression process is not independent of permanent deformation pressure (hardness) which may vary with size. Also plastic deformation tends to increase the number of dislocations in a crystal. In practice the magnitude of the permanent deformation pressure is unknown, and the particle size and shape may alter the packing density. As a consequence of these unknowns, speculations on the effect of particle size on the strength of a tablet is questionable [12].

The materials compressed in pharmacy are nonmetallic and are generally mixtures of organic compounds. The relative significance of each event in the process of compression depends on the mechanical properties (plastic behavior, crushing strength) of the mixture, its chemical nature and surface effects (friction, adsorbed films, lubrication).

II. PROPERTIES OF TABLETS INFLUENCED BY COMPRESSION

Higuchi [22] and Train [23] were probably the first pharmaceutical scientists to study the effect of compression on tablet characteristics (density, disintegration, hardness, porosity, and specific surface) and on distribution of pressure. The relationship between applied pressure and weight, thickness, density, and the force of ejection are relatively independent of the material being compressed [24]. Hardness, tensile strength, friability, disintegration, and dissolution are properties that depend predominately on the formulation. However, the developmental scientist should realize that processing and formulation are integrated disciplines, and the effect of one on a pharmaceutical product can not be totally separated from the other.

A. Density and Porosity

The apparent density of a tablet is the quotient of the weight and the geometric volume. The apparent density of a tablet is exponentially related to the applied pressure (or compressional force), as shown in Figure 2, until the limiting density of the material is approached [3]. As shown in Figure 7, a plot of the apparent density against the logarithm of applied pressure is linear except at high pressures.

As the porosity and apparent density are inversely proportional, the plot of porosity against the logarithm of applied pressure is linear with a negative slope [25], as shown in Figure 8.

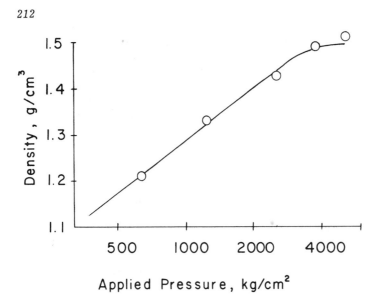

Figure 7 The effect of applied pressure on the apparent density of sulfathiazole tablets. (From Ref. 3, with permission of the copyright owner,
The American Pharmaceutical Association.)

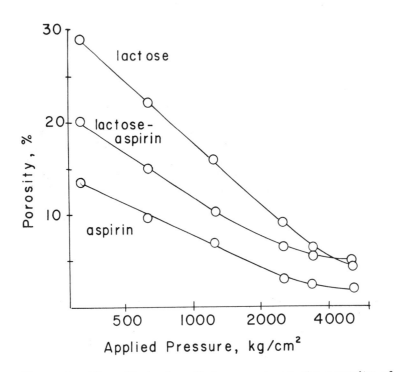

Figure 8 The effect of applied pressure on the porosity of various
tablets. (From Ref. 25, with permission of the copyright owner, The
American Pharmaceutical Association.)

When equal weights of aspirin and lactose are compressed with 10% starch, the porosity of the lactose – aspirin tablet, as indicated in Figure 8, is of a magnitude between that of the individual lactose and aspirin tablets at corresponding pressure. Thus, in tablet formulation it may be anticipated that a change in percent composition will have a corresponding arithmetic (or averaging) effect on porosity and apparent density.

B. Hardness and Tensile Strength

The ability of a tablet to withstand mechanical handling and transport has been evaluated by various types of tests (abrasion, bending, identation, hardness, diametral crushing) [26]; however, the data from these tests seldom can be correlated in a precise manner. Although hardness is not a fundamental property, diametral crushing is most frequently used for in-process control because of its simplicity. There is a linear relationship between tablet hardness and the logarithm of applied pressure except at high pressures. As shown in Figure 9 for lactose – aspirin tablets, compressed mixtures have hardness values between those of tablets composed of the individual ingredients.

The strength of a tablet may be expressed as a tensile strength (breaking stress of a solid unit cross section in kg/cm^2). As shown in Figure 10, the radial tensile strength is proportional to the applied pressure. For an isotropic, homogeneous tablet, the radial and axial tensile strengths are equal. In practice the distribution of pressure, differences in density within the tablet, and the mixture of several ingredients contribute to the nonhomogeneity of the tablet and to the nonuniformity of tensile strength. When a brittle material is compressed axially, the stress upon each

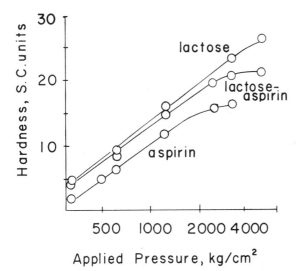

Figure 9   The effect of applied pressure on the hardness of various tablets. (From Ref. 25, with permission of the copyright owner, The American Pharmaceutical Association.)

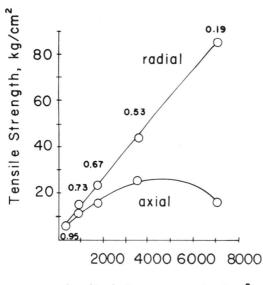

Figure 10   The effect of applied pressure on tensile strengths of tablets of dibasic calcium phosphate dihydrate granulated with 1.2% starch.   At each applied pressure, the value is given for σ_z/σ_x.   (From Ref. 10, with permission of the copyright owner, The American Pharmaceutical Association.)

particle does not necessarily compress the particles along the axial direction because of random packing and alignment of the particles toward each other during the events of compression.   A greater probability exists for vertical stress on the particles during the arrangement and fragmentation events due to the movement of the punch.   The overall result is that more clean surfaces are created when they are normal to the radial direction. As applied pressure is increased, fragmentation results in a stronger, radial tensile strength than axial tensile strength as shown in Figure 10. If more bonds are formed in the radial direction, the potential for the presence of cracks or dislocations is greater in the axial than in the radial direction.

The radial tensile strength σ_x is determined by a diametral compression test in which the maximum force F_σ to cause tensile failure (fracture) is measured.   The radial tensile strength is then calculated by

$$\sigma_x = \frac{2\,F_\sigma}{Dt\,\pi} \tag{6}$$

in which D is the diameter, and t is the thickness of the tablet.

The axial tensile strength is determined by measurement of the maximum force F_σ to pull the tablet apart in tensile failure.   The axial tensile strength is then calculated by

$$\sigma_z = \frac{4 F_\sigma}{D^2 \pi} \tag{7}$$

A blend of powders may be granulated with a granulating solution to increase the adhesiveness of a formulation. The influence of the concentration of povidone on the tensile strengths of hydrous lactose is shown in Figure 11. The radial strength is little effected by the concentration of povidone, but the axial tensile strength is increased by increased concentrations of povidone to a strength greater than the radial strength. The influence of applied pressure on the tensile strengths of lactose with 1 and 9% povidone is shown in Figure 12.

The relationship [27] of the crushing strength of granulations of lactose with povidone to the axial and radial tensile strengths of tablets compressed at 890 kg/cm^2 from the granulations is shown in Figure 13. The tensile strengths of the tablet are increased as the resistance to crushing of the granules is increased. The strength of the granule is increased as the concentration of the binder is increased; thus, the effect of the strength of the granule on the tensile strengths of the tablet is inseparable from the effect of concentration. Although the crushing strength of granules is important in the handling of the granulation in the tableting

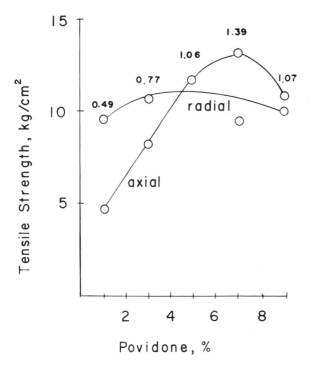

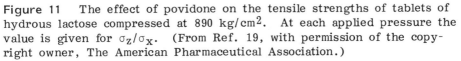

Figure 11   The effect of povidone on the tensile strengths of tablets of hydrous lactose compressed at 890 kg/cm^2. At each applied pressure the value is given for σ_z/σ_x. (From Ref. 19, with permission of the copyright owner, The American Pharmaceutical Association.)

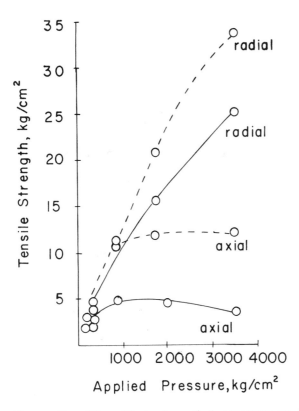

Figure 12   The effect of applied pressure on the tensile strengths of tablets of hydrous lactose granulated with 1% (————) and 9% (— — — — —) povidone.   (From Ref. 19, with permission of the copyright owner, The American Pharmaceutical Association.)

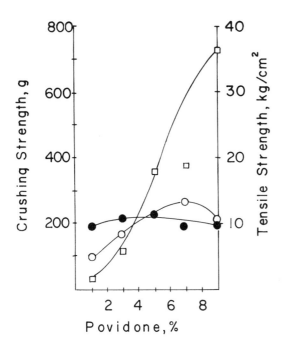

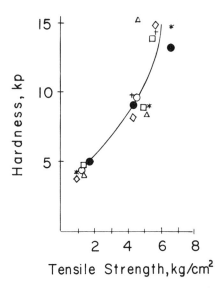

Figure 14   The relationship of hardness and axial tensile strength for di-basic calcium phosphate dihydrate with various concentrations of magnesium stearate. (●) 0%, (△) 0.075%, (□) 0.125%, (○) 0.25%, (◇) 0.5%, (*) 1.0%, and (+) 2.0%. (From Ref. 28, with permission of the copyright owner, The American Pharmaceutical Association.)

process, the applied pressure and the concentration of the binder determine the tensile strengths of a tablet.

With a hardness tester of the diametral compression type, weak tablets tend to fail due to tensile stresses, and strong tablets tend to fail due to compressive stresses. Hardness is proportional to radial tensile strength [28]. As shown in Figure 14, the relationship of hardness to axial tensile strength is nonlinear. As the hardness is increased, at higher values of hardness, there is a progressive lessening of the rate of increase of the axial tensile strength until a limiting axial tensile strength is attained. Thus, if the mechanical strength of a tablet is considered only in terms of its hardness, nothing is known of its axial strength; and if the axial tensile strength were weak, the tablet would laminate under stress.

C. Specific Surface

Specific surface is the surface area of 1 g of material. The influence of applied pressure on the specific surface area of a tablet is typified by

---

Figure 13   Relationship of binder concentration to granule strength and tensile strengths of tablets compressed at 890 kg/cm^2 from lactose monohydrate granulated with povidone. (□) granule strength, (○) axial, and (●) radial tensile strength. (From Ref. 27, with permission of the copyright owner, The American Pharmaceutical Association.)

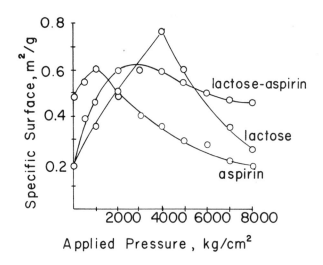

Figure 15   The effect of applied pressure on the specific surface of various tablets. (From Ref. 25, with permission of the copyright owner, The American Pharmaceutical Association.)

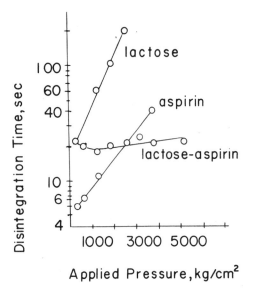

Figure 16   The effect of applied pressure on disintegration time of various tablets. (From Ref. 25, with permission of the copyright owner, The American Pharmaceutical Association.)

Figure 15. As the lactose granules, which were granulated by adding 10%
starch paste, are compressed, the specific surface is increased to a maximal value (four times that of the initial granules), indicating the formation
of new surfaces due to fragmentation of the granules. Further increases
in applied pressure produce a progressive decrease in specific surface as
the particles bond. A similar relation is shown for aspirin containing 10%
starch. When a equal weight of aspirin and lactose is blended with 10%
starch and then compressed, the specific surface is between that of the
aspirin and lactose tablets individually [25]. As the relationship between
applied pressure and apparent density is independent of the material being
compressed, the influence of starch on the specific surface and porosity is
not significant.

   For these aspirin, lactose, and aspirin–lactose tablets, the maximum
specific surface occurs at a porosity of approximately 10%, even though the
applied pressures at which the maxima occur vary with the different materials [25].

D. Disintegration

Usually, as the applied pressure used to prepare a tablet is increased,
the disintegration time is longer [29]. Frequently, there is an exponential
relationship between the disintegration time and the applied pressure, as
shown for aspirin and lactose in Figure 16.

   In other formulations there is a minimum value when the applied pressure is plotted against the logarithm of disintegration time, as shown in
Figures 16 and 17 with 10% starch. For tablets compressed at low pressures, there is a large void, and the contact of starch grains in the

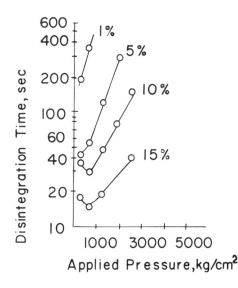

Figure 17   The effect of applied pressure on the disintegration time of
sulfadiazine tablets with various percentages of dried corn starch. (From
Ref. 25, with permission of the copyright owner, The American Pharmaceutical Association.)

interparticular space is discontinuous. Thus, there is a lag time before
the starch grains, which are swelling due to imbitition of water, contact
and exert a force on the surrounding tablet structure. For tablets compressed at a certain applied pressure, the contact of the starch grains is
continuous with the tablet structure, and the swelling of the starch grains
immediately exerts pressure, causing the most rapid disintegration, as demonstrated by a minimum in a plot of applied pressure against the logarithm
of disintegration time. For tablets compressed at pressures greater than
that producing the minimum disintegration time, the porosity is such that
more time is required for the penetration of water into the tablet, with a
resulting increase in disintegration time.

    As shown in Figure 17 for sulfadiazine tablets, the concentration of a
disintegrating agent influences the relationship between applied pressure
and disintegration time. For low starch concentrations, a small change in
the applied pressure causes a large change in disintegration time. Thus,
for formulations containing a small percent of starch, fluctuations in applied pressure during tablet production cause a large variance in disintegration time.

E. Dissolution

The effect of applied pressure on dissolution rate may be considered from
the viewpoint of nondisintegrating tablets and disintegrating tablets. Shah
and Parrott [30] have shown that under sink conditions, the dissolution
rate is independent of applied pressures from 53 to 2170 kg/cm^2 for nondisintegrating spheres of aspirin, benzoic acid, salicylic acid, an equimolar
mixture of aspirin and salicylic acid, and an equimolar mixture of aspirin
and caffeine. Mitchell and Savill [31] found the dissolution rate of aspirin
disks to be independent of the pressure over the range 2000 to 13,000 kg/cm^2 and independent of the particle size of the granules used to prepare
the disks. Kanke and Sekiguchi [32] reported that the dissolution rate of
benzoic acid disks is independent of particle size and applied pressure.

    The effect of applied pressure on the dissolution of disintegrating
tablets is difficult to predict; however, for a conventional tablet it is
dependent on the pressure range, the dissolution medium, and the properties of the medicinal compound and the excipients. If fragmentation of
the granules occurs during compression, the dissolution is faster as the
applied pressure is increased, and the fragmentation increases the specific
surface. If the bonding of the particles is the predominate phenomena in
compression, the increase in applied pressure causes a decrease in dissolution [33].

    The four most common dissolution-pressure relations are:

1. The dissolution is more rapid as the applied pressure is increased.
2. The dissolution is slowed as the applied pressure is increased.
3. The dissolution is faster, to a maximum, as the applied force is
   increased, and then a further increase in applied pressure slows
   dissolution.
4. The dissolution is slowed to a minimum as the applied pressure is
   increased, and then further an increase in applied pressure speeds
   dissolution.

Table 1 Effect of Compressional Force on Dissolution of Sulfadimide Tablets Prepared with Various Granulating Agents

Pressure (MN/m^2)	$t_{50\%}$ (min)		
	Starch paste	Methylcellulose solution	Gelatin solution
200	54.0	0.5	10.0
400	42.0	0.8	4.5
600	35.0	1.1	3.0
800	10.0	1.2	4.6
1000	7.0	1.4	4.9
2000	3.3	1.8	6.5

Source: Ref. 34.

The complexity of the release of a medicinal compound from a tablet is demonstrated in Table 1 for sulfadimidine tablets prepared by wet granulation using three different granulating agents [34]. When starch paste was used as the granulating agent, dissolution was faster as the applied pressure was increased. When a methylcellulose solution was used as the granulating agent, dissolution was slowed as the applied pressure was increased. When a gelatin solution was used as a granulating agent, the dissolution became faster as the applied pressure was increased to a maximum, and then further increases in applied pressure slowed dissolution.

III. MEASUREMENT OF COMPRESSIONAL FORCE

Instrumented tablet presses are designed on the principle that the force on a punch is proportional to the force transmitted to other parts of the tablet machine. Early instrumented tablet presses had strain gages at some practical position of the machine that would undergo a force proportional to the force exerted by the upper punch.

A strain gage is a coil of highly resistant wire mounted on paper backing. During compression the force applied causes a very small, elastic deformation of the two punches. If a suitable strain gage is firmly bound to the punch shank as close to the compression site as practical, it is deformed as the punch is deformed. With the deformation, the length of the resistance wire is decreased and its diameter is increased. The resulting decrease in electrical resistance is measured by a Wheatstone bridge used with a recording device. If a reference strain gage is placed in the opposite arm of the Wheatstone bridge, temperature fluctuation is compensated. Torsional movement of the punch may be compensated by multiple gages mounted at the periphery of the punch.

In their early work, Higuchi et al. [35] instrumented a Stokes A-3 single-punch tablet machine and as a function of time simultaneously recorded any two of the three variables—upper punch force, force transmitted to the lower punch, and displacement of the upper punch during actual operating conditions. A schematic diagram is shown in Figure 18.

The upper punch displacement is measured by a linear variable differential transformer (A) bolted to the side of the frame. The transformer consists of three coaxial windings on a hollow ceramic cylinder. One winding is placed at the middle of the form and acts as the primary of the transformer. The two secondaries are placed adjacent to and on each side of the primary. The movable core of the transformer is linked to the upper punch assembly by a threaded rod and cross-arm (D). The primary of the differential transformer is excited by a 2500-Hz signal from an oscillator integral to strain gage amplifiers. The secondaries of the transformer are connected in series opposition, so that when the core is as much in the field on one secondary as it is in the field of the other, there is no net voltage output. Displacement of the core from this zero position produces a voltage across the connected secondaries. The magnitude of the voltage is directly proportional to the distance moved by the core. The output voltage is amplified and then actuates the recording device of the oscillograph.

The force transmitted to the lower punch is measured by a load cell (C), which is placed between the base of the machine and the platform and

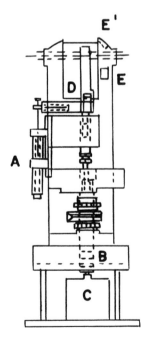

Figure 18   Diagrammatic representation of instrumentation of Stokes A-3 single-punch tablet machine. A = differential transformer, B = lower plunger extension, C = load cell, D = linkage to transformer core, E and E' = strain gages. (From Ref. 35, with permission of the copyright owner, The American Pharmaceutical Association.)

directly below the lower punch assembly. An expandable pin (B) is placed between the loading button of the cell and the lower plunger assembly, so that the entire plunger assembly rests on the cell. Thus, the upper punch force transmitted through the tablet to the lower punch is sensed directly by the load cell. A load cell consists of a centrally positioned steel column in a cylindrical heavy steel case. Strain gages are bonded to the column, and when stress is applied, the resulting strain in the column is shared by the strain gages. The gages are connected in a Wheatstone bridge circuit, so that any strain on the column causes a change in resistance of the gages and consequently an unbalance in the bridge. The unbalanced potential is directly proportional to the force applied to the loading button of the load cell. The Wheatstone bridge is excited by a 2500-Hz signal provided by the strain gage amplifier. The voltage output of the bridge resulting from the application of force to the load cell is amplified and actuates the recording device of the oscillograph.

The force exerted by the upper punch is determined by two strain gages (E and E') mounted on the frame of the tablet machine. The strain gage E is mounted on the underside of the yoke supporting the drive shaft. The strain gage E' is bonded to the same yoke on the side near its upper edge. Force exerted by the upper punch has its reaction on the drive shaft and tends to straighten the yoke that holds it and consequently stretches strain gage E. Strain gage E' is compressed in a similar manner. Strain gages E and E' are arranged in opposite arms of a Wheatstone bridge so that the response to measured force is due to the sum of the two resistance changes of the two gages. The Wheatstone bridge circuit is excited by a 2500-Hz signal from an oscillator. The output signal is treated in the same manner as that described for the lower punch force arrangement.

When the tablet resists ejection from the die by the lower punch, the resulting strain in the lift rod causes the yoke to tend to bend downward, compressing the strain gage E on the underside of the yoke and stretching strain gage E' on the other side. This permits measurement of the ejection force. Details of other instrumented single-punch tablet machines have been published [31,33,36].

A typical force-time curve for the upper and lower punches is shown in Figure 19. The segment AB of the upper punch curve is transcribed as the upper punch descends, and transitional repacking, deformation at points of contact, fragmentation, and/or deformation and bonding occur. At B consolidation of the tablet has occurred. Subsequently as the upper punch ascends, the segment BC is transcribed during the events of decompression. The drop below the baseline is a measure of the force required to remove the upper punch from the die. As the lower punch rises and ejects the tablet from the die, the segment CD is transcribed; the recorder line drops below the zero baseline, measuring the force of ejection. The segment EF of the lower punch curve is transcribed as the upper punch force is transmitted to the stationary lower punch. The segment FG is a measure of the force exerted by the tablet on the die wall. It prevents relaxation of the lower punch assembly (the upper punch is exerting no force). This is the minimum force required to eject the tablet.

The instrumentation of rotary tablet presses has been by means of bonding strain gages to the upper and lower punch and transmitting signals form the strain gages with a radio link or by means of bonding strain gages to stationary locations near the site of compression.

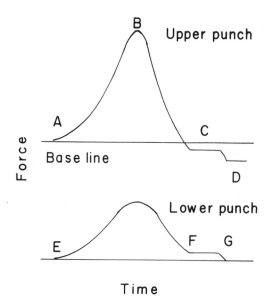

Figure 19 Diagrammatic representation of a typical record of upper and lower punch force for compression of unlibricated granulation.

In the remote instrumentation method [37] strain gages are bonded to parts (upper and lower compression release systems) remote from the punch face. A schematic representation of the instrumentation of a Stokes BB-2 rotary tablet machine is shown in Figure 20. The ejection force is measured by instrumentation of a bolt supporting a modified ejection cam, as

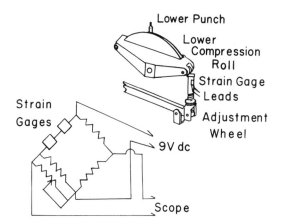

Figure 20 Diagrammatic representation of instrumentation of Stokes BB-2 rotary tablet machine for measurement of compressional force. (From Ref. 37, with permission of the copyright owner, The American Pharmaceutical Association.)

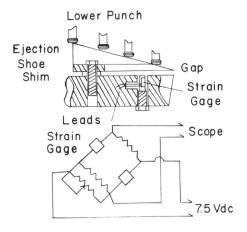

Figure 21   Diagrammatic representation of instrumentation of Stokes BB-2 rotary tablet machine for measurement of ejection force. (From Ref. 37, with permission of the copyright owner, The American Pharmaceutical Association.)

illustrated in Figure 21. The remote instrumentation method has been criticized because (a) signals received from the remote gages may not truly represent the compressional force due to distortion of various parts of the machine transmitting the force, (b) signals received may not be limited only to the signal of a single desired event because of the fast succession of events in compression, and (c) the supporting cam during the ejection bears more than one punch at a time and may not represent the ejection force. To be assured that a remote instrument machine is functioning properly, it should be verified by comparison with data obtained by an instrument-punch radio system.

The remote instrumentation method can be used at normal production speed. If the pressure-related system is instrumented, each punch is monitored and can be set up in a reproducible manner. Also, for in-process control, any discrepancy during operation is detected, so that the press may be stopped for adjustment.

In the punch instrumentation method [38], the radio transmitter is placed into several punch holders and one upper and lower punch is instrumented. Signals are obtained for upper and lower punch forces and for lower punch forces on ejection. Keyed punches are required to prevent rotation of the punch and the breaking of the electrical connections. Several strain gages are bonded to the shank of the punch and connected in series. The change in resistance is measured by an external Wheatstone bridge. With recent technological advances, the problem of space limitation has been surmounted, and the entire Wheatstone bridge may be bonded to the punch shank in the form of four strain gages (one for each arm of the bridge). Two are bonded parallel and two are bonded perpendicular to the major axis to compensate for temperature variation. With the proper selection of resistance gages, amplification of the signal is unnecessary.

IV. ENERGY EXPENDITURE

As the upper punch enters the die and begins to apply a force to the
granulation, a small quantity of energy is used to rearrange the particles
to a packing with less void. As the process of compression continues,
energy is expended to overcome die wall friction and to increase the specific surface as fragmentation and/or deformation occurs. After the tablet
has been consolidated, energy is required to overcome die wall friction as
the upper punch is withdrawn. Energy is then expended in the ejection
of the tablet from the die. The energy expenditure is the sum of the
energy dissipated as heat, the energy of reversible elastic strain, and the
energy retained in the tablet as increased surface energy. The useful
energy of compression

$$E_{compression} = E_{total} - E_{heat} - E_{elastic} \qquad (8)$$

The energy expended in the compression of granules to reduce the void
and to form a tablet is the product of the force and the distance through
which it acts. This energy may be determined by measuring the lower
punch force and the displacement of the upper punch, and then plotting
the compressional force a function of the displacement. The energy used
to compress the tablet and to overcome die wall friction is equivalent to
the area under the force-displacement curve (1 g cm = 2.3 × 10^{-5} cal).

If the granules are lubricated, the die wall friction is thus reduced
and less force is required to produce a given displacement. With the use
of a lubricant, less force is wasted to overcome friction, and as more of
the upper punch force can then be transmitted to the lower punch, the
difference between the upper and lower punch force is less than for an
unlubricated granulation. Thus, the difference between the maximum
value of force of the upper and lower punch can be a measure of the efficiency of a lubricant in overcoming die wall friction.

In Figure 22, the difference between the area under the curve for the
compression of 0.4 g of lubricated and unlubricated sulfathiazole granules
compressed at 1700 kg/cm^2 is equal to 0.8 cal, which were required to
overcome die wall friction. The 1.5 cal, as represented by the area under
the curve of the lubricated granules, was used to compress the granules
into a tablet. After compression of the unlubricated granules, 1.2 cal was
required to withdraw the upper punch. With a lubricant, the energy to
overcome die wall friction and to withdrawn the upper punch was negligible.
The energy required to eject the finished tablet was 5.1 cal. With a
lubricant, the energy for ejection was only 0.5 cal. The energy expenditure
for preparing the lubricated tablet and the unlubricated tablet is summarized
in Table 2.

By assuming that only energy expended in the process of forming the
tablet caused a temperature rise, Higuchi [39] estimated the temperature
rise to be approximately 5°C. The energy expended in the process of
tablet ejection —that needed to overcome die wall friction and that were
used to remove the upper punch from the die — were summed for a single-
punch machine operating at 100 tablets per min, and approximately 43 kcal/
hr[1] were required for unlubricated granules. Wurster and Creekmore
[41] by use of an internal temperature probe found a 2 to 5°C rise in the
temperature of tablets compressed from microcrystalline cellulose, calcium
carbonate, starch, and sulfathiazole.

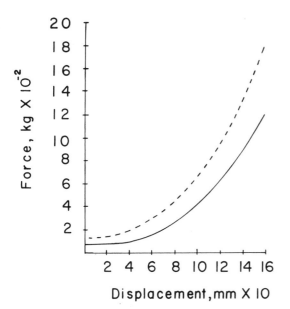

Figure 22 Diagrammatic representation of record of punch force against displacement in the compression of unlubricated and lubricated sulfathiazole granulation. (– – – –) upper punch force using unlubricated granulation. (————) lower punch force for lubricated or unlubricated granulation. (From Ref. 39, with permission of the copyright owner, The American Pharmaceutical Association.)

Table 2 Energy Expended in Compression of 0.4 g of Sulfthiazole Granulation in a Single-Punch Tablet Machine[a]

	Energy expended (cal)	
Compression	Unlubricated	Lubricated
Compression	1.5	1.5
Overcoming die wall friction	0.8	–
Upper punch withdrawal	1.2	–
Tablet ejection	5.1	0.5
Total	8.6	2.0

[a]Force of 1200 kg on lower punch using 3/8-in. (9.525 mm) flat-faced punches.
Source: Ref. 39.

The temperature of compressed tablets is affected by the pressure and speed of the tablet machine. In a noninstrumented single-punch tablet machine set at minimum pressure, the compression of 0.7 g of sodium chloride caused a temperature increase of 1.5°C; when the machine was set near maximum pressure, the temperature increase was 11.1°C [42]. When the machine was operating at 26 and 140 rpm, the increase in temperature was 2.7 and 7.1°C, respectively. When the machine was operating at 26 and 140 rpm to compress 0.5 g of calcium carbonate, the increase in temperature was 16.3 and 22.2°C, respectively.

Since heating is unwanted because of wear of the punch and die and possible degradation of the tablet ingredients, lubricants are added. The chief purpose of a lubricant is to minimize friction at the die wall, although a lubricant often enhances flow of the granules by decreasing interparticular friction. Lubrication may result from the adherence of the polar portion of the lubricant to the oxide–metal surface and the interposing of a film of low shear strength at the interface between the die wall and the tablet. A lubricant reduces the ejection force, which is directly related to the force lost to the die wall during the final event in compression process. The force lost to the die wall is dependent on the area of the tablet in contact with the die wall. It is for this reason that pharmaceutical tablets are designed with a convex surface to lessen the area of tablet in contact with the die wall.

Although a lubricant is added to facilitate the operation of tableting, its presence affects several properties of the tablet. The effect of a lubricant on mechanical strength depends on the mechanism of bonding. The strongest bonds are formed between clean, new surfaces; and for materials that undergo plastic and/or elastic deformation, the presence of the lubricant acts as a physical barrier between the new surfaces. A tablet of microcrystalline cellulose, whose bonding occurs primarily through plastic deformation and flow, is mechanically weakened by lubricants. As shown in Figure 23, the addition of magnesium stearate markedly decreases the axial and radial tensile strengths. Magnesium stearate produces the same effect in lactose tablets.

For materials that are brittle and fragment, new, clean surfaces are formed and readily bond during compression, and the lubricant has little detrimental effect on the strength of a tablet. Dibasic calcium phosphate dihydrate is consolidated by brittle fraction [6] and its axial and radial tensile strengths are not changed significantly by the presence of as much as 3% magnesium stearate, as shown in Figure 24. Stearic acid, hydrogenated vegetable oil, talc, and polyethylene glycol 4000 may be used in concentrations as great as 8% for brittle materials with only a slight to moderate change in tensile strengths [43].

Rees and co-workers [44,45] utilized force-displacement curves obtained while measuring tensile strengths to express the ease with which a tablet failed. They defined the area under the force-displacement curve as the work of failure, and they suggested that the work of failure provides a quantitative comparison of the resistance of various tablets to failure. As shown in Figure 25, magnesium stearate reduces the work of axial failure from 856 g cm for tablets of microcrystalline cellulose to 28 g cm for tablets containing 0.25% magnesium stearate [46]. The incorporation of 0.25 and 2.0% magnesium stearate reduced the work of radial failure to 48 and 20%, respectively, of that of a pure microcrystalline cellulose tablet.

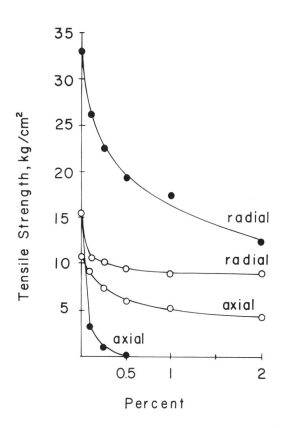

Figure 23   The effect of concentration of magnesium stearate on the tensile strengths of (●) microcrystalline cellulose and (○) anhydrous lactose tablets compressed at 355 and 710 kg/cm^2, respectively.   (From Ref. 43.)

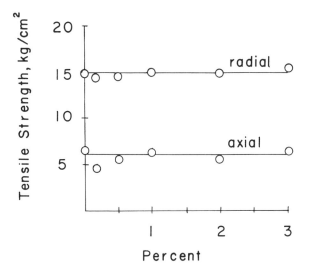

Figure 24   The effect of concentration of magnesium stearate on the tensile strengths of dibasic calcium phosphate dihydrate tables compressed at 1776 kg/cm^2.   (From Ref. 43.)

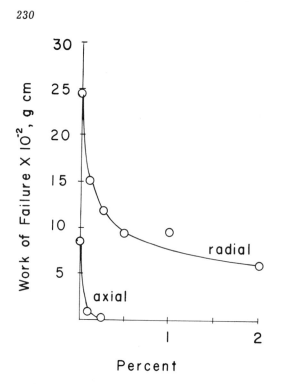

Figure 25   The effect of concentration of magnesium stearate on the work of failure of microcrystalline cellulose tablets compressed at 356 kg/cm^2. (From Ref. 46.)

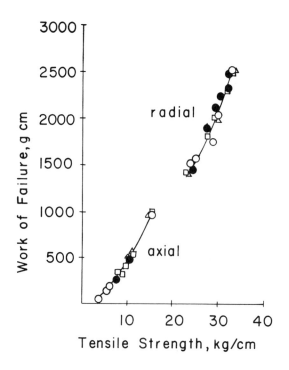

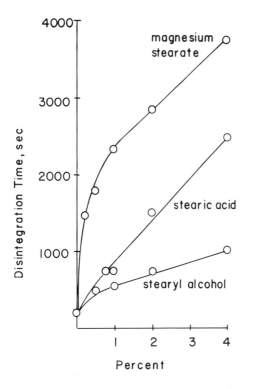

Figure 27 Disintegration time against percent of lubricant for sodium bi-carbonate tablets compressed at 1300 kg/cm^2. (From Ref. 47, with permission of the copyright owner, The American Pharmaceutical Association.)

Obviously, if a small amount of work causes failure, the tablet is unsatisfactory for handling and transport. Stearic acid, hydrogenated vegetable oil, talc, and polyethylene glycol produced the same effect. In Figure 26, the plot of work of axial and radial failure against the tensile strengths of the tablet clearly shows that considerably less work need be accomplished to cause failure (lamination) in the axial direction.

The disintegration time of a tablet may be significantly prolonged by the incorporation of a lubricant [47], as shown in Figure 27. Most lubricants are hydrophobic and excessive amounts tend to make a tablet water-resistant.

Dissolution may be affected by the incorporation of a lubricant, as shown in Figure 28. Talc in concentrations from 0.1 to 5% does not alter the dissolution rates of compressed, nondisintegrating salicylic acid, aspirin, and aspirin—salicylic acid disks. Although it is water-soluble,

Figure 26 The relationship of work of failure to axial and radial tensile strength of microcrystalline cellulose tablets containing various lubricants. (○) polyethylene glycol 4000, (△) talc, (●) hydrogenated vegetable oil, and (□) stearic acid. (From Ref. 46.)

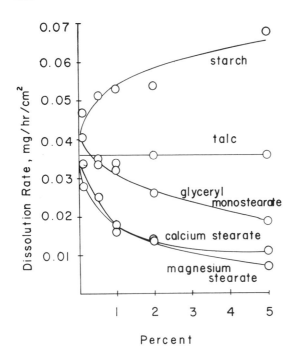

Figure 28   The effect of several lubricants in various concentrations on the dissolution rate of aspirin from a tablet composed of 0.5 M aspirin and 0.5 M salicylic acid compressed at 900 kg/cm^2. (From Ref. 48, with permission of the copyright owner, The American Pharmaceutical Association.)

polyethylene glycol does not alter the dissolution rate of these disks. The dissolution rates of aspirin–salicylic acid disks are slowed by the incorporation of calcium stearate, glyceryl monstearate, hydrogenated castor oil, magnesium stearate, and stearic acid as a lubricant in concentrations from 0.1 to 5%.

The addition of from 0.1 to 5% corn starch to aspirin–salicylic acid disks increased the dissolution, because in addition to acting as a lubricant, the starch acts as a distintegrating agent, causing flaking and increasing the effective surface.

The efficiency of a lubricant may be quantitatively expressed as the ratio R of the maximum lower punch force to the maximum upper punch force [49]. A comparison of some R values of various lubricants is shown in Table 3. In addition to the comparison of various lubricants, the R value is helpful in the determination of the concentration of a lubricant that provides an optimum lubricant effect, which for most pharmaceutical lubricants does not exceed 1%.

Table 3   Effects of Various Substances as a Lubricant for
Compression of a Sulfathiazole Granulation

Lubricant	Percent	Maximum lower punch force / Maximum upper punch force
None (control)	–	0.63
Calcium stearate	0.5	0.96
	1.0	0.98
	2.0	0.99
Sodium stearate	0.5	0.86
	1.0	0.94
	2.0	0.95
Spermaceti	0.5	0.56
	1.0	0.66
	2.0	0.68
Veegum	0.5	0.62
	1.0	0.63
	2.0	0.59
Polyethylene glycol 4000	0.5	0.76
	1.0	0.79
	2.0	0.74
Talc	0.5	0.60
	1.0	0.60
	2.0	0.63
Magnesium stearate	0.5	0.83
	1.0	0.86
	2.0	0.88

Source: Ref. 49.

V. TRANSMISSION OF FORCE

In a single-punch tablet press, the compressional force on the upper
punch is greater than the force on the lower punch. During compression
of a given weight of granules, the relationship between the upper and
lower punch is almost linear. Because of friction, the force (or pressure)
distribution is not uniform in the die cavity during compression.

As a result of the nonuniform pressure distribution during compression, there are variations in density and mechanical strength within a
tablet. Train [50] measured the distribution of pressure in a magnesium
carbonate mass while compression was occurring; and after sectioning the
extruded mass, he determined the relative densities of the sections, as
illustrated in Figure 29.

The initial pressure of the upper punch produces a peripheral region
of high density. As the upper punch descends, its initial pressure is

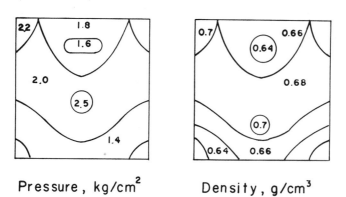

Pressure, kg/cm²   Density, g/cm³

Figure 29   Contours of pressure and density in a compact. (From Ref. 50.)

progressively lessened with the increasing friction force at the face of the
die wall. Consequently, less pressure is transmitted to the particles adjacent to the die wall, and the region at the bottom periphery is less
dense than at the top edges. On the other hand, with no die wall friction and only interparticular friction, the material at the center is relatively free to move. Thus, with a greater pressure being transmitted, the
center is compressed to a greater density. After compression there remains a residual die wall pressure, which must be overcome to eject the
tablet.

A mean value for the die wall pressure may be measured by strain
gages bonded to the outer wall of the die [51]. The die wall must be thin
to obtain a measurable response. As shown in Figure 30, a part of the

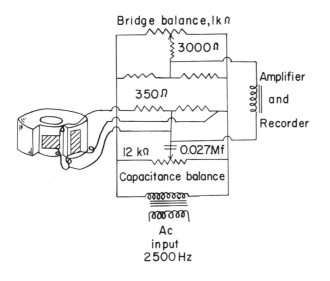

Figure 30   Diagrammatic representation of instrumentation of a single-
punch tablet machine for measurement of die wall pressure. (From Ref.
51, with permission of the copyright owner, the American Pharmaceutical
Association.)

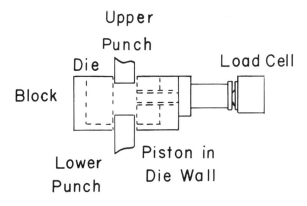

Figure 31 Diagrammatic representation of instrumentation of a single-punch tablet machine for measurement of die wall pressure. (From Ref. 52, with permission of the copyright owner, The American Pharmaceutical Association.)

die wall may be ground out to increase sensitivity. One strain gage is bonded on the die wall normal to the bore of the die, and one strain gage is bonded parallel to compensate for temperature change during compression. The strain gages form a part of a Wheatstone bridge, as shown in Figure 30. Such a system does not alter the internal die bore and does not depend on the extrusion characteristics of the material being compressed.

Die wall pressure at exact points may be measured by another technique [52]. The apparatus consists of a die in which holes perpendicular to the bore of the die have been drilled and fitted with pistons, as shown in Figure 31. The die wall pressure exerted on the piston is transmitted by mechanical linkage to a local cell, which activates a recording device.

The simultaneous measurement of die wall pressure and upper punch pressure may aid in defining the behavior of compressed materials. Axial pressure is that force per unit area being applied in the direction in which the punch moves during compression; its application causes a decrease in volume of the material being compressed. The radial pressure is the force per unit area developed and transmitted at right angles from the longitudinal axis of punch. The radial pressure is a shearing factor causing deformation.

Just as a Heckel plot characterizes the behavior of a material in bonding, a plot of the radial pressure (or force) against uniaxial pressure (or force) characterizes the behavior of a solid body. The compression characteristics [53, 54] of solids under uniaxial compression may be defined as (a) a perfect elastic body, (b) a body with a constant yield stress in shear, and (c) a Mohr body. The assumptions are that the die is perfectly rigid, there is no die wall friction, and the material is a solid body.

For a perfectly elastic body, when an axial force is applied, the transmitted radial force is of the same magnitude, and the ratio of the axial force σ to the radial force τ is constant

$$\frac{\sigma}{\tau} = \upsilon \tag{9}$$

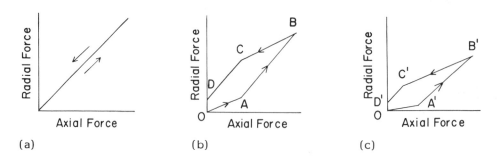

Figure 32   Theoretical pressure cycles under uniaxial compression within a rigid, frictionless die.

where υ is known as the Poisson ratio. As shown in Figure 32a as the axial force is decreased, the radial force dissipates along the same line, and when it returns to zero there is no residual radial force exerted on the die wall and the body is free to move from the die. Crystalline phenacetin had been reported to behave similarly to an elastic body [55]. It appears that few pharmaceutical tablets are a perfectly elastic body, as force is required to eject the tablet and the ejected tablet cannot be fitted back into the die cavity.

The compression cycle of a body with a constant yield stress in shear is defined in Figure 32b. In practice, segment AO may not pass through the origin, and then segment AO may be represented as [54]

$$\tau = \frac{\upsilon}{1 - \upsilon}\ \sigma \tag{10}$$

Along AO the material is within its elastic limit and Hookes law is valid. At point A (the yield stress in shear) the body begins to deform plastically, and thereafter the material fails along a shear plane. The yield stress in shear is independent of the magnitude of the principal stress. Along segment AB the body behaves as if $\sigma = \tau$, and if the yield stress in shear is S, the equation along segment AB is

$$\tau = \sigma - S \tag{11}$$

The maximum applied (axial) pressure σ_{max} is attained at point B. After point B has been reached, and the axial force is decreased, the body is no longer forced to yield. The slopes of BC and AO are equal. As the axial force is decreasing along BC, decompression and relaxation occur. The equation of segment BC is

$$\tau = \left(\frac{\upsilon}{1 - \upsilon}\right)\sigma + \left[1 - \frac{\upsilon}{1 - \upsilon}\right]\ \sigma_{max} - S \tag{12}$$

if the maximum axial force has been sufficiently large, point C is attained at which the radial force is greater than the axial force by the yield stress. Along segment CD the slope is unity, and the difference between the radial and the axial force is constant

$$\tau = \sigma + S \tag{13}$$

After the upper punch has been withdrawn, the tablet exerts a residual radial force of S on the die wall and is restrained in the die. The area under OABCD is proportional to the maximum axial pressure applied.

The compression cycle shown in Figure 32c defines a Mohr body. The Mohr body is also rigid, but after the elastic limit is exceeded, along A'B' brittle fracture or fragmentation occurs. The shearing stress in a plane of slip is a linear function of the normal stress σ_n acting in the same plane. When the body yields

$$\text{shearing stress} = S + \sigma_n \mu \tag{14}$$

in which μ is a frictional coefficient. The normal stress on the plane of shear is $\frac{1}{2}(\sigma + \tau)$, and the shearing stress is $\frac{1}{2}(\sigma - \tau)$. Substituting into Equation 14 and rearranging, after yield the radial force along segment A'B' is

$$\tau = \frac{(1 - \mu)\sigma - 2S}{1 + \mu} \tag{15}$$

With decomposition and relaxation along segment B'C', which is parallel to A'O, the radial force is

$$\tau = \left[\frac{\upsilon}{1 - \upsilon} (\sigma - \sigma_{max}) \right] + \frac{(1 - \mu) \sigma_{max} - 2S}{1 + \mu} \tag{16}$$

With decreased axial force, provided that the axial force has been sufficient, the radial force along segment C'D' is

$$\tau = \frac{(1 + \mu) \sigma - 2S}{1 - \mu} \tag{17}$$

The residual die wall force is

$$\tau = \frac{2S}{1 - \mu} \tag{18}$$

The area under A'B'C'D'O is a function of the square of the maximum axial force.

An acetaminophen granulation prepared using acetone behaves as a Mohr body [53]. The slope C'D' is 1, and the slope A'B' is 0.4. Acetaminophen granulated with 3% povidone behaves as a body with a constant yield stress in shear. The slopes CD and AB are 0.4. Acetaminophen on compression tends to cap and laminate; however, if granulated with 3% povidone, no capping is observed. For acetaminophen, the change from a capping tablet to a solid one is associated with the transformation from a Mohr body type to one with a constant yield stress in shear. This suggests that the analyses of the pressure cycles of materials may be indicative of the formation of a satisfactory or unsatisfactory compressed tablet.

VI. NATURE OF MATERIAL

A. Chemical

Jaffe and Foss [56] investigated the role of crystal properties on the
ability of materials to form tablets. They found that compounds (ammonium
halides, potassium halides, methanamine) that have cubic crystal lattice
often could be compressed directly, and that substances (ferrous sulfate,
magnesium sulfate, sodium phosphate) having water of crystallization could
be compressed directly but did not form a tablet if the water of crystallization was removed.

The compressibility of material may be expressed in terms of the slope
of a plot of the logarithm of compressional force (or pressure) against porosity. In Figure 33 the slope $d\varepsilon/d(\log P)$ is greater for methacetin than
for phenacetin, indicating that methacetin is more compressible than phenacetin. The chemical nature of phenacetin and methacetin is very similar,
yet phenacetin caps readily and is less compressible; thus, there is no
correlation between their chemical structure and compressional behavior
[57]. A general similarity of compressional behavior among formulations
of the sulfa drugs and the alkali halides has been reported [3, 49, 51].

Unfortunately, no general relationship that would allow the prediction
of compressibility of a formulation based on the chemical nature and
crystalline structure of its constituents has been demonstrated.

The applied pressure may influence reaction kinetics in the solid state.
As the applied pressure is increased through the various events of the
process of compression, a maximum specific surface that provides the most
reaction sites for the reactants, is attained. Additional pressure

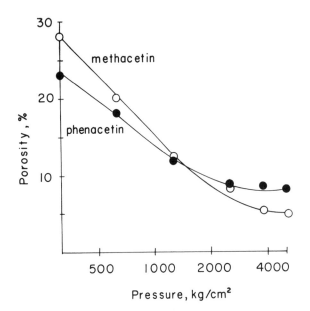

Figure 33   The effect of applied pressure on the porosity of methacetin
and phenacetin tablets. (From Ref. 57, with permission of the copyright
owner, The American Pharmaceutical Association.)

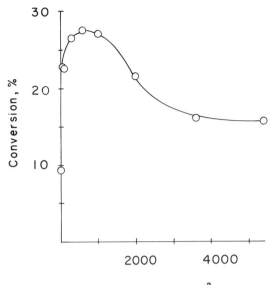

Figure 34　The effect of applied pressure on the conversion of sulfacetamide after 3 hours at 90°C. (From Ref. 58, with permission of the
copyright owner, The American Pharmaceutical Association.)

consolidates the mass with a reduction in porosity, and the rate of transport of the reactants by diffusion, surface migration or sublimation is decreased. Both effects slow the rate of reaction.

The influence of applied pressure on the addition of sulfacetamide and
succinic anhydride is shown in Figure 34. In tablets compressed at 600
kg/cm^2, 27.5% of the sulfacetamide was converted to succinylsulfacetamide
under the experimental conditions, but at 3580 kg/cm^2 only 16% of the
sulfacetamide was converted [58]. Perhaps in pharmaceutical tablets
containing compounds that interact in the solid state, there is a critical
applied pressure that would provide the optimum conditions for the unde-
sired reaction, and consequently, other pressures could be selected to
enhance stability.

B. Mechanical Properties

There is a direct proportionality between bonding and the contact area of
the solid surfaces on which intermolecular forces act. Solids, which
undergo plastic deformation to a large extent, have a greater area of contact for a given pressure and, consequently, a greater degree of bonding.
The plasticity of a crystal lattice contributes to bonding regardless of the
mechanism involved.

Sodium chloride is compressed by particle rearrangement and plastic
deformation without significant fragmentation [59]. With sodium chloride
at a given pressure, the smaller granules form a mechanically stronger
tablet than do the larger granules [60]. When the tablet is crushed, it

fractures across the crystals, indicating that the bonding between the granules is as strong as the bonding in the bulk of the solid. With sodium chloride, axial recovery is completed before ejection from the die.

Lactose, dicalcium phosphate dihydrate, and sucrose [7,20,59] fragment during compression. When fragmentation is the chief mechanism in compression, tablet strength, or the ability to form a tablet, is independent of the size of the granules. Heckel [16] used sodium chloride and lactose as examples to distinguish between the mechanism of bonding.

Capping, which occurs after the upper punch has been withdrawn, has been attributed to the effect of entrapped air. Shear at the die wall and punch may prevent the escape of air, which is then compressed within the tablet structure by the applied pressure. Upon withdrawal of the upper punch, the compressed air expands and cracks the tablet. Capping may occur by this mechanism for waxy materials and fine powders. Mechanically capping is minimized by the use of dies in which the upper punch has been tapered several thousandths of an inch to facilitate the escape of air. In some high-speed rotary presses, the use of several pressure rolls allows a gradual increase in pressure with a slower release of the air before the final compression.

In tablet production the particle size distribution of the granulation is controlled so that fine powder is not present. With the proper control of the size of the granulation and proper adjustment and operation of the tablet press, any capping that occurs is probably not caused by entrapped air but by the behavior of the material. It has been demonstrated that the capping of methanamine tablets under a vacuum is the same as that under atmospheric pressure [61].

The elastic property of a material is responsible for splitting of a tablet during decompression. A material resistant to crushing will undergo deformation under applied pressure. When the pressure is released the material tends to return to its original form, breaking any bonds that may have formed under pressure, and as the tablet is confined by the die, it exerts a pressure on the die wall because it tends to expand on decomposition. During ejection, a portion of the tablet is outside of the die, while a portion of the tablet within the die is under strain. Under these stresses a tablet may laminate in the regions of its lower density (or tensile strength).

Phenacetin is a classical example of an elastic material that caps readily [62]. In the initial stage of compression, only a small force is transmitted to the die wall, owing to the difficulty of particle rearrangement. Force-displacement curves for the compression of phenacetin indicate that at low pressure the energy is largely expended in elastic deformation and that no further increase in tablet strength is expected with increase in pressure. In the decompression phase, the residual die wall pressure is small, indicating that the phenacetin tends to recover axially and contract radially. As the movement of the tablet is restricted by the residual die wall pressure and the friction with the die wall, the stress from its axial elastic recovery and the radial contraction causes splitting.

Binders are excipients used to strengthen bonding; and thus, they reduce the tendency to cap. Binders undergo plastic deformation under pressure. As the concentration of the binder is increased, a greater portion of the energy of compression is absorbed by the binder, and less is absorbed by the elastically deformed material. Upon removal of the applied pressure, there is less elastic recovery by the whole compact, and capping is reduced.

Usually the axial tensile strength of a tablet is weaker than the radial tensile strength. As shown in Figure 10 for dibasic calcium phosphate dihydrate granulation with 1.2% starch, the radial tensile strength increases linearly as the applied pressure is increased. However, as the applied pressure is increased, the axial tensile strength attains its maximum strength at a pressure of 3130 kg/cm^2. A difference in the axial and radial tensile strengths indicates that the tablet is not homogeneous and does not have a uniform mechanical strength. As the axial and radial tensile strengths are measures of bonding, it appears that the ratio σ_z/σ_x could be used as an index of capping. The ratio would be unity for a homogeneous tablet. In Figure 10 for each applied pressure the value of σ_z/σ_x is given. As the applied pressure is increased, the ratio is smaller indicating that the tendency to cap is increased. At very low applied pressure the ratio is 0.95 and at higher pressures the ratio becomes smaller. After the maximum axial tensile strength has been attained, further increases in pressure decrease its strength. It is an erroneous concept that the strength of a tablet may be continuously increased by the application of greater pressure, and in fact, high pressures often cause capping.

As shown in Figure 12 there is a maximum axial tensile strength attained at a low concentration of binder with an observed tendency for capping at high applied pressures. At the highest applied pressure (3570 kg/cm^2) for lactose tablets containing 1 and 9% povidone, the ratio is 0.14 and 0.36, respectively. At low pressure the concentration of povidone has little effect on the radial tensile strength as demonstrated in Figure 11, but an increase in the concentration of povidone increases the axial tensile strength. At an applied pressure of 900 kg/cm^2, a 4.5 and 9% povidone granulation produces a tablet with a ratio of 1.06 indicating that bonding is approximately the same in both axes, and capping is unlikely. An examination of Figures 11 and 12 shows that for a lactose and povidone formulation, the use of a formulation containing 9% povidone and an applied pressure of 900 kg/cm^2 would produce a tablet least likely to cap.

REFERENCES

1. Griffith, A. A., *Phil. Trans. Roy. Soc. London, Serv. A, 221*:163 (1921).
2. Orowna, E., in *Dislocations in Metals* (M. Cohen, ed.), American Institute of Minerals and Petroleum Engineers, New York, 1954, Chap. 3.
3. Higuchi, T., Rao, A. N., Busse, L. W., and Swintosky, J. V., *J. Amer. Pharm. Assoc., Sci. Ed., 42*:194−200 (1953).
4. Goetzel, C. G., *Treatise on Powder Metallurgy*, Vol. 1, Interscience, New York, 1949, pp. 259−312.
5. Reier, G. E. and Shangraw, R. E., *J. Pharm. Sci., 55*:510−514 (1966).
6. Khan, D. A. and Rhodes, C. T., *J. Pharm. Sci., 64*:444−446 (1975).
7. Skotnicky, J., *Czechoslov. J. Phys., 3*:225 (1953).

8. Rankell, A. S. and Higuchi, T., *J. Pharm. Sci.*, 57:574–577 (1968).
9. Carslaw, H. S. and Jaeger, J. C., *Conduction of Heat in Solids*, 2nd Ed., Oxford University Press, London, 1959, p. 75.
10. Train, D. and Lewis, C. J., *Trans. Inst. Chem. Eng.*, 40:235 (1962).
11. Sheth, P. and Munzel, K., *Pharm. Ind.*, 21:9 (1959).
12. Hiestand, E. N., Peot, C. B., and Ochs, J. E., *J. Pharm. Sci.*, 66:510 (1977).
13. Rue, P. J., Barkworth, P. M. R., Ridgway-Watt, P., Rought, P., Sharland, D. C., Seager, H., and Fisher, H., *Int. J. Pharm. Technol. Prod. Manuf.*, 1:2–5 (1979).
14. Amidon, G. E., Smith, D. P., and Hiestand, E. N., *J. Pharm. Sci.*, 70:613–617 (1981).
15. Carstensen, J. T., Alcorn, G. J., Hussain, S. A., and Zoglio, M. A., *J. Pharm. Sci.*, 74:1239–1241 (1985).
16. Heckl, R. W., *Trans. Metall. Sco.*, *AIME*, 221:1001 (1961).
17. York, R., *J. Pharm. Pharmacol.*, 30:6 (1978).
18. York, P. and Pilpel, N., *J. Pharm. Pharmacol.*, *Suppl.*, 25:1P (1973).
19. Jarosz, P. J. and Parrott, E. L., *J. Pharm. Sci.*, 71:607–614 (1982).
20. Hersey, J. A., Rees, J. E., and Cole, E. T., *J. Pharm. Sci.*, 62:2060 (1973).
21. Ryshkewitch, E., *J. Am. Ceramic Soc.*, 36:65 (1953).
22. Higuchi, T., Arnold, R. D., Tucker, S. J., and Busse, L. W., *J. Amer. Pharm. Assoc.*, *Sci. Ed.*, 41:93–96 (1952).
23. Train, D. and Hersey, J. A., *Powder Metall.*, 6:20 (1960).
24. Knoechel, E. L., Sperry, C. C., and Linter, C. J., *J. Pharm. Sci.*, 56:116–130 (1967).
25. Higuchi, T., Elowe, L. N., and Busse, L. W., *J. Amer. Pharm. Assoc.*, *Sci. Ed.*, 43:685–689 (1954).
26. Ritter, A. and Sucker, H., *Pharm. Tech.*, *No. 9*, 4:108 (1980).
27. Jarosz, P. J. and Parrott, E. L., *J. Pharm. Sci.*, 72:530–534 (1983).
28. Jarosz, P. J. and Parrott, E. L., *J. Pharm. Sci.*, 71:705–707 (1982).
29. Lowenthal, W., *J. Pharm. Sci.*, 61:1695–1711 (1972).
30. Shah, S. A. and Parrott, E. L., *J. Pharm. Sci.*, 65:1784–1790 (1976).
31. Mitchell, A. G. and Saville, D. J., *J. Pharm. Pharmacol.*, 19:729 (1967).
32. Kanke, M. and Sekiguchi, D., *Chem. Pharm. Bull.*, 21:871 (1973).
33. Leeson, L. J. and Cartstensen, J. T., eds., *Dissolution Technology*, Industrial Pharmaceutical Technology Section, Academy of Pharmaceutical Sciences, Washington, D.C., p. 133.
34. van Oudtshorn, M. C. B., Potgieter, F. J., de Blaey, C. J., and Polderman, J., *J. Pharm. Pharmacol.*, 23:583 (1971).
35. Higuchi, T., Nelson, E., and Busse, L. W., *J. Amer. Pharm. Assoc.*, *Sci. Ed.*, 43:344–348 (1954).
36. Shotton, E. and Ganderton, D. J., *J. Pharm. Pharmacol.*, 12:87T (1960).
37. Knoechel, E. L., Sperry, C. C., Ross, H. E., and Lintner, C. J., *J. Pharm. Sci.*, 56:109–115 (1967).
38. Shotton, E., Deer, J. J., and Gandearton, D. J., *J. Pharm. Pharmacol.*, 15:106T (1963).
39. Nelson, E., Busse, L. W., and Higuchi, T., *J. Amer. Pharm. Assoc.*, *Sci. Ed.*, 44:223–225 (1955).

40. Bogs, V. and Lenhardt, E., *Pharm. Ind.*, *33*:850 (1971).
41. Wurster, D. E. and Creekmore, J. R., *Drug Devel. and Ind. Pharm.*, *12*:1511−1528 (1986).
42. Hanls, E. J. and King, L. D., *J. Pharm. Sci.*, 57:677−684 (1968).
43. Jarosz, P. J. and Parrott, E. L., *Drug Devel. and Ind. Pharm.*, *10*: 259−273 (1984).
44. Rees, J. E. and Rue, P. J., *Drug Devel. and Ind. Pharm.*, *4*: 131−156 (1978).
45. Rees, J. E., Rue, P. J., and Richardson, S. C., *J. Pharm. Pharmacol.*, *29*:38P (1977).
46. Jarosz, P. J. and Parrott, E. L., *Drug Devel. and Ind. Pharm.*, *8*: 445−453 (1982).
47. Stickland, W. A., Nelson, E., Busse, L. W., and Higuchi, T., *J. Amer. Pharm. Assoc.*, *Sci. Ed.*, 45:51−55 (1956).
48. Iranloye, T. A. and Parrott, E. L., *J. Pharm. Sci.*, 67:535−539 (1978).
49. Nelson, E., Naqvi, S. M., Busse, L. W., and Higuchi, T., *J. Amer. Pharm. Assoc.*, *Sci. Ed.*, 43:596−602 (1954).
50. Train, D., *J. Pharm. Pharmacol.*, 8:745 (1956).
51. Windheuser, J. J., Misra, J., Eriksen, S. P., and Higuchi, T., *J. Pharm. Sci.*, 52:767−772 (1963).
52. Nelson, E., *J. Amer. Assoc.*, *Sci. Ed.*, 44:494−497 (1955).
53. Leigh, S., Carless, J. E., and Burt, B. W., *J. Pharm. Sci.*, 56: 888−892 (1967).
54. Carstensen, J. T., Solid pharmaceutics, in *Mechanical Properties and Rate Phenomena*, Academic Press, New York, 1980, pp. 206−211.
55. Shotton, E. and Obiorah, B. A., *J. Pharm. Sci.*, 64:1213−1216 (1975).
56. Jaffe, J. and Foss, N. E., *J. Amer. Pharm. Assoc.*, *Sci. Ed.*, 48: 26−29 (1959).
57. Elowe, L. N., Higuchi, T., and Busse, L. W., *J. Amer. Pharm. Assoc.*, *Sci. Ed.*, 43:718−721 (1954).
58. Weng, H. and Parrott, E. L., *Powd. Technol.*, *39*:1−5 (1984).
59. Hardman, J. S. and Lilley, B. A., *Nature (Lond.)*, *228*:353 (1970).
60. Hersey, J. A., Bayraktar, G., and Shotton, E., *J. Pharm. Pharmacol.*, *19*:245 (1967).
61. Long, M. W., *Powder Metall.*, *6*:73 (1960).
62. de Blaey, C. J., de Rijk, W., and Polderman, J., *Pharm. Ind.*, *33*: 897 (1971).

5

Granulation Technology and Tablet Characterization

Roger E. Gordon, Thomas W. Rosanske, * and Dale E. Fonner

The Upjohn Company, Kalamazoo, Michigan

Neil R. Anderson

Merrell—Dow Research Institute, Indianapolis, Indiana

Gilbert S. Banker

University of Minnesota, Minneapolis, Minnesota

PART ONE: CHARACTERIZATION OF
GRANULATION[†]

Greater than 90% of all therapeutic compounds are administered via the oral route, of which the tablet dosage form is by far the most popular. The quality of this solid oral dosage form is, as a general rule, primarily governed by the physicochemical propert.es of the powder/ granulation from which the tablets are composed. For decades, however, the granulation process evolved purely on an empirical basis. Provided the finished dosage form met all registration specifications and the granulation did not significantly alter scheduling in production, extreme variability in granule physicochemical properties was tolerated. With the advent of product validation, as delineated in the Current Good Manufacturing Practices (CGMPs), the granulation process has had to become more structured, namely, documentation that systems and processes are performing as they are intended in a reproducible manner and are controllable.

To be able to monitor and to control the critical processing variables associated with the granulation unit operation may require more definitive or quantitative measurements be utilized. It is with these ideas in mind that certain topics have been included in the following discussion:

Current affiliation: Marion Laboratories, Inc., Kansas City, Missouri.

[†]Part One is contributed by Roger E. Gordon and Dale E. Fonner.

Fundamental principles governing particle size enlargement
Factors affecting granule size and potential implications to process and
    dosage form
Particle size measurement and interpretation
Shape determinations
Surface area
Densities and packings
Granule strength and friability
Electrostatic properties
Flow properties
Ease of consolidation and mechanisms

The granulation characteristics that are probably of most immediate
interest to developmental pharmacists and therefore the most universally
measured are those of bulk density, some assessment of flow, particle size
distribution, and some assessment of successful compaction into tablets.
These basic measurements of the granulation have been used to develop
and monitor the manufacture of many successful pharmaceutical solid dosage
forms.   Conceivably, then, some of the topics that will be discussed in
the sections to follow may appear purely theoretical and of little or no
practical value.   It is not uncommon, however, to encounter problems in
the formulation, design, or manufacture of tablets where a knowledge of
granulation characteristics and their measurement, beyond the routine
methods described above, may be of value.   In some cases the resolution
of tableting problems may, in fact, be satisfactorily resolved only if the
source of the problem is first identified by in-depth studies of granulation
characteristics, beyond what the basic measurements can provide.

I. FUNDAMENTAL PRINCIPLES GOVERNING
PARTICLE SIZE ENLARGEMENT

A. Introduction

Agglomerate and granule are descriptive terms that refer to the accumulation of small particles into larger aggregates.   Although both terms are
similarly defined, inspection of the manufacturing process provides an easy
method of differentiating the two aggregation phenomena, namely, agglomeration refers to the buildup of small particles into larger aggregates
without the addition of a binding agent or use of mechanical force, while
granulation refers to the buildup of small particles into larger aggregates
with the aid of a binding agent or mechanical force —water, starch paste,
roller compaction, etc.   Thus, agglomeration often occurs without intention
during such manufacturing operations as dense powder conveying, sieving,
sifting, mixing, and grinding.   Granulation, on the other hand, is a
planned operation.   Obviously, the intentional incorporation of a granulation operation into a manufacturing process must yield some intrinsic worth
to the product.   As outlined in Table 1, the granulation of small particles
into larger aggregates has the potential of changing the completion of any
formulation development project.   Thus, an understanding behind the
fundamental mechanisms essential for granule formation and growth is
desirable.

Table 1 Potential Benefits Associated with
Pharmaceutical Granulation

An improvement in powder flow

An increase in bulk density

A more uniform particle size

A reduction in punch face adherence (sticking)

A reduction in capping tendencies

An improvement in operator safety

The initial particle–particle interaction and the continued accumulation of particles into the granule requires the activation and expression of adhesive forces between particles such that sufficient strength is achieved in the granule to resist the destructive shear forces exerted by the agitation process. To this end, an overview of the possible forces responsible for the particle–particle adhesion and growth is presented below.

This section is not intended to explore in depth the theoretical derivations presented by Rumph, Capes, Sherrington, and Oliver, but to qualitatively introduce the reader to conclusions drawn by these authors. The inquisitive reader should consult the references if a further theoretical perspective is sought [1–4].

B. Intermolecular Forces

London dispersion forces are primarily the forces taken into consideration when describing particle–particle adhesion due to intermolecular forces. As a result, several investigators have, depending on the geometrical model and theoretical approach, developed relationships which are reported to describe the intermolecular dispersion forces role in the adhesion of particles [5–7]. Simplification of these complex relationships requires the acceptance of one critical assumption — the system is composed of molecularly smooth spherical particles [4]. This assumption is obviously invalid for real systems and thus hinders the quantitative accuracy of these models. Nonetheless, despite this shortcoming, these models aid in understanding the conditions under which intermolecular forces may possibly play a role in the granulation process; in particular, London dispersion forces are partly responsible for the adhesive forces between particles or between particles and surfaces when the separation distances are less than 10^3 A^o [8]. For this reason it thus seems reasonable to conclude that intermolecular forces originating from unadulterated particulate systems in and by themselves are not a significant factor governing initial particle attraction and growth. Exceptions to this statement do exist. For example, Rumpf [9] was able to demonstrate intermolecular forces were primarily responsible for the formation and survival of granules produced via a slugging operation. During compaction, particles were compressed together with separation distances approaching 10 A; thus, London dispersion forces were primarily responsible for the existence of the granule.

C. Electrostatic Forces

Electrostatic forces arise in almost every particulate system, either as a result of interparticulate friction or through the generation of contact potentials [7,10,11]. Typical charge densities range from 10^{-10} to 10^{-6} cm^{-3} [12]. For large particles in the dry state, electrostatic effects are instrumental in the initial adhesion of the particles and the generation of agglomerates. Further decreasing the surface roughness of the particles will, in fact, elevate the importance of the electrostatic forces in regards to intermolecular forces [7,13].

D. Liquid and Solid Bridges

Dispersing a liquid into a powdery mass will generally result in a significant increase in the formation and strength of particle—particle aggregates. The degree to which granules form and grow, however, is governed by the quantity of liquid added, the mobility of the liquid, the granulating equipment utilized, and the particle size of the powdery mass. Considering for the moment the state of liquid dispersion, three physical categories have been reported to increase the level of cohesion exhibited between particles [1,15]:

1. The adsorbed immobile liquid state
2. The mobile liquid state
3. The viscous liquid state

With the adsorbed immobile liquid state, the magnitude of the adhesive bonds established between two particles in close proximity is influenced in two ways [1,14]:

1. "The surface imperfections are smoothed out, increasing the available particle—particle contact area."
2. "van der Waal's and electrostatic forces assume a greater role in the granulating process as a result of a reduction in interparticle separation."

Thus, although the adsorbed surface film increases [5] the magnitude of adhesive forces between particles, these forces by themselves are generally insufficient to survive the deleterious effects of agitation or handling. With the addition of larger quantities of liquid, however, liquid bridges are established between the particles, and thus a significant increase in granule strength is observed. To a large extent, the strength of the granule is now governed by the amount of liquid occupying the interstitial pore volume of the granule. Assuming the granulating medium wets the particles, namely, the contact angle is zero, the primary forces responsible for maintaining granule integrity are the surface tension of the liquid and the negative pressures associated with the curvature of the liquid menisci at the air—liquid interface. Newitt and Conway-Jones [15] have observed three unique states of mobile liquid:

1. The pendular state
2. The funicular state
3. The capillary state

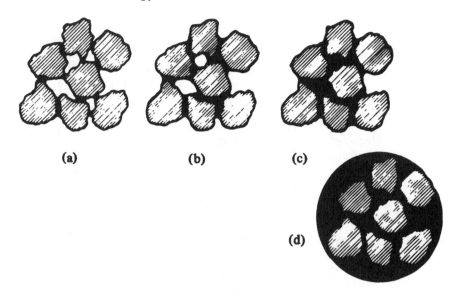

Figure 1 Three states of liquid distribution in moist aggregates: (a) pendular state, (b) funicular state, (c) capillary state, and (d) liquid droplet with particles inside or at its surface. (From Ref. 2.)

These three states are distinguished by the relative amounts of liquid occupying the interstitial pore volume, S, of the granule (Fig. 1).

The pendicular state is characterized by the formation of liquid bridges between adjacent particles at point contacts (Fig. 1a). The eventual degree to which contact is established between any two particles is a function of the size, shape, and surface roughness of the particles [16,17]. By gradually increasing the quantity of liquid in the system (S ⩾ 25%), the funicular state is achieved (Fig. 1b). This state is recognized by localized areas of complete void space saturation, along with bridge formation. With further liquid addition (S ⩾ 80%), the capillary state is reached where all the interstitial pores are completely filled with granulating medium and a concave menisci develops around the surface of the granule (Fig. 1c).

Regardless of the liquid state, the cohesive forces arising in the granule are the result of capillary forces. The pendicular state, for example, acquires its strength from the surface tension of the granulating medium and the observed pressure differential across the liquid menisci. Rumpf [14], Pietsch et al. [18], and Sherrington et al. [4] have derived theoretical mathematical relationships that summarize the contribution of each of these capillary forces to granulate strength. Although the numerical accuracy of these models is questionable, qualitative conclusions can, nonetheless, be drawn, namely, as the bridge volume decreases, the strength of the granule either remains constant or gradually decreases [18,19]. Further work by Rumpf [13] indicates capillary pressure is the primary force responsible for granule strength when the capillary state is reached. Obviously, between these two extremes is the funicular state, which acquires its strength via both mechanisms.

From a practical standpoint, if a developmental scientist were dealing
with a system where the surface tension of the granulating medium is held
constant and the particle size of the powder mixture remains unaltered,
the tensile strength of a granule in the pendicular state would be approximately one-third that of the capillary state, while the funicular state
would be intermediate.

Thus, the following conclusions can be drawn when considering mobile
liquid bridges: the cohesive forces responsible for granule strength arise
from the granulating medium's surface tension, the observed pressure differential across the menisci and van der Waal's forces; further these forces
must be sufficient to withstand the detrimental effects of agitation during
granulation to obtain suitable granules.

The mere addition of a granulating fluid into a powdery mass promotes
the initial adhesive forces between irregular particles and is responsible
for granule growth. Nevertheless, a granulation operation developed without regard to other physicochemical characteristics will, on drying, often
be soft and easily broken down on further handling and/or transportation.
This, of course, assumes constituents of the powder mass are not solubilized
by the granulating medium. The strength and quality of the final granulation can be dramatically improved with the addition of a viscosity-inducing
agent. The viscosity of the system, assuming a consistent solvent vehicle
is employed, will be governed by the addition of binding agents, which
may be added to the system either in the dry state or in the granulating
medium. In either case, a change in pressure and/or temperature sufficient
to cause a phase change in the liquid medium will result in the crystallization of the dissolved and/or suspended binders. Solid bridges thus form
between adjacent particles and the strength of the granule increases dramatically. Five mechanisms are reported to be responsible for the formation of solid bridges [1,3,20-22]:

1. Crystallization of dissolved binders
2. Hardening binders
3. Particle melting or localized fusion welding
4. Particle deformation followed by sintering
5. Chemical reaction

Of these five mechanisms, the pharmaceutical industry primarily utilizes
methods one and two for wet granulation and methods 3 and 4 for roller
compaction.

From a practical perspective, Pietsch [23] demonstrated that, while
binder and binder concentration contribute to the final strength of the
granule, drying conditions are also a critical parameter to consider. Figures 2a and 2b show the development of salt bridges that were obtained
at different drying temperatures. Visual examination of the beads indicates drying temperature is an important parameter in the development of
granule strength, even if all other parameters remain constant. Conversely, the drying process is greatly influenced by the distribution of
the binding agent. For example, as the granulating medium begins to
evaporate at the surface of the granule, the liquid flows to the surface by
means of capillary forces. The binder crystallizes and forms a crust
which may hinder further drying of the porous granule. Thus, with
higher degrees of void saturation and binder concentration, binder

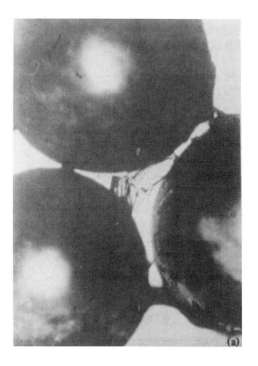 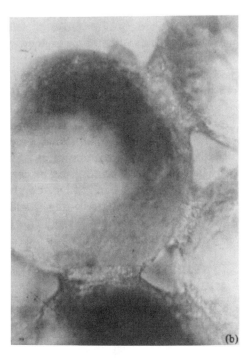

Figure 2   Crystallization rate of sodium chloride between glass bead (model experiment):   (a) drying at room temperature and (b) drying at 110°C. (From Ref. 2.)

encrustations may form at the surface of the particles and/or granule, thus retarding further drying.

As illustrated in Figure 3, the tensile strength of granules formed on the addition of a nearly saturated salt solution to a sieve cut of limestone powder is dependent on two primary variables: crystallization velocity (drying temperature) and quantity of binding agent forming the bridges. When the interstitial pore volume in this example assumed a level of less than 20% (curves a and b), crust formation did not develop and the tensile strength of the granule increased with drying temperature.   Comparing the tensile strength of curves a and b reveals the rise in tensile strength is caused first by the increasing crystallization rate and second by a pro- portional addition of salt.   At an interstitial pore saturation level of 20%, a thin crust begins to form, which influences the granules' tensile strength slightly.   At higher void saturations (S $\geq$ 45% curves e and f), a dense crust governs further drying of the granules and the further formation of solid bridges.   Thus, granules formed in this example with at least 45% void space occupied by granulating medium will have low tensile strength. Notice curve d, however; high tensile strength granules were obtained when the granulation was dried above 350°C.   This result was achieved due to small hair-like fractures in the crust, which allowed a greater dry- ing rate and thus an increase in the velocity of crystallization.   This

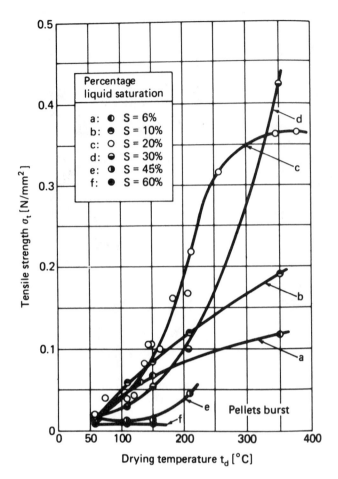

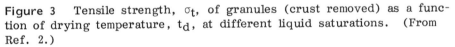

Figure 3   Tensile strength, σ_t, of granules (crust removed) as a function of drying temperature, t_d, at different liquid saturations.   (From Ref. 2.)

suggests an optimum drying temperature exists where the granules dry quickly but do not build up sufficient internal pressure to cause cracking or disintegration.

Replotting the data from Figure 3 illustrates that around 20% void saturation the granules generally acquire their maximum strength regardless of temperature (Fig. 4).   Curve e further serves to document the importance of selecting the proper drying temperature.

Although this example serves to illustrate the importance of drying temperature, void saturation and binder concentration, the reader is cautioned about generalizing from this experiment to pharmaceutical formulations.   For, in this example, the crust was removed from the granules before the tensile strength was obtained.   Chare [24] was able to document that the strength of granules increased in proportion to void saturation when the crust was not removed (Fig. 5).

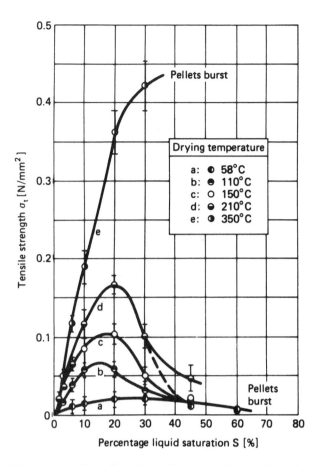

Figure 4   Tensile strength, σ_t, of granules (crust removed) as a function of liquid saturation, S, before drying at different drying temperatures. (From Ref. 2.)

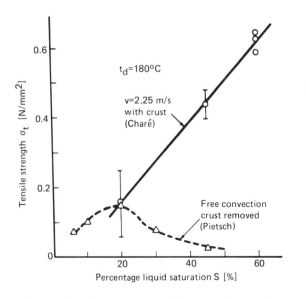

Figure 5   Tensile strength, σ_t, of granules as a function of the liquid saturation, S, before drying with and without the crust. (From Ref. 2.)

Thus, while the examples employed in Figures 3 and 4 are not representative of pharmaceutical operations, the examples do serve to point out that binder concentration, void saturation, and drying temperature all play a critical role in the success of the granulation operation. Further, to obtain a strong granule, the concentration of the binding agent in the granulating medium and the drying temperature should be selected as high as possible.

II. PARTICLE SIZE MEASUREMENT AND INTERPRETATION

The principal intent of particle size measurement is to establish the true particle size frequency distribution. Although the concept is simple, there are basic problems in defining both size and distribution. If powders or granulations contained only spherical particles, there would be no difficulty in defining particle size, because the size of a sphere is uniquely determined by its diameter. But particles are rarely spherical in shape and, more often than not, are quite irregular in shape. Experimental methods vary greatly, and the observed particle size distribution is dependent upon the methodology and technique employed. In addition, powders and granulations pose some unique sampling problems. The amount of material subjected to a particle size analysis usually represents only a very small part of the particulate material in question. Therefore, it is essential that the sample(s) selected be unbiased and representative of the total material. In spite of these problems, it is possible to establish valid frequency distributions of particle size. The observed distribution then serves as the basis for establishing descriptive characteristics or constants, such as median diameter (by weight or number), percent by weight greater than a stated size, or standard deviation. Several good reference sources are available on particle size measurement and interpretation [25-29]. This discussion begins by covering the various methods of data presentation.

A. Methods of Data Presentation

Tabular Presentation

Note that the frequency data in Table 2 are presented by weight rather than by number. The size distribution can be defined in terms of the weight or number of particles within a given size range. For pharmaceutical granulations, size distributions are normally described by weight. For example, it is far simpler to weigh the amount of granulation retained on a sieve as opposed to counting individual particles. For the granulation represented in Table 2, 5% by weight of the particles are from 0 to 100 μm, 17% by weight are in the range 100 to 200 μm, and so forth. From the cumulative percent distribution, 22% of the particles by weight are less than 200 μm in size, 40 by weight are less than 300 μm in size, and so forth. It should be pointed out that the weight distribution data of Table 2 are hypothetical, since standard sieves do not exist that produce an even 100 μm size fractions shown in the table.

Table 2 Size Distribution Data for a Hypothetical
Tablet Granulation

Size (μm)	Percent frequency distribution by weight	Cumulative % by weight less than stated size
0 – 100	5.0	5.0
100 – 200	17.0	22.0
200 – 300	18.0	40.0
300 – 400	15.0	55.0
400 – 500	11.0	66.0
500 – 600	8.0	74.0
600 – 700	6.0	80.0
700 – 800	4.0	84.0
800 – 900	3.0	87.0
900 – 1000	2.0	89.0
≥1000	11.0	100.0
	100.0	

Graphical Presentation

Although the most precise and explicit way of presenting size distribution data is by tabular form, there are several compelling reasons for presenting size distribution data graphically. Graphs are more concise than are long tables, and in some cases, numerical measurements or constants can be obtained which further describe the distribution of particle sizes. Also, skewness of the distribution and location of the mean particle size can readily be approximated. Further, graphical presentation offers a clear and concise way to compare size distribution data from two or more samples. Histograms, size frequency curves, and cumulative frequency plots represent the most common ways of graphically illustrating size distribution data. Any elementary book on statistical analysis [30] will provide the reader with additional background information concerning these types of graphical analyses.

FREQUENCY HISTOGRAMS. The simplest graphical form is a histogram plot in which frequency of occurrence is plotted as a function of the size range. A histogram plot of the data represented in Table 2 is shown in Figure 6. Note that the height of each rectangle corresponds to the frequency percent for the size range indicated. For example, the height of the rectangle in the range 0 to 100 μm is 5% on the frequency scale, indicating that 5% by weight of the particles are in the size range 0 to 100 μm.

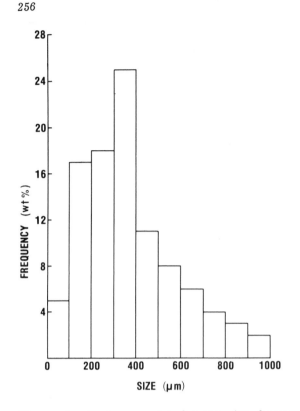

Figure 6   Histogram plot for the size frequency data given in Table 2.

SIZE FREQUENCY CURVES.   A size frequency curve can be drawn from the histogram; this is shown in Figure 7.   A size frequency curve is nothing more than a smoothed-out histogram and is obtained by drawing a continuous line through the midpoints of the top of the rectangles.   In other words, it can be seen that the tops of the rectangles form a smooth curve.   Some words of caution are in order concerning size frequency curves.   These curves are valid only if a large number of points are utilized.   Considerable error is introduced when trying to draw a size frequency curve from a small number of points.   Also, the shape of the size frequency curve can become quite irregular if uneven size ranges are used.   Therefore, it is preferable to draw size frequency curves employing many points and equal size intervals.   Often, it is not practical to obtain size intervals in a regular progression.   This is especially true when using sieving as a method of particle size analysis.   In these instances, the cumulative percent plot is valuable and is discussed next.

CUMULATIVE FREQUENCY CURVES.   Cumulative frequency curves are arrived at by plotting the percent of particles less than (or greater than) a given particle size versus particle size.   A cumulative frequency plot of the data is contained in Figure 8.   If the summation is carried out from the top downward, as in Table 2, the result is the percent of particles smaller than the upper limit of the successive size intervals.

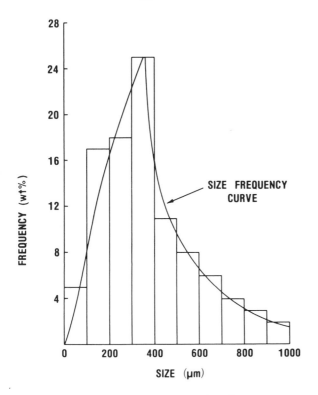

Figure 7   Illustration of the size frequency curve for the data given in Table 2.

The cumulative frequency data in Table 2 could just as easily have been summed from the bottom upward, yielding the percentage of particles greater than the lower limit of the successive size intervals. A cumulative frequency plot of percent greater than stated size could then be drawn. The choice of whether to use percent less than, or greater than, a stated size is largely arbitrary but may be based on whether the researcher is most interested in directly identifying the fraction of particles that are "oversize" or "undersize" vis-a-vis, a particular cutoff point. It should also be clear that these graphical methods are just as applicable for size frequency data generated on a number basis.

From a mathematical standpoint, integration of the size frequency curve (Fig. 7) will give the cumulative frequency curve (Fig. 8). In a like manner, differentiation of the cumulative frequency curve will yield a smooth size frequency curve. The latter point is of practical value, as the cumulative frequency curve can be drawn from data with unequal size intervals. As was mentioned before, drawing a size frequency distribution curve from frequency data in uneven size intervals will often yield a very irregular curve. This can be overcome by first plotting the cumulative frequency curve and then deriving the size frequency curve from a differentiation of this plot over equal size intervals.

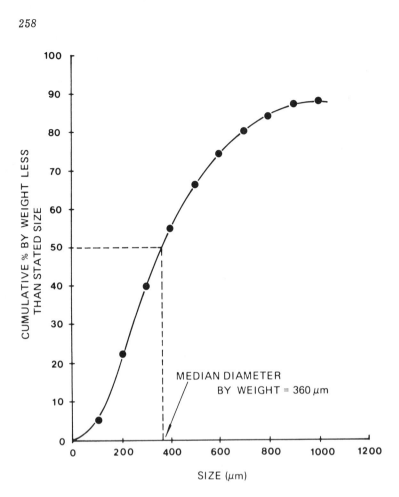

The useful constant or descriptive characteristic that can be obtained from the cumulative frequency curve is the median diameter by weight (or number). On a weight basis, the median diameter is that particle size value above and below which half the total weight of particles is found. In Figure 8, it can be seen that the median diameter by weight is equal to approximately 360 μm.

B. Distribution Functions

Log-Normal Law

Perhaps the most important statistical law in nature is the log-normal distribution law [25, 26, 31, 32]. With this law it is the logarithm of the variant that is distributed normally rather than the variant itself. Note that the size frequency curve in Figure 7 is skewed and has a long "tail" of large particles. This skewness is characteristic of many, if not most, particulate systems. Thus, the normal distribution law is not applicable to most

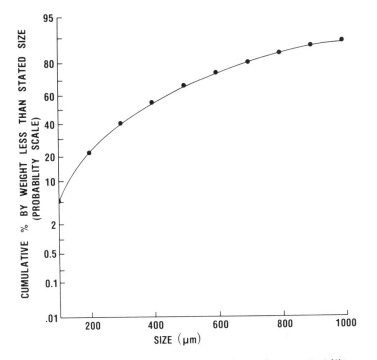

Figure 9 Cumulative frequency plot using probability paper for the data presented in Table 2.

particulate systems. Figure 9 contains a cumulative frequency plot on probability paper for the data contained in Table 2.

Had the data followed a normal distribution, the points would have resulted in a straight line. However, when the cumulative percent data contained in Table 2 are plotted against the log of particle size (Fig. 10), a straight line results. The graph paper used in Figure 10 is termed log-probability paper and can be used to determine if particle size distribution data follows a log-normal distribution. The straight-line relationship shown in Figure 10 indicates that these particle size data follow the log-normal law.

To reiterate, most particulate systems will approximate the log-normal distribution rather than the normal distribution. When constructing the log-probability plot, it is not uncommon to find that experimental data are scattered, with the apparent degree of scattering being greater at the extremities (the very small and very large particles). When determining the best straight line, greater weight should be given to those points lying closest to the 50% cumulative point [33]. Because of the distortion created by the probability axis at the extremities, some authors recommend that when fitting the best straight line, only experimental points within the 20 to 80% range be used.

Further, to minimize human error in determining the best straight line, it is suggested that regression analysis be employed if significant "scatter" is observed in the experimental data. Again, if the particle size distribution

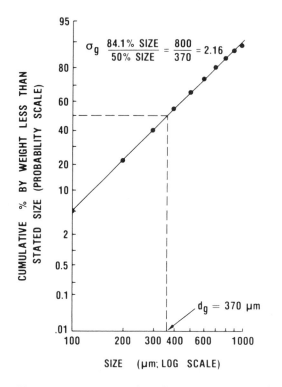

Figure 10   Cumulative frequency plot using log-probability paper for the data presented in Table 2.

follows a log-normal distribution, it will always be represented by a straight line on log-probability paper.

Two useful constants can be derived from Figure 10 and these are the geometric mean diameter d_g and the geometric standard deviation σ_g. The value of d_g is equal to the median or 50% diameter:

$$d_g = \text{antilog} = \frac{\sum\limits_{i=1}^{n} n_i \log d_i}{\sum\limits_{i=1}^{n} n_i} = 50\% \text{ size} \tag{1}$$

where d_i are diameters and are equal to the midpoints of the particle size intervals employed, and n_i are the number or weight of particles having these respective diameters. d_g is usually determined graphically, and from the plot of Figure 10, d_g is found to be approximately 370 μm. The geometric standard deviation σ_g can be found by dividing the diameter at the 84.1% size by the 50% diameter, d_g. Mathematically,

$$\sigma_g = \text{antilog} = \frac{\displaystyle\sum_{i=1}^{n} n_i (\log d_i - \log d_g)^2}{\displaystyle\sum_{i=1}^{n} n_i}$$

$$= \frac{84.1\% \text{ size}}{50.0\% \text{ size}} = \frac{50.0\% \text{ size}}{15.9\% \text{ size}} \tag{2}$$

In the case of both d_g and σ_g, it is generally easier to obtain these values from a graphical plot on log-probability paper as opposed to employing their mathematicl counterparts [Eqs. (1) and (2)]. The derivation of the fact that σ_g = 84.1% size/50.0% size = 50.0% size/15.9% size follows from integration of the probability curve describing the log-normal distribution. The derivation will not be presented here and the interested reader is referred to the literature [35]. Again, σ_g is usually determined graphically, and from Figure 10, σ_g is found to be 2.16. Note that σ_g and d_g describe completely the distribution of particle sizes and are, therefore, useful when comparing size distribution data from several samples.

Equations (1) and (2) are applicable for size frequency data derived on a number or weight basis. That is, n_i can represent either the number or weight of particles having a diameter d_i. For purposes of clarity in future discussions, d_g will be used to represent the median particle size derived on a weight basis and d'_g will be used to represent this parameter derived on a number basis. It can be shown that if the particle size distribution gives a straight line on a weight basis when plotted on log probability paper, the size distribution by number will be a parallel straight line on the same coordinates [34,35]. Thus, for a particular sample of particles, the geometric standard deviation by weight equals the geometric standard deviation by number. Therefore, only the term σ_g will be used in future discussions. It is also possible to convert the geometric mean diameter by weight to a number basis as follows [28]:

$$\log d'_g = \log d_g - 6.908 \log^2 \sigma_g \tag{3}$$

Diameters on a number basis will generally be considerably smaller than those on a weight basis. For example, if one substitutes d_g = 370 μm and σ_g = 2.16 (obtained from Fig. 10) into Eq. (3), d'_g = 62.4 μm. In a like manner, Fonner et al. [36] found that for a granulation prepared by the hand screen method (No. 12 mesh), d_g and σ_g on a weight basis were 900 μm and 4.12, respectively. From Eq. (3) the geometric mean diameter by number of this sample was equal to 2.19 μm. On a weight basis d_g = 900 μm, and on a number basis, d'_g = 2.19 μm. Thus, it can be seen that the contribution by smaller particles on a number basis is enormous.

Normal Law

If the data follow a normal distribution, one should get a straight line from cumulative plots made on probability paper. The arithmetic mean d_a and standard deviation σ can be obtained from such a plot as follows:

$$d_a = \frac{\sum_{i=1}^{n} n_i d_i}{\sum_{i=1}^{n} n_i} = 50\% \text{ size} \tag{4}$$

$$\sigma = \frac{\sum_{i=1}^{n} n_i (d_i - d_a)^2}{\sum_{i=1}^{n} n_i} = 84.1\% \text{ size} - 50\% \text{ size} \tag{5}$$

If the particle size data follow a normal distribution, d_a and σ completely describe the distribution of particle sizes and are valuable for comparison purposes. As with the log-normal distribution, d_a and σ can be determined from a graphical plot on probability paper, as opposed to using cumbersome equations [Eqs. (4) and (5)]. Should particle size data not fit either the normal or log-normal distribution law, there are other distributions, such as modified log-normal distributions and empirical equations, that may be considered [25]. However, it may be well to just present the data as shown in Table 2 or Figures 6 to 8 should data not follow a normal or log-normal distribution.

C. Average Particle Size

The average particle size or mean diameter for a population of particles can be defined in many ways. We have already been exposed to two of these, the geometric mean diameter and the arithmetic mean diameter. Numerous other ways exist for calculating mean diameters, and Edmundson defines a total of 11 different ways in which a mean diameter can be computed [28]. Of these, perhaps the most important is the mean volume surface diameter d_{vs}, which is defined as follows:

$$d_{vs} = \frac{\sum_{i=1}^{n} n_i d_i^3}{\sum_{i=1}^{n} n_i d_i^2} \tag{6}$$

The mean volume surface diameter is often of value and interest because it is inversely proportional to the specific surface area of the sample. Therefore, if the physical or chemical properties of the particulate sample are dependent upon surface area, the mean volume surface diameter should be used to describe the mean particle size. It should be noted that d_g and d_a are of value for comparative purposes only and are not relatable or proportional to any physical properties of the particles in question. However, this is often not a serious drawback, as most studies involving pharmaceutical granulations are of a comparative nature. In other words, we are usually interested in the effect of various processing variables (e.g., granulating equipment, granulation solution, processing time, etc.) on the size distribution of granules produced. On the other hand, the surface area of the granules produced may affect dissolution rate, ease of compaction, flowability, and so on. If such characteristics are related to granule surface area and of importance to the investigator, then d_{vs} should be used to define the average particle size of the sample. Although Eq. (6) can be used to compute d_{vs}, if the particle size distribution obeys the log-normal law, d_{vs} can be obtained from a knowledge of d_g [37]:

$$\log d_{vs} = \log d_g - 1.151 \log^2 \sigma_g \tag{7}$$

For the data shown in Figure 10 ($d_g = 370$ µm and $\sigma_g = 2.16$), d_{vs} is found to be equal to 275 µm through the use of Eq. (7). Thus, for the size frequency data contained in Table 2, we have now computed the mean particle diameter by three methods, with the following results:

d_g = geometric mean diameter by weight = 370 µm

d'_g = geometric mean diameter by number = 62.4 µm

d_{vs} = mean volume surface diameter by weight = 275 µm

Each of the above is a valid way of computing and expressing the average particle size for a sample. Of these diameters, d_{vs} has the most practical significance in that it is related to specific surface area. Opankunle et al. [38] have illustrated the use of d_{vs} as applied to drying-rate studies on lactose and sulfathiazole granulations.

D. Methods of Particle Size Determination

Sieving represents by far the simplest and most widely used method for the determination of particle size for pharmaceutical granulations and powders. For this reason, sieving will be considered in detail.

Sieving

Factors involved in sieving of pharmaceutical powders have been investigated [36] and an extensive study of the physical laws that govern the sieving of particles has been published by Whitby [40]. It was shown by Whitby that the sieving curve can be divided into two distinctly different regions, with a transition range in between. The sieving curve can be obtained by plotting the cumulative percent by weight passing the sieve versus time. Plots may be made on log–log paper or on log-probability paper.

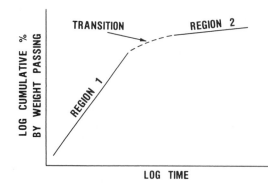

Figure 11   Typical plot of cumulative percent by weight of material passing through a sieve as a function of time.

A typical example of the former case is given in Figure 11. Whitby found that the rate at which material passes a sieve in region 1 is a constant and closely follows the following relationship:

$$\% \text{ Passing} = at^b \tag{8}$$

where t is the sieving time, b is a constant, and a is a sieving-rate constant. Region 2 was found to follow the log-normal law. In this region all of the particles much smaller than the mesh size have already passed the sieve; consequently, particles now passing through the sieve are of a constant mesh size. Exact equations for determining the amount of material passing through a sieve are given in Whitby's paper.

For all practical purposes, the sieve is considered to be at equilibrium at the time when region 2 begins, since the slight positive slope of the line is due mostly to attrition of larger-than-mesh-size particles. To minimize experimental error, it is important when determining a sieve time for a stack of sieves that one be in region 2.

Sieves are made with woven-wire cloth and have square openings. Two standard series are utilized in the United States, the Tyler Standard Scale and the United States Sieve Series. The relationship between mesh number and aperture dimensions are given in Table 3 for both of these standard sieves.

Sieves are normally used for coarse particles. However, depending upon the material, they traditionally have been employed down to a particle size of about 37 µm (400 mesh). Recent developments in screen fabrication technology and the employment of an oscillating air column for particle movement through sieves allows one to go as low as 5 µm in sieving separations. These developments greatly extend the utility and versatility of the sieving method for particle size analysis.

Sieves are calibrated by manufacturers according to National Bureau of Standards specifications. Sieves, especially shopworn sieves, should be checked periodically for proper calibration. Care should be exercised in

Table 3 Relationship Between Sieve Mesh and Aperture for Tyler Standard Scale and United States Sieve Series

United States		Tyler	
Mesh number	Aperture (mm)	Mesh number	Aperture (mm)
3½	5.66	3½	5.613
4	4.76	4	4.699
5	4.00	5	3.962
6	3.36	6	3.372
7	2.83	7	2.794
8	2.38	8	2.362
10	2.00	9	1.981
12	1.68	10	1.651
14	1.41	12	1.397
16	1.19	14	1.168
18	1.00	16	0.991
20	0.840	20	0.833
25	0.710	24	0.701
30	0.590	28	0.589
40	0.420	35	0.417
45	0.350	42	0.351
50	0.297	48	0.295
60	0.250	60	0.246
70	0.210	65	0.208
80	0.177	80	0.175
100	0.149	100	0.147
120	0.125	115	0.124
140	0.105	150	0.104
170	0.088	170	0.088
200	0.074	200	0.074
230	0.062	250	0.061
270	0.053	270	0.053
325	0.044	325	0.043
400	0.037	400	0.038

Table 4   Presentation of Particle Size Data for Sieving Analysis Problem

Mesh number	Aperture (μm)	Weight retained on sieve (g)	Size range (μm)	Percent frequency distribution	Cumulative % (less than)
16	991	20.0	>991	10.0	–
28	589	30.0	589 – 991	15.0	90.0
42	351	38.0	351 – 589	19.0	75.0
60	246	28.0	246 – 351	14.0	56.0
100	147	44.0	147 – 246	22.0	42.0
200	74	24.0	74 – 147	12.0	20.0
270	53	9.0	53 – 74	4.5	8.0
Pan	–	7.0	<53	3.5	3.5
		200.0		100.0	

the use and particularly in the cleaning of sieves that are employed for particle size fractionation. Brushes should be avoided in cleaning sieves, because brushing may cause disorientation of the screen wires. Soluble components should be dissolved or gently washed out of the screen surface. Insoluble materials may best be removed by running a gentle stream of water against the back side of the screen and/or by driving a compressed airstream against the reverse side of the screen surface.

Stainless or corrosion-resistant steel is recommended as a material of construction for screens. Carefully sized fractions of glass beads are available from the National Bureau of Standards for calibration purposes.

In sieve analysis, an accurately weighed sample is placed on the top sieve of a nest or stack of sieves. Each sieve has a smaller size opening in the wire cloth than the one immediately above it. The same is then shaken through the various sieves and thereby separated into a series of fractions on the individual sieves. The amount of material retained on each sieve is then weighed. This figure can then be divided by the initial sample weight to arrive at the percent frequency for the described size range. For example, consider a nest of sieves as shown in the first column of Table 4. Assume a 200 g sample of a granulation is then shaken through these sieves, with the results being as shown in Table 4.

The first column in Table 4 indicates the mesh number of the sieve and the order in which they were stacked from top to bottom. The second column gives the aperture opening for each sieve in microns. The third column gives the weight retained on each sieve in grams. Note that the total of the individual sample weights on each sieve equals 200 g, the size of the sample taken for analysis. The fourth column gives the theoretical size ranges for the particles on each sieve in the stack, respectively. The fifth column gives the percent frequency distribution which is computed by dividing individual sample weights on each sieve by the initial sample weight of 200 g. The last column then gives the cumulative percent by weight less than stated size. This is arrived at by summing, from the bottom up, the results in the percent frequency distribution column (the fifth column). The data contained in Table 4 can then be presented graphically by any one of the methods previously described. Note, however, that the range of any midpoint between the various size ranges in Table 4 are not equal, as is typical for such sieve data.

These are numerous factors that can affect the screening operation. An awareness of these factors is important in minimizing the magnitude of sieving errors and assuring reproducibility. The more notable factors influencing the performance of the sieving operation are given below:

Sieve load and sieving time
Screen movement, particle orientation, and particle shape
Aperture size and variations
Sampling of material

From an examination of the sieving curve (Fig. 11), it is clear that different sieving times will give different results. The effect of sieving time on d_g for lactose granulation has been studied [36]. As expected, as sieving time increases, d_g decreases. A straight line with a negative slope was obtained when log d_g was plotted against time. There is no absolute end point, but rather an arbitrary time is chosen. It has been shown that sieving rate decreases as the initial sieve load increases [36, 39, 40]. Therefore, at constant sieving times, different size loads of the same material will give different particle size distributions. Thus, sieving analysis methods should be established to accommodate the material being evaluated, and thereafter closely standardized for subsequent analysis.

The type and intensity of screen movement can affect the resultant size distribution. Common screen motions are circular, resonant, or linear, and the mode chosen will affect the results [41, 43]. The orientation that particles present to sieve apertures are quite random. There is only a certain probability that a particle oriented in a certain fashion will pass an aperture and a certain probability that it will reach the aperture in that orientation [44].

Studies have shown that as the particle size approaches the aperture size, the rate of material passing the sieve decreases rapidly [36, 39, 45]. Furthermore, the aperture sizes in a sieve are not absolutely uniform, but form a normal distribution about a mean value. During the sieving process, the more irregular the particle, the longer the time interval before peak blinding occurs [45]. Finally, if a number of samples of the same weight are withdrawn from the same material and these are sieved on the same equipment at the same speed setting for the same length of time, the sieving results will differ because of random variations in the composition of the samples. The homogeneity of the sample is determined by the extent of mixing. From a statistical sampling standpoint, one should use large samples. At the same time, the researcher is often interested in differences in particle size distribution in various regions of a powder or granulation blend, and will run several analyses rather than one composite analysis, to determine this information. As the initial sieve load is increased, in attempting to run more representative samples, the researcher must remember that the sieving efficiency decreases, and attrition affects may be accentuated.

It has been stated that the optimal sieving load is one that results in a powder depth of one to two particle diameters. Therefore, obtaining a representative sample must be balanced against sieving efficiency. For further details on the factors affecting sieving, the reader is referred to Jansen and Glastonbury [46].

Other Methods for Determining Particle
Size Distributions

There are many other methods for determining the particle size distribution of powders. Some of the more common methods are as follows:

1. Microscopy
2. Sedimentation
3. Light scattering
4. Adsorption methods [Brunauer−Emmett−Teller (BET) apparatus]
5. Electrolytic resistivity (Coulter counter)
6. Permeametry

When dealing with granulated powders, sieving is the preferred method for determining particle size distribution. However, when dealing with fine powders, such as a direct-compression powder system, one or more of the foregoing methods may be of value in particle size determinations. The chief limitation of sieving is that of particle size. When the size distribution of the powder in question is in the range 0 to 100 μm, one of the foregoing methods may be better suited than sieving. The reader is referred to the literature [25,28,47,48] for an in-depth review of the various methodologies available for determining particle size.

E. Factors Affecting Granule Size and Potential Implications to Process and Dosage Form Design

If the frequency of articles published over the last five years is indicative of the state of granulation technology, the pharmaceutical industry seems to be converging on two primary methods of granulation (a) fluid bed and (b) high shear. This of course does not preclude the use of planetary mixers, sigma blades, pony tubs, and extruders; nonetheless, the virtues of the fluid bed and high shear mixer are formidable; i.e., increased manufacturing efficiency, improved batch to batch reproducibility, and improved safety.

This section will be primarily limited to but not restricted to summarizing those formulation and process variables reported to influence granule size and granule size distribution for fluid bed granulators and high shear mixers.

Granulations processed in a fluid bed granulator generally are quite sensitive to bed moisture. If the powder bed, for example, becomes over wet, the system becomes unstable and the granules resist fluidization. If, on the other hand, the powder blend is insufficiently wetted, aggregation fails to progress to a significant degree and small, friable granules are obtained. Based on these observations, many investigators have concluded granule size is influenced by the establishment of a critical dynamic equilibrium between moisture addition and vaporization [2, 49–56]. Thus, granule size has been reported to be influenced by the following fluid bed process variables:

1. Quantity of granulating agent (binder) added [49, 51, 57–59]
2. Binder concentration [4, 40–42]
3. Flow rate of granulating medium [50, 56]
4. Air inlet temperature [56–59]
5. Atomization pressure [49, 51, 57–59]
6. Nozzle height above the distribution grid [57–59]

To fully characterize, describe, and validate the role of each of these parameters on granule size and/or granule size distribution, statistically designed studies are recommended. Meshali et al. [60] employed a full factorial design to investigate the influence of parameters, 2 through 5 above, in addition to air velocity, X_7, on sulfadiazine granulations. From this study, the following order of main effects on granule size was established $X_5 > X_3 > X_2 > X_4$. First order interactions were also significant X_2X_7 and X_4X_7 (see Tables 5 and 6).

It can thus be concluded that granule size and size distribution from a fluid bed granulator are the net result of many formulation and process variables. If the mean granule size is found to be critical (e.g., granule

Table 5 Tabular Display of the Significant Factorial Coefficients Obtained From a Statistically Designed Study Investigating Factors Influencing Granule Size

Coefficient	Numerical value
b_0	0.598
b_2	0.205
b_3	0.220
b_4	−0.133
b_5	−0.290
b_7	−
b_{24}	−0.075
b_{27}	−0.0123

Regression equation:

$$Y = b_0 + b_2X_2 + b_3X_3 + b_4X_4 + b_5X_5 + b_7X_7 + b_{37}X_3X_7 + b_{24}X_2X_7$$

Source: Ref. 60

Table 6   Actual Versus Predicted Granule Size

Trial no.	Experimental	Predicted[a]
1	0.830	0.838
2	0.369	0.378
3	0.070	0.064
4	1.646	1.644
5	0.375	0.388
6	0.775	0.778
7	0.290	0.282
8	0.414	0.402

[a]Predicted values are calculated from the regression equation.
Source: Ref. 60.

size directly affects granulation flowability and tablet weight variation),
then an appreciation and understanding of the factors discussed previously
are important.

Unlike the fluid bed granulator, the high shear mixer mechanically consolidates the particulate system through an impeller and a chopper mixing arrangement. Although both contribute force to the system, impeller speed has been documented as the critical process parameter for dicalcium phosphate systems [61,62]. Lactose granulations, on the other hand, were not similarly affected by either the impeller or the chopper speed [63,64]. Initially confusing, Schaefer et al. [61], were able to demonstrate that lactose, unlike dicalcium phosphate, easily densifies on liquid addition; thus, an increase in impeller speed and/or longer process times did not increase particle consolidation and subsequently liquid saturation, while for dicalcium phosphate the opposite was observed.

Further binder concentration-like impeller speed may play a key role in granule growth; however, growth is dependent on the binder selected [62].

Also, contrary to the fluid bed granulator, Timko et al. [64] was able to document that the rate of introduction of the granulating medium had little, if any, effect on granule size. Kristensen et al. [56], nonetheless, suggests it might still be advantageous to introduce the binder solution into the bowl in an atomized state to obtain a homogeneous liquid distribution [65,66].

Thus, these results seem to indicate high shear mixers should be equipped with variable speed motors and spray nozzles to aid in the control and the optimization of the granulation processes.

Finally, Chalmers and Elworthy [67–69], utilizing an oscillating granulator, noted the effects of various formulation and processing variables on granule size of oxytetracycline tablet granulations. They found that when

changing from water to 1.25% polyvinylpyrrolidone (PVP) as the granulating solution, average granule size decreased (360 μm versus 210 μm).
As the volume of granulating solution was increased, granule size increased dramatically. In all cases, inclusion of the excipients alginic acid
and/or microcrystalline cellulose reduced mean granule size of the granulations produced both by slugging and wet granulation techniques. These
authors further found that as the wet mixing time was increased, mean
granule size increased. The particle size of the oxytetracycline had a dramatic effect on granule size. For example, for material wet massed for a
total of 15 min, the mean granule size for granulations produced from
oxytetracycline having a particle size of 15 and 1.9 μm was 235 and 535
μm, respectively.

The discussion thus far has centered primarily on the critical process
parameters of the granulation equipment. Other formulation and processing
factors that can affect granule size are the type and amount of binder
used, the particle size of the ingredients, and the method of granulation.
Nonetheless, the factor having perhaps the largest effect on mean granule
size is the mesh size of the screen utilized during dry sizing.

In summary, the critical formulation and process parameters influencing
granule size and size distribution may either contribute to or detract from
the quality of the product, i.e., fluctuation in granule size and size distribution have been shown to affect the average tablet weight [70, 71],
tablet weight and variation [71, 71], disintegration time [72], granule
friability [71], granulation flowability [71], and the drying rate kinetics
of wet granulations [23, 73, 74]. The exact effect of granule size and size
distribution on processing requirements, bulk granulation characteristics,
and final tablet characteristics is dependent upon formulation ingredients
and their concentration as well as the type of granulating equipment and
processing conditions employed. Therefore, it is up to the formulator to
determine for each formulation and manufacturing process the effects of
granule size and size distribution and whether they are important or not.

III. CHARACTERIZATION OF GRANULE SHAPE

Prior to the 1970s, morphological analysis experienced the slow and meth-
odical evolutionary change associated with any new scientific concept;
however, of late, the field has rapidly expanded due to major break-
throughs in computer imaging and analysis and the establishment of a
cause and effect relationship between particle shape and the internal
angle of power friction, flow times, coatability, particle packing, and ease
of compaction [44, 75, 76].

Over the developmental course of morphological analysis, many methods
have evolved to quantitatively describe via mathematical descriptors the
shape of a particle population (see Table 7). Of these seven methods, only
four will be discussed further: volume shape factor, surface shape factor,
shape coefficient, and morphological descriptors.

The volume shape, surface shape, and shape coefficient factors are all
based on ascribing shape to deviation from spherocity. These methods
thus suffer the inability to describe rugosity; nonetheless, these methods
are routinely utilized due to time and cost constraints and the ease with
which the data may be interpreted and understood. Morphic descriptors,

Table 7   Methods Utilized in Shape
Determination

---

1. Heywood, L, B, T:

    M = flatness ratio = B/ T

    N = elongation ratio = L/ B

2. Sphericity

    a. Volume of an equivalent sphere
    b. Projected area of an equivalent sphere
    c. Statistical particle diameters

3. Surface shape factor

4. Volume shape factor

5. Shape coefficient

6. Morphic descriptors

7. Fractiles

---

on the other hand, yields a set of quantitative values which can be used
to regenerate the original two-dimensional shape; however, the meaning of
the morphological descriptors is not quite as clear-cut as the volume shape,
surface shape, and shape coefficient factors.

A. Volume Shape Factor Relative to a Sphere

The volume of a spherical particle is proportional to the cube of the particle's diameter. Thus, the volume occupied by a spherical particle may
be easily calculated by

$$V = \alpha_v d^3 \tag{9}$$

where d is the diameter of the sphere and α_v equals $\pi/6$. The proportionality constant α_v is known as the volume shape factor. Thus, for a
sphere, α_v and d are easy to come by.

For irregularly shaped particles, one computes α_v [by rearrangement
of Eq. (9)] employing the following equation [29,77]:

$$\alpha_v = \frac{V}{d_p^3} \tag{10}$$

where d_p is the equivalent projected diameter, defined as the diameter of
a sphere having the same projected area as the particle when placed in its
most stable position on a horizontal plane and viewed from above and V is

the average particle volume. Average particle volume is generally determined by counting out a specific number of particles and weighing them. Thus,

$$V = \frac{M_n}{\rho_g n} \tag{11}$$

where n is the number of particles weighed, M_n is the mass of n particles, and ρ_g is normally computed using the pycnometer method.

The equivalent projected diameter is normally arrived at by photographing or tracing the outline of particles that have been magnified and then determining the diameter of a sphere that has the same projected area. The area of the magnified images can be obtained using a planimeter [44], by cutting out projected images from photographs and weighing them [75], or by computer analysis. In either case, computed areas from enlarged images must be reduced to true areas by dividing by p^2, where p is the power of magnification. Thus, it can be shown that

$$\frac{A}{p^2} = \frac{\pi d_p^2}{4} \tag{12}$$

or

$$d_p = \frac{4A}{\pi p^2} \tag{13}$$

where A is the average area of the magnified images.

When computing average particle volume V and average equivalent projected diameter d_p, at least 100 or more particles should probably be used. As mentioned, $\alpha_v = \pi/6 \backsim 0.52$ for a sphere, and as the particle becomes irregular, the value of α_v changes. Some values of α_v for lactose granulations in the 20- to 30-mesh range that were prepared by different methods of granulating are shown in Table 8. These authors also found that as the volume shape factor increased, bulk density increased (Table 8 and Fig. 12). This is as would be expected, because more spherical or

Table 8 Volume Shape Factors (α_v) and Bulk Densities (ρ_b) for 20- to 30-Mesh Particles Prepared by Various Granulation Methods

	Colton upright	Oscillating granulator	Hand screen	Fitzpatrick comminutor	Liquid – solid V-shaped blender
α_v	0.15	0.18	0.16	0.22	0.25
ρ_b	0.37	0.39	0.40	0.43	0.51

Source: Data from Ref. 44.

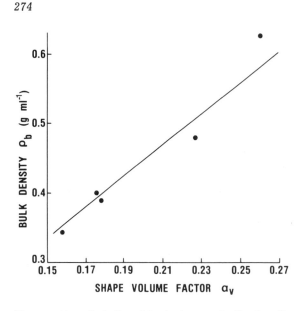

Figure 12   Relationship between bulk density and shape volume factor of
20- to 30-mesh particles prepared by five different granulation methods.
(From Ref. 44.)

more regular-shaped particles produce the closest packing arrangements
and hence the greater bulk density.

One can readily check the accuracy of experimentally determined α_v
values through the use of the following equation [12]:

$$N = \frac{1}{\alpha_v \rho_g d_p^3} \tag{14}$$

where N is the number of particles per gram and ρ_g the particle density.
One can compute N and compare it with values obtained through the actual
counting and weighing procedure.   The more accurate α_v, ρ_g, and d_p
are, the closer the computed value of N will be to actual values.

In summary, the volume shape factor is a measure of particle shape.
It has been used to describe shape differences in pharmaceutical granulations [44].

B.   Surface Shape Factor

The surface area of a spherical particle is proportional to the square of
the particle's diameter.   Thus, the surface area of a spherical particle
can be easily calculated by

$$S = \alpha_s d^2 \tag{15}$$

where S is the surface area of the particle, d the particle's diameter, and α_S a proportionality constant. The proportionality constant α^S is termed the surface shape factor and in the case of a sphere, $\alpha_S = \pi \sim 3.14$. For irregularly shaped particles, one computes α_S [by rearrangement of Eq. (15)] in the following manner [29,77]:

$$\alpha_S = \frac{S}{d_p^2} \tag{16}$$

where d_p is again the average equivalent projected diameter. The determination of d_p has been discussed previously. The average surface area per particle must, therefore, be determined by gas adsorption, air permeability, and so on. Methods for estimating surface area are discussed later in this chapter. Since the method of determining surface area can have a pronounced effect upon the results (e.g., gas adsorption may give surface area values 10 to 100 times greater than results obtained by air permeability), the method of determining S must be stated when presenting or comparing values of α_S. Some values of α_S for various mesh sizes of sand are presented in Table 9.

C. Shape Coefficient

The volume shape factor α_V and the surface shape factor α_S may be combined as a ratio α_S/α_V. This ratio is called the shape coefficient α_{vs}, and is defined as follows [78]:

$$\alpha_{vs} = \frac{\alpha_S}{\alpha_V} \tag{17}$$

Table 9   Surface Shape Factors for Various Mesh Sizes of Natural Uncrushed Sand

Mesh size	Sample no.	Surface shape factor
44 – 60	1	3.03
	2	2.68
30 – 36	1	3.28
	2	2.89
18 – 20	1	3.54
	2	3.39

Source: Data from Ref. 75.

For a perfect sphere,

$$\alpha_{vs} = \frac{\pi}{\pi/6} = 6.0 \tag{18}$$

As particle shape becomes more irregular, the value of α_{vs} increases. For example, the α_{vs} for a cube can be calculated.

Using Eq. (13) without the magnification term, the projected diameter of a cube with sides of length a is

$$d_p = \sqrt{\frac{4A}{\pi}} = \sqrt{\frac{4a2}{\pi}} = \frac{2a}{\sqrt{\pi}} \tag{19}$$

The volume of the cube $V = a^3$ and the surface of the cube $S = 6a^2$. From Eq. (10),

$$\alpha_v = \frac{V}{\sqrt{d_p^3}} = \frac{a^3}{8a^3/\pi\sqrt{\pi}} = \frac{\pi\sqrt{\pi}}{8} = 0.696 \tag{20}$$

From Eq. (16),

$$\alpha_s = \frac{S}{d_p^2} = \frac{6a^2}{4a^2/\pi} = \frac{6\pi}{4} = 4.71 \tag{21}$$

Substituting into Eq. (17), we obtain

$$\alpha_{vs} = \frac{\alpha_s}{\alpha_v} = \frac{4.71}{0.696} = 6.8 \tag{22}$$

The effect on the α_{vs} when various sections of a cube of width b are taken is shown in Figure 13. Ridgway and Shotton [80] found that as the shape coefficient of sand particles increased, the mean weight of die fill on a tablet machine decreased and the coefficient of variation of die fill increased. The latter effect is shown in Figure 14. Ridgway and Rupp [75] found that as the shape coefficient increased, bulk density decreased and angle of repose increased. The effect of the shape coefficient on bulk density is shown in Figure 15.

D. Morphic Descriptors

Unlike the three previously described shape descriptors, morphic descriptors are invariant mathematical quantities which can be utilized to regenerate the two-dimensional shape of any particle. This technique, however, requires the use of a particle imaging system in combination with computer analysis (see Figs. 16 and 17). Thus, the system is capable of visualizing, collecting, analyzing, and evaluating the data in an unbiased mechanical fashion.

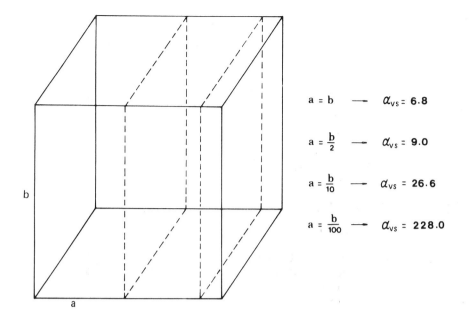

$a = b \quad \longrightarrow \quad \alpha_{vs} = \mathbf{6.8}$

$a = \dfrac{b}{2} \quad \longrightarrow \quad \alpha_{vs} = \mathbf{9.0}$

$a = \dfrac{b}{10} \quad \longrightarrow \quad \alpha_{vs} = \mathbf{26.6}$

$a = \dfrac{b}{100} \quad \longrightarrow \quad \alpha_{vs} = \mathbf{228.0}$

Figure 13   Shape coefficients for sections of a cube.   (From Ref. 79.)

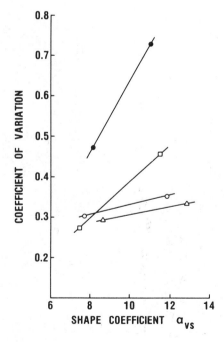

Figure 14   Effect of shape coefficient on the coefficient of variation of the die fill for different sizes of sand. ●, d_p = 805 μm; □, d_p = 461 μm; △, d_p = 302 μm; ○, crushed sand having d_p = 213 μm. (From Ref. 78.)

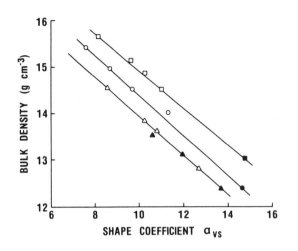

Figure 15 Bulk density as a function of shape coefficient for three sizes of sand. □, Mean projected diameter 805 μm; ○, mean projected diameter 461 μm; △, mean projected diameter 302 μm; ■, ●, and ▲ refer to crushed sand of the same mean diameter. (From Ref. 75.)

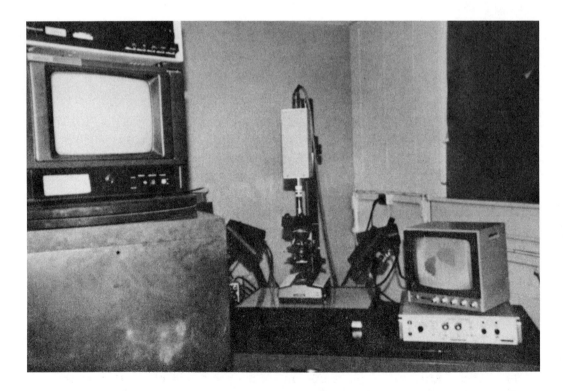

Figure 16   Particle image analyzing system (PIAS).   (From Ref. 85.)

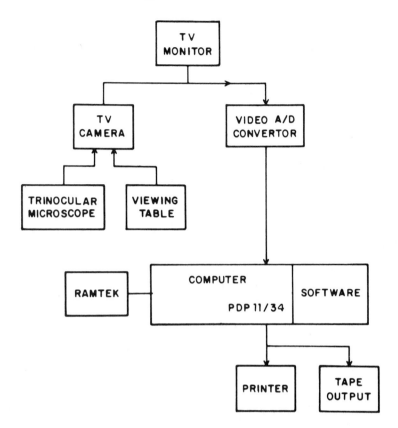

Figure 17   Schematic representation of the PIAS.   (From Ref. 85.)

Although several methodologies or software programs are currently available to analyze the data, work by Beddow and Vetter and Luerkin et al. [81,82], has indicated Fourier analysis provides results that are primarily invariant of axis placement and are reproducible.

Once the data has been collected and manipulated, a series of morphic descriptors are obtained (Table 10).   These, in effect, represent via mathematical values the features or profile pattern of the particle.

The reader is encouraged to study the work of Beddow [83] if a more rigorous presentation of the theoretical derivation is required.

The utility of the morphic descriptors in describing shape and its influence on processing properties is best realized by a review of literature (Table 11).

As way of illustration of the power of this technique, samples of adipic acid were analyzed after atomization, comminution, and crystallization from an aqueous solution (Table 12).   Visual illustration of the typical form particles possessed from these different operations is displayed in Figure 18 and a plot of μ_2 vs μ_3 is shown in Figure 19.   Inspection of Figure 19 reveals the presence of three unique populations which correspond to the three different unit operations.

Table 10   Set of Morphological Descriptors

R_o = equivalent radius

$\mu2_o$ = mean radius

μ_2 = radial standard deviation (the radiance)

μ_3 = radial skewness

r = rugosity coefficient

L_o

$\left.\begin{array}{c} L_{2(m)} \\ L_{3(m,n)} \end{array}\right\}$ Shape terms

---

Source: Particle characterization, in *Technology, Volume II. Morphological Analysis*, CRC Press, Boca Raton, Florida.

Table 11   Established Morphic Descriptors Correlation with Processing Properties

Material investigated	Property investigated	Ref.
Sand	Abrasiveness	84
Adipic acid	Morphology after atomizing comminution and crystallization	85
Spherical steel Atomized iron Electrolytic iron	Morphology and sieving	86
Isometric particles	Sedimentation rate	87
Agricultural grains	Angle of friction	88
PVC	Angle of friction	88
Sands	Flow	88

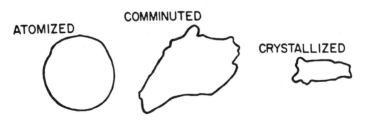

Figure 18   Representative shapes of adipic acid.   (From Ref. 85.)

Table 12 Morphic Descriptors of Adipic Acid as a Function
of Particle Size Reduction Method

	Atomized	Comminuted	Crystallized
R_o	3.0115×10^1	3.7047×10^1	2.6428×10^1
L_o	9.9972×10^1	9.9579×10^1	8.8253×10^1
Radance	2.4029×10^2	7.7573×10^2	2.1279×10^1
Skewness	0.5694×10^5	1.2239×10^2	2.0465×10^1
L2(1)	7.7067×10^{-7}	1.8195×10^{-3}	2.8373×10^{-3}
L2(2)	2.5623×10^{-4}	5.8642×10^{-2}	1.2358×10^{-1}
L2(3)	9.3942×10^{-5}	6.2347×10^3	2.1098×10^{-3}
L2(4)	4.8729×10^{-5}	4.5173×10^{-3}	4.0936×10^{-2}
L2(5)	2.2268×10^{-5}	2.4086×10^3	2.6239×10^{-3}
L2(6)	1.5830×10^{-5}	1.3420×10^{-4}	1.6135×10^{-2}

Source: Particle characterization, in *Technology, Volume II.
Morphological Analysis*, CRC Press, Boca Raton, Florida.

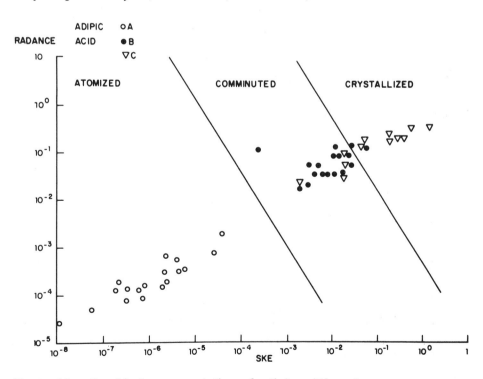

Figure 19 Graphical representation of adipic acid's radance versus
skewness obtained with the PIAS. (From Ref. 85.)

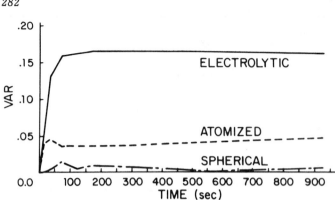

Figure 20 Particle radance (VAR) versus sieving time for different powders. (From Ref. 85.)

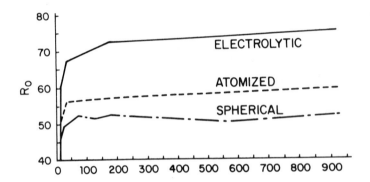

Figure 21 Equivalent radius of the powders as a function of sieving time for different powders. (From Ref. 85.)

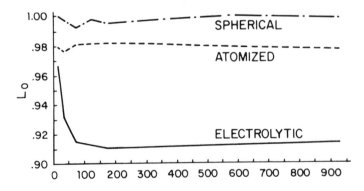

Figure 22 Morphic descriptor obtained with the PIA system as a function of sieving time for different powders. (From Ref. 85.)

Further, Beddow et al. have demonstrated that sieving time and shape are, as expected, related. These investigators were able, with quantitative values for shape of the particles, to develop a model which, within reason, was predictive of a real system (Figs. 20, 21, and 22).

Thus, morphic descriptors are capable of quantating the shape of a particle and have been shown to influence further processing times and functions.

E. Other Measures of Shape

There are many other measurements of particle shape available and readers are referred to Pahl et al. [89] and Davies [90] for an extensive review of this literature.

IV. SURFACE AREA

It is fairly common practice to determine the surface area of finely milled drug powders. This is especially true with drugs that exhibit limited water solubility. In these cases, particle size or available surface area of the drug can have a significant effect upon dissolution rate. It is uncommon to determine the surface area of granulations. Generally, if one is interested in the effects of granulation surface area upon measurable properties of the final dosage form, the particle size of the granulation is employed. Thus, it is normally assumed that there is an inverse relationship between particle size and surface area. Furthermore, technology available for determining the surface area of coarse powders is not as advanced as it is for fine powders. Thus, available methods for determining surface areas of a solid are better suited for fine powders. For these reasons, only the fundamentals will be covered here, and the reader will be referred to reference texts for more in-depth information.

The term that is used to describe the surface area for a bed of powder or granules is the specific surface area, S_w, which is the surface area per unit weight. Thus,

$$S_w = \frac{\text{total surface area of particles}}{\text{total weight of particles}} \qquad (23)$$

S_w is usually expressed in cm^2/g^{-1} or m^2/g^{-1}. The S_w measurement of a powder can be used for quality control purposes, and many pharmaceutical companies specify acceptable S_w values for the tablet lubricant magnesium stearate. For example, the tablet lubricant, magnesium stearate, may be purchased having a specific surface as high as 25 m^2/g^{-1}.

A. Experimental Determination of Surface Area

The two most commonly utilized methods for determining surface area of a solid are gas adsorption and air permeability. In the first method (gas adsorption), the amount of gas that is adsorbed onto the powder to form a monolayer is a function of the surface area of the powder sample. In the latter, the rate at which air permeates through a bed of powder depends upon the surface area of the powder sample and is the basis of the measurement. For further details on gas adsorption, the reader is referred to Martin et al. [91], Fries [92], Shaw [93], and Adamson [94]. For more details on permeametry, the reader is referred to Edmundson [28], Herdan [26], Martin et al. [91], Irani and Callis [25], Rigden [95], and Carman [96,97].

V. DENSITY AND PACKING

Particles may be dense, smooth, and spherical in one case and rough, spongy, and irregular in another. It stands to reason from these two cases that dissimilar particle packing arrangements will, in all likelihood, be quite different. Measurements are discussed in this section that help describe these characteristics and assist in describing individual particles or granules, as well as how they behave en masse. Thus, this section covers such topics as granule density, granule porosity, bulk density, and bed porosity. Granule density, porosity, and hardness are often interrelated properties. In addition, granule density may influence compressibility, tablet porosity, dissolution, and other properties. Dense, hard granules may require higher compression loads to produce a cohesive compact, let alone acceptable-appearing tablets free of visible granule boundries. The higher compression load, in turn, has the potential of increasing the disintegration time. Even if the tablets disintegrate readily, the harder, denser granules may dissolve at a slower rate. At the same time, harder, more dense granules will generally be less friable. Thus, moderation or trade-off analysis is required to insure an acceptable, aesthetically appealing tablet is obtained.

A. Granule Density

Granulations typically exhibit surface cracks or fissures and are quite porous. To insure proper interpretation and avoid confusion with similarly defined density measurements, the nomenclature of Heywood [29] will be employed:

> *True density*: The mass of a particle(s) divided by the volume of the particle(s), excluding open and closed pores
> *Apparent particle density*: The mass of a particle(s) divided by the volume of the particle(s), excluding open pores but including closed pores
> *Effective particle density*: The mass of a particle(s) divided by the volume of the particle(s), including open and closed pores

Regardless of the type of granule density being pursued, a pycnometer is capable of obtaining all three densities. For true density, a helium pycnometer is suitable; for effective density, a liquid pycnometer utilizing mercury intrusion is suitable; and for apparent density, a liquid pycnometer utilizing a low surface tension solvent (e.g., benzene) in which the granules are not soluble is appropriate.

The mercury displacement method described by Stickland et al. [98] provides an approximation of the granules' effective density. This method is able to differentiate intergranular versus intragranular pore volumes

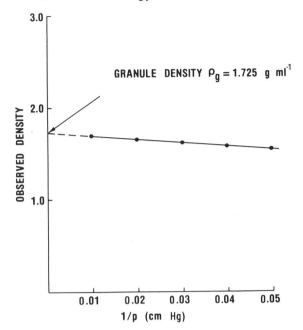

Figure 23   Mercury displacement method for determining granule density. (Data from Ref. 97.)

and thus provides an accurate estimate of the granules' effective density with the aid of the following relationship:

$$D = \frac{1892}{p} \tag{24}$$

where p is the pressure of mercury applied in dyn cm^{-2} and D equals the minimum pore diameter in centimeters through which mercury will enter at pressure p. The effective granule density, p_g, is thus obtained by plotting observed density versus 1/P and extrapolating the linear portion of the curve back to the density axis. As a result, this method includes both open and closed pores. Figure 23 illustrates this graphical process.

Other authors have used the pycnometer method, employing an organic solvent in which the granules are insoluble [44,57–59]. Details of this method are outlined by Weissberger [99]. In this method of determining granule density, most open pores are excluded from the density determination and granule density approximates the apparent particle density described earlier by Heywood. When employing this method, the following equation applies:

$$g = \frac{G}{C - B/F} \tag{25}$$

where G is the weight of granules in grams, C the capacity of the pycnometer in milliliters, B the weight of the intrusion fluid in grams, and F the specific gravity of the intrusion fluid.

Davies and Gloor [57−59] have studied the effects of various formulation and processing variables in lactose granulations produced in a fluid-bed dryer. The results of their investigation indicate process variables have the following impact: (a) as the addition rate of water was increased, granule density increased; (b) as inlet air temperature was increased, granule density tended to increase slightly; and (c) as nozzle height above the grid was increased, granule density tended to decrease. These authors further reported as the formula weight of binder was increased, the granule density tended to increase. The latter effect was observed for the binders povidone, NF; hydroxypropylcellulose; Gelatin, USP; and Acacia, USP.

Strickland et al. [98] determined ρ_g for a number of different tablet granulations. Their studies included granulations that were prepared with starch paste as well as one that was prepared by slugging. Fonner et al. [44] determined the granule density for a lactose granulation that was produced from several different types of granulation equipment. In general, they found that granules produced from an oscillating granulator were the most dense (ρ_g = 1.54) and those produced from a Fitz mill and liquid−solid V-shaped blender were the least dense (ρ_g = 1.42 to 1.45). Armstrong and March [100] compared granule density of granulations prepared from various diluents that were wet-screened through an oscillating granulator and dried in a fluid-bed dryer. Chalmers and Elworthy [67−69] studied the effects of various formulation and processing variables on granule density of oxytetracycline formulations. Granules produced by slugging were significantly more dense than granules produced by the wet granulation technique. They also found that increasing the wet mixing time increased granule density for granulations produced by the wet granulation technique.

B. Granule Porosity

Granule porosity (intragranular porosity) is computed from a knowledge of p_g and the true particle density:

$$\varepsilon_g = 1 - \frac{\rho_g}{\rho} \times 100 \tag{26}$$

where ε_g is the granule porosity in percent. The method of determining ε_g should be specified so that one knows whether ε_g includes or excludes open pores in the granules.

Some studies involving granule porosity have been reported in the literature [101,102]. These authors found that ε_g decreased as the amount of water used to granulate lactose powder was increased. This effect is shown in Figure 24. These authors also found that lengthening the massing time also decreased ε_g, but the effect was not as dramatic as that produced by varying the amount of water used to granulate. These authors also studied effects of initial lactose particle size and amount of water used to granulate on macropore size (10−80 μm) distribution in lactose granules. In general, the distribution of pores is related to the initial particle size of the lactose. Those granulations made with coarser grades of lactose had a greater percentage of large pores. Also, increasing the amount of water used to granulate lactose causes densification by rapidly eliminating larger pores, thus reducing mean pore diameter and

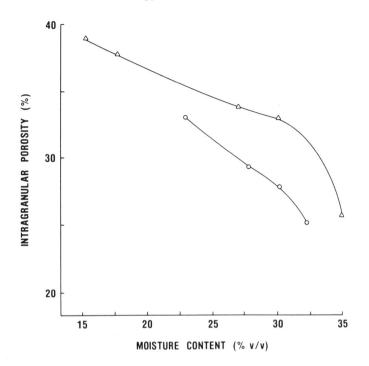

Figure 24 Intragranular porosity as a function of moisture content in a 12- to 16-mesh lactose system. ○, pan-granulation; △, massed and screened. (From Ref. 100.)

increasing granule strength. The same authors [103], working with a calcium phosphate granulation, found that granule porosity increased as the amount of water used to granulate was increased. This unusual result was felt to be due to the assertion that calcium phosphate is not readily consolidated by capillary forces during wet massing because the irregular particles cannot easily rearrange to form a closely packed system. In fact, pendular or capillary liquid bonds tend to maintain a rigid, open structure. These authors further found that as massing was increased, granule porosity decreased for the three types of massing equipment evaluated. Strickland et al. [98] determined ε_g for a number of pharmaceutical granulations. For those cases where granulations were prepared with starch paste, $\varepsilon_g \sim 30\%$. For a slugged aspirin granulation, they found that $\varepsilon_g \sim 3\%$. Chalmers and Elworthy [68,69] found that granules produced by slugging had much lower granule porosity values than did those produced by wet granulation. For oxytetracycline granulated with water, $\varepsilon_g = 38.9\%$; for granules produced by slugging, $\varepsilon_g = 17.8\%$. In the former case, the mean pore size was 0.97 μm, and in the latter, 0.10 μm. They also found that as wet mixing time was increased, granule porosity and mean pore size decreased. The studies conducted by these investigators demonstrate that granule density and/or porosity could be used as the characteristic(s) with which to evaluate granulation techniques, formula changes, equipment changes, and the like. Granule density and/or porosity could even be used as the measurable characteristic by which to control a granulation process.

C. Characteristics of Packing

The geometrical arrangement of mono-sized spheres will be the basis of understanding the general state of packing of granules. When considering this ideal system, the spheres will form geometrically stable configurations if the four center points of the spheres position themselves at the corners of a square all on the same plane, and the three spheres in contact make a triangle. Six stable arrangements of this theme are possible and are illustrated in Figure 25. The void volume, void fraction, and coordination number of these arrangements are listed in Table 13. Close inspection of the arrangements in Figure 25 reveals, with the exception of the void directions, the second and third square arrangement are equivalent to the fourth and sixth arrangement.

Thus, it has been inferred that in general the void fraction decreases and the coordination number increases as the degree of deformation of the unit cell increases [3].

In heterogeneous systems, packing arrangements can become quite complicated. For example, smaller particles can fill the interstical spaces between large particles, thus reducing void volume. On the other hand.

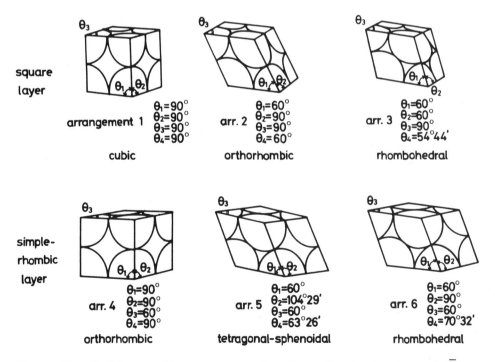

Figure 25   Cellular packing arrangements of equally sized spheres ($\bar{\Theta}_4$ indicates the inclined angle between right side of the plane and the horizontal plane). (From Ref. 2.)

Table 13 Packing Properties of Unit Cell

Arrange-ment no.	Bulk volume	Void volume	Void fraction	Coordination no.
1	1	0.4764	0.4764	6
2	$\sqrt{3/2}$	0.3424	0.3954	8
3	$1/\sqrt{2}$	0.1834	0.2594	12
4	$\sqrt{3/2}$	0.3424	0.3954	8
5	3/4	0.2264	0.3019	10
6	$1/\sqrt{2}$	0.1834	0.2595	12

Source: Ref. 2.

this reduction in void space may be nullified by the fact that fine particles tend to form stable arches or bridges that result in an increase in void space. For example, a very fine powder such as carbon black may have a voidage as high as 96 to 98% [104]. In the case of large particles, where cohesion effects are negligible, voidage is decreased when the particles extend over a wide range of sizes.

The arrangement of particles when poured or dropped into a container cannot be predetermined. However, it is possible to describe certain characteristics of packings once formed. Thus, such terms as bulk density and bed porosity are measures used to describe the packing of particles or granules. To date, it has not been possible to relate these measures of packings to other superficial features of the particles themselves. Particles in a container may be in a state of open packing, or the bed of particles may have been "tapped" to facilitate rearrangement and a closer packing. To attain good reproducibility, bulk density and bed porosity should be reported on the tapped product.

D. Bulk Density and Bed Porosity

The equation for determining bulk density ρ_b is

$$\rho_b = \frac{M}{V_b} \tag{27}$$

where M is the mass of the particles and V_b the total volume of packing. Another measure often used is bulk volume, which is the reciprocal of bulk density. The volume of the packing should be determined in an apparatus similar to that described by Neumann [105]. This device consists of a graduated cylinder mounted on a mechanical tapping device consisting of a specially cut cam that is rotated. An accurately weighed sample of powder or granulation is carefully added to the cylinder with the aid of a funnel.

Typically, the initial volume is noted and the sample is then tapped until
no further reduction in volume is noted. The volume obtained at this
tightest packing is then used in Eq. (27) to compute bulk density ρ_b.
Considerable variation exists in the literature as to the length of tapping
or number of taps employed [44,106-108]. However, the important point
is not the number of taps required to obtain the tightest packing, but
that the tightest packing is dependent upon the material or granulation
under study. Therefore, a sufficient number of taps should be employed
to assure reproducibility for the material in question. Further, the tapping
should not produce particle attrition or a change in the particle size distribution of the material under test.

Several empirical equations have also been developed to describe the
consolidation of a powder bed due to tapping [109-111]:

$$\rho_{b,fn} - \rho_{b,n} = (\rho_{b,fn} - \rho_{b,o}) \exp(-k,n_{tp}) \tag{28}$$

$$\frac{V_o - n_{tp}}{V_o - V_{nt}} = \frac{1}{k_2 k_3} + \frac{n_{to}}{k_2} \tag{29}$$

where $\rho_{b,fn}$ is the final constant bulk density, $\rho_{b,o}$ is the initial bulk
density, V_o is initial bulk volume, V_{nt} is the powder volume after n_{tp}
taps, n_{tp} is the number of taps, and k_1, k_2, and k_3 are constants. If
Eq. (28) is plotted on semilogrimech graph paper, a straight line should
result. Oftentimes, however, a biphasic profile is achieved, especially
with fine cohesive powders, as shown in Figure 26. For white alundum
(Fig. 26), k_2 is observed to increase with decreasing particle size, while
k_3 assumes a minimum value around 3 μm [111].

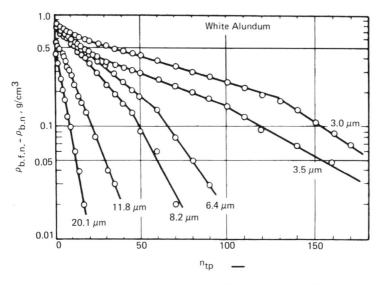

Figure 26   Graphical illustration of the number of taps on bulk density.
(From Ref. 2.)

Carr [112] has been able to demonstrate that the percent compressibility, C, of a powder bed gives an indication of the flow characteristics of the powder:

$$C = \frac{\rho_f - \rho_o}{\rho_f} \times 100 \qquad (30)$$

where ρ_o is the initial bulk density and ρ_f is the final constant bulk density.

Often, it is of interest to know bed porosity or percentage of void space in a packing. Bed porosity ε_b, in percent, is determined by the equation

$$\varepsilon_b = 1 - \frac{\rho_h}{\rho_g} \times 100 \qquad (31)$$

Bed porosity is often referred to as percent voids, void porosity, void space, interspace porosity, or extragranular porosity. As with granule density and porosity, bulk density and bed porosity may be used as granulation-characterizing measurements for quality control specifications, for equipment evaluations, for raw material evaluations, for process changes, and for new product development. Fonner et al. [44] compared the bulk density of 20−30 mesh lactose granulations prepared by five different granulation methods (Table 8). Over this narrow size range, bulk density was found to be largely dependent upon particle shape (see Fig. 12). As the particles became more spherical in shape, bulk density increased. Ridgway and Rupp [75], working with sand particles, found this same dependency of bulk density upon particle shape (see Fig. 10). Harwood and Pilpel [113] investigated the effect of granule size and shape on the bulk density of griseofulvin granulations. As granule size increased, bulk density was found to decrease. The smaller granules were able to form a closer, more intimate packing than were larger granules. Granule shape had a very great impact on bulk density. As noted previously, the bulk density for irregularly shaped granules is generally lower than the bulk density for the more spherical particles.

Nouh [50], Meshali et al. [60], and Davies and Gloor [57−59] investigated the effects of various formulation and processing variables on bulk density and bed porosity of granulations produced in a fluid bed dryer, as noted, in part, previously. Table 14 summarizes the observed effects of water addition rate and inlet air temperature variations on bulk density as observed by Davies and Gloor. Nouh and Meshali et al. were able to corroborate Davies and Gloor observation that as the amount of water increased or the concentration of binder in the granulating medium decreased, bulk density increased and bed porosity decreased. Although the mixing action and dynamics of the fluid bed granulator is entirely different than the high shear mixer, Timko et al. [64] reached similar conclusions for a 4:1 lactose−microcrystalline cellulose-PVP granulation manufactured in a high shear mixer. Further, Chalmers and Elworthy [68] noted a decrease in bulk density and an increase in bed porosity as the level of microcrystalline cellulose and/or alginic acid was increased in the granulation blend. The bulk density values of granules produced by

Table 14   Effect of Processing Variables on the Bulk Density and Porosity of Granulations Produced in a Fluid Bed Dryer

Processing variables	Level	Bulk density $(q\ ml^{-1})$	Porosity (%)
Addition rate (g H_2O/min)	85	0.41	72.4
	100	0.44	70.5
	115	0.46	69.1
	130	0.46	69.1
	145	0.48	67.9
Inlet air temperature (°C)	25°	0.54	63.8
	40°	0.50	66.6
	50°	0.44	70.7
	55°	0.41	72.6

Source: Data from Ref. 57.

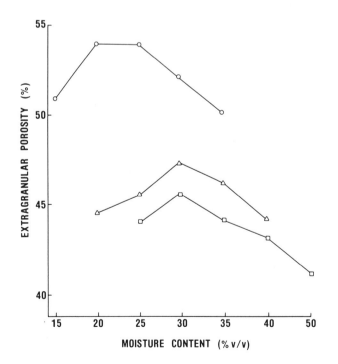

Figure 27   Extragranular porosity as a function of moisture content in a 12- to 16-mesh lactose system. □, Mean particle diameter d_m = 26 μm; △, d_m = 70 μm; ○, d_m = 140 μm. (From Ref. 100.)

slugging and traditional wet granulation methods generally exhibit a greater bulk density than those obtained through fluid bed granulation [68,114].

Hunter and Ganderton [102] found that as the amount of water used to granulate lactose powder was increased, bed porosity went through a maximum value, as shown in Figure 27. This region of poor packing was found at the lower end of the "useful granulation range" and is the result of overall shape effects resulting from irregular or "fluffy" granules. The authors also found that at a given moisture content, the finer grades of lactose formed granules with more regular surfaces, promoting closer packing and a reduction in bed or extragranular porosity. In a similar study [101], these authors determined bed porosity for calcium phosphate and lactose granulations that were prepared by a rotating pan and oscillating granulator. With both lactose and calcium phosphate, those granulations that were prepared in a rotating pan had the lowest bed porosity. The granulated lactose material that had an almost spherical shape and a dense packing had a bed porosity of 36 to 42%. On the other hand, granules from the oscillator were irregular in shape and had a bed porosity of about 50%. Their results for lactose granulations are shown in Table 15.

Eaves and Jones [114] describe the effects of increasing moisture content on the packing properties of various particulate materials. These authors found that the inherent cohesiveness of the bulk solid plays an important role in determining the effect of moisture on packing properties and tensile strength of moist beds. Their experiments covered the effect of consolidation of moist beds, which is of relevance to the granulation process. These authors concluded that aggregate size is usually dependent upon tensile strength of the moist granule. For example, granules will disintegrate before or during drying if tensile forces are weak. In addition, final granule density is largely dependent upon the density of the

Table 15   Effect of Granulating Method on the Extragranulor Porosity of 12−16 Mesh Lactose Granules

Granulating method	Amount of H_2O used to granulate (% v/v)	Extragranular porosity
Pan	23.0	39.0
	28.3	39.5
	30.6	41.0
	32.1	42.0
Oscillator	15.3	48.5
	18.4	49.5
	27.5	50.5
	30.6	50.0
	33.7	50.0

Source: Data from Ref. 100.

moist granular bed, although some density changes may be expected during drying. At a fixed moisture content, increasing the consolidation stress produces a decrease in specific volume and an increase in tensile strength. Therefore, granulation methods that employ a consolidation step (e.g., an oscillating granulator, a high shear mixer, etc.) can be expected to produce denser granules than those that do not (e.g., rotating pan method).

Recent work in the area of particle packings is aimed at establishing a quantitative geometric description of packing [115,116]. These authors describe radiological techniques needed to obtain a geometric description of a packing involving particles of any shape and a large range of sizes.

VI. ELECTROSTATIC PROPERTIES

Only the contact and separation of solids is necessary to induce electrostatic charges. Static electrification is perhaps best known for its potential fire and explosion hazards, and the importance of proper "grounding" of pharmaceutical processing equipment cannot be overemphasized. Electrostatic forces are also well known for the detrimental effect they may have on the mixing process. The mixing action often results in generation of static surface charges, as evidenced by a tendency for powders to agglomerate following a period of agitation. Thus, the generation of electrostatic charges during solids blending is one of the principal factors responsible for the phenomenon of unblending. In a general sense, such unit operations as mixing, milling, sizing, and tablet compression do induce static electrification. All these operations lead to the overall charge development on granules and finished tablets, which can cause difficulties in the efficient operation of processing equipment [117].

Electrostatic forces probably do not play a significant role in the flow behavior of granules produced by the wet granulation method or slugging. The magnitude of these forces are negligible when compared to the weight of individual granules [118].

Further, electrostatic forces contribute very little to the overall strength of a granule; however, it is not unreasonable to assume that these forces play a part in the initial formation of aggregates [119]. Also, electrostatic forces may influence the behavior of direct compression formulations [120].

Early work on the electrification of particles dealt with atmospheric dust [121]. In the early 1900s, it was assumed that electrification of particles was produced by friction or contact with dissimilar substances. In 1927, it was demonstrated [122] that charges could be produced by friction and contact between particles themselves, even though similar in composition. Later, Kunkel [123] demonstrated that while a powder mass may be essentially neutral, the majority of individual particles will carry a charge. Finally, in 1959, it was established that friction was not a prerequisite—that only contact and separation were necessary to charge particles electrostatically [124]. There is evidence to indicate that the mechanism of contact charging involves the transfer of electrons from one solid to another [125,126]. For an in-depth review of electrostatic forces, the interested reader is referred to Krupp [127] and Hiestand [128]. Only a few reports appear in the pharmaceutical literature that deal with electrostatic forces, and these are reviewed as follows.

Gold and Palermo [120] utilized a commercially available ionostat to measure hopper flow electrostatics of acetaminophen formulations. Fine crystalline and crystalline acetaminophen exhibited higher induced static charges than did acetaminophen granulations prepared from ethylcellulose, starch paste, or syrup. Tablet excipients were found to have an effect on hopper flow static charge of fine crystalline acetaminophen. Lubricants such as talc and magnesium stearate at a 2% concentration level were found to dramatically reduce static charge. The addition of 0.5% water was also found to dramatically reduce hopper flow static charge. In a follow-up article, the authors [129] evaluated antistatic properties of tablet lubricants. Ten tablet lubricants at 1% concentrations were investigated and their ability to reduce static charge of anhydrous citric acid. Magnesium stearate, polyethylene glycol (PEG) 4000, sodium lauryl sulfate, and talc significantly lowered static charge. Liquid petrolatum, fumed silicon dioxide, stearic acid, and hydrogenated vegetable oil were found to have no antistatic properties. The antistatic properties of the lubricant were not altered by the material to which they were added to acetaminophen and ascorbic acid. In a subsequent article [130], the effect of powder flow rates on static charge potential of selected organic acids was studied. A summary of their data is shown in Table 16. As expected, increasing the powder flow rate resulted in a significant increase in induced static charge. Of the materials tested, tartaric acid resulted in the largest hopper flow static charge.

Lachman and Lin [131] describe the design and operating principles of an apparatus capable of measuring the inherent static charge on materials as well as the relative static electrification tendencies of materials. The basic equipment consists of an electrostatic tester, an X−Y recorder, and a humidifying chamber. The electrostatic tester is composed of three parts: a dual-polarity high-voltage power supply unit, a modified Faraday cage, and an electrostatic voltage-sensing pistol. The sample to be evaluated is placed in the Faraday cage, and voltage accumulation or decay

Table 16 Flow Rates and Static Charges of Selected Organic Acids as Obtained with Different Hopper Orifices

| | Orifice diameter | | | |
| | 8.0 mm | | 15.0 mm | |
	Flow rate ($g\ sec^{-1}$)	Static charge ($V\ cm^{-1}$)	Flow rate ($g\ sec^{-1}$)	Static charge ($V\ cm^{-1}$)
Aspirin	4.77	239	37.77	600
Ascorbic acid	4.41	472	36.11	744
Citric acid, anhydrous	3.77	533	44.22	1039
Tartaric acid	5.99	1306	49.37	2289

Source: Ref. 130.

Table 17   Equilibrium Potential (%) on
Powders at Applied Potential of 6000 V

Materials	Polarity of applied potential	
	+	−
Sodium chloride	85.0	90.0
Stearic acid	55.0	45.0
Sulfisomidine	60.0	48.0
Iodochlorhydroxyquin	50.2	50.3

Source: Ref. 131.

can be read on the ammeter of the voltage sensing pistol or displayed on
the X-Y recorder. The authors report on the relative static electrification tendencies of sodium chloride, stearic acid, sulfisomidine, and iodochlor-
hydroxyquin. The equilibrium potential as a percent of applied potential
is shown in Table 17. The equilibrium potential of sodium chloride is much
greater than that for other materials tested, which is in agreement with
the concept that charge flows faster in a good conductor (e.g., sodium
chloride). In the steady state, only sulfisomidine exhibited an inherent
electrostatic charge (+240 V). No measurable inherent static charge was
detectable for the other materials tested. The authors further obtained
charge accumulation and decay data and these were plotted according to
first-order kinetics. Results for stearic acid are shown in Figure 28.
As noted in the figure, there are two slopes, the first being steeper than
the second. The authors feel that the initial slope is due to inherent tendencies of the material to be polarized by the applied potential; and the
second slope represents the saturation of the surface of the material with
the applied potential, as well as a loss of charge from the material due to
radiation and conduction to the surrounding air. The rate constants
derived from the plots for stearic acid (Fig. 28) are shown in Table 18.
Thus, it is possible to rate static electrification tendencies of materials
through use of this equipment and treatment of data in accordance with
first-order kinetic principles. It should, therefore, be possible to acquire fundamental knowledge that will permit a scientific approach toward
alleviating static charge problems in pharmaceutical systems.

In summary, electrostatic charges may play a role in initial granule
formation that may be beneficial or harmful, depending upon the extent of
attractive and repulsive charges. In pharmaceutical processing systems,
static charges can cause detrimental effects ranging from unblending in
mixing operations to fire and explosion hazards. Several methods have
been suggested to minimize the effects of electrostatic charges [117,128].
These include modification of the crystalline habit, use of antistatic agents,
and humidity control. Static charge problems are most apparent with non-
conductive materials that accumulate charges. The problem can usually
be overcome by increasing the surface conductivity of powders or granules.
Thus, in addition of glidants, surfactants, other antistatic agents, and

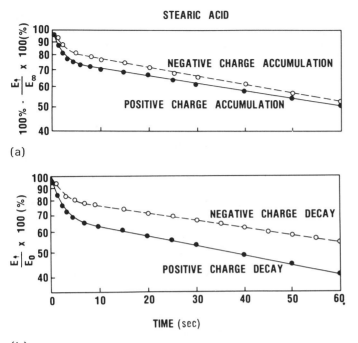

Figure 28 First-order plot of charge accumulation and decay data for stearic acid at a positive (————) and negative (– – – – –) applied potential of 600 V. (From Ref. 131.)

increased humidity are capable of dissipating accumulated static charges in nonconductors. All of the previous produce a conductive path that will allow the charge to drain off or otherwise be neutralized. This can also be accomplished by making the air around the surface conductive by breaking up the air into positively and negatively charged particles. This is the principle upon which nuclear static elimination devices are

Table 18 Accumulation and Decay of Negative and Positive Electrification for Stearic Acid at Applied Potential of 6000 V

Charge	Accumulation rate (sec^{-1})		Decay rate (sec^{-1})	
	k_1	k_2	k_1	k_2
+	8.92×10^{-2}	5.90×10^{-3}	1.06×10^{-1}	8.35×10^{-3}
−	7.90×10^{-2}	6.37×10^{-3}	5.36×10^{-2}	6.96×10^{-3}

Source: Data from Ref. 131.

based. Typically, a radioisotope such as polonium 219 (a pure α particle emitter) is used to ionize the air. As the α particles streak through the air, they interact with electrons in the air, causing them to float as free as electrons, leaving the rest of the molecule positively charged.

VII. RHEOLOGICAL PROPERTIES

Solid particles attract one another, and forces acting between particles when they are in contact are predominantly surface forces. There are many types of forces that can act between solid particles. Pilpel [118] identifies five types: (1) frictional forces, (2) surface-tension forces, (3) mechanical forces caused by interlocking of particles of irregular shape, (4) electrostatic forces, and (5) cohesive or van der Waals forces. All of these forces can affect the flow properties of a solid. With fine powders (≤150 μm), the magnitude of frictional and van der Waals forces usually predominate [118]. However, surface-tension forces between particles can be significant where capillary condensation has occurred [138]. Thus, small liquid bridges can be formed between particles if moisture content is high or particles are exposed to high humidities (≥60% relative humidity). Surface-tension forces resulting from absorbed films of gasses are generally quite small and not significant in comparison to other forces acting between particles. Although electrostatic forces of a magnitude greater than van der Waals forces are theoretically possible, the usual presence of even minute quantities of water are sufficient to minimize the effect of electrostatic forces. For larger particles (≥150 μm), such as granules produced by a wet granulation technique, frictional forces normally predominate over van der Waals forces. Thus, when evaluating interparticle forces of granules, agglomerates, or other large particles, cohesive or van der Waals forces are often assumed to be insignificant or equal to zero. The gravitational effect of large particles will normally overwhelm any effects due to van der Waals forces. Also, as particles increase in size, mechanical or physical properties of particles and their packings become important. The packing density of the mass of particles and bed expansion required to develop a shear plane are important considerations with larger particles. Many methods are available to measure the extent of interparticle forces. Such measures are then commonly employed as an index of flow. Some of the more common methods that will be discussed are: (a) repose angle, (b) shear strength determinations, and (c) hopper flow rate measurements. However, before undertaking a detailed discussion of these methods, the fundamental properties of solid particles that influence mass powder flow will be addressed. Such properties as particle size, particle size distribution, particle shape, surface texture or roughness, residual surface energy, and surface area affect the type and extent of particle–particle interactions. Studies involving the effect of some of these properties on flow of solids are summarized in previous sections.

A. Repose Angle

Many different types of angular properties have been employed to assess flowability [111,132,133]. For example, the following angular properties have been identified: (a) angle of repose, (b) angle of slide or friction,

(c) angle of rupture, (d) angle of spatula, and (e) angle of internal friction. Of these, angle of repose and angle of internal friction are perhaps
the most relevant to predict particle flow. The angle of internal friction
will be discussed later under shear strength measurements.

The more common procedures of determining angle of repose are illustrated in Figure 29. In the fixed-funnel and free-standing cone method,
a funnel is secured with its tip a given height, H, above a flat horizontal
surface to which graph paper is attached. Powder or granulation is carefully poured through the funnel until the apex of the conical pile just
touches the tip of the funnel; thus,

$$\tan \alpha = \frac{H}{R} \tag{32}$$

or

$$\alpha = \arctan \frac{H}{R} \tag{33}$$

where α is the angle of repose. In the fixed-cone method, the diameter
of the base is fixed by using a circular dish with sharp edges. Powder is
poured onto the center of the dish from a funnel that can be raised
vertically until a maximum cone height, H, is obtained. The repose angle
is calculated as before. In the tilting box method, a rectangular box is
filled with powder and tipped until the contents begin to slide. In the
revolving cylinder method, a cylinder with one end transparent is made to

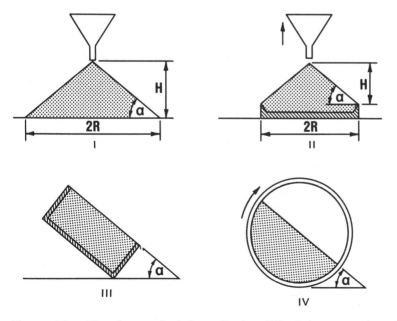

Figure 29 The four principle methods utilized in measuring the angle of
repose. I, Fixed-funnel and free-standing cone; II, fixed bed cone; III,
tilting box; IV, revolving cylinder. (From Ref. 134.)

revolve horizontally when half filled with powder. The maximum angle that the plane of powder makes with the horizon on rotation is taken as the angle of repose. Angles determined by the first three methods (Fig. 29) are often referred to as the static angle of repose, and the angle arrived at in Method IV is commonly called the kinetic angle of repose. Usually, the kinetic angle of repose is smaller than the static angle of repose. Other methods of determining the repose angle are given by Pathirana and Gupta [135] and Pilpel [118]. For a discussion of the forces involved in the formation of a conical pile of particles, including cohesion and friction, see Refs. 128, 135, and 137.

The angle of repose is best suited for particles $\geqslant 150$ µm [138]. In this size range, cohesive effects will be minimal and the coefficient of friction will be largely dependent upon the normal component of the weight of the test specimen. Values for angles of repose $\leqslant 30°$ generally indicate a free-flowing material, and angles $\geqslant 40°$ suggest a poorly flowing material [118]. The value of the angle of repose for a given material is dependent upon particulate surface properties that will also affect flowability [107]. However, as mentioned previously, the flow of coarse particles will also be related to packing densities and mechanical arrangements of particles. For this reason, a good auxiliary test to run in conjunction with repose angle is the compressibility test. The measurement of this value was discussed previously and is given in Eq. (3). From the angle of repose and compressibility values, a reasonable indication of a material's inherent flow properties should be possible. Carr [111] employs these two measurements together with the angle of internal friction to arrive at a flow index value for a particular material. The important point is that one can be misled if a judgment on flowability is based entirely on angle-of-repose measurements.

Several factors and granule characteristics have been studied for their effect on the angle of repose. Among them are particle size, use of glidants, moisture effects, and particle shape. Numerous authors have investigated the effect of particle size on the angle of repose. In a general sense, the repose angle normally increases as particle size is reduced, and this effect is usually quite dramatic in the small particle size range [139–142]. This effect is shown in Figure 30 for magnesia particles. It has also occasionally been observed that a plot of repose angle versus particle size goes through a minimum value [139–141,143]. Figure 31 illustrates this effect for a sulfathiazole granulation that was fractioned into various sieve cuts. The repose angle goes through a minimum at about 500 µm.

Another area that has been heavily investigated deals with the effect of glidants and "fines" on angle of repose. Craik [144] and Craik and Miller [145] studied the effect of magnesium oxide fines on the angle of repose of starch and found that with this system the repose angle went through a minimum at about a 1% concentration of magnesium oxide. Nelson [140] found that as the percentage of fines (100 mesh) was increased the repose angle increased, as would be expected from the discussion above. Pilpel [118] found that for mixtures of two sieve cuts of magnesia particles, the angle of repose was inversely proportional to the size of the fine particles but was directly proportional to their weight fraction.

The effect of glidants on the repose angle of various materials has been reported in detail. In general, the angle of repose goes through a minimum and then increases as glidant concentration increases, as

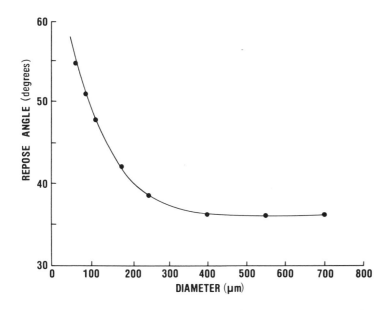

Figure 30 Angles of repose for different sieve cuts of magnesia. (From Ref. 118.)

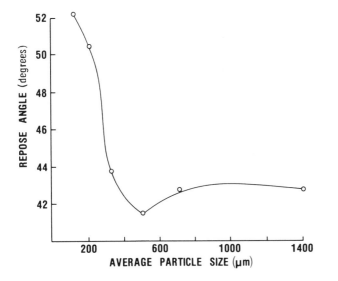

Figure 31 Repose angle as a function of sulfathiazole granule average particle size. (From Ref. 140.)

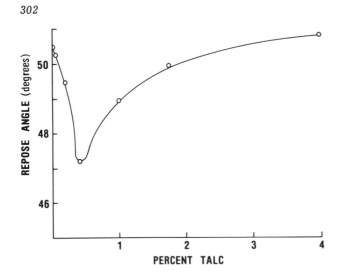

Figure 32   Effect of talc on repose angle of 60- to 80-mesh sulfathiazole
granules. (From Ref. 140.)

illustrated by the effect of small concentrations of talc on the repose angle
of 60- to 80-mesh sulfathiazole granules in Figure 32. In addition to talc,
investigators have tested the effects of colloidal silica on the angle of repose of lactose [145], magnesium oxide, titanium dioxide, zinc oxide,
cornstarch, and magnesium carbonate [147]. Gold et al. [148] reported on
the effect of small concentrations of talc, magnesium stearate, silicon dioxide, and starch on the repose angle of aspirin, calcium sulfate granules,
and spray-dried lactose particles. Other reports of interest are those of
Nash et al. [149], Awada et al. [150], Dawes [151], Carstensen and Chan
[152], and Carr [111].

When materials that take up moisture from the atmosphere are exposed
to high humidities, the materials generally become more cohesive, cake in
their containers, and exhibit very poor flow characteristics. It would appear from such observations that moisture and humidity affect the angle
of repose. Figure 33 illustrates the effect 24 hours of exposure to various relative humidities has on the observed angle of repose for starch
mixtures. As noted in Figure 33, as the storage humidity is increased,
repose angle increases. This effect of moisture on repose angle has been
noted by others [107,137,147,152].

It is generally recognized that particle shape has an effect upon the
angle of repose, and this has been illustrated by Ridgway and Rupp [75].
They found that as the shape coefficient of sand particles increased
(particles becoming more irregular), repose angle increased. The effect
of various pieces of granulating equipment on the repose angle of 20 – 30
mesh lactose granulations has been reported [44]. Comparisons of hopper-
flow-rate values of various materials with their respective repose angle
measurements have been published [138,139,146]. In dealing with angle
of repose of particles, it should be remembered that, in general, "the
angle of repose is *not* an inherent property of a solid, but a result of the
interplay of properties, equipment-design parameters, and the history of
the material" [154]. As mentioned previously, repose-angle measurements

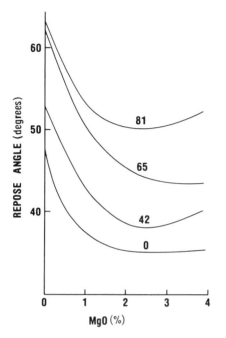

Figure 33 Angle of repose of starch and mixtures with light magnesium oxide after 24 hours of exposure to atmospheric moisture of 0, 42, 65, and 81% relative humidity at 30°C. (From Ref. 145.)

are applicable to relatively free flowing powders greater than 150-μm-diameter particle size; with cohesive powders, however, repose angles become inaccurate [107]. In efforts to assess the flow characteristics of cohesive powders, powder failure testing equipment (i.e., shear cells for shear strength measurements) has been used.

B. Shear Strength Measurements

A simplified schematic diagram of a shear cell apparatus is illustrated in Figure 34. Reference articles by Jenike [155–158] and others [138,159] describe in detail this type of biaxial translatory shear tester, often called the Jenike shear cell. The Jenike shear cell is the one in most common use, but other types of shear cells have been used [149,160,161]. To use the shear cell (Fig. 34), the bulk solid specimen is compacted to a specific state of consolidation inside the powder chamber. A normal load, P, which is less than the original consolidating load, is then applied to the cover. The powder bed is sheared by a translatory movement of the top half of the cell over the base at a constant shear strain rate. Shear force, S, is continuously measured by a transducer and results are plotted in the form of a stress/strain curve, shown in Figure 35. The degree of original consolidation is critical. If the consolidating force is too great, a curve such as C will result; and if the powder specimen is under compacted, a curve such as A will result. If the correct amount

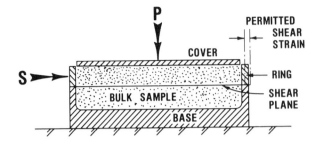

Figure 34   Schematic cross section of a shear cell ready for shear-strength measurement.

of consolidating force is applied, a curve such as B will result. Note that curve B reaches a limiting value that is termed the shear stress at failure, τ_f. The shear stress at failure is then obtained for a number of different reduced loads. Results are then plotted to give a so-called yield locus, and this is illustrated in Figure 35. This is generally referred to as a Mohr's shear diagram. The reader should refer to Hiestand et al. [161] for a discussion of the basic concepts involved with shear cell measurements and shear diagrams. Since the shear stress data obtained may be limited, a linear regression line may be drawn as an estimate of the yield locus.

From the yield locus, two useful measures describing particle–particle interaction influencing flow characteristics can be obtained: the cohesion

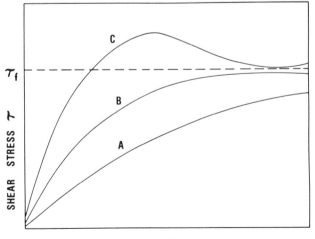

Figure 35   Typical stress/strain curves for powders; τ_f, shear stress at failure. [From N. Pilpel, in *Advances in Pharmaceutical Sciences*, Vol. 3 (H. S. Bean, X. X. Beckett, and J. E. Corless, eds.), Academic, New York, 1971.]

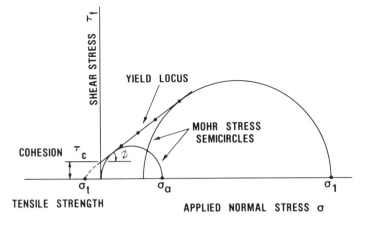

Figure 36   Typical Mohr's shear diagram.

value of the powder τ_c, and the angle of internal friction ϕ. The cohesion value of the powder is defined as the value of the shear stress at
zero applied load and is obtained by extrapolating the yield locus curve
back to the τ_f axis. The angle that the yield locus curve makes with the
τ_f axis gives a rough approximation of the angle of internal friction for
the powder. The angle of internal friction is a measure of the difficulty
of maintaining a constant volume flow [162]. By employing tensile strength
measurements, the tensile strength, σ_t, of the powder can be determined.
Hiestand and Peot [163] discuss methodology for accurately determining
σ_t.

Another parameter of interest in predicting flow properties of a material is a quantity known as the material's flow factor, FF [146,156,158].
To arrive at this quantity, shear-cell testing is done, the yield locus is
plotted, and two Mohr's stress circles are drawn with their centers on the
σ axis, tangently to the yield locus (see Fig. 36). The smaller semicircle
is constructed to pass through the origin and defines the unconfined yield
stress σ_α. The larger semicircle is drawn to pass through the end point
of the yield locus and defines the major normal stress σ_1. A graph is
then made by plotting σ_α versus σ_1 obtained from several yield loci. The
graph is often rectilinear, but if not, then FF is defined as the reciprocal
slope of the tangent to the graph at the origin of the axes [138].

York [146] has used the FF measurements from shear cell testing for
assessing the effect of glidants on the flowability of cohesive pharmaceutical
powders. As an example, the effect of magnesium stearate concentration
on the flowability of lactose and calcium phosphate is shown in Figure 37.
The optimum glidant level for lactose is 1.75% and for calcium phosphate
is 2.2%.

Other investigators have made use of shear cell testing in assessing
the flowability of cohesive powders that have not been covered in this section. The reader is referred to the literature for a more in-depth study
[160, 164−166].

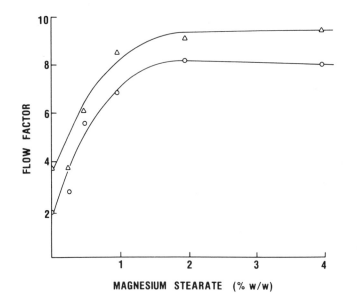

Figure 37   Magnesium stearate effects on the flow factor of host powders.
○, Lactose−magnesium stearate mixtures; △, calcium hydrogen phosphate−
magnesium stearate mixtures.   (From Ref. 146.)

C. Hopper Flow Rates

Hopper flow rates have been employed by numerous authors as a method of
assessing flowability. In addition, in some production operations, tablet
weight variation may be influenced by hopper flow rates, especially if
material flow to the feed frame of the tablet press is not consistent. Most
of the instrumentation employed is a variation of that described by Gold
et al. [130,146,167,168], and basically involves a recording balance.
Instrumentation is generally quite simple and results are easy to interpret,
making the method attractive from a practical standpoint. These authors
compared hopper-flow-rate data with repose angle for glidant studies, investigated factors affecting the flow rate of lactose granules, and presented
methods for determining uniformity of flow. The degree of correlation between hopper flow rate and repose angle was judged to be low. Talc was
found to be a poor glidant for the materials studied, as it decreased flow
rates at all concentrations tested. For the glidants magnesium stearate,
fumed silicon dioxide, and cornstarch, optimum concentrations were 1% or
lower, with flow rates decreasing at higher concentrations. When studying
lactose granules, these authors found that the percent fines, the amount
and type of granulating agent, particle size distribution, and the type of
glidant all had a measurable effect on flow rate. In their last article, the
authors describe instrumentation necessary for qualitative and quantitative
evaluation of flow uniformity through a hopper orifice, and examples are
presented to illustrate the utility of the instrumentation.

        Davies and Gloor [57−59], in a series of publications, have described
the effect of various formulation and process variables on hopper flow

rates of granulations produced in a fluid bed dryer. Increasing the addition rate of water and decreasing the inlet air temperature were found to increase hopper flow rates. The authors conclude that the reason for this enhanced flow is because these conditions result in better wetting of the solids and more robust granules. Increasing the formula weight (% w/w) of binder was found to decrease hopper flow rates for the three binders tested. For example, with gelatin as a binder, the flow rate for granules containing 2% w/w gelatin was 168.8 g min⁻¹. The authors conclude that the decreased hopper flow rates are a result of the increase in average particle size that occurs as formula weight of binder was increased. At a constant formula weight of binder, increasing the amount of water used to granulate resulted in granules that gave a higher hopper flow rate. Marks and Sciarra [105] and Harwood and Pilpel [112] also found that hopper rate was inversely proportional to average granule size. Others [139, 143] have reported that a plot of flow rate versus particle size goes through a maximum. This is illustrated in Figure 38 for lactose granules.

Jones [169] presents an excellent review of the effect of glidant addition on the flow rate of bulk particulate solids. He concludes that many glidants can improve the flowability of bulk solids and that several mechanisms of action may be involved. Glidants may act by one or more of the following mechanisms: reduction of interparticulate friction, change in surface rugosity, separation of coarse particles, reduction of liquid or solid

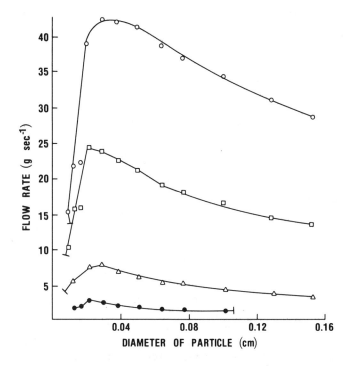

Figure 38   Flow rate of various sizes of lactose granulation through circular orifices with diameters: ○, 1.905 cm; □, 1.428 cm; △, 0.925 cm; ●, 0.6530 cm; b, blocked. (From Ref. 139.)

briding, and minimization of static charge. Many glidants are lubricants
and often possess a coefficient of friction less than that of the bulk solid
to which they are added. Such lubricants may also act by reducing surface rugosity, which will minimize mechanical interlocking of the particles
and thereby reduce rolling friction. The glidant may also function by
providing a physical separation of coarse particles in the bulk solid.
Agglomerated glidant particles may adhere to the surface of coarse particles and thereby provide this physical separation. This is thought to
reduce the action of capillary adhesion forces and also prevents formation
of solid bridges between particles.

VIII. GRANULE STRENGTH AND FRIABILITY

A granule is an aggregation of component particles that is held together by
the presence of bonds of finite strength [119]. The strength of a wet
granule is due mainly to the surface tension of liquid and capillary forces.
These forces are responsible for initial aggregation of the wet powder.
Upon drying, the dried granule will have strong bonds resulting from
fusion or recrystallization of particles and curing of the adhesive or binder.
Under these conditions, van der Waals forces are of sufficient strength to
produce a strong, dry granule. Measurements of granule strength are,
therefore, aimed at estimating the relative magnitude of attractive forces
seeking to hold the granule together. The resultant strength of a granule
is, of course, dependent upon the base material, the kind and amount of
granulating agent used, the granulating equipment used, and so on.
Factors affecting granule strength will be discussed in this section.
Granule strength and friability are important, as they affect changes in
particle size distribution of granulations and consequently compressibility
into cohesive tablets. Less appreciated is the fact that granule friability
can also affect unit dose precision in some tablet systems. This is especially true for hydrophobic drugs that are poorly wetted by the granulating
agent and are not firmly bound into the granulation. When such granulations break down, the drug may preferentially separate from the granules
and, as particle size separation occurs, the tablets containing a higher
level of fines also contain a higher concentration of drug. In addition,
the measurement of granule hardness and friability can be used as a characterizing tool, together with granule size, density, and porosity, in an
effort to quantitatively characterize a granulation to the extent that
processing parameters can be set and controlled so that highly reproducible
granulations can be manufactured. The more that is known about a process,
the better that process can be controlled or problems solved and eliminated
from the process. The ability to produce reproducible tablets, batch-to-
batch and lot-to-lot, is directly related to the ability to produce reproducible granulations.

When determining a relative measure of granule strength, three distinct
types of measurements can be made. The one that is perhaps the most
commonly used is that of compression strength. In this test, a granule is
placed between anvils and the force required to break the granule is
measured. An example of this type of apparatus is shown in Figure 39. A
lab jack is used to raise the granule until it is in contact with an upper
flat plate that is mounted to the bottom of a balance pan. Lead shot is
then added until the granule breaks; the amount of lead shot added is

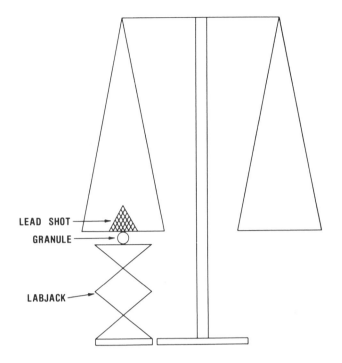

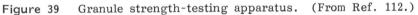

Figure 39   Granule strength-testing apparatus.   (From Ref. 112.)

termed the breaking load and taken as a measure of granule strength.   A
more sophisticated variation of the compression strength test was employed
by Gold et al. [170] and Ganderton and Hunter [100].   In the latter case,
the authors used a miniature press in which the lower platen was driven
upward at a constant rate.   A sensitive load cell was employed with the
electrical output being fed to a recording galvanometer to give a continuous record of the signal.

Other common methods of studying granule strength are those that relate to friability measurements [45,57,105,171].   Most of these methods are
a variation of the American Society for Testing and Materials (ASTM)
tumbler test for the friability of coal (ASTM Designation, D441-45, 1945).
These methods provide a means of measuring the propensity of granules to
break into smaller pieces when subjected to disruptive forces.   The method
typically involves taking granules that are known to be greater than a
particular mesh size, say m*.   The granules are then placed in a container
that is then tumbled or shaken for a predetermined period.   The material
is then shaken on a screen of mesh size m*.   The percentage of material
passing is then taken as a measure of granule friability or strength.

A third type of measurement involves determining the indentation hardness of a granule [79,172].   The equipment consists of a pneumatic micro-
indentation apparatus that employs a spherical sapphire as the indenter.
The diameter of the impression is determined, and from this the Brinell
hardness number can be determined.   This methodology for determining
granule strength has limited application.   One must be able to accurately

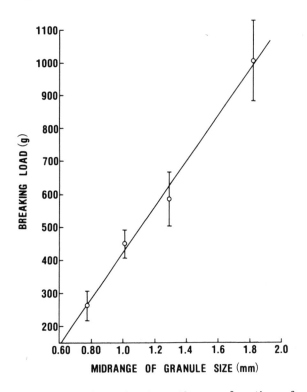

Figure 40   Granule strength as a function of aspirin granule size. (From
Ref. 170.)

determine the diameter of the impression; and to do this, regularly shaped
granules having a smooth surface must be used. Most granulations do not
fall into this category.

In a batch of granules, it would appear that the larger granules
possess more strength than the smaller ones [105,112,170], as illustrated
in Figure 40. It would appear that smaller granules are more poorly
formed and thus less robust than are their larger counterparts.

Numerous reports exist in the literature to show that increasing
amounts of binder produce granules of greater strength [58,99,102,112,
173,174]. Figure 41 illustrates this effect with dibasic calcium phosphate
granules and various binding agents.

In lactose and sucrose granulations using water as the granulating
fluid, granule strength was found to increase as the amount of water used
to granulate was increased [173]. This same dependency of granule
strength upon the amount of water used was reported for lactose granulations that had been produced on three different pieces of mixing—massing
equipment [102]. However, with calcium phosphate granulations, granule
strength went through a maximum as the amount of water used to granulate
was increased.

Hunter and Ganderton [101] conducted a revealing study on the effect
of the amount of water used to granulate and initial particle size on granule
strength of lactose granulations. Their results are illustrated in Figure 42.

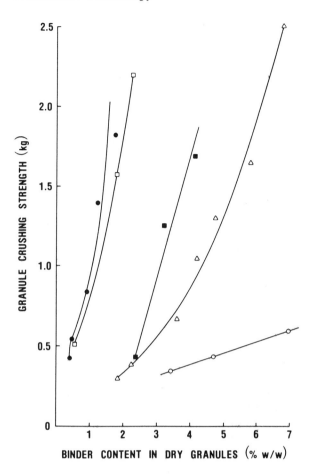

Figure 41 Crushing strength of dibasic calcium phosphate granules prepared with various binding agents. ●, Gelatin; □, potato starch mucilage; ■, acacia; △, povidone; ○, polyethylene glycol 4000. (From Ref. 99.)

Four different particle size grades of lactose were used. As shown in Figure 42, granule strength was found to be inversely related to the initial mean particle size of the lactose, with the increase being dramatic for the finest grade of lactose used. Granules produced from grade A lactose were much stronger, owing to the large number of bonds formed per unit volume. Essentially, the number of bonds formed with the fine grades of lactose is a function of particle size. Thus, with the finer grades of lactose, more bonds were formed during granulation and granule strength was therefore greater for these granules than for those produced from the coarse grades of lactose. As has been noted previously, as the amount of water used to granulate was increased, granule porosity decreased and granule strength increased. As the amount of water used to granulate is increased, the number of points at which liquid bonds form increases, resulting in less porous and greater strength granules upon drying.

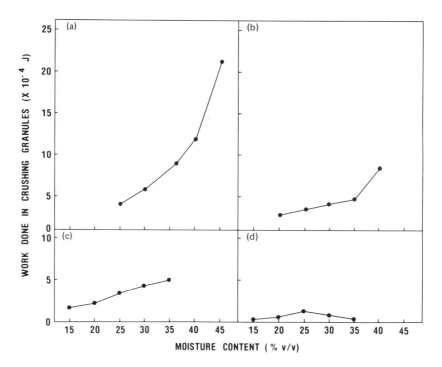

Figure 42 Moisture content utilized to form the granulation on the mean work performed (joules) in crushing 14- to 16-mesh granules prepared from four grades of lactose. Grade A, d_m = 26 µm; Grade B, d_m = 70 µm; Grade C, d_m = 140 µm; Grade D, d_m = 340 µ. (From Ref. 101.)

At a constant binder concentration in the final formula, dilution of the binder solution increases granule strength or reduces granule friability [59,175]. This was found true for a lactose granulation prepared in a fluid-bed dryer using gelatin as a binder, as well as a lactose granulation using starch paste and produced on conventional granulating equipment.

The effect of processing variables on granule strength has been reported on by numerous authors. Processing variables of the fluid bed technique were found to have a large impact on granule strength [57]. These included water addition rate, inlet air temperature, air pressure to the binary nozzle, and nozzle height. Fonner et al. [44] compared the granule strength of lactose granulations prepared from five different pieces of granulating equipment. Of the five pieces of equipment studied, granules produced from the oscillating granulator were the strongest and those produced in a liquid–solid V-shaped blender were the weakest. Working with a granulation of calcium phosphate, Ganderton and Hunter [100] found that granules that were massed and screened were stronger than those produced in a rotating pan. When lactose was used in place of calcium phosphate, these authors found that the strength of granules from massing and screening was about equal to those produced by the rotating pan method. Chalmers and Elworthy [69] investigated the effect of wet mixing time on granule strength for oxytetracycline granulations. In general, as wet mixing time increased, granule strength increased.

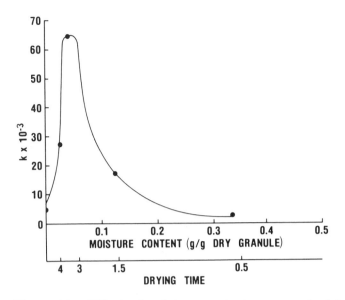

Figure 43 Effect of moisture content on granule friability. k is the gradient of the straight line representing the attrition time against the logarithm of the percentage weight intact for granules shaken in the multiple-attrition-cell apparatus. (From Ref. 172.)

Ridgway and Rubinstein [172] studied solute migration during granule drying. They worked with a magnesium carbonate granulation that utilized PVP as the binder. Material was massed and screened and then rotated in a coating pan to produce spherical granules. Selected granules were then dried in a special drying tunnel. The effect of moisture content on granule friability is shown in Figure 43. The attrition rate k is plotted against drying time and granule moisture content. Initially, the wet particles are held together by liquid-surface-tension forces and the granules are quite resistant to attrition. As drying proceeds, the granules become more friable and reach a maximum at the point when the granule surface is just dry. After this point, the interior of the granule starts to dry and granule strength increases. Working with dried granules, the authors determined granule strength as a function of depth from the granule surface. They found that Brindell hardness decreased linearly as measurements were taken from the outer surface toward the center of the granule. Finally, a point is reached where no further decrease in granule hardness occurs. This point provides a measure of crust thickness residing on the outer surface of the granule. During the initial stages of drying, PVP migrates to the granule surface and upon evaporation is deposited, forming a crust of finite thickness.

IX. EASE OF CONSOLIDATION AND MECHANISM

The process of consolidation and compact formulation is complex owing to numerous internal events that are acting simultaneously [176]. These

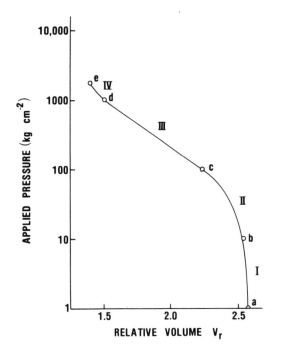

Figure 44   Relation between applied pressure and relative volume of a
compact.   (Data from Ref. 177.)

events include (a) particle rearrangement (consolidation), (b) particle
fracture, and (c) plastic deformation.   Particle rearrangement occurs
mostly at low compression pressures and plastic deformation occurs at high
pressures.   All these events lead to a greater area of true interparticle
contact, with high compression pressure, resulting in extensive areas of
true particle contact.   At these true areas of contact, van der Waals
forces act to provide strong bonds that maintain the integrity of the
compact.   A simplistic view of the consolidation process can be achieved
by considering the effect of pressure on the relative volume of a compact
V_r, as shown in Figure 44.   It was concluded that the consolidation
process proceeded in stages.   During stage I (point a to b in Fig. 44),
the decrease in V_r arises through interparticulate slippage of powder,
leading to a closer packing.   This rearrangement of particles continues
until they become immobile relative to each other.   Stage II (b to c) is
characterized by the formation of temporary struts, columns, and vaults
arising through interparticular contact points.   These temporary structures
in effect support the compressive load.   In state III (c to d), the increasing compressive load brings about a failure of the aforementioned
temporary structures by fracture or plastic flow.   The true area of particle
contact begins to increase, and bonding occurs at these points.   The
generation of fresh surfaces has been illustrated by Higuchi [178] using
nitrogen absorption methods to measure specific surface areas of sulfadiazine tablets.   From Figure 45 it can be seen that the surface area of
the compact goes through a maximal value as the compressive force is increased.   The authors attribute this phenomenon to particle fragmentation

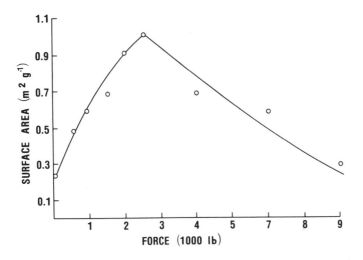

Figure 45   Effect of compressional force on the specific surface area of sulfadiazine tablets. (Data from Ref. 178.)

at the lower compressive loads, with subsequent rebounding at higher compressive loads. In stage IV (d to e) of the compression cycle, rebonding is probably occurring more rapidly than is fragmentation. Plastic flow may also occur in this region.

Rubinstein [179] has studied granule consolidation during compaction by measuring the deformation of small cylindrical aggregates of dibasic calcium phosphate containing 10% by weight of radiographic barium sulfate. Spherical granules were lightly compressed (15 MN m^{-2}) with 3.2-mm-diameter flat-faced punches into small cylindrical aggregates. These aggregates were placed diametrically in the middle of a bed of sucrose granules and compacts were prepared at various pressure settings. X-rays were taken of the compacts, and from the radiographs, diameter and thickness measurements of dibasic calcium phosphate aggregates were determined using a traveling microscope. Also, these aggregates could be recovered from the compact by dissolving out the sucrose with water. The authors interpretation of their experimental data is shown in the following paragraph.

Up to 200 MN m^{-2}, there is an increase in aggregate diameter accompanied by a corresponding reduction in thickness. The result is that there is only a relatively small reduction in aggregate volume. This phase may be attributable to interparticulate slippage, which leads to a closer packed arrangement. The increase in diameter is the result of granules being squeezed outward by the descending upper punch. At about 2000 MN m^{-2}, the aggregate diameter no longer increases because solid bridges are formed between the particles making up the granules and the die walls, preventing any further squeezing out of the granules. From 200 to 420 MN m^{-2}, failure of the granular material occurs by plastic deformation and a consolidation occurs by a reduction in aggregate thickness only. Finally, from 420 to 800 MN m^{-2}, a structure is formed that can support the applied load without further consolidation. This structure behaves elastically, since the aggregates increase in size when removed from the compacts.

Hiestand et al. [176,180] state that during compaction, particles undergo sufficient plastic deformation to produce die wall pressures greater than can be relieved by elastic recovery when the punch pressure is removed. This die wall pressure causes enough internal stress in some materials to cause a crack to propagate and initiate fracture of the compact in the die. If the excess stresses do not initiate fracture upon decompression in the die, the compact will laminate or "cap" upon ejection from the die. As the compact is ejected, the die wall pressure is allowed to go to zero. The emerging compact will expand while the confined portion cannot, thus concentrating shear stresses at the edge of the die and initiating fracture.

Compacted materials that do not fracture have the ability to relieve the shear stresses developed during decompression and/or ejection by plastic deformation. This stress relaxation is time-dependent, and therefore the occurrence of compact fracture is also time-dependent. Intact compacts of acetaminophen, methenamine, and erythromycin were made when the decompression was extended for several hours. If rapidly decompressed, the compacts fracture. Stress relaxation could be the explanation for some practical tableting problems. Tablet lamination or capping problems are often eliminated by precompression, slowing the tableting rate and reducing the final compression pressure. In each adjustment, the stress relaxation time is increased or the amount of stress needing to be relieved is reduced, allowing an intact compact to be formed.

In many cases, deep concave punches produce tablets that cap. In this case, the curved part of the tablet expands radially whereas the body of the tablet cannot, which establishes a shear stress that initiates the fracture. Flat punches avoid this additional shear stress.

X. SUMMARY: CHARACTERIZATION OF GRANULATION

As noted in the introduction of this section on the characterization of granulations, the various physical and physicochemical properties of granulations affect many quality features of tablets, such as compressibility, unit dose accuracy, porosity, hardness, friability, capping tendency, disintegration, and dissolution rate. Unfortunately, a single granulation property can influence many different tablet properties, improving some tablet properties while degrading others, as the granulation property is systematically changed in a given direction. In addition, adding to the complexity of property relationships is the fact that many different granulation properties, along and as interaction effects, often influence a single tablet property. Nevertheless, optimization procedures [181] have been employed to optimize tablet properties, such as dissolution rate [182]. As granulation properties are more clearly defined and the exact relationships of these properties to tablet quality features are established, optimization of the properties of tablets will become more realistic and feasible.

PART TWO: EVALUATION OF TABLETS*

Pharmaceutical tablets are evaluated for their chemical, physical, and biological (bioavailability and drug performance) properties. These properties in consort, describe the total quality of any given tablet or tablet formulation, according to its particular method of manufacture, in its package/container, and under fixed storage or a range of storage conditions (including possible and reasonable environmental exposures under conditions of use). In the case of physical or chemical properties, a series of characteristics are generally required to fully identify the particular property. All three property classes — chemical, physical, and biological — may be interrelated. For example, chemical breakdown of or interactions between tablet components may alter physical tablet properties in such a way that the biological properties are significantly changed. Even without chemical breakdown, various physical properties of tablets can undergo change under environmental or artificial stress conditions, and these changes may be of more significance and concern in some tablet systems than chemical stability. Evaluation of a particular formulation or establishment of an expiration date for a product requires that the stability of all three classes of properties be addressed.

The development of a tablet formulation goes through several phases, with an increasing number of tablet evaluations performed as each new phase is entered. During an initial formulation screening phase, the concept or feasibility of a new dosage form may be evaluated as to its behavior in vivo. Generally a prototype formulation is used for this evaluation and few tablet characteristics are of great concern.

Following a successful screening phase, a more intense development phase is begun. In the development phase, the tablet formula is perfected into a safe, efficacious, and reliable dosage form. A formulation optimization is generally conducted in this phase on relatively small scale lots. It is during this optimization that the effects of variations in formulation ingredients and often processing steps on critical tablet characteristics are studied. Where possible, attempts are made to quantitate these effects.

Once developed and optimized, a tablet formulation and process is scaled up to production scale and other operational units are given the opportunity to work with and comment on the production suitability in their operations. Operational areas also considered in this phase are packaging and shipping. Finally, production begins and quality assurance/quality control releases the new tablet for consumer use.

As the development of a tablet moves through each phase, the formulator becomes concerned about an increasing number of specific aspects of

---

*Part Two is contributed by Thomas W. Rosanske, Neil R. Anderson, and Gilbert S. Banker.

the tablet formula and evaluates the tablet for those properties. Therefore, as the project progresses, the total cumulative number of tablet evaluations performed increases. Following is a description of those tablet
properties considered critical by a formulator and evaluated at various
stages of development. Keep in mind that the evaluations are cumulative
with each development phase.

XI. SCREENING AND FEASIBILITY

During the initial formulation screening for a new tablet product, only a
minimum number of measurable tablet properties are involved. These may
include such properties as tablet size and shape, thickness, color, and
sometimes any unique identification markings to be placed on the tablets.

A. Size and Shape

Several factors contribute to the overall size and shape of a tablet.
Among the most significant factors are drug dosage, density of the final
granulation mix, and overall tablet weight. Once an overall, or perhaps
even a prototype, formulation is established, considerations of tablet shape
and size in terms of physical dimensions begin. In considering the shape
and size for a particular tablet formulation, the formulator needs input
from other sources such as Marketing and Production. With the competitive nature of the pharmaceutical industry, marketing considerations often
focus on unique tablet designs that have consumer appeal and can easily
be distinguished from other products of a similar nature or used for the
same indication. Production, on the other hand, is more concerned that
tablets be manufactured consistently and at a rapid rate.

The size and shape of a tablet can influence the particle size of the
granulation that can be used, the type of tablet press required, production lot sizes, the type of tablet processing that can be used, packaging
operations, and overall production costs. The shape of the tablet alone
can influence the choice of tablet machine that can be used. For example,
because of the nonuniform forces experienced within a tablet during compression, the more convex the tablet surface, the more likely one is to
observe capping problems, thus necessitating the use of a slower tablet
press or one with precompression capabilities [176].

It is essential from the perspective of consumer acceptance, tablet-to-
tablet uniformity, and lot-to-lot uniformity, and manufacturability that a
high degree of control over the shape and size is maintained. This requires that tablet tooling be uniform and within established specifications
[183]. In 1981, the IPT Section of the Academy of Pharmaceutical Sciences published a revised Tablet Specification Manual [184]. This publication describes dimensional and tolerance specifications for commonly
used tableting tools, and also includes recommendations for the inspection
and control of the tools.

B. Tablet Thickness

Once the tablet size (weight) and shape have been established, tablet
thickness remains the only overall dimension variable. Although thickness

specifications may be set on an individual product basis, as a general rule, the thickness should be controlled to within 5% or less of an established standard value. Excessive variation in tablet thickness can result in problems with packaging as well as consumer acceptance. Difficulties may be encountered in the use of unit dose and various other types of packaging equipment if the volume of the material being packaged is not consistent. In multi-unit packages such as bottles, variations in tablet thickness may result in differences in fill levels for a given number of dosage units. In order to maintain product acceptance by the consumer, variations in tablet thickness must not be visible to the unaided eye. Other tablet quality properties that may be related to tablet thickness include drug release and bioavailability (particularly in sustained release preparations), and tablet friability.

Variations in tablet thickness can also indicate formulation or processing problems. At a constant compressive load, variations in tablet thickness are indicative of changes in die fill and, consequently, tablet weight, whereas with a constant die fill, thickness variations reflect changes in compressive force. Several factors influence tablet thickness and tablet thickness control. These include (a) the physical properties of the raw materials, including crystal form and true and bulk density; (b) the granulation properties, including bulk density, particle size, and particle size distribution; (c) the physical and mechanical properties of the final compressing mix, including powder flow; and (d) consistency of the upper and lower punch lengths, which should be appropriately standardized. Since tablet thickness cannot be independently adjusted because of the interrelationships between thickness, weight, compressional force, tablet porosity, etc., it is obvious that appropriate control of raw materials, granulation and final mix properties, and machine operation are fundamental to the satisfactory control of the tablet thickness in practice. Tablet thickness is often used as one of several in-process tests and is monitored at regular intervals during the compressing stage of tablet manufacture. If appropriate, adjustments can then be made by machine operators to maintain tablet thickness within specifications.

The thickness of individual tablets are generally measured with a micrometer, which permits very accurate measurements and provides information on the tablet-to-tablet variation. Digital readout calipers have recently been introduced which provide accurate single tablet thickness measurements to one one-hundredth of a millimeter. Another technique, employed less often in production control involves placing 5 or 10 tablets in a holding tray and measuring the total thickness with a sliding caliper scale. This method is perhaps a more rapid way to provide an estimate of tablet thickness but does not provide information on the variability between tablets. If the punch and die tooling have been adequately standardized and the tablet machine is functioning properly, this latter method may be considered satisfactory for production control.

Aside from production control, measurement of tablet thickness is also useful in determining the density of tablet compacts. This is of interest to the formulator in evaluating the consolidation characteristics of various materials or tablet formulations by measuring the density of the tablet compacts under standard pressures and pressure loading conditions. The volume of a standard flat face tablet can be calculated from the formula for the volume of a cylinder ($V = \pi r^2 h$, where r is the radius of the tablet surface and h the tablet thickness). Density equals mass per unit volume, where mass is determined by weighing the individual tablets. Formula or processing modifications of a particular drug that produce a greater tablet density under given compression-loading conditions generally reflect improved consolidation of the formula and may be expected to yield a more cohesive tablet compact. The resultant tablets may be expected to have improved mechanical strength and friability characteristics, but perhaps at the expense of increased disintegration and dissolution times.

C. Color

Most pharmaceutical companies use variations in tablet color as a means of identifying distinct products as well as different strengths within a given product line. Tablet colors are generally selected such that the tablets have an aesthetic appeal to consumers, thus requiring that the color of a product be uniform (a) within a single tablet (nonuniformity is generally referred to as "mottling"), (b) from tablet to tablet, and (c) from lot to lot. Nonuniformity of coloring not only lacks aesthetic appeal but could be associated by the consumer with nonuniformity of content and general poor quality of the product [185].

The evaluation of color in tablets is usually a subjective test, depending on the ability of the tablet inspector to discriminate color differences visually. But because the unaided eye is not an analytical instrument, it has shortcomings in the evaluation of surface color, and storage of visually acquired data is often very difficult. The eye cannot discriminate between small differences in color of two similar substances, nor can it precisely define color. In addition, the eye has limited memory-storage capacity for color. Different people will perceive the same color differently, and often even one person will describe the same color differently at different times. Generally, visual comparisons require that a sample be compared against some standard. However, color standards are subject to change with time, thus forcing a redefinition of standards, which can ultimately lead to a gradual but significant change in an acceptable color [186].

Spectrophotometric techniques were used to analytically evaluate color uniformity between tablets as early as 1957 [187]. Among the techniques used are reflectance spectrophotometry [188–197] and tristimulus colorimetric measurements [186,196,198,199]. The use of a microreflectance photometer has been used to measure the color uniformity and gloss on a tablet surface [185].

A different approach was taken by Armstrong and March [200] to evaluate the problem of mottling. In their studies, photographs were taken of mottled sample tablet surfaces. The photographic negatives were then scanned by a microdensitometer, which was designed to produce a graphic record of the changes in absorbance along a path across the transparent negative.

Many dyes are particularly susceptible to fading over time, particularly when exposed to periods of direct sunlight or artificial light (particularly shorter wavelength). When a dye is selected for use with a particular formulation, the formulator should evaluate the susceptibility to fading. This is most often done using a Fadeometer [197,199] or a Xenotest [199], in which the tablets are subjected to a controlled amount of light for a given period of time. The instruments described above are then used to detect changes in color.

D. Unique Identification Markings

In addition to color, companies producing tablets very often use some type
of unique marking on the tablet to aid in the rapid identification of their
product. These markings generally take the form of embossing, engraving,
printing, or unique and novel shapes. A browse through the product
identification section of the current *Physician's Desk Reference* [201] will
give the interested reader an idea of the many variations that are used in
the pharmaceutical industry. Film-coated tablets are generally printed.
However, with the advent of new film-coating systems and equipment, many
engraved or embossed tablets have been film coated without compromising
the quality of the tablet detail.

The type of information placed on a tablet generally includes any number or combination of the following: company name or symbol, a product
code such as that from the NDC number, the product name, and the potency. The amount of information that can be placed on a tablet will depend on such factors as the tablet size and formulation. If a formulator
tries to put too much information on a tablet via engraving or embossing,
he may encounter such problems as sticking and picking in the fine detail.
A great deal of care must be taken in the design, manufacture, and use of
very intricate tooling.

XII. DEVELOPMENT/OPTIMIZATION

Once the feasibility studies have indicated a likelihood for success, a more
formal development program is initiated. During the development phase,
significant attention is paid to critical quality characteristics of the tablet.
This phase is often characterized by use of statistical design or other
means to evaluate and, where possible, quantify those formulation and
frequently process variables that have a significant effect on the established tablet quality characteristics. In addition to those discussed above,
tablet properties often considered in this phase of development include general appearance, potency/content uniformity, weight variation, hardness,
friability, disintegration, dissolution, porosity, film coating, and stability.

A. General Appearance

General appearance of the tablets is a highly important quality parameter as
viewed by the consumer. As such, all tablets should have an aesthetic
appearance that is free of any kind of visual defect.

B. Potency and Content Uniformity

The potency of tablets is generally expressed in terms of grams (g),
milligrams (mg), or micrograms (μg) (for some very potent drugs) of drug
per tablet, and is given as the label strength of the product. Compendial
or other standards provide an acceptable potency range around the label
potency. For very potent, low-dose drugs such as digitoxin, this range
is usually not less than 90% and not more than 110% of the labeled amount.
For most drugs in tablet form, the stated compendial range for acceptability

is not less than 95% and not more than 105% of the labeled amount. The usual method of determining potency of tablet products (average assay content) involves taking 20 tablets, powdering them, taking an accurately weighed sample of the powder, analyzing that powder sample by an appropriate analytical technique, and calculating the average assay content of the product. For very potent drugs, 20 tablets may not provide an adequate sample for potency determination. For example, with digitoxin the monograph specifies that a counted number of tablets be taken to represent about 5 mg of drug. The digitoxin assay goes on to specify that the tablets are finely powdered, and a powdered sample representing about 2 mg of drug is taken for assay. For any product, the amount of powder required depends on the accuracy and precision of the analytical method used for the assay. The assay results thus obtained will disclose, *on average*, how close the tablets are to the labeled potency and if they are within the specified potency range. For example, in the case of the digitoxin tablets at 50 μg labeled potency, let us assume that the assay results indicate 1.9 mg rather than 2.0 mg in the powder sample — thus 4.75 mg in the total 100-tablet sample (representing 5 mg of drug), or an average tablet potency of 47.5 μg/tablet. Since the compendial monograph permits an average potency as low as 90% of label, or 45 μg/tablet, the product is within specified potency limits, *on average*. However, in such composite assays, resulting in an average content, individual tablet variations can be masked by the use of the blended, powdered samples. In the hypothetical case of the digitoxin tablets described above, if 50 of the tablets averaged 42.5 μg, and the remaining 50 tablets averaged 50 μg, the overall average would be an acceptable 47.5 μg, yet half of the tablets would be subpotent (less than 45 μg). Therefore, even though the average assay result looks acceptable, it could be the result of a wide variation in individual tablet potency, with the result that a patient could be variably underdosed or overdosed. With a drug such as digitoxin, for which the safe and effective level and the toxic level are close (or even overlapping), exceeding the official or accepted potency range is not only undesirable but could be dangerous. Thus, tablets must be subjected to additional testing that relate to or quantify the range in potency from tablet to tablet.

To assure uniform potency for tablets of low-dose drugs, a Content Uniformity Test is applied. In this test, not less than 30 tablets are randomly selected for the sample, and at least 10 of them are assayed individually. Nine of the 10 tablets must contain not less than 85% or not more than 115% of the label claim, and the Relative Standard Deviation must be less than or equal to 6.0%. The tenth tablet may not contain less than 75% or more than 125% of the labeled amount. If either of these conditions are not met, an additional 20 tablets must be individually assayed. None of the additional 20 tablets may fall outside of the 85% to 115% range and the overall Relative Standard Deviation of the 30 tablets may not exceed 7.8% [202]. In evaluating a particular lot of tablets, several samples of tablets should be taken from various parts of the production run in order to satisfy statistical procedures.

What appears to be a wide acceptance range (85 to 115%) for content uniformity can often be difficult to achieve for low-dose tablet formulations. Three factors can contribute directly to content uniformity problems in tablets: (a) nonuniform distribution of the drug substance throughout the powder mixture or granulation, (b) segregation of the powder mixture or

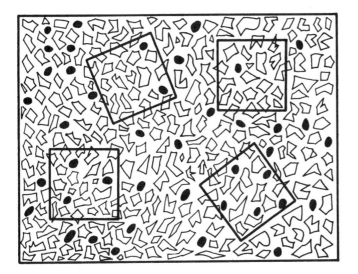

Figure 46 A powder mixture, angular open particles represent excipient, dark circles represent drug. The squares represent identical-size powder samples, which contain as few as one to as many as five drug particles. Solid dosage forms represent similar powder or granule "samples." The presence of a large number of drug particles per dose is critical to low-dose variation between tablets. [From G. S. Banker, in *Sprowl's American Pharmacy*, 7th Ed. (L. W. Dittert, ed.), Lippincott, Philadelphia, 1974, p. 376.]

granulation during the various manufacturing processes, and (c) tablet weight variation. The precision and variation of the assay used in the content uniformity test is also a factor that enters as an error factor in the determination of content uniformity.

The problem of nonuniform distribution is illustrated in Figure 46. The irregularly shaped drug particles are dispersed in irregularly shaped diluent particles of various sizes, and it is not difficult to comprehend why a perfect physical mixture never occurs geometrically (uniform physical placement of the drug particles) or statistically (equal probability that all sections of the mix will contain a certain number of drug particles). The squares drawn in the picture illustrate various possible random samples that might be drawn from the mixture and represent the amount of mixture required for one tablet. The squares contain as many as five particles and as few as one drug particle.

It is obvious that, to achieve a reasonable content uniformity, there must be a large number of drug particles in every sample taken. For example, if there are only three particles, on the average, of drug in a particular weight sample, an error or plus or minus one particle will constitute an error of 33% in the dose. If, on the other hand, there are an average of 100 particles of drug in every sample taken, an error of plus or minus one particle per sample is an error of only 1%. Even 100 particles of drug per dosage unit might not be adequate in practice, however, because statistical sampling might result in as many as 110 or as few

as 90 particles much of the time. It would be more reasonable to have
1000 or more particles per dosage unit sample weight if acceptable content
uniformity is to be achieved. Increasing the number of particles, however, requires a reduction in drug particle size. This approach to improving dose uniformity is often offset, however, by increased electrostatic effects and potential for segregation, as well as a decrease in flow
properties of the final mix.

The greatest potential for drug-diluent segregation in a tablet system
occurs with powder or particulate mixtures intended for direct compression or with wet granulations in which drug migration is likely. In the
first case, segregation is promoted by such actions as vibration of the
feed hopper or other parts of the compressing machine, where differences
in particle size and density of the drug and excipient will cause a consistent movement of the drug throughout the bulk of the mixture. In
such a situation, smaller, denser particles will sift through the bulk of
the granulation and move downward, while larger or lighter particles will
tend to float to the top of the bed. With wet granulations, segregation is
most likely to occur if the drug is very soluble in the granulating fluid
and if a static drying method is employed. As the granulating fluid (drug
solvent) evaporates, the drug tends to be carried to the surface of the
drying granulation. This migration destroys the homogeneous mix and
reduces the chances of good content uniformity in the tablet, because the
uniformity is dependent on the mixing in the lubrication step [203].

The uniformity of drug distribution in tablets generally cannot be
better than that of the granulation from which the tablets are made.
Therefore, it is advisable to determine the drug content uniformity of the
granulation or tablet mix *before* compression, especially with new production runs of a product with which there is little experience, or in tableting
systems where uniformity problems are known to exist. Many pharmaceutical companies have in-place formalized validation programs that examine final mix uniformity prior to transfer of the product to production.
Once the tablets are made, corrections such as grinding and recompressing
may not be possible if the tablets are found to be outside of the specification limits. Corrective steps that are taken before tablet compression are
simpler, less expensive, and less likely to have adverse effects on tablet
quality characteristics such as dissolution rate or in vivo drug availability.

Although potency and content uniformity are routinely measured and
controlled properties of tablets, the results of these tests do not necessarily reflect the effective drug content of the product. The effective
drug content is not the amount of drug that is determinable by assay, but
rather the amount of drug in the product that is present in an absorbable
or bioavailable form. Many controlled studies [204−211] indicate that the
effective drug content of solid dosage forms is frequently not 100% of the
assayable drug content of the product, but may be as low as 50% or less
of the labeled and assayed drug content. In addition, if certain manufacturing variables such as compressive load influence bioavailability, the
effective drug content and the effective drug content uniformity of a
batch of tablets may be dependent upon both the actual drug content per
tablet and the processing method and its variables employed to make that
particular batch of product. The variation in effective drug content
uniformity is undoubtedly much greater in most cases than the chemical
content uniformity indicates. This factor could be critical in the case of
drugs that are subject to significantly reduced effective content and which

may be further influenced by manufacturing methodology. For example, with low-dose drugs such as the anticoagulants, extreme care in product control operations is required during manufacturing to minimize variations in content.

The purity of tablets is usually assured by utilizing raw materials, both active drug and all excipients, that meet official or other rigid specifications for quality. Extraneous substances present in a raw material or drug which are not specifically allowed by compendial or well-defined manufacturer's specifications may render the product unacceptable for pharmaceutical use. These extraneous substances may be toxic on acute or long term use or may have an unpredictable or deleterious effect on product stability or efficacy. Certain well-defined impurities will often appear in the specification of raw materials or drug substances, or if they are the product of unavoidable decomposition of the drug, may be listed with an upper tolerance limit. For example, Aspirin Tablets USP may contain no more than 0.15% of free salicylic acid relative to the amount of aspirin present.

C. Weight/Weight Variation

A tablet is designed to contain a specific amount of drug in specific amount of tablet formula. As a check that a tablet contains the proper amount of drug, tablet weight is routinely measured. Composite samples (usually 10) are taken and weighed throughout the compression process. This weight, however, is an average and contains the usual problems of average values. Within the composite sample weighed, there could be tablets that are excessively overweight and tablets that are excessively underweight but with an average value that is acceptable.

Weight uniformity can be considered indicative of dosage uniformity provided: (a) the major component of the tablet is active drug and (b) the uniformity of drug distribution of the granulation or powder from which the tablets are made is perfect. The *United States Pharmacopeia* [202] allows the use of a Weight Variation Test as a measure of uniformity of dosage units provided the tablet being tested contains 50 mg or more of a single active ingredient comprising 50% or more, by weight, of the dosage form unit. To perform the USP Weight Variation Test, 10 tablets are selected from a sample of not less than 30 tablets and individually weighed. From the assay result, the content of drug is calculated for each of the 10 tablets, assuming homogeneous distribution of the drug substance in the tablets. Requirements for dose uniformity are met if the calculated amount of active drug in each of the 10 dosage units tested lies between 85% and 115% of the label claim and the relative standard deviation of the 10 tablets is less than or equal to 6%.

Granulation as well as mechanical problems can contribute to tablet weight variation. The actual weight of the tablet is related to the geometry of the die and the position of the lower punch in the die as dictated by the weight adjustment cam. If everything is working well mechanically, the weight can be caused to vary by a poorly flowing granulation, which causes spasmodic filling of the dies. The improper mixing of the glidant into the granulation can influence the weight variation by not allowing for uniform flow. If the granulation particle size is too large for the die size, the dies will not be uniformly filled, resulting in weight variation [212]. Granulations having a wide particle size distribution may have a localized nonuniformity of density within the granulation. With the geometry being fixed, nonuniform densities will cause varying amounts of granulation to fill the dies, resulting in variation in tablet weights. A wide particle size distribution can also be produced when a granulation has not been thoroughly mixed with extragranular excipients and/or when a granulation or final tablet mix has been stored in an area where vibrations were present to cause particle segregation. Ridgway and Williams [213] found for a uniform size granulation that as the particle shape became more angular, the weight variation increased.

Mechanical problems can cause weight variation with a good granulation. A set of lower punches with nonuniform length will cause weight variations, and will lower punches that are dirty enough to restrict their movement to their lowest point during die fill. A cupped lower punch that becomes filled in with a sticking granulation will also cause weight variation. Also, for a given granulation, Delonca et al. [212] found that as the tablet itself increased, the weight variation also increased.

Advances in tablet machine technology have had several effects on tablet weight variation, and vice versa. Although tablet machines have been designed to operate at ever-increasing speeds and higher production rates (up to 10,000 to 15,000 tablets per min theoretical maximum rate), the practical maximum production rate is often limited by tablet weight variation, caused by an inability to adequately and consistently feed granulation to the rapidly circulating die cavities. When the demand for material by a tablet machine approaches or exceeds the flow capacity of the hopper or feed frame, tablet weight variation will increase greatly.

Induced-die feeding systems have been developed to permit higher production speed while achieving satisfactory weight variation control. Automated tablet weight control devices, such as the Thomas Tablet Sentinel (Thomas Engineering, Inc., Hoffman Estates, Illinois), has made improved weight variation possible with high speed equipment. The Sentinel is one commercial result of many studies on instrumenting tablet compressors. This device continuously measures the compression load using force transducers (strain gauges) and is capable of maintaining a preset compressional force by adjusting, as necessary, the weight cam on the machine. The weight cam is turned through a synchronous-drive motor which is controlled by impulses from a "black box" according to the information sent from the force transducers. Thus, if the particle size of the granulation being compressed is reasonably consistent as it is fed from the hopper, the compressive load is a function of the volume fill in the die cavity.

There are currently several commercially available automated tablet presses (see Chap. 1, Vol. 3). These automated presses have several advantages in addition to reducing tablet weight variation. Such machines *continuously* monitor tablet weight and provide assurance of total lot conformity. The Sentinel and similar units can be set to automatically turn a machine off and sound an alarm when it goes too far out of control or goes out of control too often.

Rapid and automatic weighing balances such as instruments available from Cahn (Cahn Instrument Div., Ventron Corp., Cerritos, California), Mettler (Mettler Instrument Corp., Hightstown, New Jersey), and Scientech (Scientech, Inc., Boulder, Colorado) have greatly expedited tablet weight variation measurements. These instruments can be coupled

to a computer to provide various statistical control values as a data print-
out. Ritschel [214] described such an installation and its application to
automated tablet weight analysis and dosage accuracy calculation.

D. Hardness

Once ejected from the compressing machine, a tablet requires a certain
amount of mechanical strength to withstand the shocks of handling in its
manufacture, packing, shipping, and dispensing. The tablets may also be
able to withstand a reasonable amount of abuse imparted by the consumer,
e.g., a partially filled bottle bounding around in a purse or pocket.
Hardness and friability (discussed in a following section) are the most
common measures used to evaluate tablet strength.

Tablet hardness must be an important consideration to a formulator
from the early stages of formulation development, as it can have a significant influence on such quality tablet parameters as disintegration and
dissolution properties. It is important to know the relationships between
tablet hardness and critical tablet quality characteristics and also the
formulation or processing variables that significantly affect the tablet
hardness. It may be especially important to monitor the tablet hardness
for sustained release drug products or other products that possess real or
potential bioavailability problems or are sensitive to variations in drug release profiles.

The definition and measurement of tablet hardness have evolved over
the years. Historically, tablet strength was determined by breaking a
tablet between the second and third fingers using the thumb as a fulcrum.
If there was a sharp "snap," the tablet was considered to have acceptable
strength [215]. This provided a very crude measure of the flexure of
tablets, but suffered from some obvious limitations such as tablet size and
shape and operator subjectivity. Attempts have been made to instrument
the flexure test and provide a more versatile and reproducible way of
measuring the flexing or bending properties of tablets [216,217]. Although variations on the flexure test continue to be used for research
purposes [218], the pharmaceutical industry generally accepts the definition of tablet hardness as being the force required to break a tablet in a
diametrial compression test. This test consists of placing the tablet between two anvils and applying pressure to the anvils until the tablet
breaks. The crushing strength that just causes the tablet to break is
recorded. Hardness is thus sometimes referred to as "tablet crushing
strength." Several instruments have been developed for measuring
tablet hardness in this manner. These include the Stokes (Monsanto)
tester [219], the Strong-Cobb tester [220], the Pfizer tester [221], the
Erweka tester [222], the Heberlein (or Schleuniger) tester [223,224], the
Key tester [225], and the Van der Kamp tester [226].

One of the first instruments designed to measure tablet hardness was
the Stokes, or Monsanto, tester. This device was developed approximately
50 years ago and consisted of a barrel containing a compressible spring
held between two plungers. The lower plunger was placed in contact with
the tablet and a zero reading was taken. The upper plunger was then
forced against a spring by turning a threaded bolt until the tablet fractured. As the spring was compressed, a pointer rode along a gauge in
the barrel to indicate pressure. The pressure of fracture was recorded

and the zero pressure deducted from it. The zero pressure was the gauge reading at which the lower plunger barely contacted the tablet when it was initially placed in the instrument. To overcome the manual nature of this first tester and decrease the time (1 min or longer) required to test a single tablet, the Strong-Cobb tester was developed about 20 years later. In the original Strong-Cobb tester, a plunger was activated by pumping a lever arm that forced an anvil against a stationary platform using hydraulic pressure. The force required to fracture the tablet was read from the hydraulic gauge. In later modifications of this instrument, the force could be applied by a pressure-operated air pump rather than manually. The dial was calibrated to 30 kg in^{-2}.

About another decade later, the Pfizer hardness tester was developed and made available to the pharmaceutical industry. This instrument operates on the same mechanical principle as a pair of pliers. As the handles of the pliers are squeezed, the tablet is compressed between a holding anvil and a piston connected to a direct-force reading gauge. The dial indicator remains at the reading where the tablet breaks. A reset button is used to return the indicator to zero. This tester was extensively preferred over the previous testers because of its simplicity, low cost, and speed.

The older testers described above suffered from several disadvantages. The Stokes and Pfizer instruments both exhibited considerable spring fatigue over time, and all three suffered from non-uniform loading rates as well as ease of operation and instrument variability. The more recent generation of tablet testers were developed to eliminate some of these disadvantages. In an early version of the Erweka tester, the tablet is placed on the lower anvil, and the anvil is then adjusted so that the tablet just touches the upper test anvil. A motor driven suspended weight moves along a rail and slowly and uniformly transmits pressure to the tablet. A pointer moving along a scale provides an indication of the breaking strength. A more modern version of the Erweka tester allows for horizontal loading of tablets. The Schleuniger, or Heberlein, design tester is based on a counterweight principle. In this tester, a moving anvil driven by a speed-controlled electric motor presses the tablet against a stationary anvil connected to a counterweight. The applied pressure is proportional to the time that the counterweight is lifted. The Key and Van der Kamp hardness testers both use strain gauges to determine the linear force needed to fracture a tablet. Most of the modern hardness testers are equipped with microprocessors providing digital readouts and simple statistical analyses of the data. Also, most modern instruments have the capabilities of providing data in any one of the several hardness unit systems (e.g., kP, SCU, kN) used in the industry.

Although the modern hardness testing equipment is a dramatic improvement of the first testers, the several types of testers available do not produce the same results for essentially the same tablet. To some degree, operator variation, lack of calibration, spring fatigue, and manufacturer variation still contribute significantly to the lack of uniformity [223,227]. It is therefore important that the formulator be aware of these variations, especially when the tablets are to be evaluated by other persons or in other labs. For accurate comparison, each instrument should be carefully calibrated against a known standard.

Because of the lack of precision with the commonly used hardness testers, investigators doing work in the fields of compaction physics or

[handwritten note: *I would interpret that to mean GMPs for finished pharmaceuticals simply based on the chronology of questions*]

tablet-breaking t... means to determine the strength
of compacts. Fo... ment instrumentation such as
the Instron teste... ngth tester [228], work of failure measurement... essed square compacts [163],
impact testing [2... asurements [231].

The hardness... of many things all working together. The fac... he preceding section as being
sources of variat... ay also produce variations in
tablet hardness... of applied compressional force and
is therefore a fu... at cause the force to vary. As
additional force i... tablet, the tablet hardness will
increase. This r... to a maximum value beyond
which increases i... e an increase in hardness, but
will cause the tab... thus destroying its integrity.
The influence of... e force on tablet hardness and
critical product q... ould be established for all new
potential formulat... mportant in the selection of an
optimum formulati...

Tablet size, ... the tester will also affect the
measured hardnes... mulation. Large tablets require a
greater force to ... herefore often considered "harder"
than small tablets... ion, flat-face tooling will produce
a harder tablet tl...

Factors that may alter tablet hardness in the course of a production
run are substantial alterations in machine speed, a dirty or worn cam
track, and changes in the particle size distribution of the granulation mix
during the course of the compressing run. These latter changes affect
the die fills. Dies having a light fill (large particles, low density) will
produce a softer tablet than dies receiving a heavy fill (small particles,
high density).

It is the die fill/compressional force relationship, provided tooling is
uniform, that makes tablet hardness a useful tool for physically controlling
tablet properties during a production operation, particularly when this
measurement is combined with tablet thickness. The fill/force relationship
is also the basis for instrumenting tablet machines. Tablet hardness is
often monitored as an in-process test during a compressing run, although
tablets are often harder several hours after compression than they are
immediately after compression.

Lubricants can have a significant affect on tablet hardness when used
in too high a concentration or when mixed too long. The lubricants will
coat the granulation particles and interfere with tablet bonding [232,233].
The effect of lubricant level and lubrication time on tablet hardness needs
to be evaluated by the formulator as part of the development process.

The optimum hardness for a given tablet formulation will depend to
some degree on the intended use for the tablet. For tablets intended to
be directly packaged and eventually swallowed by a consumer, disintegration and dissolution properties may be prime considerations for tablet
hardness, so long as the tablets can withstand packaging. For a chewable
tablet, a softer tablet may be desirable. If a tablet is to be coated, it
must be made hard enough to withstand the rigors of coating pans. An
appropriate balance between a minimally acceptable tablet hardness to
produce an adequate friability value and a maximally accepted hardness
to achieve adequate dissolution may be required.

E. Friability

As mentioned in an earlier section of this chapter, another measure (in addition to hardness) of a tablet's strength is its friability. Friability is a measure of the tablet's ability to withstand both shock and abrasion without crumbling during the handling of manufacturing, packaging, shipping, and consumer use. Tablets that tend to powder, chip, and fragment when handled lack elegance and, hence, consumer acceptance. These tablets can also create excessive dust and dirt in processing areas such as compressing, coating, and packaging, and can add to a tablet's weight variation or result in content uniformity problems. Historically, friability was subjectively measured by visually inspecting tablets after they had been shaken together for a few seconds in the operator's cupped hands. Tablets that did not cap or have excessively worn edges were considered acceptable. At one time, indications of tablet friability were obtained from field trials which involved shipping tablets in their usual containers and shipping cartons to various parts of the country. The problem with this approach is that it is uncontrolled, with no real indications of the actual exposures to which the tablets may have been subjected.

As a means of controlling, and even quantitating, the measurement of friability, a laboratory device, known as the Roche Friabilator, was developed [234]. This device subjects a number of tablets to the combined effects of shock and abrasion by utilizing a plastic chamber which revolves at 25 rpm, dropping the tablets a distance of 6 inches with each revolution. Normally, a preweighed tablet sample is placed in the Friabilator chamber which is then rotated for 100 revolutions. The tablets are removed from the chamber, dusted, and reweighed. Conventional tablets that lose less than 0.5 to 1.0% in weight are generally considered acceptable. Some chewable tablets and most effervescent tablets would have higher friability weight losses. When capping is observed during the friability testing, tablets should not be considered acceptable, regardless of the percentage weight loss.

When concave, especially deep concave, punches are used in tableting, and especially if the punches are in poor condition or worn at their surface edges, the tablets produced could exhibit "whiskering" at the tablet edge. Such tablets will result in higher than normal friability values, because the "whiskers" will be removed during the testing. Tablet friability may also be influenced by the moisture content of the tablet granulation in the finished tablets. A low but acceptable moisture level frequently serves as a binder. Very dry granulations that contain only fractional percentages of moisture will often produce more friable tablets than will granulations containing 2 to 4% moisture. The manufacture of hydrolyzable drugs into tablets having maximum chemical stability and mechanical soundness is often very difficult.

F. Disintegration

It is generally accepted that in order for a drug to be available to the body, it must first be in solution. Figure 47 illustrates a scheme of the ways in which drugs formulated into a tablet become available to the systemic circulation. For most conventional tablets, the first important step in the sequence is the breakdown of the tablet into smaller particles or

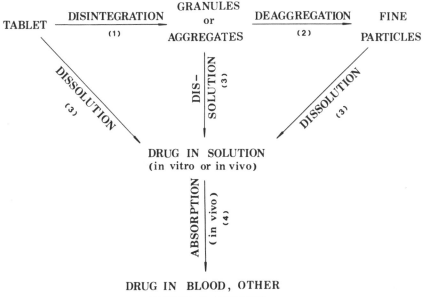

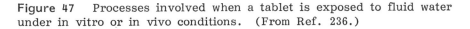

DRUG IN BLOOD, OTHER
FLUIDS, & TISSUES

Figure 47   Processes involved when a tablet is exposed to fluid water under in vitro or in vivo conditions.   (From Ref. 236.)

granules.   This process is known as disintegration.   The time it takes for a tablet to disintegrate in aqueous medium is measured using a device described in the United States Pharmacopeia [235].   Wagner [236] has written an excellent review of the disintegration test and the reader is referred to that reference for a more in-depth study.

Several researchers have in recent years studied the phenomenon of disintegration, and various mechanisms have been proposed for the process [237–244].   One cannot *a priori* expect a correlation between disintegration and dissolution [245], but often the disintegration of a tablet is a limiting factor of drug dissolution, particularly for drugs with low aqueous solubility [244].   Because of this, disintegration is still used as a guide to the formulator in preparation of an optimum formulation and to the production and control operators in monitoring the production process and ensure lot-to-lot uniformity [246].

Several methods other than the official USP method have been used to measure disintegration.   Rubenstein and Wells [247] followed the disintegration of phenylbutazone tablets by the measurement of the surface area of the generated particles in a Coulter Counter.   Thermal analysis has been used by Nakai et al. [248] not only to measure the disintegration of sugar-coated tablets but also to follow the dissolution of the sugar components, the inhibitive action of the barrier coat, the release of vitamins from the core, the reaction of the calcium carbonate in the tablet with acid media, and the reaction of ascorbic acid with metal ions in solution.

The *United States Pharmacopeia* [235] has long had a device to measure disintegration of tablets in a controlled fashion.   The device consists of a

basket rack assembly containing six glass tubes, 7.75 cm long, open at
the top, and with a 10-mesh screen attached to the bottom. To measure
disintegration time, one tablet is placed in each tube, and the basket rack
assembly is positioned in a 1-liter beaker of water, simulated gastric fluid,
or simulated intestinal fluid maintained at 37 ± 2°C. A standard motor-
driven device is used to move the basket assembly up and down through a
distance of 5.3 to 5.7 cm at a rate of 29 to 32 cycles per min. During
this movement of the basket assembly, the tablets in the tubes must remain 2.5 cm below the surface of the liquid on their upward movement and
must not descend closer than 2.5 cm from the bottom of the beaker. Perforated disks may also be used in the test. These are placed on top of
the tablets and impart an abrasive action to the tablets. The disks may
or may not be meaningful or impart more sensitivity to the test, but they
are useful for tablets that float.

Compliance with the USP standards or other specifications means that
the tablets must disintegrate and all particles pass through the 10-mesh
screen in the time specified. If any residue remains, it must have a soft
mass with no palpably firm core. The USP contains procedures for testing
disintegration of uncoated tablets, plain coated tablets, enteric coated
tablets, buccal tablets, sublingual tablets, and hard gelatin capsules.
Uncoated USP tablets may have disintegration times as low as 5 min, but
the majority of tablets have a maximum disintegration time of 30 min.
Enteric coated tablets are to show no evidence of disintegration after 1 hr
in simulated gastric fluid. The same tablets then tested in simulated
intestinal fluid are to disintegrate in 2 hr plus the time specified in the
monograph. If only the enteric coated tablet is recognized in the USP,
the disintegration in the simulated intestinal fluid must occur within the
time specified in the monograph.

The medium used, the temperature of the medium, and the operator
performing the test all can have a significant effect on the recorded disintegration times [236]. In addition, many factors involved with a tablet's
formulation and method of manufacture can affect the disintegration. The
disintegration times can be affected by the nature of the drug, the
diluents used [249], the binders or amount of binder, as well as the manner in which these are incorporated into the tablet [236,247]. The type
and amount of disintegrating agent can profoundly affect disintegration
times [236]. The presence of excess amounts of lubricants or excessive
lubrication times can increase disintegration times. The compaction pressure used to compress the tablets also influences disintegration, with an
increase in pressure generally resulting in an increase in disintegration
times [248–252].

G. Dissolution

In our discussion of disintegration, a scheme (Fig. 47) was presented to
show the processes involved in making a drug administered as a solid
dosage form available for absorption. It was pointed out that the original
rationale for using tablet disintegration tests was that as the tablet broke
down into small particles, a greater surface area was exposed to the dissolving medium, and therefore disintegration must be related to the
availability of the drug to the body. However, the disintegration tests
offer no assurance that the formulation will release the drug, even in the
form of small particles.

Since a drug must normally be in solution before absorption can take place, drugs given via orally administered tablets must dissolve in the contents of the gastrointestinal tract before systemic absorption can occur. Often, the rate of drug absorption is determined by the rate of dissolution from the tablet. Therefore, if it is important to achieve peak blood levels quickly, it will usually be important to obtain rapid drug dissolution from the tablet. For drugs that are absorbed in the upper part of the gastrointestinal tract, i.e., acidic drugs, rapid dissolution may be especially important. In such cases, the design of the tablet and the dissolution profiles may determine the total amount of drug absorbed as well as the rate of absorption. Thus, the rate of dissolution may be directly related to the efficacy of the tablet product. The most direct assessment of drug release obviously would be in vivo bioavailability studies. However, such studies are not always practical for reasons that include a lengthy time required to perform the studies, highly skilled personnel required to perform the studies, and assumed correlations with the diseases state and data obtained from healthy subjects or animals.

The utility of using in vitro data has been presented extensively in the literature over the past 15 – 20 years. Only a brief introduction to dissolution testing is presented in this section; the interested reader is referred to the literature for more in-depth information [253 – 256].

The primary objectives of an in vitro dissolution test are to demonstrate that (a) essentially 100% of the drug can be released from the dosage form, and (b) the rate of drug release is uniform from batch to batch and is the same as the release rate from those batches proven to be bioavailable and clinically effective.

In designing a dissolution test, several requirements should be kept in mind. The dissolution test should be designed to be suitable for use with a wide range of drugs and dosage forms. The test should be able to meaningfully discriminate between formulations of the same drug. There should be a reliable and reproducible assay for the drug being tested. The test should also be simple to do and easily amenable to automation. Many different dissolution apparatus have been reported in the literature. This section, however, will be limited to discussions concerning the current USP Apparatus 1 and Apparatus 2 [257].

Various parameters of the dissolution testing apparatus can affect results. The dissolution medium used is extremely important. Water has been used as the preferred medium in many cases, but it is hardly a universal medium because of solubility restrictions and pH changes as the drug dissolves. In the latter case, addition of buffers can remedy the problem. The pH of the medium is an important factor regarding the solubility and stability of most drugs and formulations. It is also important when trying to make the medium reflect the medium at the site of systemic absorption or above it in the gastrointestinal tract. For example, solubility allowing, acidic drugs are generally best tested in acidic medium, since it is likely that they will be best absorbed (and hence must dissolve) in the stomach or upper part of the small intestine. Dissolution testing of such drugs in a medium of pH 7.4, such as simulated intestinal fluid, would perhaps serve little purpose, since the acidic drugs would be nearly completely ionized and absorption would be inhibited at that pH.

The volume of dissolution medium, in theory, should be sufficient to maintain sink conditions throughout the test. To maintain sink conditions, it is suggested that the volume of the medium be at least three to five times the saturation volume. For low solubility drugs, this could conceivably be several liters. In practice, however, the volume used is usually determined by the particular apparatus used. The compendial testing apparatus specify use of a 100 mL round bottom flask for dissolution testing. The most commonly used volume with a USP apparatus is 900 mL. Thus, maintaining sink conditions often means adjusting the pH of the medium such that the drug solubility is maximized, or using a hydroalcoholic or mixed solvent medium. Nonaqueous dissolution media have the disadvantage, however, of rapid evaporation and too little resemblance to the aqueous environment encountered by the drug in the body.

The temperature of the medium is generally $37 \pm 0.5°C$ maintained throughout the test. Both the dissolution vessel and the water bath used to warm the dissolution medium should be covered to minimize losses to evaporation. This is particularly true when testing sustained release formulations, as evaporative losses can be substantial over a 12 or 24 hr testing period, thus imparting a bias to the test results. In some cases, removal of dissolved gases from the medium may be required prior to the start of the test. This is particularly true with USP Method I, where the basket can be covered with bubbles, thus retarding the dissolution medium from coming in contact with the dosage form.

The agitation of the dissolution medium should be widely variable but highly controlled. Both high and low agitation speeds can cause problems in dissolution testing. High-speed agitation may result in excessively fast dissolution of drug and hence a loss in discriminating power between formulations or batches. Low-speed agitation, on the other hand, may produce a very discriminating dissolution test but could suffer from inhomogeneous mixing in the dissolution vessel. Without homogeneous mixing, areas of differing drug concentration can occur in the vessel, thus making the position from which the sample is drawn for assay very important in obtaining consistent and meaningful data.

A compendial dissolution test apparatus is constructed such that "no part of the assembly, including the environment in which the assembly is placed, contributes significant motion, agitation, or vibration beyond that due to the smoothly rotating stirring element" [257]. This extra agitation can cause differences in mean dissolution rates and increase the differences between dissolution vessels. The vibrations can come from the dissolution test equipment itself, such as the water bath and its agitator/pump, as well as from external sources such as the benchtop on which the test equipment is placed or heavy machinery operating in close proximity. A further source of extra medium agitation or movement can come from currents set up by the sampling pump or probes in a continuous-flow automated dissolution test apparatus.

The dissolution apparatus should permit a convenient method of placing a tablet into the dissolution medium and holding it there for the duration of the test while retaining the ability for the test operator to observe the tablet throughout the test. The dissolution vessel itself must be exactly specified as to its dimensions, especially with multi-vessel test apparatus. Significant differences in dissolution rates have been found for products tested in different vessels [258].

Dissolution samples removed for assay are generally filtered to remove solid particles that may interfere with the assay. Care must be taken to choose a filter that does not adsorb drug from solution (particularly for low dose (drugs) or release substances that can interfere with the assay.

Dissolution testing may employ intermittent sampling or continuous analysis of the dissolution medium. When intermittent sampling is employed, corrections may be necessary to account for the volume and drug content of the samples removed for analysis or for dilution resulting from the addition of fresh medium to maintain volume. When the dissolution medium is analyzed continuously, the volume corrections are usually not necessary, since the medium is returned to the vessel after it is analyzed. However, as mentioned earlier, the sampling pump should be such that it does not induce any additional agitation by setting up currents inside the vessel. Important in any dissolution test is that the analytical method employed be highly reliable and reproducible. Simple, direct analytical methods are preferred, but care must be taken to make sure that tablet excipients do not interfere with the assay method.

Equally important as running the dissolution test properly is proper interpretation of the resulting data. Dissolution results may be expressed in terms of the concentration of drug in the dissolution medium versus time, the amount of drug (mg or % of label) released from the dosage form versus time, the amount of drug remaining unreleased from the dosage form versus time, or the time required for a stated amount of the drug to dissolve. For conventional, immediate releasing formulations, the latter is the most common way of expressing dissolution data. For example, for Hydrochlorothiazide Tablets USP, the USP specifies that not less than 60% of the labeled amount of drug dissolves in 30 min. The primary disadvantage of this expression of dissolution results is that it does not account for the portion of the drug remaining unreleased. For example, it is entirely possible that 60% of the labeled amount of hydrochlorothiazide could be released in 5 min and also that 10% or more would never be released from the same tablet. Alternatively, it is possible for 60% to be released rapidly and for the remaining 40% to be released very slowly. Thus, the description of a dissolution process in terms of a single time point is inherently risky. Such expressions are useful, however, for quality control purposes once the dissolution characteristics of a drug and dosage form are well understood.

For sustained-release tablet preparations in which the dissolution test duration is several hours, three dissolution time points are generally reported based on the dosing interval, D. The first is an early time point, usually 0.25D, which conveys an assurance that the tablets are not dose-dumping. The second is an intermediate time point, usually 0.5D, which demonstrates that the drug release is sustained. The final time point is late in the dosing interval, often 1.0D, and is used to demonstrate that most or all of the drug is released from the dosage form within the normal dosing period. Implied in this type of reporting scheme is that the in vitro drug release environment adequately simulates the in vivo release environment in terms of overall length of time to release all of the drug from the dosage form. Since over an extended period, the dosage form will encounter several different environments in vivo, use of a USP dissolution test will require that the drug release not be sensitive to changes in such environmental factors as pH. Over the last several years, significant attention has been given to the subject of in vitro/in vivo correlation [259-270].

H. Porosity

Porosity measurements are not routinely performed as an indication of
tablet quality. However, since many of the traditionally measured physical
characteristics of tablets may perhaps relate to tablet porosity, there has
been significant interest in recent years in porosity structure determination
and characterization.

The major parameters associated with the porous nature of solids is the
volume of the void space, designated as the porosity or pore volume; the
size of the pores, characterized by their diameters; and the distribution of
the pore size [271]. Methods used to measure pore size include air
permeametry [272−274], adsorption isotherms [275,276], and mercury intrusion [277−280].

Higuchi et al. [281] hypothesized in 1952 that "it seems reasonable to
assume that the volume of void space in a given tablet would greatly influence its disintegrating property." Taking this lead, several investigators
have used a measure of porosity in attempts to determine the effects of
tablet porosity on tablet disintegration and to study the mechanism of disintegrant action [279,282].

Stanley-Wood and Johansson [276] evaluated the surface area, pore
size, and total voidage in an effort to get some insight into the mechanisms
of tablet compaction. By evaluating the contact areas between particles,
the authors were able to show particle rearrangement or plastic flow bonding. Duberg and Nystrom [283] obtained porosity-pressure function data
for several pharmaceutical substances and related the data to bonding
properties of the materials and compact strength.

From the standpoint of stability, especially when dealing with hydrolyzable drugs, a physical description of the porous state of tablets may be of
fundamental importance if the porosity and pore size distribution affect the
accessibility of water and water vapor into the pore system of the tablet.

Gucluyildiz et al. [278], using the mercury intrusion technique for
porosity determinations, found that the stability of aspirin tablets increased
when the porosity of the tablets was decreased by the addition of silicon
dioxide. The increase in stability was explained in terms of the silicon
dioxide reducing the porosity by reducing the size and volume of the
coarser pores, thereby reducing the accessibility of moisture to the aspirin
component of the tablet.

I. Film-Coating Tests

Many tablet products currently marketed appear as film-coated tablets.
Film coating is used extensively for purposes of taste and odor masking,
aesthetic appearance, protection of unstable core materials, and the like.
Film coating is discussed extensively elsewhere in this series of volumes
and the reader is referred there for more details [284]. The development
of a film coating for tablets may require an investigation of the adhesion
of the polymeric film to the tablet surface and adhesion prediction models.
Actual adhesive forces have been measured using a tensile-strength
measuring device to measure either the peel strength [285,286] of the film
or the actual adhesive force [287]. Using these force measuring devices,
several parameters were investigated as possible predictive measures:
surface tension of the film coating solution, contact angle of the film

coating solution placed on the tablet surface [285,286], surface roughness of the tablet [286,288,289], and the porosity of the tablet [288,290]. Rowe [289] concluded that there are direct relationships between porosity and roughness of the tablet surface, between porosity and adhesion, and between roughness and adhesion [286]. Rowe [289] therefore argues that a measurement of the average surface roughness is the measure to be used in optimizing film coatings for adhesion.

J. Physical Stability

Stability is one of the most important factors to consider in evaluating tablet products. Stability is important not only from the standpoint of aesthetics and customer acceptance (color changes and fading), but also in maintaining uniform drug strength, identity, quality, and purity as exemplified by the inclusion of a stability section in the CGMPs (21 CFR, part 211, Section 211.6) and a section of "Stability Considerations in Dispensing Practice" in the USP [291]. It is recognized that physical characteristics of tablets have stability profiles, just as do chemical characteristics. Since some of the physical properties of tablets may have a profound influence on a product's in vivo as well as in vitro drug release characteristics, changes in these properties may result in corresponding changes in, for example, bioavailability. In establishing expiration dates for solid dosage forms, it is essential that the physical characteristics and the bioavailability properties be given equal consideration with the chemical characteristics, since all of these properties may change with product age and exposure. Therefore, many of the physical parameters, such as hardness, disintegration, and dissolution, are routinely evaluated within the framework of a stability program for a solid dosage form.

XIII. SCALE-UP/FINALIZATION PHASE

Following the intensive development/optimization phase, the overall formulation and process must be scaled-up to production scale and validated to insure that specifications established for the critical tablet quality characteristics established can be met in a large scale operation. It is also during this finalization phase that a new tablet formulation should be tested for its durability during the handling associated with such operations as coating, packaging, and shipping. The traditional evaluations performed on tablets involve only a small sample of tablets. How the tablets will withstand the mechanical shocks of a production environment is a function of the large number of tablets involved, production equipment, and production personnel. Rough-handling tests can be performed to give an indication of how well the new tablet will hold up in its specified package and shipping container during shipment. Rough-handling tests generally include a vibration test, a drop test, and an inclined-plane impact test [292–294]. Some investigators have actually shipped bottled product across the country and back again to get an idea of the strength of the new tablet product in shipment.

Problems can and do arise with new tablets in the packaging operation. Tablets undergo a number of mechanical shocks during the packaging operation, such as dumping into the packaging machine hopper, rectification into the filling slats, dropping into bottles, compression by the cottoning operation, and squeezing by the labeling operation. Perhaps the best way to test a new tablet is to allow the packaging personnel to package a large number of tablets under normal operating conditions and to evaluate the tablet's performance in comparison to how other tablets run under the same conditions. This same approach should be carried out with the printing of coated tablets by letting the production operators comment on how the new tablet functions under normal production conditions.

XIV. PRODUCTION/RELEASE PHASE

The majority of in-process tests performed by Production personnel and the drug release tests performed by Quality Control/Quality Assurance are tests used by the formulator to develop the new tablet. In fact, data supplied by the formulator is generally acted on by Quality Control or Quality Assurance to establish the product/release specifications.

As additional checks for identity, strength, quality, and purity, several other evaluations can be made during and after tablet production. Many companies are now using automated force/weight monitoring devices with automatic weight control feedback mechanisms to reduce tablet weight variation (some modern tablet presses are instrumented with systems that will automatically discard tablets that are out of weight specifications). Metal detection devices have been used for on-line metal detection in tablets. Coated tablets are mechanically sorted or visually inspected to eliminate out-of-size tablets, tablets with poor printing, or tablets with other defects. Some quality assurance release specifications also include microbial contamination tests.

XV. SUMMARY: EVALUATION OF TABLETS

As noted earlier in the chapter, the quality of pharmaceutical tablets can be no higher than the quality of the granulation from which the tablets are made. It is for this reason that a fairly detailed section was included on the characterization of granulations. An oft-repeated axiom in pharmaceutical research, development, and manufacture is that quality must be built into a product; it cannot be assayed in. This is certainly true in tablet product design and manufacture. A critical element in building quality into tablet products is thus in the design of the granulation or direct compression systems from which the tablets are made. The quality of the tablets can, of course, be much lower than the quality of the granulation source, depending on the processing conditions, the equipment used, and the skills of the personnel employed in the manufacturing step.

Tablets are the most widely used and most frequently used of all dosage form classes. They are, however, heterogeneous systems, and as such, they are one of the most complex classes of drug products from a physical sense. They have a range of mechanical properties not seen in other dosage forms because they are compressed systems. Achieving satisfactory drug dissolution profiles is more difficult from tablets than from any other class of oral dosage form. It is increasingly recognized that the physical and mechanical properties of tablets may undergo change on aging or on exposure to environmental stresses, thus having a stability profile that affects bioavailability and other fundamental tablet properties. Thus, it can be seen that the physical and mechanical property stability profiles can be as important as, if not more important than, the chemical stability of a tablet product. It is also apparent that attempts at optimizing tablet formulations and dosage forms can only be as successful as the accuracy and adequacy of the physical methods used in the product evaluation. This chapter has provided comprehensive listings and descriptions (with full reference to the literature) of test methods used for granulations and tablets throughout the development and production of tablet dosage forms.

REFERENCES

1. Rumpf, H., in *Agglomeration* (W. A. Knepper, ed.), Interscience, New York, 1962, pp. 379−413.
2. Capes, C. E., in *Handbook of Power Science and Technology* (M. E. Fay and L. Otten, eds.), Van Nostrand Reinhold, New York, 1984.
3. Capes, C. E., *Particle Size Enlargement*, Elsevier, New York, 1980.
4. Scherrington, P. J. and Oliver, R., in *Granulation* (A. S. Goldberg, ed.), Heyden and Sons, Philadelphia, 1981, pp. 7−60.
5. Hamaker, H. C., *Physic.*, 4:1058 (1937).
6. Corn, M., in *Aerosol Science* (C. N. Davies, ed.), Academic, New York, 1966.
7. Knupp, H., in *Particle Adhesion Advances in Colloid Interface Science*, I, III, 1967.
8. Lennard-Jones, J. E., *Proc. Phys. Soc. London*, 43:461 (1931).
9. Rumpf, H., *J. Res. Assoc. Japan Powder Technol.*, 9:13 (1972).
10. Pariff, G. D., *Dispersion of Powders in Liquids*, 2nd Ed., Applied Science, Berking, 1973.
11. Rumpf, H., in *Agglomeration 77* (K. V. S. Sastry, ed.), AIME, New York, p. 101, 1977.
12. Turner, S. A., Balasubromarian, M., and Otten, L., *Powder Technol.*, 15:97 (1976).
13. Rumpf, H., *Chem. Ing. Tech.*, 46:1 (1974).
14. Rumpf, H., *Chem. Ing. Tech.*, 30:144 (1958).
15. Newitt, D. W. and Conway-Jones, J. M., *Trans. Inst. Chem. Eng.*, 36:422 (1958).
16. Fisher, R. A., *J. Agric. Sci.*, 16:492 (1926).
17. Fisher, R. A., *J. Agric. Sci.*, 18:406 (1928).
18. Pietsch, W. B. and Rumpf, H., *Chem. Ing. Tech.*, 39:885 (1967).
19. Pietsch, W. B., *Nature*, 213:1158 (1969).
20. Pietsch, W. B., *Trans. ASME*, B91(2):435 (1969).
21. Orr, C., *Particle Technology*, Macmillan, London, 1966.
22. Pietsch, W. B., *Rev. Tech. Luxenberg*, 2:53 (1967).
23. Pietsch, W. B., *Car. J. Chem. Eng.*, 47:403 (1969).
24. Clare, I., Ph.D. Thesis, University (TH) Karlsruhe, 1976/77.
25. Irani, R. R. and Callis, C. F., *Particle Size: Measurement, Interpretation and Application*, Wiley, New York, 1963.
26. Herdan, G., *Small Particle Statistics*, Elsevier, New York, 1953.
27. Dallavalle, J. M., *Micromeretics*, Pitman, New York, 1948.

28. Edmundson, I. C., in *Advances in Pharmaceutical Sciences*, Vol. 2 (H. S. Bean, A. H. Beckett, and J. E. Corless, eds.), Academic, New York, 1967, pp. 95−129.
29. Heywood, H. J., *Pharm. Pharmacol.*, *15*:56T (1963).
30. Wilks, S. S., *Elementary Statistical Analysis*, Princeton University Press, Princeton, New Jersey, 1961.
31. Smith, J. E. and Jordan, M. L., *J. Colloid. Sci.*, *19*:549 (1964).
32. Aitchison, J. and Brown, J. A. C., *The Log-Norma Distribution*, Cambridge University Press, Cambridge, Massachusetts, 1957.
33. Kottler, F., *J. Franklin Inst.*, *250*:339, 419 (1950).
34. Ames, D. P., Irani, R. R., and Callis, C. F., *J. Phys. Chem.*, *63*: 531 (1959).
35. Hatch, T., *J. Franklin Inst.*, *215*:27 (1933).
36. Fonner, D. E., Barker, G. S., and Swarbrick, J., *J. Pharm. Sci.*, *55*:576 (1966).
37. Hatch, T. and Choate, S. P., *J. Franklin Inst.*, *207*:369 (1929).
38. Opankunle, W. O., Bhutani, B. R., and Bhatia, N., *J. Pharm. Sci.*, *64*:1023 (1975).
39. Whitby, K. T., *ASTM Spec. Tech. Publ.*, No. 235 (1958).
40. Shergold, F. A., *J. Soc. Chem. Ind.*, *65*:245 (1946).
41. Davis, R. F., *Trans. Inst. Chem. Eng.*, *18*:76 (1940).
42. Kluge, W., *Quarry Manager's J.*, p. 506 (March 1953).
43. Wolff, E. R., *Ind. Eng. Chem.*, *46*:1778 (1954).
44. Fonner, D. E., Banker, G. S., and Swarbrick, J., *J. Pharm. Sci.*, *55*:181 (1966).
45. Roberts, T. A. and Beddow, J. K., *Powder Technol.*, *2*:121 (1968/1969).
46. Jansen, M. L. and Glastonbury, J. R., *Powder Technol.*, *1*:334 (1967/1968).
47. Lapple, C. E., *Chem. Eng.*, *75*:149 (May 1968).
48. Laws, E. Q., *Analyst*, *88*:156 (1963).
49. Andreev, B. V., Gorodnichev, V. I., Minina, S. A., and El-Benna, H. M., *Pharm. Ind.*, *42*:1304 (1980).
50. Nouh, A. T. I., *Pharm. Ind.*, *48*:670 (1986).
51. Alkan, M. H. and Yuksel, A., *Drug Develop. Indust. Pharm.*, *12*(10): 1529 (1986).
52. Schaefer, T. and Woerts, O., *Arch. Pharm. Chem. Sci. Ed.*, *6*:1 (1978).
53. Ormos, Z., Pataki, K., and Csukas, B., *Hung. J. Ind. Chem.*, *1*: 463 (1973).
54. Ormos, Z., Pataki, K., and Csukas, B., *Hung. Ind. Chem.*, *1*:307 (1973).
55. Schaefer, T. and Woerts, O., *Arch. Pharm. Chem. Sci. Ed.*, *5*:178 (1977).
56. Kristensen, H. G. and Schaefer, T., *Drug Develop. Ind. Pharm.*, *13*(4&5):803 (1987).
57. Davies, W. L. and Gloor, W. T., *J. Pharm. Sci.*, *60*:1869 (1971).
58. Davies, W. L. and Gloor, W. T., *J. Pharm. Sci.*, *61*:618 (1972).
59. Davies, W. L. and Gloor, W. T., *J. Pharm. Sci.*, *62*:170 (1973).
60. Meshali, M., El-Banna, H. M., and El-Sabbagh, H., *Pharmazie*, *38*: 323 (1983).

61. Schaefer, T., Holm, P., and Kristensen, H. G., *Arch. Pharm. Chem. Sci. Ed.*, *14*:1 (1986).

62. Ritala, M., Jungersen, O., Holm, P., Schaefer, T., and Kristensen, H. G., *Drug Develop. Ind. Pharm.*, *12*(11&13):1685 (1986).

63. Holm, P., Schaefer, T., and Kristensen, H. G., *Powder Technol.*, *43*: 225 (1985).

64. Timko, R. J., Barrett, J. S., Mettach, P. A., Chen, S. T., and Rosenberg, H. A., *Drug Develop. Ind. Pharm.*, *13*(3):405 (1987).

65. Schaefer, T., Bak, H. H., Jaegerskou, A., Kristensen, A., Sevensson, J. R., Holm, P., and Kristensen, H. G., *Pharm. Ind.*, *48*:1083 (1986).

66. Holm, P., Jungersen, O., Schaefer, T., and Kristensen, H. G., *Pharm. Ind.*, *45*:806 (1983).

67. Chalmers, A. A. and Elworthy, P. H., *J. Pharm. Pharmacol.*, *28*:228 (1976).

68. Chalmers, A. A. and Elworthy, P. H., *J. Pharm. Pharmacol.*, *28*:234 (1976).

69. Chalmers, A. A. and Elworthy, P. H., *J. Pharm. Pharmacol.*, *28*:239 (1976).

70. Arambulo, A. S. and Deardorff, D. L., *J. Am. Pharm. Assoc., Sci. Ed.*, *42*:690 (1953).

71. Marks, A. M. and Sciarra, J. J., *J. Pharm. Sci.*, *57*:497 (1968).

72. Forlano, A. J. and Chaukin, L., *J. Am. Pharm. Assoc., Sci. Ed.*, *49*:67 (1960).

73. Opankuale, W. O., Bhutari, B. R., and Bhatia, V. N., *J. Pharm. Sic.*, *64*:1023 (1975).

74. Pitkin, C. and Carstensen, J., *J. Pharm. Sci.*, *62*:1215 (1973).

75. Ridgway, K. and Rupp, R., *J. Pharm. Pharmacol.*, *21*:30S (1969).

76. Shotton, E. and Obiorah, B. A., *J. Pharm. Sci.*, *64*:1213 (1975).

77. Rose, H. E., *The Measurement of Particle Size in Very Fine Powders*, Chemical Publishing Co., New York, 19--.

78. Fair, G. M. and Hatch, L. P., *J. Am. Water Works Assoc.*, *25*:1551 (1933).

79. Rupp, R., *Boll. Chem. Farm.*, *116*:251 (1977).

80. Ridgway, K. and Shotton, J. B., *J. Pharm. Pharmacol.*, *22*:24S (1970).

81. Beddow, J. K. and Vetter, A. F., *J. Powder Bulk Solids Technol.*, *1*:42 (1977).

82. Luekin, D. W., Beddow, J. K., and Vetter, A. F., *Powder Technol.*, *31*(2):209 (1981).

83. Beddow, J. K., *Particle Characterization in Technology*, Vols. I and II, CRC Press, Boca Raton, Florida, 1984.

84. Vetter, A. F. and Swanson, P., in *Particle Characterization in Technology*, Vol. II, CRC Press, Boca Raton, Florida, 1984, p. 173.

85. Guo, A., Ram Akrishnan, P., and Beddow, J. K., in *Particle Characterization in Technology*, Vol. II, CRC Press, Boca Raton, Florida, 1984, p. 173.

86. Rajpal, S., Hua, L., Chang, C. R., and Beddow, J. K., in *Particle Characterization in Technology*, Vol. II, CRC Press, Boca Raton, Florida, 1984, p. 193.

87. Carmichael, G. R., in *Particle Characterization in Technology*,
     Vol. II (J. K. Beddow, ed.), CRC Press, Boca Raton, Florida,
     1984, p. 205.

88. Chang, C. R., Beddow, J. K., Yin, J., Vetter, A. F., Butters, G.,
     and Smith, D. L., in *Particle Characterization in Technology*,
     Vol. II, CRC Press, Boca Raton, Florida, 1984, p. 223.

89. Pahl, M. H., Shadel, G., and Rumpf, H., *Aufbercit. Tech.*, *14*:
     Secs. 5, 10, 11 (1973).

90. Davies, R., *Power Technol.*, *12*:111 (1975).

91. Martin, A. W., Swarbrick, J., and Cammarata, A., *Physical
     Pharmacy*, Lea & Febiger, Philadelphia, 1969.

92. Fries, J., *The Determination of Particle Size by Adsorption Methods*,
     ASTM Spec. Tech. Publ. No. 234 (1958).

93. Shaw, D. J., *Introduction to Colloid and Surface Chemistry*, Butter-
     worths, Washington, D.C., 1966.

94. Adamson, A. W., *Physical Chemistry of Surfaces*, Interscience, New
     York, 1960.

95. Rigden, P. J., *J. Soc. Chem. Ind.*, *66*:130 (1947).

96. Carman, P. C., *J. Soc. Chem. Ind.*, *57*:225 (1938).

97. Carman, P. C., *Flow of Gases Through Porous Media*, Butterworths,
     Washington, D.C., 1956.

98. Stickland, W. A., Busse, L. W., and Higuchi, T., *J. Am. Phar.
     Assoc.*, *2nd Ed.*, *45*:482 (1956).

99. Weissberg, A., *Techniques of Organic Chemistry: Physical Methods*,
     Part 1, 3rd Ed., Interscience, New York, 1959.

100. Armstrong, N. A. and March, G. A., *J. Pharm. Sci.*, *65*:198
     (1976).

101. Ganderton, D. and Hunter, B. M., *J. Pharm. Pharmacol.*, *23*:1S
     (1971).

102. Hunter, B. M. and Ganderton, D., *J. Pharm. Pharmacol.*, *24*:17P
     (1972).

103. Hunter, B. M. and Ganderton, D. J., *Pharm. Pharmacol.*, *25*:71P
     (1973).

104. Heywood, H., *J. Imp. Coll. Chem. Eng. Soc.*, *2*:9 (1946).

105. Neumann, B. S., in *Flow Properties of Disperse Systems* (J. J.
     Hermons, ed.), North-Holland, Amsterdam, 1953, Chap. 10.

106. Marks, A. M. and Sciarra, J. J., *J. Pharm. Sic.*, *57*:497 (1968).

107. Butler, Q. A. and Ramsey, J. C., *Drug Stand.*, *20*:217 (1952).

108. Neumann, B. S., in *Advances in Pharmaceutical Sciences*, Vol. 2
     (H. S. Bean, A. H. Beckett, and J. E. Carless, eds.), Academic,
     New York, 1967, pp. 182–221.

109. Shinohara, K., in *Handbook of Powder Science and Technology*
     (M. E. Fayed and L. Otten, eds.), VanNostrand Reinhold, New
     York, 1984, Chap. 5, pp. 143–145.

110. Kuno, H., *Proc. Fac. Eng. Keioh Univ.* *11*(41):1 (1958).

111. Arakawa, M., Okada, T., and Suito, E., *Zairgo*, *15*:151 (1966).

112. Carr, R. L., *Chem. Eng.*, *72*:163 (Jan. 1965).

113. Harwood, C. F. and Pilpel, N., *J. Pharm. Sci.*, *57*:478 (1968).

114. Eaves, T. and Jones, T. M., *J. Pharm. Pharmacol.*, *25*:729 (1973).

115. Arthur, J. R. F. and Dunsten, T., *Nature (Hand.)*, *223*:464
     (1969).

116. Arthur, J. R. F. and Dunsten, T., *Powder Technol.*, *3*:195 (1969/1970).
117. Milosovich, G., *Drug Cosmet. Ind.*, *92*:557 (1963).
118. Pilpel, N., *J. Pharm. Pharmacol.*, *16*:705 (1964).
119. Barlow, C. G., *Chem. Eng. (Lond.)*, *220*:196 (1968).
120. Gold, G. and Palermo, B. T., *J. Pharm. Sci.*, *54*:310 (1965).
121. Ridge, W. A. D., *Philos. Mag.*, *25*:481 (1913).
122. Boning, P., *Z. Tech. Phys.*, *8*:385 (1927).
123. Kunkel, W. B., *J. Appl. Phys.*, *21*:820, 833 (1950).
124. Jefimenko, O., *Am. J. Phys.*, *27*:604 (1959).
125. Harper, W. R., *Adv. Phys. (Suppl. to Philos. Mag.)*, *6*:365 (1957).
126. Harper, W. R., *Soc. Chem. Ind. (Lond.)*, *Mongr.*, *14*:115 (1961).
127. Krupp, H., *Adv. Colloid Interface Sci.*, *1*:11 (1967).
128. Hiestand, E. N., *J. Pharm. Sci.*, *55*:1325 (1966).
129. Gold, G. and Palermo, B. T., *J. Pharm. Sci.*, *54*:1517 (1965).
130. Gold, G., Duvall, R. N., and Palermo, B. T., *J. Pharm. Sci.*, *55*: 1133 (1966).
131. Lachman, L. and Lin, S., *J. Pharm. Sci.*, *57*:504 (1968).
132. Pilpel, N., *Br. Chem. Eng.*, *11*:699 (1966).
133. Zenz, F. A. and Othmer, D. F., *Fluidization and Fluid Particle Systems*, Van Nostrand Reinhold, New York, 1960.
134. Train, D., *J. Pharm. Pharmacol.*, *10*:127T (1958).
135. Pathirana, W. K. and Gupta, B. L., *Can. J. Pharm. Sci.*, *11*:30 (1976).
136. Loews, T. M., *Fuel Soc. J. Univ Sheffield*, *16*:35 (1965).
137. Lowes, T. M. and Perry, M. G., *Rheol. Acta*, *4*:166 (1965).
138. Pilpel, N., in *Advances in Pharmaceutical Sciences*, Vol. 3 (H. S. Bean, A. H. Beckett, and J. E. Carless, eds.), Academic, New York, 1971, pp. 173−219.
139. Danish, F. Q. and Parrott, E. L., *J. Pharm. Sci.*, *60*:548 (1971).
140. Nelson, E., *J. Am. Pharm. Assoc.*, *Sci. Ed.*, *44*:435 (1955).
141. Kelley, J. J., *J. Soc. Cosmet. Chem.*, *21*:37 (1970).
142. Jones, T. M. and Pilpel, N., *J. Pharm. Pharmacol.*, *18*:18S (1966).
143. Jones, T. M. and Pilpel, N., *J. Pharm. Pharmacol.*, *17*:440 (1965).
144. Craik, D. J., *J. Pharm. Pharmacol.*, *10*:73 (1958).
145. Craik, D. J. and Miller, B. F., *J. Pharm. Pharmacol.*, *10*:136T (1958).
146. York, P., *J. Pharm. Sci.*, *64*:1216 (1975).
147. Tawashi, R., *Drug Cosmet. Ind.*, *106*:46 (1970).
148. Gold, G., Duvall, R. N., Palermo, B. T., and Slater, J. G., *J. Pharm. Sci.*, *55*:1291 (1961).
149. Nash, J. H., Leiter, G. G., and Johnson, A. P., *Ind. Chem. Prod. Res. Dev.*, *4*:140 (1965).
150. Awada, E., Nakajimi, E., Morioka, T., Ikegami, Y., and Yoshizumi, M., *J. Pharm. Soc. Jpn.*, *80*:1657 (1960).
151. Dawes, J. G., *Min. Fuel Power (Br.) Safety Mines Res. Estab.*, No. 36 (1952).
152. Carstensen, J. T. and Chan, P. C., *J. Pharm. Sci.*, *65*:1235 (1977).
153. Fowler, R. T. and Wyatt, F. A., *Aust. J. Chem.*, *1*:5 (June 1960).
154. Johanson, J. R., *Chem. Eng.*, *85*:9 (Oct. 30, 1978).

155. Jenike, A. W., Elsey, P. J., and Wooley, R. H., *Proc. ASTM, 60*: 1168 (1960).
156. Jenike, A. W., *Utah Eng. Exp. Sta. Bull.*, No. 108, University of Utah (1961).
157. Jenike, A. W., *Trans. Inst. Chem. Eng., 40*:264 (1962).
158. Jenike, A. W., *Utah Eng. Exp. Sta. Bull.*, No. 123, University of Utah (1964).
159. Williams, J. C., *Chem. Proces Eng., 46*(4):173 (1965).
160. Carr, J. F. and Walker, D. M., *Power Technol., 1*:369 (1967/1968).
161. Heistand, E. N., Valvani, S. C., Peot, C. B., Strzelinski, E. P., and Glasscock, J. F., *J. Pharm. Sci., 62*:1513 (1973).
162. Williams, J. C. and Birks, A. H., *Power Technol., 1*:199 (1967).
163. Hiestand, E. N. and Peot, C. B., *J. Pharm. Sci., 63*:605 (1974).
164. Peleg, M. and Mannheim, C. H., *Powder Technol., 7*:45 (1973).
165. Kurup, T. R. R. and Pilpel, N., *Powder Technol., 14*:115 (1976).
166. Farley, R. and Valentin, F. H. H., *Power Technol., 1*:344 (1967/1968).
167. Gold, G., Duvall, R. N., Palermo, B. T., and Slater, J. G., *J. Pharm. Sci., 57*:667 (1968).
168. Gold, G., Duvall, R. N., Palermo, B. T., and Slater, J. G., *J. Pharm. Sci., 57*:2153 (1968).
169. Jones, T. M., *J. Soc. Cosmet. Chem., 21*:483 (1970).
170. Gold, G., Duvall, R. N., Palermo, B. T., and Hurtle, R. L., *J. Pharm. Sci., 60*:922 (1971).
171. Mehta, A., Zoglio, M. A., and Carstensen, J. T., *J. Pharm. Sci., 67*:905 (1978).
172. Ridgway, K. and Rubinstein, M. H., *J. Pharm. Pharmacol., 23*:11S (1971).
173. Ganderton, D. and Selkirk, A. A., *J. Pharm. Pharmacol., 22*:345 (1970).
174. Jaiyeoba, K. T. and Spring, M. S., *J. Pharm. Pharmacol., 31*:192 (1978).
175. Hill, P. M., *J. Pharm. Sci., 65*:313 (1976).
176. Hiestand, E. N., Wells, J. E., Peot, C. B., and Ochs, J. F., *J. Pharm. Sci., 66*:510 (1977).
177. Train, D., *J. Pharm. Pharmacol., 8*:45T (1956).
178. Higuchi, T., Rao, A. N., Busse, L. W., and Swintosky, J. V., *J. Am. Pharm. Assoc., Sci. Ed., 42*:194 (1953).
179. Rubinstein, M. H., *J. Pharm. Sci., 65*:376 (1976).
180. Hiestand, E. N., paper presented at International Conference on Powder Technology and Pharmacy, Basel, Switzerland, 1978.
181. Buck, J. R., Peck, G. E., and Banker, G. S., *Drug. Dev. Commun., 1*(2):89 (1974/1975).
182. Fonner, D. E., Banker, G. S., and Buck, J. R., *J. Pharm. Sci., 59*:1587 (1970).
183. Ling, W. C., *J. Pharm. Sci., 62*:2007 (1973).
184. *IPT Standard Specifications for Tableting Tools*, Tableting Specification Manual, Academy of Pharmaceutical Sciences, Washington, D.C., 1981.
185. Matthews, B. A., Matsumota, S., and Shibata, M., *Drug Dev. Commun., 1*:303 (1974/1975).

186. Bogdansky, F. M., *J. Pharm. Sci.*, *64*:323 (1975).
187. McKeehan, C. W. and Christian, J. E., *J. Am. Pharm. Assoc.*, *Sci. Ed.*, *46*:631 (1957).
188. Lachman, L. and Cooper, J., *J. Am. Pharm. Assoc.*, *Sci. Ed.*, *48*: 226 (1959).
189. Urbanyi, T., Swartz, C. J., and Lachman, L., *J. Am. Pharm. Assoc.*, *Sci. Ed.*, *49*:163 (1960).
190. Lachman, L., Swartz, C. J., Urbanyi, T., and Cooper, J., *J. Am. Pharm. Assoc.*, *Sci. Ed.*, *49*:165 (1960).
191. Lachman, L., Swartz, C. J., and Cooper, J., *J. Am. Pharm. Assoc.*, *Sci. Ed.*, *49*:213 (1960).
192. Lachman, L., Weinstein, S., Swartz, C. J., Urbanyi, T., and Cooper, J., *J. Pharm. Sci.*, *50*:141 (1961).
193. Swartz, C. J., Lachman, L., Urbanyi, T., and Cooper, J., *J. Pharm. Sci.*, *50*:145 (1961).
194. Swartz, C. J., Lachman, L., Urbanyi, T., Weinstein, S., and Cooper, J., *J. Pharm. Sci.*, *51*:326 (1962).
195. Everhard, M. E. and Goodhart, F. W., *J. Pharm. Sci.*, *52*:281 (1963).
196. Goodhart, F. W., Everhard, M. E., and Dickcius, D. A., *J. Pharm. Sci.*, *53*:338 (1964).
197. Turi, P., Brusco, D., Maulding, H. V., Tausendfreund, R. A., and Michaelis, A. F., *J. Pharm. Sci.*, *61*:1811 (1972).
198. Goodhart, F. W., Lieberman, H. A., Mody, D. S., and Nimger, F. C., *J. Pharm. Sci.*, *56*:63 (1967).
199. Nyqvist, H., *Acta Pharm. Suec.*, *21*:245 (1984).
200. Armstrong, N. A. and March, G. A., *J. Pharm. Sci.*, *63*:126 (1974).
201. *Physician's Desk Reference*, 42nd Ed., Medical Economics, Inc., Oradell, New Jersey, 1988, pp. 403ff.
202. *United States Pharmacopeia*, 21st Rev., Mack, Easton, Pennsylvania, 1985, pp. 1277–1278.
203. Warren, J. W. Jr. and Price, J. C., *J. Pharm. Sci.*, *66*:1409 (1977).
204. Caminetsky, S., *Can. Med. Assoc. J.*, *88*:950 (1963).
205. Campagna, F. A., Cureton, G., Mirigian, R. A., and Nelson, E., *J. Pharm. Sci.*, *52*:605 (1963).
206. Catz, B., Ginsberg, E., and Salenger, S., *N. Engl. J. Med.*, *266*: 136 (1962).
207. Engle, G. B., *Australas J. Pharm.*, *47(Suppl 39)*:S22 (1966).
208. Glasko, A. J., Kinkel, A. W., Alegnani, W., and Holmes, E. L., *Clin. Pharmacol. Ther.*, *9*:472 (1968).
209. Levy, G., Hall, N., and Nelson, E., *Am. J. Hosp. Pharm.*, *21*:402 (1964).
210. Lozinski, E., *Can. Med. Assoc. J.*, *83*:177 (1960).
211. Searl, R. and Pernarowski, M., *Can. Med. Assoc. J.*, *96*:1513 (1967).
212. Delonca, H., Puech, A., Youakin, Y., and Segura, G., *Pharm. Acta Helv.*, *44*:464 (1969).
213. Ridgway, K. and Williams, I. E., *J. Pharm. Pharmacol.*, *29*:57P (1977).
214. Ritschel, W. A., *Pharm. Ind.*, *26*:757 (1964).

215. Gunsel, W. C. and Kanig, J. L., in *The Theory and Practice of Industrial Pharmacy*, 2nd Ed. (L. Lachman, H. A. Lieberman, and J. L. Kanig, eds.), Lea and Febiger, Philadelphia, 1976, p. 347.

216. David, S. T. and Augsburger, L. L., *J. Pharm. Sci.*, *63*:933 (1974).

217. Gold, G., Duval, R. N., and Palermo, B. T., *J. Pharm. Sci.*, *69*: 384 (1980).

218. Gold, G., Pandya, H. B., Duvall, R. N., and Palermo, B. T., *Pharm. Technol.*, *7*(12):30 (1983).

219. Smith, F. D. and Grosch, D., U.S. Patent 2,041,869 (1936).

220. Albrecht, R., U.S. Patent 2,645,936 (1953).

221. Michel, F., U.S. Patent 2,975,630 (1961).

222. Brook, D.B. and Marchall, K., *J. Pharm. Sci.*, *57*:481 (1968).

223. Goodhart, F. W., Draper, J. R., Dancz, D., and Ninger, F. C., *J. Pharm. Sci.*, *62*:297 (1973).

224. Dr. Schleuniger Productronic AG, Solothurn, Switzerland.

225. Key International, Inc., Englishtown, New Jersey.

226. Van-Kel Industries, Inc., Edison, New Jersey.

227. Newton, J. M. and Stanley, P., *J. Pharm. Pharmacol.*, *29*:41P (1977).

228. Nystrom, C., Alex, W., and Malmquist, K., *Acta Pharm. Suec.*, *14*: 317 (1977).

229. Rees, P. J. and Richardson, S. C., *J. Pharm. Pharmacol.*, *29*:38P (1977).

230. Hiestand, E. N., Bane, J. M., and Strzelinski, E. P., *J. Pharm. Sci.*, *60*:758 (1971).

231. Bhata, R. P. and Lordi, N. G., *J. Pharm. Sci.*, *68*:898 (1979).

232. Lerk, C. F. and Bolhuis, G. K., *Pharm. Acta Helv.*, *52*:39 (1977).

233. Shah, A. C. and Mlodozeniec, A. R., *J. Pharm. Sci.*, *66*:1377 (1977).

234. Shafer, E. G. E., Wollish, E. G., and Engel, C. E., *J. Am. Pharm. Assoc.*, *Sci. Ed.*, *45*:114 (1956).

235. *The United States Pharmacopeia*, 21st Rev., Mack, Easton, Pennsylvania, 1985, pp. 1242–1243.

236. Wagner, J. G., *Biopharmaceutics and Relevant Pharmacokinetics*, Drug Intelligence Publications, Hamilton, Illinois, 1971, pp. 64–97.

237. Bolhuis, G. K., VanKamp, H. V., Lerk, C. F., and Sessink, G. M., *Acta Pharm. Technol.*, *28*:111 (1982).

238. Colombo, P., Conte, U., Carmella, C., LaManna, A., Guyot-Herman, A. M., and Ringard, J., *Il. Farm. Ed. Prat.*, *35*:391 (1980).

239. Colombo, P., Conte, U., Carmella, C., Geddo, M., and LaManna, A., *J. Pharm. Sci.*, *73*:701 (1984).

240. Kanig, J. L. and Rudnic, E. M., *Pharm. Technol.*, *8*:50 (1984).

241. Shangraw, R., Mitrevej, A., and Shah, M., *Pharm. Technol.*, *4*:49 (1980).

242. Carmella, C., Colombo, P., Conte, U., Gazzaniga, A., and LaManna, A., *J. Pharm. Technol. Prod. Manuf.*, *5*:1 (1984).

243. Ringard, J. and Guyot-Herman, A. M., *Drug Dev. Ind. Pharm.*, *7*: 155 (1981).

244. Carmella, C., Colombo, P., Conte, U., Ferrari, F., Gazzaniga, A., LaManna, A., and Peppas, N. A., *Int. J. Pharm.*, *44*:17 (1988).

245. Alam and Parrott, E. L., *J. Pharm. Sci.*, *60*:795 (1971).
246. Madan, P. L., *Can. J. Pharm. Sci.*, *13*:12 (1978).
247. Rubinstein, M. H. and Wells, J. I., *J. Pharm. Pharmacol.*, *29*:363 (1977).
248. Nakai, Y., Nakajima, S., and Kakizawa, H., *Chem. Pharm. Bull.*, *22*:2910 (1974).
249. Lerk, C. F., Bolhuis, G. K., and DeBoer, A. H., *Pharm. Weekbl.*, *109*:945 (1974).
250. Kitazawa, S., Johno, I., Ito, Y., Teramura, S., and Okada, J., *J. Pharm. Pharmacol.*, *27*:765 (1975).
251. Suren, G., *Acta Pharm. Suec.*, *7*:483 (1970).
252. Bolhuis, G. K. and Lerk, C. F., *Pharm. Weekbl.*, *108*:469 (1974).
253. Hersey, J. A., *Manuf. Chem. Aerosol News*, *40*:32 (1969).
254. Wagner, J. G., *Biopharmaceutics and Relevant Pharmacokinetics*, Drug Intelligence Publications, Hamilton, Illinois, 1971, pp. 98–147.
255. Cooper, J. and Rees, J. E., *J. Pharm. Sci.*, *61*:1511 (1972).
256. Leeson, L. J. and Carstensen, J. T., eds., *Dissolution Technology*, Industrial Pharmaceutical Technology Section, Academy of Pharmaceutical Sciences, Washington, D.C., 1974.
257. *Unites States Pharmacopeia*, 21st Rev., Mack, Easton, Pennsylvania, 1985, pp. 1243–1244.
258. Cox, D. C., Doyle, C. C., Furman, W. B., Kirchoeffer, R. D., Wyrick, J. W., and Wells, C. C., *Pharm. Technol.*, *2*:41 (1978).
259. Tanigawara, Y., Yamaoka, K., Nakagawa, T., and Uno, T., *J. Pharm. Sci.*, *71*:1129 (1982).
260. Kingsfore, M., Eggers, N. J., Soteros, G., Maling, T. J. B., and Shirkey, R. j., *J. Pharm. Pharmacol.*, *36*:536 (1984).
261. Riegelman, S. and Upton, R. A., in *Drug Absorption* (L. F. Prescott and W. S. Nimmo, eds.), 1981, p. 297.
262. Tanigawara, Y., Yamaoka, K., Nakagawa, T., Nakagawa, M., and Uno, T., *J. Pharm. Dyn.*, *5*:370 (1982).
263. Moller, H. and Langenbucher, F., *Pharm. Ind.*, *44*:1065 (1982).
264. Dakkuri, A. and Shah, A. C., *Pharm. Technol.*, *6*(9):67 (1982).
265. Voegele, D., *Meth. Find. Exptl. Elin. Pharmacol.*, *6*:597 (1984).
266. Lathia, C. D. and Banakar, U. V., *Drug Dev. Ind. Pharm.*, *12*:71 (1986).
267. Skelly, J. P., Yau, M. K., Elkins, J. S., Yamamoto, L. A., Shah, V. P., and Barr, W. H., *Drug Dev. Ind. Pharm.*, *12*:1177 (1986).
268. Concheiro, A., Vila-Jato, J. L., Martinez-Pacheco, R., Seijo, B., and Ramos, T., *Drug Dev. Ind. Pharm.*, *13*:501 (1987).
269. Chung, B.-H. and Shim, C.-K., *J. Pharm. Sci.*, *76*:784 (1987).
270. Lin, S.-Y. and Yang, J.-C., *Drug Dev. Ind. Pharm.*, *14*:805 (1988).
271. Swartz, J. B., *J. Pharm. Sci.*, *63*:774 (1974).
272. Nogami, H., Fukusawa, H., and Nakai, Y., *Chem. Pharm. Bull.*, *11*:1389 (1963).
273. Lowenthal, W. and Burruss, R. A., *J. Pharm. Sci.*, *60*:1325 (1971).
274. Rispin, W. T., Selkirk, A. B., and Stones, P. W., *J. Pharm. Pharmacol.*, *23*(*Suppl*):215S (1971).
275. Matusmaru, H., *Yakugaku Zasshi*, *78*:1198 (1958).

276. Stanley-Wood, N. G. and Johansson, M. E., *Drug Dev. Ind. Pharm.*, 4:69 (1978).
277. Selkirk, A. B. and Ganderton, D., *J. Pharm. Pharmacol.*, *22(Suppl)*: 79S (1970).
278. Gucluyildiz, H., Banker, G. S., and Peck, G. E., *J. Pharm. Sci.*, *66*:407 (1977).
279. Dees, P. J., Jr., Dubois, F. L., Oomen, J. J. J., and Polderman, J., *Pharm. Weekbl.*, *113*:1297 (1978).
280. Lowenthal, W., *J. Pharm. Sci.*, *61*:303 (1972).
281. Higuchi, T., Arnold, R. D., Tucker, S. J., and Busse, L. W., *J. Am. Pharm. Assoc., Sci. Ed.*, *41*:93 (1952).
282. Lowenthal, W., *J. Pharm. Sci.*, *61*:1695 (1972).
283. Duberg, M. and Nystrom, C., *Powder Technol.*, *46*:67 (1986).
284. Porter, S. C., Bruno, C. H., and Jackson, G. J., in *Pharmaceutical Dosage Forms: Tablets*, Vol. 3 (H. A. Lieberman and L. Lachman, eds.), Marcel Dekker, New York, 1982, pp. 73–117.
285. Wood, J. A. and Harder, S. W., *Can. J. Pharm. Sci.*, *5*:18 (1970).
286. Nadkarni, P. D., Kildsig, D. O., Kramer, P. A., and Banker, G. S., *J. Pharm. Sci.*, *64*:1554 (1975).
287. Fisher, D. G. and Rowe, R. C., *J. Pharm. Pharmacol.*, *28*:866 (1976).
288. Rowe, R. C., *J. Pharm. Pharmacol.*, *29*:723 (1977).
289. Rowe, R. C., *J. Pharm. Pharmacol.*, *30*:473 (1979).
290. Rowe, R. C., *J. Pharm. Pharmacol.*, *30*:343 (1978).
291. *United States Pharmacopeia*, 21st Rev., Mack, Easton, Pennsylvania, 1985, pp. 1345–1347.
292. *Drop Test for Shipping Containers*, D880, Annual Book of ASTM Standard, Part 20, American Society for Testing and Mateials, Philadelphia, 1978, pp. 180–187.
293. *Incline Impact Test for Shipping Containers*, D880, Annual Book of ASTM Standards, Part 20, American Society for Testing and Materials, Philadelphia, 1978, pp. 229–233.
294. *Vibration Testing of Shipping Containers*, D999, Annual Book of ASTM Standards, Part 20, American Society for Testing and Materials, Philadelphia, 1978, pp. 282–285.

6

Bioavailability in Tablet Technology

Salomon A. Stavchansky and James W. McGinity

University of Texas at Austin, Austin, Texas

I. GENERAL CONSIDERATIONS

Drugs are administered locally for protective action, antisepsis, local anesthetic, and antibiotic effects, and they are given systemically for action on the cells and organs of the body or to counter the effects of invading organisms. A number of physiological and chemical factors are important in the absorption, distribution, and elimination of drugs in the body. Some of the properties of the buccal cavity, stomach, and small and large intestines that influence drug therapy are found in Tables 1 and 2.

When drugs are given for systemic action, a number of routes are available, including oral, rectal, parenteral, sublingual, and inhalation. After absorption into the body, a drug is distributed by the blood and lymphatic system and passes into the extracellular fluids of various tissues. The drug molecules may enter cells immediately and exert their pharmacological action in this way or be stored as a reservoir in muscle and fatty tissue for prolonged action. The drug may also be bound to albumin and other components of the plasma, altering tissue distribution and elimination from the body.

Drugs are metabolized by enzyme systems of the body, and this process is given the general term "biotransformation." The net effect may be inactivation or detoxification of the compound, or the drug may be converted from an inactive or prodrug form into the pharmacologically active species. For example, the azo dye Prontosil is reduced in the body to sulfanilamide, and the discovery of this conversion led to the development and use of sulfonamides as medicinal agents. Biotransformation is mainly handled in the liver, but the process also occurs in the kidneys, intestines, muscles, and blood.

Table 1 Physiological and Chemical Characteristics of Gastrointestinal Fluids in the Gastrointestinal Tract

Factors	Stomach	Small intestine
Properties of fluids[a]		
pH value	1–3	5–8
Volume of fluid available (ml)	50–250	25–125
Surface tension (dyn cm^{-1})	35–50	32–45
Viscosity (cP)	0.8–2.5	0.7–1.2
Buffer capacity[b]		
β (NaOH)	30–60	4–8
β (HCl)	600	8–16
Δt (°C)	0.3–0.8	0.62
Density	1.01	1.01
Water (%)	98	98
Juice secretion (liter day^{-1})	2–4	0.2–0.8
Water circulation (liter day^{-1})	1–5	1.5–5
Enzymes and electrolytes	Variable	Variable

[a]Fasting subjects, temperature 37°C.
[b]= mmol NaOH or HCl/liter × ΔpH × pH (stomach fluid 1.5 ± 0.1).
Source: Modified from Ref. 121.

Table 2 Buccal, Gastric, and Intestinal Fluids

	Daily volume (ml)	pH
Saliva	1200	6.0–7.0
Gastric secretion	2000	1.0–3.5
Pancreatic secretion	1200	8.0–8.3
Bile	700	7.8
Succus entericus	2000	7.8–8.0
Brunner's gland secretion	50	8.0–8.9
Larger intestinal secretion	60	7.5–8.0

Source: Modified from Ref. 121.

KIDNEY

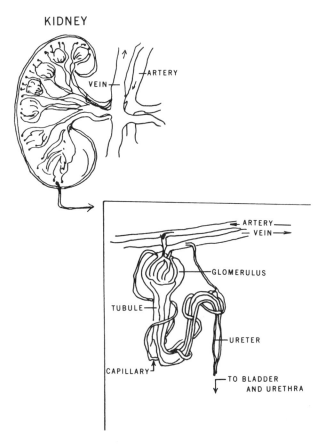

Figure 1   Schematic diagram of kidney.   A glomerulus and associated structure are enlarged and shown in the insert.

Whether biotransformed or not, the drug molecules must finally be eliminated from the body.   The kidneys are the principal organs of excretion, but foreign compounds may be eliminated from the lungs or in bile, saliva, and sweat.   The kidney (Fig. 1) is composed of millions of units consisting of a filtering capsule or glomerulus.   The liquid, which contains soluble excrement that is filtered through the glomerulus into the kidney tubules, is referred to as the glomerular filtrate.   The tubules are surrounded by capillaries, and some solute molecules present in the glomerular filtrate may be reabsorbed and returned to the bloodstream. Molecules of physiological importance, such as glucose, water, chloride, potassium, and sodium sions, are reabsorbed at various segments of the tubules.   Some drugs, such as penicillin G, do not pass through the glomerular apparatus but rather are actively transported from capillaries directly to the tubules where they are excreted in the urine.   Thus, owing to pH, active transport mechanisms, solubility, and ionic characteristics, drug molecules may be eliminated in the glomerular filtrate or directly absorbed into the tubules and excreted, and may be reabsorbed

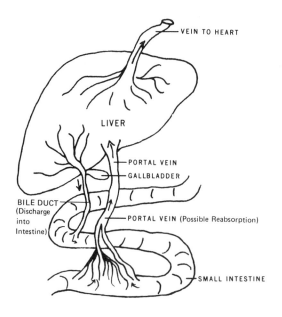

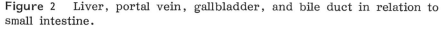

Figure 2   Liver, portal vein, gallbladder, and bile duct in relation to small intestine.

from the tubules into the systemic circulation for recycling through the body. The excretion of weakly acidic and basic drugs is influenced by the pH of the urine, and elimination of these compounds may be altered by controlling urinary pH. Alkalinizing the urine results in reabsorption of quinidine and may result in sufficiently high plasma levels of the drug as to manifest toxicity.

Biliary excretion has been found to be an important elimination route for some drugs (see Fig. 2). The drug present in the bile is discharged into the intestines and may be eliminated in the feces or into the vascular system from a region lower in the intestinal tract. Thus, as in kidney excretion, biliary passage may involve a cycle of elimination and reabsorption. This process, which occurs with morphine, penicillins, and a number of dyes, is called enterohepatic circulation; the process tends to promote higher and prolonged concentrations of the drug and its metabolites in the body than would be expected were the recycling process not involved. However, repeated passage through the liver may lead to significant metabolism of the drug.

The processes of diffusion and the partitioning of drug molecules across membranes as a function of pH, pK_a, and other factors will be discussed in later sections of this chapter.

The kinetics of absorption, distribution, and excretion of drugs following administration was first set forth by Teorell [1] in 1937 (Fig. 3).

A. Biopharmaceutics and Pharmacokinetics

A drug administered as a tablet or another dosage form must be released and reach its site of action in an active state before it can exert a

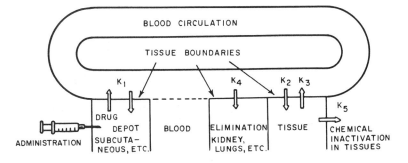

Figure 3 Schematic description of drug absorption, distribution, and elimination. (After Ref. 1.)

pharmacological response. The physical chemical properties of the drug, the characteristics of the dosage form in which the drug is administered, and the physiological factors controlling absorption, distribution, metabolism, and elimination of the drug must all be considered in order to formulate and manufacture effective and safe therapeutic agents. This wide range of considerations comprise the subject called biopharmaceutics.

Pharmacokinetics is a branch of biopharmaceutics and encompasses in a quantitative way the kinetics of absorption, distribution, metabolism, and excretion, often called ADME, of therapeutic agents and related chemical substances. The time course of passage of intact drugs and metabolites in various body tissues and fluids and the models constructed to interpret these data, which comprise the subjects of pharmacokinetics, will be introduced as elementary mathamatical expressions and graphs of data early in the chapter and elaborated upon in later sections. The final part of the chapter considers the elements of pharmacokinetics in some detail. The subject is presented step by step with worked examples, so that a reader with a background in pharmacy, chemistry, or biology but minimal grounding in mathematics can follow the treatment with relative ease.

At the beginning it is well to define some of the terms to be used throughout the chapter, particularly the words biopharmaceutics, pharmacokinetics, and bioequivalency. Some of the terms, as defined in the 1977 Bioequivalence Requirements and In Vitro Bioavailability Procedures of the FDA [2], are found in Table 3.

B. Bioequivalence

The forces that have led in the last decade to the concept of bioavailability were principally those due to the generic equivalence (bioequivalence) issue. Specifically, it is of the utmost importance to be assured that chemically equivalent drug products from different manufacturers result in essentially the same degree of therapeutic action.

An examination of the definitions as outlined in Table 3 shows that emphasis has been placed on the ability of two or more drug products to produce essentially identical blood levels in the same individual. The dosage form is a drug delivery system; it can be a good one or a poor one in its role of releasing the drug efficiently for absorption into the systemic circulation or site of action. Thus, appropriate testing of generic products

Table 3 Definition of Terms Dealing with Bioavailability and
Bioequivalence

Drug	Active therapeutic moiety.
Drug product	Delivery system, tablet, capsule, suspension (e.g., containing the therpeutic moiety), generally but not necessarily in association with inactive ingredients.
Bioavailability	The rate and extent to which the active drug ingredient or therapeutic moiety is absorbed from a drug product and beocmes available at the site of action.
Bioequivalent drug products	Pharmaceutical equivalents or alternatives whose rate and extent of absorption are not significantly different when administered to humans at the same molar dose under similar conditions.
Pharmaceutical equivalents	Drug products identical in amount of active drug ingredient and dosage form, and meeting compendial or other standards for identity, strength, quality, and purity. They may not be identical in terms of inactive ingredients. An example is erythromycin stearate tablets (Brand X and Brand Y).
Pharmaceutical alternatives	Drug products that contain the identical therapeutic moiety or its precursor but not necessarily in the same amount or dosage form and not necessarily as the same salt or ester. Examples are erythromycin stearate versus erythromycin ester; chlorpheniramine maleate chewable tablets versus chlorpheniramine maleate capsules.
Bioequivalence requirements	A requirement imposed by the FDA for in vitro and/or in vivo testing of specified drug products which must be satisfied as a condition of marketing.

must be conducted. These tests are not done only through clinical trials of efficacy since it is ordinarily not the drug that is in question but the dosage form; the latter primarily influencing the absorption step. It is the absorption process or factors connected with the delivery system that must be studied to assure proper bioavailability of the drug and bioequivalence of products from one manufacturer to another and from batch to batch.

A number of studies of marketed drug products containing the same chemical ingredient have revealed differences in bioavailability. Examples of problems with chemically equivalent drug products include tetracycline [3,4], chloramphenicol [5], digoxin [6,7], phenylbutazone [8,9], and oxytetracycline [10,11]. In addition, variations in bioavailability of different batches of digoxin from the same company have been demonstrated [7]. In one report, a thyroid preparation that met compendial standards was found to be therapeutically inactive [12]. Since lack of bioequivalence in these examples involves marketed products, it can be concluded that neither standards for testing the finished product nor specifications for materials, manufacturing processes, and controls are presently adequate to ensure that drug products are bioequivalent. Good Laboratory Practice and Good Manufacturing Practice regulations promulgated by the U.S. Food and Drug Administration (FDA) will assist in correcting the problem, but specific actions regarding bioavailability must be taken to assure equivalent marketed products. In most instances it is concluded that therapeutic inequivalence is a result of variations in the bioavailability of drug products.

C. Relative Bioavailability and Drug Performance

If a drug is administered at a dosage level that does not greatly exceed the minimum effective blood concentration (MEC) required, the availability of the drug from the dosage form may greatly influence the drug's performance. Figure 4 schematically illustrates this case. In curve I the product formulation causes the drug to have a good therapeutic response. In curve II, because of a delayed rate of absorption, the effective response is more transient. The slow absorption process of curve III leads to a lack of pharmacological response, even through the amount absorbed as determined by the total area under the curve is equal to the other two. This example illustrates that although the amount of drug absorbed may not differ, the rate of absorption of three products may be quite different, leading to variations in therapeutic action. A real example is presented in Figure 5, illustrating the work by Sullivan et al. [13]. It shows average

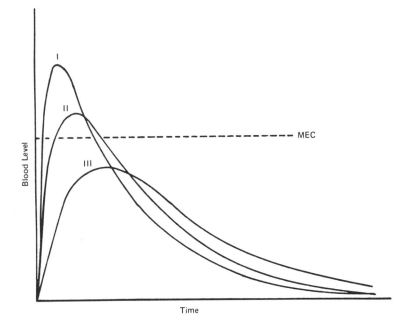

Figure 4   Blood levels from three products, illustrating differences in the rate of absorption but not in the total amount of drug absorbed.

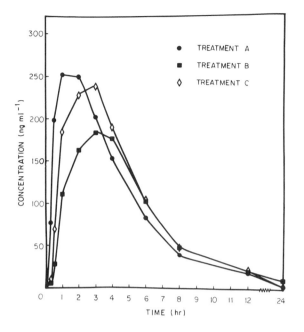

Figure 5 Average plasma levels of prednisone in nine adult volunteers following oral administration of 10 mg of prednisone (as two 5-mg tablets). (From Ref. 13.)

plasma levels of prednisone obtained in nine adult volunteers in a three-way crossover study when a 10-mg dose of prednisone was administered as two 5-mg tablets made by three different manufacturers.   Treatment A gave the fastest absorption and highest plasma levels.   Treatments B and C were two generic prednisone tablets that had a history of clinical failure and did not pass the USP tablet dissolution test.   Treatment A passed all compendial tests in the laboratories of the FDA.   In this case the rate of appearance of prednisone in plasma was different for the three tablets, although the average areas under the plasma concentration-time curves of individual subjects did not differ significantly.   This is a case in which documented evidence of clinical failure with generic tablets can be related to differences in rates of absorption.

Figure 6 illustrates the results obtained by Glazko et al. [5] when testing four capsules of chloramphenicol in human subjects.   Here the principal difference, as indicated by the area under the curve, is that the four products differ in the total amount of chloramphenicol absorbed. Product A gave an excellent blood level curve in subjects, whereas the other three formulations gave poor plasma levels.   Because of these data, the FDA had products B, C, and D recalled and reformulated, and then instituted requirements that have brought the problem of chloramphenicol products under control.   The significance of this finding is that all the products were chemically equivalent.   That is, they contained the correct amount of chloramphenicol, and the particle size of the drug in each of the products was similar.   Figure 7 illustrates the results obtained by

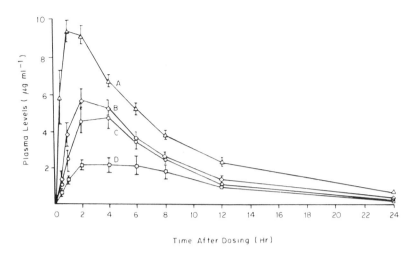

Figure 6 Mean plasma levels for groups of 10 human subjects receiving single 0.5-g oral doses of chloramphenicol capsules. Vertical lines represent one standard error on either side of the mean. Capsule A, △; capsule B, ◇; capsule C, ○; capsule D, □. (From Ref. 5.)

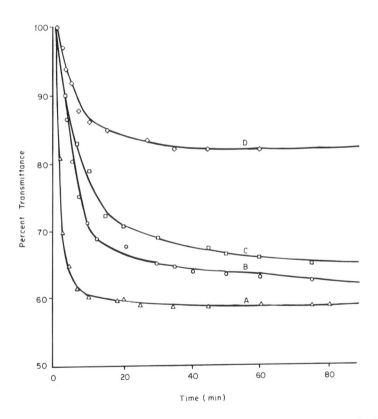

Figure 7 Relative disintegration rates of chloramphenicol capsules in simulated gastric fluid. Capsule A, △; capsule B, ○; capsule C, □; capsule D, ◇. (From Ref. 14.)

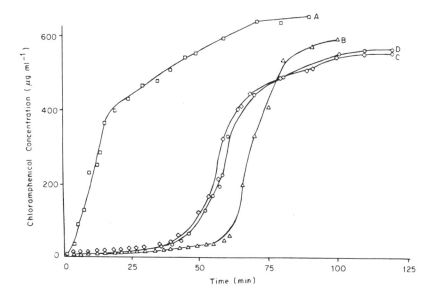

Figure 8 Dissolution rates of chloramphenicol capsules in simulated gastric fluid. Capsule A, □; capsule B, △; capsule C, ◇; capsule D, ○. (From Ref. 14.)

Aguiar, showing that the disintegration rates of the four products differed greatly [14]. Product A, the one that produced the highest plasma level in the study by Glazko, had excellent disintegration characteristics, whereas products B and C showed poor rates, and product D, the product having the poorest plasma level in patients, exhibited the poorest disintegration rate. In fact, product D had such poor disintegration properties that the powder mass maintained its capsule shape in simulated gastric fluid after the gelatin capsule had dissolved. The results in Figure 8 demonstrate the performance of the four products in a dissolution rate test. When product A was placed in simulated gastric fluid, it dissolved rapidly, whereas products B, C, and D showed greater lag times prior to dissolution, principally because of the time required for deaggregation [14].

Dissolution tests and disintegration tests in some cases have been shown to correlate well with human bioavailability tests, as evidenced by the previous example. Lindenbaum's work on digoxin is another example of in vivo/in vitro correlations [7].

The FDA, in its bioequivalence preamble, stated [2]:

> Advances in pharmaceutical technology have made bioequivalence a most precise and reproducible method for determining drug product variability. These bioequivalence techniques are not inadequately defined or reachless concepts. They are scientifically valid methods of comparing different drug products as well as different batches of the same drug products.

It is indeed fortunate that dissolution methodology frequently provides a measure of variability among drug dosage forms. The conclusion that can be drawn from the bioequivalence requirements and in vivo bioavailability procedures of the FDA, published in the *Federal Register* of January 1977, is that dissolution testing will more than likely become the most frequently used means of testing and assuring bioequivalence [2]. Although it will probably not be the only criterion for obtaining marketing approval, the FDA report states that "a dissolution test may constitute a proper element in reaching the decision to approve an NDA or supplemental application for a drug product with a bioequivalence problem." In another section of this chapter we discuss some of the methodology presently available for dissolution testing.

The digoxin tablet problem is an example of a situation that led to establishment by the FDA of a dissolution rate certification requirement and adoption of a dissolution specification by the USP. Digoxin is a drug in which the effective blood level is close to the toxic concentration. Product formulation may greatly influence the rate and extent of absorption, and consequently the therapeutic activity and toxicity of digoxin.

D. Federal Regulations Covering Bioavailability and Bioequivalence

In the *Federal Register* of January 1973 [15], the FDA published proposed bioavailability requirements for new drugs and for generic drug products. These proposals became regulations as published in the *Federal Register* of January 1977 [2], with appropriate modifications as suggested by various individuals and groups. The regulations clearly establish that studies must be undertaken with new drugs or new dosage forms to assure that optimal absorption characteristics are achieved.

The selection of the reference material (standard drug sample) as stated by the FDA is an important consideration. It depends upon the scientific questions to be answered, the data needed to establish comparability with a currently marketed drug product, and the data needed to establish dosage regimens. The reference material should be taken from a current batch of a drug product that is the subject of an approved new drug application and that contains the same active drug ingredient or therapeutic moiety. Thus, tetracycline hydrochloride cannot be the reference product for tetracycline phosphate; salts cannot be compared against esters, capsules cannot be compared with tablets.

In the report of the Office of Technology Assessment (OTA), Drug Bioequivalence Study Panel [16], it was concluded that studies on bioavailability are neither feasible nor desirable for all drugs or drug products. According to OTA, certain classes of drug should be identified for which evidence of bioequivalence is critical. Selection of these classes would be based on clinical importance, ratio of therapeutic to toxic concentration in blood, and certain pharmaceutical characteristics. The panel believed, however, that bioavailability studies should be required for products if the active ingredient in the product had not yet been introduced into the market.

A large number of drug products are available on the market, and for only a few of these are there adequate data documenting bioavailability in humans. Thus, many bioavailability studies would be required; this involves large numbers of human volunteers and the expense of clinical investigators and other scientific personnel. Consequently, it is not feasible and justifiable to carry out studies of bioavailability in humans for all drug products. In asserting that studies of bioavailability will not be required for all drug products, it becomes important to set general criteria to guide the selection of those products whose bioavailability should be documented by testing in humans, those requiring no testing, and those few in which in vitro methodology would be deemed adequate. The report of the OTA study panel concluded that for drugs with a wide therapeutic range, moderate differences in drug blood levels, owing to differences in bioavailability of chemically equivalent products, would be tolerated. Conversely, drugs that have a relatively narrow therapeutic range would be candidates for testing of bioavailability on human subjects. Examples of drugs that fall into this category include cardioactive agents (digitalis glycosides), anticonvulsants (diphenylhydantoin), some corticosteroids, and certain antibiotics (chloramphenicol and cephalosporins). In summary, drug products will be considered candidates for human bioavailability studies if they:

Are used for treatment or prevention of serious illness
Have steep dose-response curves or unfavorable therapeutic indices
Contain active ingredients that are relatively insoluble or are converted to insoluble forms in the gastrointestinal fluids

In the *Federal Register* of January 1977, the FDA [2] published criteria for waiver of evidence of bioavailability. The requirement for submission of in vivo bioavailability data will be waived if:

1. The drug product meets both of the following conditions:
   a. It is a solution intended solely for intravenous administration.
   b. It contains an active drug ingredient or therapeutic moiety in the same solvent and concentration as an intravenous solution that is the subject of an approved full new drug application.
2. The drug product is a topically applied preparation (e.g., a cream, ointment, or gel) intended for local therapeutic effect.
3. The drug product is an oral dosage form that is not intended to be absorbed (e.g., an antacid or a radiopaque medium).
4. The drug product meets both of the following conditions:
   a. It is an oral solution, elixir, syrup, tincture, or similar other solubilized form.
   b. It contains an active drug ingredient or therapeutic moiety in the same concentration as a drug product that is the subject of an approved full new drug application.
   c. It contains no inactive ingredient that is known to significantly affect absorption of the active drug ingredient or therapeutic moiety.

The regulations proceed to list drugs for which in vivo bioavailability data of solid oral dosage forms need not be submitted to the FDA.

For certain drug products, bioavailability may be demonstrated by evidence obtained in vitro in lieu of in vivo data. The FDA waives the requirements for the submission of evidence obtained in vivo demonstrating the bioavailability of the drug product if the drug product meets one of the following criteria:

1. The drug product is subjected to the bioequivalence requirement established by the Food and Drug Administration under Subpart C of this part that specifies only an in vitro testing requirement.

2. The drug product is in the same dosage form, but in a different strength, and is proportionally similar in its active and inactive ingredients to another drug product made by the same manufacturer and the following conditions are met:
   a. The bioavailability of this other drug product has been demonstrated.
   b. Both drug products meet an appropriate in vitro test approved by the Food and Drug Administration.
   c. The applicant submits evidence showing that both drug products are proportionally similar in their active and inactive ingredients.

3. The drug product is, on the basis of scientific evidence submitted in the application, shown to meet an in vitro test that assures bioavailability (i.e., an in vitro test that has been correlated with in vivo data).

4. The drug product is a reformulated product that is identical, except for color, flavor, or preservative, to another drug product made by the same manufacturer and both of the following conditions are met:
   a. The bioavailability of the other product has been demonstrated.
   b. Both drug products meet an appropriate in vitro test approved by the Food and Drug Administration.

5. The drug product contains the same active drug ingredient or therapeutic moiety and is in the same strength and dosage form as a drug product that is the subject of an approved full or abbreviated new drug application, and both drug products meet an appropriate in vitro test that has been approved by the Food and Drug Administration.

The FDA, for good cause, may defer or waive a requirement for the submission of evidence of in vivo bioavailability if deferral or waiver is compatible with the protection of the public health.

In the 1970s the FDA developed what is now known as the Approved Drug Products with Therapeutic Evaluation Publication [17] (referred to in text as the List). The List was distributed as a proposal in January 1979. It included only currently marketed prescription drug products approved by FDA through new drug applications (NDAs) or abbreviated new drug applications (ANDAs) under the provisions of Section 505 or 507 of the Federal Food, Drug, and Cosmetic Act (the Act). The therapeutic equivalence evaluations in the List reflect FDA's application of specific criteria to the approved multisource prescription drug products on the List. These evaluations are presented in the form of code letters that indicate the basis for the evaluation made.

A complete discussion of the background and basis of FDA's therapeutic equivalence evaluation policy was published in the *Federal Register* on January 12, 1979 (44 FR 2932). The final rule, which includes FDA's responses to the public comments on the proposal, was published in the

Federal Register on October 31, 1980 (45 FR 72582). The first publication, October 1980, of the final version of the List incorporated appropriate corrections and additions. Each subsequent edition has included the latest approvals and data changes.

On September 24, 1984, the President signed into law the Drug Price Competition and Patent Term Restoration Act (1984 Amendments). The 1984 Amendments require that FDA, among other things, make publicly available a list of approved drug products with monthly supplements. The *Approved Drug Products with Therapeutic Equivalence Evaluations* publication and its monthly Cumulative Supplements satisfy this requirement.

The main criterion for the inclusion of any product in the List, is that the product is the subject of an approved application that has not been withdrawn for safety or efficacy reasons. Inclusion of products on the List is independent of any current regulatory action through administrative or legal means against a drug product. In addition, the List contains therapeutic equivalence evaluations for approved multisource prescription drug products.

The List is composed of four parts: approved prescription drug products with therapeutic equivalence evaluations, over-the-counter (OTC) drug products that require approved applications as a condition of marketing, drug products in the Division of Blood and Blood Products approved under Section 505 of the Act, and products discontinued from marketing or products which have had their approval withdrawn for other than safety or efficacy reasons. This publication also includes indices of prescription and OTC drug products by trade or established name and by applicant name (holder of the approved application), and a list of applicants' abbreviated name designations. In addition, a list of uniform terms is provided. An Addendum contains appropriate drug patent and exclusivity information for the Prescription, OTC, and Drug Products in the Division of Blood and Blood Products Approved Under Section 505 of the Act lists.

E. In Vitro Indexes of Bioavailability

In view of these regulations, additional research aimed at improving the assessment and prediction of bioequivalence is needed. It is important that this research include efforts to develop in vitro tests that will be valid predictors of bioavailability in humans. If in vitro dissolution properties for a drug are found to serve as a useful index of in vivo absorption, the time, expense, and difficulties of clinical studies may be reduced or eliminated. Levy et al. [18] and Wagner [19] have shown in several cases that correlations exist between in vitro testing and in vivo absorption.

In vitro dissolution rate screening has been used [20] as a sensitive quality control measure to show changes in drug release for products undergoing variable storage conditions. It is also used to warn of poor bioavailability of drugs from dosage forms that show erratic release patterns in comparative studies.

An early investigation by Nelson [21] demonstrated a correlation between in vitro dissolution rate and the speed at which tetracycline in four different dosage forms was excreted in vivo. Levy [22] showed a linear correlation between salicylate excretion following oral administration of two aspirin tablets and rate of in vitro dissolution. Levy went on to demonstrate a correlation between percent of drug absorbed and rate of dissolution. MacDonald et al. [23] found differences in in vivo availability among tetracycline capsules from various sources and attempted to correlate these differences by an in vitro method using an automated dissolution apparatus. The authors reported that they were partially successful in their goal. Bergan et al. [24] determined that in vitro dissolution rates of two tetracycline and seven oxytetracycline preparations and compared them with absorption characteristics as obtained by a crossover study on 10 volunteers. The products showed marked variations in bioavailability. The rate of dissolution was found to correlate well with absorption characteristics for some products but not for others.

Other workers [25,26] have found good correlation between dissolution rate and drug plasma levels. However, correlations cannot always be expected between in vivo and in vitro results. The failure of good correlation is the result of a number of factors, including improper in vitro stirring rate, variable gastric emptying time, rapid versus slow absorbers, failure of dissolution to be the rate-limiting step in vivo, and other problems.

F. Methodology for Conducting Bioavailability Studies

In 1972, the Academy of Pharmaceutical Sciences [27] published Guidelines for Biopharmaceutical Studies in Man. This monograph presents a systematic approach to the conduct of bioavailability studies based on analytical determination of drug in blood and/or urine.

In January 1977, the FDA [2] published in the *Federal Register* the Characteristics of good analytical methodology for an in vivo bioavailability study. They stated that the method for

metabolite(s), in body fluids or excretory products, or the method used to measure an acute pharmacological effect shall be demonstrated to be accurate and of sufficient sensitivity to measure, with appropriate precision, the actual concentration of the active drug ingredient or therapeutic moiety, or its metabolite(s), achieved in the body.

In addition, when the analytical method is not sensitive enough to measure accurately the concentration of the active drug ingredient or therapeutic moiety, or its "metabolite(s), in body fluids or excretory products produced by a single dose of the test product, two or more single doses may be given together to produce higher concentration."

It is interesting that the regulations were not more specific in their analytical requirements. For example, no distinction is made between chemical, radioactive, microbiological, and other methods. Radioactive methods are used extensively today in drug development, and the investigators must be careful to verify that the measured radioactivity is contained in the intact compound separated from its metabolites. It is also important to recognize that the dosage form containing the radioactive drug to be tested possess physical and chemical properties identical to those of the unlabeled dosage form.

The 1977 monograph of the FDA [2] listed the following general approaches for determining bioavailability:

1. Bioavailability is usually determined by measurement of:
    a. The concentration of the active drug ingredient or therapeutic moiety, or its metabolite(s), in biological fluids as a function of time; or
    b. The urinary excretion of the therapeutic moiety or its metabolite(s) as a function of time; or
    c. An appropriate acute pharmacological effect.
2. Bioavailability may be determined by several direct or indirect in vivo methods, generally involving testing in humans. The selection of the method depends upon the purpose of the study, the analytical method available, and the nature of the drug product. These limitations affect the degree to which precise pharmacokinetic studies can be applied and, in some cases, necessitate the use of other methods. Bioavailability testing shall be conducted using the most accurate, sensitive, and reproducible approach available among those set forth in paragraph (c) of this section.
3. The following in vivo approaches, in descending order of accuracy, sensititivity, and reproducibility, are acceptable for determining the bioavailability of a drug product:
    a. In vivo testing in humans in which the concentration of the active drug ingredient or therapeutic moiety or its metabolite(s), in whole blood, plasma, serum, or other appropriate biological fluid is measured as a function of time, or in which the urinary excretion of the therapeutic moiety, or its metabolite(s), is measured as a function of time. This approach is particularly applicable to dosage forms intended to deliver the active drug ingredient or therapeutic moiety to the bloodstream for systemic distribution within the body (i.e., injectable drugs, most oral dosage forms, most suppositories, certain drugs administered by inhalation, and some drugs administered by local application to mucous membranes).
    b. In vivo testing in humans in which an appropriate acute pharmacological effect of the active drug ingredient or therapeutic moiety, or metabolite(s), is measured as a function of time if such effect can be measured with sufficient accuracy, sensitivity, and reproducibility. This approach is applicable when appropriate methods are not available for measurement of the concentration of the active drug ingredient or therapeutic moiety, or its metabolite(s), in biological fluids or excretory products but a method is available for the measurement of an appropriate acute pharmacological effect. This approach is applicable to the same dosage forms listed in paragraph (3, a) of this section.
    c. Well-controlled clinical trials in humans that establish the safety and effectiveness of the drug product. This approach is the least accurate, sensitive, and reproducible of the general approaches for determining in vivo bioavailability in humans. For dosage forms intended to deliver the active drug ingredient or therapeutic moiety to the bloodstream for systemic distribution within the body, this approach shall be considered as providing a sufficiently accurate estimate of in vivo bioavailability only when analytical methods are not available to permit use of one of the approaches outlined in paragraph (3,

a and b) of this section. This approach shall also be considered as sufficiently accurate for determining the bioavailability of dosage forms intended to deliver the therapeutic moiety locally (e.g., topical preparations for the skin, eye, ear, musous membranes); oral dosage forms not intended to be absorbed (e.g., an antacid or a radiopaque medium); and bronchodilators administered by inhalation if the onset and duration of pharmacological activity are defined.

d. Any other in vivo approach approved by the Food and Drug Administration intended for special situations should include those circumstances where the in vivo bioavailability of a drug product might be determined in a suitable animal model rather than in humans or by using a radioactive or nonradioactive isotopically labeled drug product.

When a drug dosage form is administered to humans and/or animals and serial blood samples are obtained and quantified for drug content, data are obtained as a function of time. This enables one to graphically represent the results as illustrated in Figure 9. The curve can be mathematically analyzed and pharmacokinetic parameters obtained as discussed in Section IV. However, it should be noted that there are three important parameters necessary for the interpretation of bioavailability studies. These include the peak height concentration, the time of the peak concentration, and the area under the plasma concentration-time curve. The peak height is important because it gives an indication of the intensity,

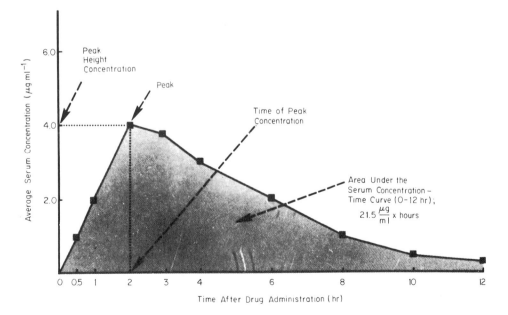

Figure 9 Serum concentration-time curve following a single dose of a drug that shows an absorption phase and an elimination phase. (From Ref. 27.)

and in conjunction with the minimum effective concentration (MEC), provides an indication of duration of action. The time for the peak to occur
is important because it is related to the rate of absorption of the drug
from dosage form after oral administration. It should only be considered
as a simple measurement of rate of absorption. The area under the curve
is perhaps one of the most important parameters. It represents, in this
case, the amount of drug absorbed following a single administration of the
drug.

Several integration techniques may be used to determine the area
under the curve, and the accuracy of the value obtained will vary depending on the integration technique selected. The following integration methods (in decreasing order of accuracy) have been employed [28]:

1. Milne fifth-order predictor-corrector
2. Range-Kutta fourth order
3. Adams second order
4. Simpson's rule
5. Trapezoidal rule
6. Rectangular rule

The trapezoid rule has gained popularity, although it is not the most
accurate method. It is described in a later section, where the trapezoidal
rule is used in a sample calculation.

Let us assume that a bioavailability study is conducted with the purpose of comparing two different formulations containing the same therapeutic moiety. The results of these studies are graphically illustrated in
Figure 10. It can be concentration and time to peak. The area under the

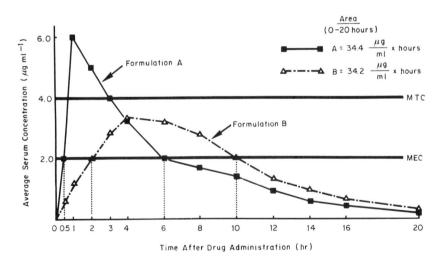

Figure 10 Serum concentration-time curves obtained for two different
formulations of the same drug given at the same dose. The relationship of
the curves to the minimum toxic concentration (MTC) and minimum effective concentration (MEC) is shown. (From Ref. 27.)

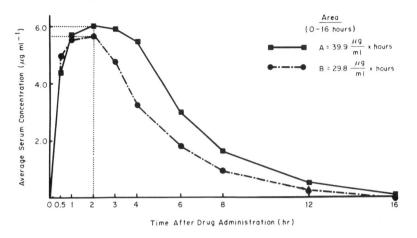

Figure 11 Serum concentration-time curves obtained for two formulations of the same drug given at the same dose, showing similar peak heights and times, but significantly different areas under the curve. (From Ref. 27.)

concentration-time curve for each formulation is the same, indicating that the extent (amount) of drug absorption is the same for both formulations. However, since disparities exist with regard to peak height and time to peak, these formulations cannot be considered to be bioequivalent. Consequently, they may not perform equivalently in terms of efficacy and toxicity. It should be emphasized that differences between formulations are reflected in rate of absorption and not in extent of obsorption. Figure 11 illustrates an example in which the rate of absorption is the same for both formulations, as observed by the same time to peak and peak concentration, but the extent of drug absorption as reflected by the areas under the respective concentration curves is different. In neither of the cases can the formulations be considered bioequivalent; these are clear examples of inequivalence in bioavailability. Wagner [29] summarized the different types of comparative bioavailability studies.

Figures 12 to 14 depict methods of estimating bioavailability based on studies in humans where blood levels, urinary excretion, or acute pharmacological response are measured. The methods can be classified depending on the measurement that is made: Figure 12 considers measurement of unchanged drug, Figure 13 a metabolite of a drug, and Figure 14, the total drug, that is, metabolite(s) plus unchanged drug. The symbol τ represents the dosing interval.

The quantitative aspects of biopharmaceutics and pharmacokinetics and associated methods are presented in later sections of the chapter. But before we can study the absorption kinetics of a drug, we should become familiar with the preparation of protocols for comparative bioavailability testing, and then examine various factors, both physiological and physical chemical, which influence the release of a drug from its dosage form and absorption into the systemic circulation.

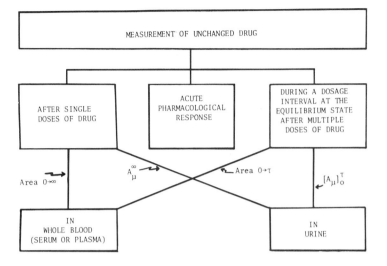

Figure 12 Measurement of unchanged drug for the estimation of bioavailability. Area 0 → ∞ = area under concentration curve from zero to
infinite time. Area 0 → τ = area under concentration curve within a dosage
interval τ. A_μ^∞ = amount of unchanged drug excreted in the urine in infinite time after a single dose. $[A_\mu]_0^\tau$ = amount of unchanged drug excreted in the urine during a dosage interval τ. (From Ref. 29.)

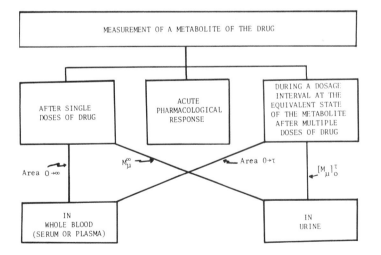

Figure 13 Measurement of a drug metabolite for the estimation of bioavailability. M_μ^∞ = the amount of a metabolite excreted in the urine in
infinite time. $[M_\mu]_0^\tau$ = the amount of metabolite excreted in the urine in a
dosage interval τ. (From Ref. 29.)

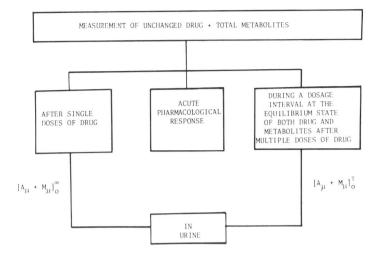

Figure 14 Measurement of unchanged drug and total metabolites for the estimation of bioavailability. $[A_\mu + M_\mu]_0^\infty$ = total amount of unchanged drug and all metabolites excreted in the urine in infinite time. $[A_\mu + M_\mu]_0^\tau$ = total amount of unchanged drug and all metabolites excreted in the urine during a dosage interval τ. (From Ref. 29.)

G. Protocols for Comparative Bioavailability Trials

The success of any experiment lies in its design. For this reason, protocols for bioavailability studies are of extreme importance. At the 13th Annual International Industrial Pharmacy Conference at Lakeway, Texas, Skelly [30] discussed the elements of a good protocol. His intent was to make it easier for the FDA and the applicant to recognize and resolve differences of opinion before a study got under way rather than after, in order to expedite the review of drugs where bioavailability is a critical requirement for approval.

The protocol guidelines for ANDA and NDA submissions as suggested by Skelly [30] include information on the drug and its clinical use; clinical facilities to be used and investigators responsible for the study; a plan of experimentation including reference to subjects involved; drugs to be administered; the treatment plan; sample collection; chemical, pharmacological, and/or clinical end points; assay methodology; and data analysis. Appendices to the protocol should include the consent form, precautions for the subject regarding possible adverse reactions, subject instruction sheet, clinical chemistry form, and an insert describing the characteristics of the drug. The reader should refer to the original paper [30] for a detailed outline of the proposed protocol.

H. Statistical Considerations of Bioavailability/ Bioequivalence Studies

Donald Schuirmann [31], in a very elegant way, discussed the statistical issue associated with the analysis of bioavailability/bioequivalence studies.

Briefly, the issue that has received the most attention in the pharmaceutical and statistical literature is the question of statistical methods for determining whether two formulations of a drug have been shown to be equivalent with respect to average bioavailability in the population. Bioavailability, in this context, is to be characterized by one or more blood concentration profile variables, such as area under the blood concentration-time curve (AUC), maximum concentration (C_{max}), etc., and possibly by urinary excretion variables as well.

Hauck and Anderson [32], in an article in which they proposed a new approach to this problem, gave a clear explanation of why the null hypothesis of *no difference* between the two averages, as tested by the "treatments" F test from the analysis of variance of a two-treatment (formulation) study, is the wrong statistical hypothesis for assessing the evidence in favor of a conclusion of equivalence. And yet, as Hauck and Anderson note, the test of the hypothesis of no difference is still utilized by many who seek to demonstrate equivalence of two formulations. In most cases those who utilize the test of the hypothesis of no difference supplement it with some assessment of what the power of the test would have been if the averages had been different enough to be considered inequivalent. This Power Approach, as it will be called, has been a standard method in bioequivalence testing, in spite of the fact that it is based on the test of an inappropriate statistical hypothesis.

Schuirmann compares this power approach to another method for assessing the equivalence of two formulations which will be called the *Two One-Sided Tests Procedure*. Then the two one-sided tests procedure was compared to the proposed method of Hauck and Anderson.

Schuirmann concluded that for the specific choice of $\alpha = 0.05$ as the nominal level of the one-sided tests, the two one-sided tests procedure has uniformly superior properties to the power approach in most cases. The only cases where the power approach has superior properties when the true averages are equivalent correspond to cases where the chance of concluding equivalence with the power approach when the true averages are not equivalent exceeds 0.05. With appropriate choice of the nominal level of significance of the one-sided tests, the two one-sided test procedure always has uniformly superior properties to the power approach.

The Two One-Sided Tests Procedure

The Two One-Sided Tests Procedure, as its name implies, consists of decomposing the interval hypothesis H_0 and H_1 into two sets of one-sided hypotheses

$$H_{01}: \quad \mu_T - \mu_R \leq \theta_1$$

$$H_{11}: \quad \mu_T - \mu_R > \theta_1$$

and

$$H_{02}: \quad \mu_T - \mu_R \geq \theta_2$$

$$H_{12}: \quad \mu_T - \mu_R < \theta_2$$

The two one-sided tests procedure consists of rejecting the interval hypothesis H_0, and thus concluding equivalence of μ_T and μ_R, if and only if both H_{01} *and* H_{02} are rejected at a chosen *nominal level of significance* α. The logic underlying the two one-sided tests procedure is that if one may conclude that $\theta_1 < \mu_T - \mu_R$, and may also conclude that $\mu_T - \mu_R \leqslant \theta_2$, then it has in effect been concluded that $\theta_1 < \mu_T - \mu_R < \theta_2$.

Under the normality assumption that has been made, the two sets of one-sided hypothesis will be tested with ordinary one-sided t tests. Thus it will be concluded that μ_T and μ_R are equivalent (for a balanced study) if

$$t_1 = \frac{(\overline{X}_T - \overline{X}_{12}) - \theta_1}{s\sqrt{2/n}} \geqslant t_{1-\alpha(v)}$$

and

$$t_2 = \frac{\theta_2 - (\overline{X}_T - \overline{X}_R)}{s\sqrt{2/n}} \geqslant t_{1-\alpha(v)}$$

where, once again, s is the square root of the "error" mean square from the crossover design analysis of variance. $t_{1-\alpha(v)}$ is the point that isolates probability α in the upper tail of the Student's t distribution with v degrees of freedom associated with the "error" mean square.

The two one-sided test procedure turns out to be operationally identical to the procedure of declaring equivalence only if the ordinary $1 - 2\alpha$ (not $1 - \alpha$) confidence interval for $\mu_T - \mu_R$ is completely contained in the equivalence interval $[\theta_1, \theta_2]$. For this reason, it is sometimes referred to as the confidence interval approach. In this form, it has been recommended by Westlake [33].

Unbalanced Crossover Studies

Schuirmann [31] discussed the statistical procedure for unbalanced studies. The assumption made previously is that the bioavailability/bioequivalence study under consideration was a balanced crossover study, that is

1. There is an equal number of subjects in each treatment-administration sequence.
2. There are no missing observations from any subject.

All of the results cited above concerning the properties of the two one-sided tests procedure and the power approach are equally true for unbalanced crossover studies. If we let *Est.* be the estimator of $\mu_T - \mu_R$, and SE be the standard error of the estimator, then the two one-sided tests procedure utilizes the two test statistics.

$$t_1 = \frac{Est. - \theta_1}{SE} \qquad \text{and} \qquad t_2 = \frac{\theta_2 - Est.}{SE}$$

In the case of balanced studies, the estimator *Est.* is in fact the difference of the *observed* means, $\overline{X}_T - \overline{X}_R$, and therefore the standard error SE is equal to $s\sqrt{2/n}$. In the case of unbalanced studies, the best unbiased (least squares) estimator of $\mu_T - \mu_R$ is *not*, in general, the difference of observed means.

For the special case of a two-treatment, two-period crossover study in which n_1 subjects receive the test formulation in period one and the reference formulation in period two, while n_2 subjects receive the reference formulation in period one and the test formulation in period two, the unbiased estimator is given by

$$Est. = \frac{\overline{X}_{T1} + \overline{X}_{T2}}{2} - \frac{\overline{X}_{R1} + \overline{X}_{R2}}{2}$$

where

$\overline{X}_{T1}$ = The observed mean of the n_1 observations on the test formulation in period one.

$\overline{X}_{T2}$ = The observed mean of the n_2 observations on the test formulation in period two.

$\overline{X}_{R1}$ = The observed mean of the n_2 observations on the reference formulation in period one.

$\overline{X}_{R2}$ = The observed mean of the n_1 observations on the reference formulation in period two.

$$Se = s\sqrt{\frac{1}{2}\left(\frac{1}{n_1} + \frac{1}{n_2}\right)}$$

where as before s is the square root of the "error" mean square from the crossover design analysis of variance, based on v degrees of freedom.

Note that if $n_1 = n_2$, these formulas reduce to *Est.* $\overline{X}_T - \overline{X}_R$ and $s\sqrt{2/n}$ (where n = total number of subjects = $n_1 + n_2$) as before.

In the case of a study with more than two treatments (formulations) and/or periods, the formulas for *Est.* and SE will depend on the particular pattern of unbalance, and can be very complicated. Usually a computer routine will be needed to obtain them. The following example will illustrate the use of the two one-sided *t*-test.

A two-way crossover bioequivalence study was conducted on 27 subjects. The study is a balance study in the statistical sense. The following data was obtained from the Division of Generic Drugs at the FDA (Personal Communication).

Test product mean = 20.69

Reference product mean = 20.51

Error degrees of freedom = 26

t-value for 26 d$_f$ = 1.7081

Error mean square = 5.41186

Number of subjects N = 27

Thus

$$20.96 - 20.51 \pm 1.708 \times \sqrt{5.41186} \times \sqrt{2/27}$$

$$0.18 \pm 1.080 \text{ or}$$

$$-0.9008 \text{ and } 1.2608$$

Using 100% as the reference value, the lower limit of confidence interval will be

$$-0.9008/20.51 = -0.0439 \text{ or } -4.39\%$$

$$100\% - 4.39\% = 95.61\% \text{ lower limit.}$$

The upper limit of the confidence interval will be

$$1.2608/20.51 = 0.0615 \text{ or } 6.15\%$$

$$100\% + 6.15\% = 106.15\% \text{ upper limit.}$$

In conclusion, the confidence interval will be

$$95.61\% - 106.15\%$$

I. Common Pitfalls in Evaluating Bioavailability Data

Shrikant Dighé [34] has discussed the current Bioavailability and Bioequivalence requirements and regulations. In his discussion he indicated that despite the progress in the conduct of bioequivalence studies the FDA has observed the following five major causes of deficient submissions:

1. Inadequate validation of analytical methodology
2. Insufficient duration of study
3. Insufficient sampling
4. Inadequate number of subjects
5. Deficient experimental design

Validation of Analytical Methodology

Once a drug assay is validated with respect to precision, accuracy, and linearity, subject samples should be measured along with a suitable standard or calibrated curve, and at least two independently prepared control samples. Ideally, controls should be run at three concentrations —low, intermediate, and high. Each should be analyzed in duplicate. The advantage of the multilevel control is that if a systematic error develops, information may be obtained as to whether the error is proportional to concentration or constant over the assay range. The duplicate analyses of controls permit assessment of within-batch imprecision. Loss of precision is often an early warning of problems in an analytical system.

The control samples should be spread evenly throughout the batch. A control sample after every 8–10 subject samples is not unreasonable, and each should be preceded by a subject sample. Good laboratories generate a standard curve daily for analysis of samples. Some laboratories even prepare a new standard curve for analysis of blood samples of each subject. Whatever the practice, a reliable standard curve and use of controls during analysis are required to assure the validity and reliability of results.

Insufficient Duration of Study

Insufficient duration of a bioavailability study is another deficiency that crops up from time to time in the submissions. In a bioequivalence study, sampling of the biological fluid should normally be conducted for 3 to 5 biological half-lives of the drug which is under investigation. A drug with an elimination of half-life of 15 hr would, thus, entail collecting blood or urine samples for at least 48 hr.

Insufficient Sampling

Insufficient number of samples and inappropriate times of sampling is a deficiency that was quite common a few years ago. However, even today the FDA occasionally see submissions with inadequate sampling times. From an analytical point of view, the blood level curve for an oral dosage form consists of two important portions — the absorptive portion and the elimination portion. It is important that for an acceptable bioavailability study that both the absorption and elimination phases are characterized properly. One can achieve this by collecting enough blood samples at regular intervals. Thus, for a study of 24-hr duration, at least four samples should characterize absorption phase and an equal number of samples, the elimination phase. In view of the fact that three samples are needed to characterize the peak as accurately as possible, the number of samples needed would be actually greater than minimal eight samples for such a study.

Experimental Design

The experimental design for bioequivalence study should preferably be randomized Latin square crossover. Although rather rare now, one does occasionally see studies with parallel or sequential treatment design when a proper design calls for a crossover.

Insufficient number of subjects in a bioequivalence study still plagues some of the studies in submissions. A bioequivalence study should have sufficient power statistically to detect at least 20% difference between the two treatments at α of 0.05 and β of 0.2. A power of 0.8 or better ensures the acceptability of the study statistically. The power of the study depends on the variability observed from subject to subject and hence, on the number of subjects employed in the study. The higher the variability, the greater the number of subjects needed for a bioequivalence study with adequate power.

Minor Deficiencies in Biopharmaceutical Submissions

Dighé [34] also pointed out minor deficiencies encountered in bioequivalence studies. Some of these are:

1. Absence of data on dropouts
2. Lack of reporting of adverse reactions
3. Absence of information of the test product lot employed in bioavailability/dissolution testing
4. Dissolution testing on 6 instead of required 12 dosage units

5. Absence of description of assay method used in dissolution testing
6. Formulations of different strengths of a dosage form not submitted
7. Reformulation Supplements: Composition of old formulation and dissolution data on it not submitted

Dighé [34] discussed in his article that investigators should be aware of the requirement of bioequivalence studies for a dosage form with multiple strengths. New products with multiple strengths subject to bioavailability requirement under ANDAs and paper NDAs will be required to conduct in vivo bioequivalence studies on the low as well as high strengths in order to obtain approval of the two strengths, and the strengths in between. In the case of controlled release products a single dose study and a multi-dose study will have to be conducted on at least one strength, and a single dose study on other strengths.

The FDA is increasingly becoming aware of the role played in therapy of metabolites which exhibit pharmacologic activity similar to that of the parent drug. In light of this information, the Division of Biopharmaceutics will require that active metabolites be also measured in addition to the parent drug in a bioavailability study. As an example, the FDA cited thioridazine hydrochloride tablets. Recently, the agency approved ANDAs from three firms for this drug product on the basis of single dose studies. The two active metabolites of thioridazine are mesoridazine and sulforidazine. The agency requires that in a bioequivalence study for thioridazine HCl tablets, the two active metabolites along the parent drug should also be measured.

Dittert and DiSanto [35] have discussed common pitfalls in evaluating bioavailability data. They indicated that perhaps the single most common error made in interpreting bioavailability data is that of "cross-study comparison." This occurs when the blood concentration-time curve of a drug product in one study is compared with the blood concentration-time curve of that drug product in another study. They stated three reasons why such cross-study comparisons are dangerous and can lead to false conclusions. The following examples used to illustrate the three points are taken from actual bioavailability data.

1. *Different Subject Populations,* Figure 15 shows serum concentration-time curves for the same lot of penicillin tablets in two subject populations. Both studies were performed with the same protocol. Study 1 was done with hospital employees, while study 2 was done with prison volunteers. There is approximately a 25% difference in both peak concentration and area (0 to 6 hr) under the serum concentration-time curve. This apparent difference in the bioavailability of the same lot of tablets conducted with identical protocols and assayed by the same technique can be attributed to the different subjects used in these studies.

2. *Different Study Conditions.* Parameters such as the food intake of the subjects before and after drug administration can have dramatic effects on the absorption of certain drugs. Figure 16 shows the results of a three-way crossover test where the subjects were fasted 12 hr overnight and 2 hr after drug administration of (a) an uncoated tablet, (b) a film-coated tablet, and (c) an enteric-coated tablet of an acid-labile antibiotic. The results of this study suggest that the unprotected tablet is superior to both the film-coated and enteric-coated tablet in terms of blood level performance. These results also suggest that neither film coating nor enteric coating is necessary for optimal blood level performance. Figure 17

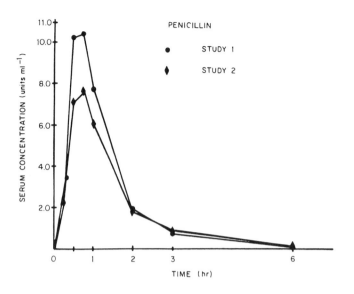

Figure 15 Average serum concentrations obtained after a single oral 500-mg dose of penicillin using the same lot of penicillin tablets in two different subject populations. (From Ref. 27.)

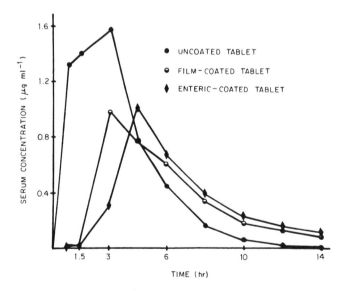

Figure 16 Serum level-time profiles of an acid-labile antibiotic administered in equal doses but as three different tablet dosage forms. The single oral dose consisted of two 250-mg tablets. Results are for 21 normal adults who fasted overnight. (From Ref. 27.)

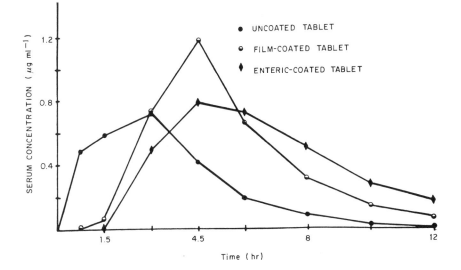

Figure 17 Serum level-time profiles of an acid-labile antibiotic administered in equal doses but as three different tablet dosage forms. The single oral dose consisted of two 250-mg tablets. Results are for 12 normal adults with only a 2-hr preadministration fast. (From Ref. 35.)

shows results with the same tablets when the study conditions were changed to only a 2-hr preadministration fast with 2 hr of fasting preadministration. In this case, the blood levels of the uncoated tablet were markedly depressed, whereas the film-coated and enteric-coated tablets showed relatively little difference in blood levels. From this second study, it might be concluded that film coating appears to impart the same degree of acid stability as does an enteric coating. This might be acceptable if only one dose of the antibiotic were required. However, Figure 18 shows the results of a multiple-dose study in which the enteric-coated tablet and the film-coated tablet were administered four times a day immediately after meals. The results show that the film coating indeed does not impart the degree of acid stability that the enteric coating does when the tablets are administered immediately after food in a typical clinical situation.

3. *Different Assay Methodology.* Depending on the drug under study, more than one assay method may be available. For example, some steroids can be assayed by a radioimmunoassay, competitive protein binding, gas—liquid chromatography, or indirectly by a 17-hydroxycorticosteroid assay. Figure 19 shows the results of a comparison of steroid tablets using a competitive protein binding method and a radioimmunoassay, respectively. Obviously, the wrong conclusion would have been reached if one product had been assayed by one method and the other product by the second method and the results had been compared. Even in cases where only one assay method is employed, there are numerous modifications with respect to technique among laboratories which could make direct comparisons hazardous.

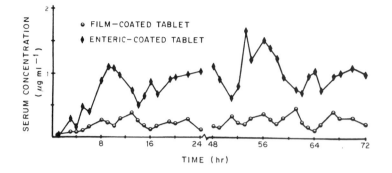

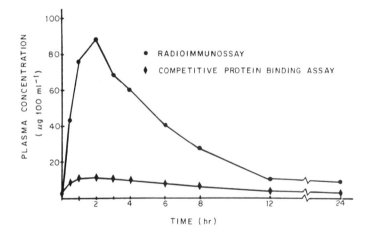

Figure 18 Average serum level-time curves for an acid-labile antibiotic administered in two different tablet dosage forms. In each case the oral tablets were tested in 24 normal adults each of whom received the medication q.i.d., with meals and at bedtime. (From Ref. 35.)

Figure 19 Average plasma level curves for a steroid administered as single oral doses to 24 normal adults. In one case plasma levels were determined by a competitive protein binding assay and in the other case by a radioimmunoassay. (From Ref. 35.)

II. DRUG ABSORPTION

A drug must transverse several biological membranes before it reaches its site of action irrespective of the route of administration. In the oral cavity there are two regions, buccal and sublingual, where the membranes are very thin and have a copious blood supply. Sublingual administration of a drug entails the placing of the drug in its dosage form (e.g., tablet) under the tongue for its ultimate absorption into the systemic circulation. Buccal administration of a drug is ordinarily accomplished by placing the drug between the cheek and the gums.

Drugs administered orally, and probably rectally, pass directly through the liver on their circulation through the body (see Figure 2). If the drug is readily biotransformed in the liver, this initial passage by way of the hepatic route can result in considerable metabolism of the drug before it arrives at the peripheral circulation. This loss of drug on first passage through the liver is called the *first pass effect*. Drugs given by intravenous, intramuscular, subcutaneous, sublingual, and buccal administration, on the other hand, enter the circulation directly and are carried to body tissues before passage through the liver, where they might be broken down. Sublingual and buccal tablets are therefore ideal for potent, low-dose drugs.

Venous drainage from the oral cavity goes directly to the heart, which makes it an excellent route for treating angina with nitroglycerin. On the other hand, toxic drugs such as nicotine also pass directly to the heart without any chance of detoxication. Once widely used as an insecticide, nicotine produced an environmental hazard because of its great toxicity.

The transport or passage of drugs across membranes in various parts of the body depends to a large degree on the selectivity and characteristics of the membrane. Pore size, membrane composition, and the presence of energy-dependent carriers may all affect drug absorption; however, most drugs pass across biological membranes by simple or passive diffusion.

A. Passive Membrane Diffusion

Passive diffusion happens when drug molecules exist in high concentration on one side of a membrane and lower concentration on the other side. Diffusion occurs in an effort to equalize drug concentration on both sides of the membrane, the rate of transport being proportional to the concentration gradient across the membrane.

When the volume of fluids are fixed, the movement of drug across a membrane can be described in terms of Fick's laws. Fick's first law states that the rate of diffusion or transport across a membrane is directly proportional to the surface area of the membrane and to the concentration gradient, and is inversely proportional to the thickness of the membrane. The expression for Fick's first law is

$$\frac{dm}{dt} = -DA \frac{dc}{dx} \tag{1}$$

where m is the quantity of drug or solute diffusing in time t, dm/dt the rate of diffusion, D the diffusion constant, A the cross-sectional area of the membrane, dc the change in concentration, and dx the thickness of the membrane. A change in any of these variables will alter the rate of transport of drug into the blood. The value of the diffusion coefficient is dependent on the chemical nature of the drug and, in particular, its degree of lipophilicity, which can be evaluated approximately from the oil−water partition coefficient. Diffusion can also be influenced by temperature, pressure, and by the nature of the solvent. Faster absorption occurs in the small intestine rather than the stomach because of the high surface area provided by villi and microvilli found in the small intestine. Drugs are rapidly absorbed through very thin membranes (e.g., the alveolar membrane of the lungs). This explains why inhaled medication is more

rapid acting than drugs in oral dosage forms. The driving force for passive diffusion in Eq. (1) is the concentration gradient between drug in the
gut and drug in the blood. According to Fick's law, the rate of diffusion
is proportional to the concentration gradient. Therefore, the rate of
change of concentration is proportional to the concentration, and since the
concentration of drug in the blood is negligible compared to that in the gut:

$$\frac{dc}{dt} = -kc \tag{2}$$

The negative sign in this first-order equation indicates that concentration
decreases with time.

If the concentration of drug at the absorption site is c_0 at $t = 0$, then
at some later time t, the concentration of drug remaining unabsorbed may
be designated as c. Integration of Eq. (2),

$$\int_{c_0}^{c} \frac{dc}{c} = -k \int_{0}^{t} dt \tag{3}$$

yields the equation

$$\ln \frac{c}{c_0} = -kt \tag{4}$$

or

$$\log \frac{c}{c_0} = \frac{-kt}{2.303} \tag{5}$$

A plot of c/c_0 on a logarithmic scale against time on a rectangular
scale should produce a straight line with a negative slope representing the
absorption rate constant k. The half-life for drug absorption is the time
required for the concentration of drug in the gut, c, to be reduced to
one-half its initial value, and for a first-order process can be calculated
by using the expression

$$t_{1/2} = \frac{0.693}{k} \tag{6}$$

B. Active Membrane Transport

Drugs absorbed via an active transport mechanism may pass from areas of
lower concentration to areas of higher concentration. The transfer is
thought to be mediated by a "carrier," and in contrast to passive diffusion,
chemical energy expended by the body is required for active transport to
occur. The carrier system may consist of an enzyme or other substance
in the gastrointestinal wall. The carrier combines with the drug and ac-
companies it through the membrane to be discharged on the other side.
The carrier-drug complex is considered to have a higher permeability
through the membrane of the gut than the drug alone. The process is

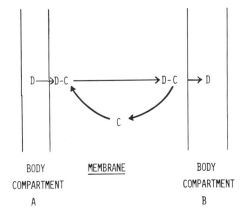

Figure 20   Action of carrier C, which facilitates passage of drug molecule D across a membrane.   C combines with the drug at the surface of compartment A and releases the drug at compartment B.   Carrier C returns to ferry the next drug molecule across the membrane.

depicted in Figure 20.   Active transport of drugs is site-specific, and the greatest absorption occurs in locations of the gastrointestinal tract, where carrier concentration is highest.   At low concentrations, the rate of drug absorption by active transport is proportional to drug concentration in the gut.   At higher levels of drug, the carrier system eventually becomes saturated and the absorption levels off at a fixed maximum rate.   Therefore, the absorption rate for substances absorbed via active transport will not increase as the dose increases, once the carrier mechanism has been saturated.   Several body nutrients and vitamins, such as amino acids, thiamine, niacin, and riboflavin, are absorbed via active transport [36, 37].   Where the structure of a drug resembles that of an actively absorbed material, a strong possibility exists for the drug to pass into the blood via active transport.   A number of organic compounds, including penicillin and phenol red, are secreted in the proximal renal tubules by active transport. Other examples include the transport of sodium ions from the gut lumen into the blood, and the secretion of hydrogen ions into the stomach [38]. Some antitumor drugs are thought to be transported actively, and these include 5-fluorouracil [39] and the serine and threonine derivatives of nitrogen mustard [40].

Facilitated diffusion is a special form of carrier transport (Fig. 20) that has many of the characteristics of active transport, but the substrate does not move against a concentration gradient.   The uptake of glucose by cells is an example of facilitated diffusion.   As with active transport, facilitated diffusion is mediated via a carrier molecule in the mucosa, is selective, saturable, and can be "poisoned" or inhibited by certain electrolytes (e.g., fluoride, and organic dinitrophenols).   The main difference between active transport and facilitated diffusion is that there is no energy expenditure by the body for the latter process to occur.

Other mechanisms of absorption include pinocytosis and ion-pair absorption.   Pinocytosis literally means "cell drinking" and is a process whereby the cell surface invaginates and takes in a small vacuole of liquid

containing the solute or drug. It is an important transport mechanism for
proteins, but its significance in drug absorption is not entirely clear.
The ion-pair absorption mechanism was postulated by Higuchi [41] to
explain the absorption of large ionized compounds (e.g., quaternary
amines and sulfonic acids), where absorption cannot be explained by the
pH/partition theory. The authors postulated that the organic ion combined
with a large ion of opposite charge to form an nonionized species. The
increased lipoidal nature of the resulting molecule would account for rapid
passage through the mucous membranes of the gastrointestinal tract.

In a recent paper by Boroujerdi [42], the kinetic relationships of the
formation of the ion pair as a function of the ion-pair agent and the type
of the biological membrane were discussed and analyzed. The author developed criteria for distinguishing the following two cases: (1) when the
absorption is the rate limiting step in the process of permeation of the
ion-pair, and (2) when the ion-pair crosses the membrane as through it
were a fine sieve. Boroujerdi also extensively reviewed several studies
where ion-pair formation improved the partition coefficient and diffusion
across synthetic and biological membranes.

C. The pH-Partition Hypothesis

Passive diffusion through a membrane is probably the most common mechanism of drug absorption in the body regardless of the location of the membrane. Therefore, the greater the lipid solubility of the nonionized moiety,
the faster and easier a drug will pass through the membrane. The pH-
partition hypothesis was developed by Brodie et al. [43–46] to explain the
absorption of ionized and nonionized drugs. The pK_a and oil/water partition ratio are two important parameters involved in the pH-partition theory
of drug absorption. For a particular pH in the gastrointestinal tract,
these parameters dictate the degree of ionization and lipoid solubility of a
drug, which, in turn, determine the rate of absorption of drugs and transport through cellular membranes in the body. The pH of the human
stomach varies from 1 to 3.5, although higher values have been recorded.
Disease and the presence of food or antacids may drastically increase
gastric pH. The duodenal pH is generally in the range 5 to 6 and the
lower ileum may approach a pH of 8. Theoretical calculations and predictions as to the amounts and sites of absorption of weakly acidic and basic
drugs have been made using the Henderson-Hasselbalch equations and the
pH-partition principle.

For acids:

$$pH = pK_a + \log \frac{[\text{ionized form}]}{[\text{nonionized acid}]} \tag{7}$$

For bases:

$$pH = pK_a + \log \frac{[\text{nonionized base}]}{[\text{ionized form}]} \tag{8}$$

From the equations, one might expect acidic drugs or very weakly basic
drugs to be absorbed predominantly from the stomach and basic drugs or
very weakly acidic drugs to be absorbed from regions of higher pH in the

intestines. These expectations are based on the premise, following the pH partition theory, that the primary mode of drug absorption is via passive diffusion of the uncharged species. Thus, the Henderson-Hasselbalch equation can be used to calculate the relative amounts of charged and neutral forms from the pK_a of the drug and the pH of the environment.

The percent ionized is given by

$$\% \text{ Ionized} = \frac{I \times 100}{I + U} \tag{9}$$

where I is the concentration of a species in the ionized conjugate form and U the concentration of unionized species. Equation (7) may be rearranged to give

$$\frac{U}{I} = \text{antilog } (pK_a - pH) \tag{10}$$

for a weak acid so that Eq. (9) becomes

$$\% \text{ Ionized} = \frac{100}{1 + \text{antilog } (pK_a - pH)} \tag{11}$$

where pK_a is the dissociation constant for the neutral or nonionized acid. For a weak base, such as atropine or morphine, the comparable expression is

$$\% \text{ Ionized} = \frac{100}{1 + \text{antilog } (pH - pK_a)} \tag{12}$$

where pK_a is the dissociation constant for the cationic acid conjugate to the molecular base.

As an example, if one considers morphine, in which the pK_a of its cationic acid form (morphine H)$^+$ is 7.87 at 25% C, the percentage ionization of morphine at a pH of 7.50 can be calculated using Eq. (12):

$$\% \text{ Ionized} = \frac{100}{1 + \text{antilog } (7.50 - 7.87)} + \frac{100}{1 + \text{antilog } (-0.37)}$$

$$= \frac{100}{1 + 0.427} = 70.10$$

The percentages of ionic (I) and molecular (U) forms of morphine ($pK_a = 7.87$) at various pH values are shown in Table 4. As observed in Figure 21, nonionized drug will distribute across the membrane so that the concentration of nonionized in fluid A will equal nonionized in fluid B. It is assumed that the ionized form of the drug cannot pass through the membrane. The pH of the fluids and the pK_a of the drug will then determine the ratio of nonionized to ionized drug in the two fluids, as seen in Figure 22. The relationship between pK_a and pH at the absorption site has been demonstrated for a variety of acids and bases. Table 5 shows the absorption of drugs from the rat stomach. The acidity of the stomach ensures that weak acids are but slightly ionized. The exceptions are

Table 4 Percentages of Morphine in
Ionized (I) and Unionized (U) Forms at
Various pH Values

pH	Percent I	Percent U
2.0	100	0.00
4.0	99.99	0.01
6.0	98.67	1.33
7.0	88.11	11.89
7.5	70.10	29.90
8.0	42.57	57.43
8.5	19.00	81.00
9.0	6.90	93.10
10.0	0.74	99.26
13.0	0.00	100.00

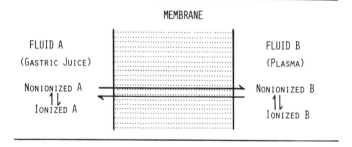

Figure 21 Partitioning of drug between gastric fluid and plasma.

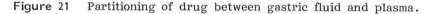
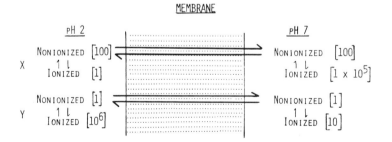

Figure 22 X, Nonionized and ionized concentrations of a weakly acidic
drug with a pK_a of 4 in fluids with a pH of 2 and 7 separated by a membrane; Y, nonionized and ionized concentrations of a weakly basic drug
with a pK_a of 8, under the same conditions as X.

Table 5   Absorption of Drugs from the Rat Stomach

Drug		pK	Absorption (%)
Acid	5-Sulphosalicylic	Strong	0
	Phenol red	Strong	2
	Salicylic	3.0	61
	Thiopental	7.6	46
	Barbital	7.8	4
	Quinalbarbitone	7.9	30
	Phenol	9.9	40
Base	Acetanilide	0.3	36
	Caffeine	0.8	24
	Aniline	4.6	6
	Dextromethorphan	9.2	0
	Mecamylamine	11.2	0
	Mepipophenidol	Strong	0
	Tetraethylammonium	Strong	0

Source: From Ref. 45.

relatively strong acids, such as phenol red, which is highly ionized even at pH 1.

The poor absorption of barbital illustrates that pK_a is not the only limiting factor, the lipid solubility of the nonionized form also being important. Very weak bases such as caffeine are well absorbed in the stomach, since these bases exist predominately in a nonionized form, even at acid pH. The varying degrees of absorption of three barbiturates have been shown by Schanker [47] to be related to the lipid–water partition coefficient, as shown in Table 6. The three barbiturates have very similar pK_a values but differ in lipid solubility, which apparently controls the degree of absorption.

The absorption of weak acids and weak bases from the rat intestine at varying pHs is shown in Table 7. As the pH of the solution in the intestinal lumen increased, the absorption of weak acids was found to decrease. The opposite was seen for weak bases: as the pH increased, the percent drug absorbed increased. It is important to realize that information in Table 4 was obtained from experiments conducted on animals under special conditions and that, as such, the data are highly idealized. Hogben et al. [44] postulated that the distribution across the gut with weak acids or bases is dependent on the "virtual" pH of the mucosal solution (i.e., the pH of a narrow microclimate adjacent to the mucosal surface rather than the pH of the bulk solution in the lumen of the gut). They

Table 6   Gastric Absorption of Barbiturates Compared
with Their pK$_a$ Values and Lipid–Water Partition
Coefficients

Barbiturate	pK$_a$	Absorption (%)	$K = \dfrac{[CHCl_3]}{[H_2O]}$
Barbital	7.8	4	0.7
Secobarbital	7.9	30	23.3
Thiopental	7.6	46	100.0

Source: From Ref. 45.

pointed out that such a microclimate of fluid with a low pH calculated to be
5.3 would lead to a relatively high concentration of nonionized acid next to
the mucosa, as compared to the concentration of nonionized species in the
bulk mucosal solution at a higher pH, normally 6.6. The high concentration of the un-ionized species would lead to increased mucosal to serosal
movement of the acid by a passive diffusion of the nonionic form. Values
greater than 1 for the steady-state concentration ratio C_{plasma}/C_{gut} of a
weak acid could be explained by this mechanism without postulating specific
active transport.

Table 7   Comparison of Intestinal Absorption in the Rat at Several
pH Values

Substance		pK$_a$	pH 4	pH 5	pH 7	pH 8
Acid	5-Nitrosalicylic	2.3	40	27	0	0
	Salicylic	3.0	64	35	30	10
	Acetylsalicylic	3.5	41	27	–	–
	Benzoic	4.2	62	36	35	5
Base	Aniline	4.6	40	48	58	61
	Amidopyrine	5.0	21	35	48	52
	p-Toluidine	5.3	30	42	65	64
	Quinine	8.4	9	11	41	54

Source: From Ref. 48.

For weak acids, ratios of C_{plasma}/C_{gut} are much higher for the stomach than for the intestine, which accounts for the generalization that weak acids are best absorbed from the stomach. The steady-state or equilibrium conditions employed by Brodie are not present in the intact animals and do not take into account the rate of absorption, which is a better determinant for the optimal absorption site than is the equilibrium ratio of C_{plasma}/C_{gut}. For weak acids the large surface area of the intestines results in a higher rate of absorption than in the stomach, and this is more important than the less favorable pH of the intestine.

Suzuki et al. [49, 50] have used theoretical models to study drug transport and absorption phenomena and have shown that pH-partition theory is a special limiting case of a more general approach. These investigators tested their models using the experimental data of Kakemi et al. [51–54]. These data included the in situ results in rats for intestinal, gastric, and rectal absorption of sulfonamides and barbituric acid derivatives. The correlations of in situ data using the models proved to be generally satisfactory, and pointed out the various diffusional coefficients and constants that should be accounted for in the study of absorption of drugs through living membranes.

D. Gastric Emptying Rate: Influence of Food and Other Factors

When a medicinal agent is preferentially absorbed in the stomach or intestine, and when absorption is site-specific in the gastrointestinal tract, the presence of food can have a profound influence on drug bioavailability. Food will slow tablet disintegration, decrease the dissolution rate of the active ingredient, and decrease intestinal absorption by reducing gastric emptying. An increase in the gut residual of certain drugs may result in several toxic side effects to the patient. Alteration in the normal microbiologic flora of the stomach by broad-spectrum antibiotics results in malabsorption of essential nutrients. The change in flora may cause infections in the tract because of the presence of foreign organisms that are usually kept under control by the natural flora. The ulcerogenic potential of potassium chloride and antiinflammatory agents, both steroidal and nonsteroidal, may be increased by lengthening gut residence time.

Among the several factors [55] that influence gastric emptying are the types of food ingested, volume, pH, temperature, osmotic pressure, and viscosity of stomach contents. The age, health, and position of the patient are also important. Davenport [55] reported that cold meals increase and hot meals decrease the emptying time of gastric contents. Levy and Jusko [56] have shown that an increase in the viscosity of the gastrointestinal fluids can decrease the absorption rate of certain drugs by retarding the diffusion of drug molecules to the absorbing membrane. However, Okuda [57] showed that a delay in gastric emptying due to high viscosity results in enhanced absorption of certain drugs (e.g., vitamin B_{12} and other vitamins).

A surfactant may also exert a specific pharmacologic effect on the gastrointestinal tract which influences drug absorption. Lish [58] reported that dioctyl sodium sulfosuccinate inhibits the propulation of a test meal in the rat, owing to the formation of an inhibitory compound when the surface-active agent came in contact with the intestinal mucosa. Gastric motility in the dog was also found to be inhibited following the introduction of certain detergents into the gastric pouch [59].

The coadministration of a number of drugs, such as anticholinergics [60], narcotic analgesics [61], nonnarcotic analgesics [62], and certain tricyclic antidepressants [63], also cause delayed stomach emptying. Studies in humans have been reported correlating drug availability and stomach emptying with L-dopa [64] and digitoxin [65].

Jaffee et al. [66] demonstrated that the type of food can influence absorption. In studies with acetaminophen, carbohydrates were found to decrease absorption, whereas proteins did not. A report [67] related to the effects of food on nitrofurantoin absorption in humans indicated that the presence of food in the stomach appreciably delayed gastric emptying. A marked enhancement in the bioavailability of both macro- and micro-crystalline nitrofurantoin from commercial solid dosage forms in nonfasting as compared to fasting subjects was also observed. These findings are consistent with the argument that a significant fraction of drug from both dosage forms dissolves in the stomach prior to being emptied into the duodenal region of the small intestine, where absorption is optimal [68]. Penicillin [69], lincomycin [70], tetracycline [71], erythromycin [72], and theophylline [73] have all shown reduced absorption efficiency when given with meals. Meals containing a high content of fats have been shown to increase the absorption of griseofulvin [74].

Drug absorption and excretion in some instances may be influenced by the quantity of fluid intake. Nogami et al. [75] followed the disintegration in vivo of calcium p-aminosalicylate tablets by X-ray. The tablets disintegrated more rapidly when ingested with water than without water. Human studies with digoxin have employed volumes of 240 ml [6] and 100 ml [7] of water administered to the patient. The effect of such gross differences in the quality of water utilized in bioavailability studies has not been extensively studied. The influence of the type of beverage administered with drugs has been studied by Levy et al. [76-78]. Theophylline absorption in the rat [76] was enhanced when administered in hydroalcoholic solutions containing 5 or 15% ethanol. Absorption was significantly decreased when theophylline was administered in 20% ethanolic solutions, as seen in Figure 23. When tested in several normal subjects, there was no significant difference in the average plasma concentrations of theophylline produced by these two solutions [77]. However, three subjects (all female) experienced nausea after taking the aqueous solution, whereas none became nauseous after taking theophylline in the hydroalcoholic solution.

A study [79] in humans showed that caffeine contained in a proprietary carbonated beverage (Coca-Cola) was absorbed much more slowly from this beverage than from coffee or tea. The sucrose and phosphoric acid contained in carbonated beverages have been shown to inhibit gastric emptying [80, 81]. On the other hand, a more recent paper by Houston and Levy [78] reported that compared to water, the carbonated beverage increased the bioavailability of riboflavin-5'-phosphate and significantly altered the metabolic rate of salicylamide when administered to healthy human adults. Sodium and calcium cyclamates have been reported to interfere markedly with the absorption of lincomycin [82]. The interference occurs both when the sweetening agent was mixed in solution and then

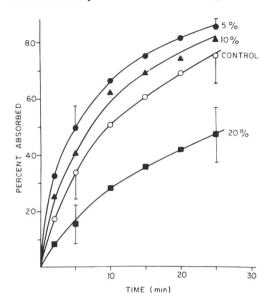

Figure 23 Effect of 0, 5, 10, and 20% (v/v) ethanol on the absorption of theophylline from a 50 mg% solution instilled into a cannulated segment of the small intestine of anesthetized rats (average of six animals per group). Vertical bars indicate one standard deviation in each direction. (From Ref. 76.)

ingested, and when the antibiotic was ingested and the sweetening agent was coadministered as a diet beverage.

Wilson and Washington [83] found that the major complication when studying the dissolution of dosage forms in vivo was the presence of food within the gastrointestinal tract. Food not only affects the rate at which the dosage form travels through the tract, but also influences the distribution of the formulation in the various segments. The size and shape of the dosage form plus the amount and type of food present at the time of administration, all influence the residence time of the dosage form in the stomach. Since food influences the gastric pH, the possibility for physical and chemical interactions between the drug and the food are possible. In addition, the food also changes the viscosity of the gastrointestinal fluid in which the drug is presented to the absorbing mucosa. Wilson and Washington [83] extensively reviewed the applications of gamma scintigraphy to study the dissolution and disintegration of tablets in vivo and drug distribution in the body. Gamma scintigraphy allows the passage of the formulation throughout the gastrointestinal tract to be monitored and stasis of the formulation can usually be detected. The position of a formulation and the degree of dispersion within the gastrointestinal tract can be related to the simultaneous plasma concentration for the drug. Since the majority of drugs are absorbed from the intestine, factors that influence the delivery of a dosage form to this region, e.g., food, can be studied using a dual isotope technique.

Thebault and co-workers [84] studied the influence of food on the bioavailability of theophylline from a slow release hydrophilic matrix tablet.

The release of drug from the tablet was independent of pH and followed zero order kinetics. A bioavailability study was conducted in volunteers who received the drug while fasting, or with a standard low fat, or high fat meal. Although several workers have previously reported the influence of food on the bioavailability of theophylline, Thebault and co-workers concluded from this study that the slight food/drug interaction which was seen with these slow release theophylline tablets seemed to be of no clinical significance.

E. Drug Interactions with Components of the Gastrointestinal Tract

Bile salts, present in the biliary secretions of the small intestine, act as surface-active agents. The influence of orally administered bile salts on the enhancement of drug absorption has been reviewed by Gibaldi and Feldmann [85]. It was suggested that the wetting action of these salts would promote the dissolution of hydrophobic and poorly soluble drugs, resulting in a faster rate of absorption. The dissolution rate of griseofulvin and hexestrol was, in fact, increased in solutions of bile salts [86]. Since the administration of a fatty meal stimulates bile production in the body, the high blood levels of griseofulvin in Figure 24 following such a meal can readily be explained [71].

However, other investigators have shown that bile salts do not enhance drug efficacy in all cases. The formation of insoluble nonabsorbable complexes have been demonstrated with neomycin and kanamycin [87]. More recent studies by Thompson et al. [88] demonstrated by analyses of aspirated intestinal content that ionized fatty acids, bile salts, and labeled cholesterol administered in a test meal were precipitated by neomycin. The precipitation of micellar lipids by the polymeric antibiotic provides an explanation for the hypocholesterolemia induced by this compound.

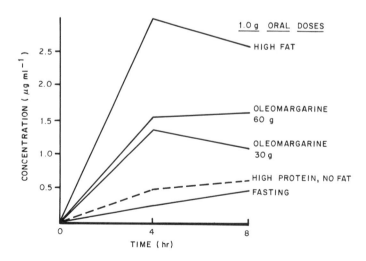

Figure 24 Effects of different types of food intake on the serum griseofulvin levels following a 1-g oral dose. (From Ref. 74.)

Neomycin had no effect on the lipase concentration in the mixed pancrease and lipases, which is called pancreatin. Neomycin was found to have no effect on the pH of intestinal contents. The loss of activity of antibacterial and antimycotic agents has been reported by Scheirson and Amsterdam [89].

Other components in the gastrointestinal tract that may influence drug activity include enzymes and proteins plus the mucopolysaccharide material called mucin, which lines the mucosal surfaces of the stomach and intestine. Enzymes found in the gastrointestinal tract transform the inactive drug moieties, chloramphenicol palmitate [90] and the acetoxymethyl ester of benzylpenicillin [91] to their active parent compounds. The binding of large quantities of dihydrostreptomycin and streptomycin [92] and quaternary ammonium compounds [93] to mycin has been suggested to explain the poor absorption seen with these compounds.

F. Absorption Enhancing Agents

In recent years, significant progress has been made in identifying agents that significantly increase the absorption of drugs that are poorly absorbed when administered alone. In an excellent review by Fix, published in 1987, compounds which have been identified as effective absorption-enhancing agents were reviewed [94]. Since many drugs are characterized by poor or highly variable absorption when administered to the GI tract, several approaches have been employed to increase drug absorption from the GI tract. These approaches include the optimization of drug release, site specific drug administration, prodrugs, modification of GI drug absorption, and vehicle optimization. Fix pointed out that all of these approaches tend to be drug specific and offer little in terms of providing general utility for increasing drug absorption. Absorption enhancing agents, which increase the absorption of coadministered drugs, provide a potential means of increasing mucosal membrane permeability in a more general manner and hence provide greater utility with a variety of compounds. Although a considerable effort has been directed towards identifying safe and effective absorption enhancing agents, little progress however, has been made in defining a mechanism of action for these compounds.

G. Cigarette Smoking and Drug Absorption

Recent studies have shown that the clinical efficacy and toxicity of benzodiazepine [95], propoxyphene [96], and chlorpromazine [97] may be influenced by cigarette smoking. An increase in the metabolism of these drugs by stimulated microsomal systems has been postulated as a possible mechanism. An increase in the rate of biotransformation of pentazocaine [98], phenacetin [99], and nicotine [100] has been demonstrated, and the effect of smoking on the disposition of theophylline was recently examined [101]. The results showed that the plasma half-life of theophylline (administered as aminophylline) in smokers was nearly half (mean value 4.3 hr) that found in nonsmokers (mean value 7.0 hr) and that the apparent volume of distribution of theophylline was larger in smokers than in nonsmokers. The authors suggested that the increase in theophylline clearance caused by smoking was probably the result of induction of drug-metabolizing enzymes, and that these enzymes do not normalize after cessation of smoking for 3 months.

H. Patient Characteristics

Considerable difference in patterns of drug absorption for some drugs have been found. Riegelman [102] and Levy [103] have reported that bioavailabilities of a drug from the same product can differ in the same person from one day to another or with the time of day. In addition, the age, posture, activity, stress, temperature, gastrointestinal pH, mobility, mucosal perfusion, gut flora, and disease state may all influence drug absorption. Drug-induced changes in portal blood flow or in hepatic function would alter the degree of biotransformation of a drug during its passage through the liver in the portal venous blood. Achlorhydria, biliary disorders, malabsorption syndromes [104], and reconstructive gastrointestinal surgery [105] can appreciably impair drug bioavailability. The drugs most influenced by patient factors are those whose bioavailability is quite incomplete under the best of circumstances.

III. PHYSICOCHEMICAL PROPERTIES OF DRUG AND DOSAGE FORM

Of prime concern to the pharmaceutical scientist involved in preformulation and dosage form design is a knowledge of the various properties of dosage forms that influence the biological effectiveness of medicinal agents.

A. Release of Drug from its Dosage Form

When a drug is administered orally in tablet dosage form, the rate of absorption is often controlled by the slowest step in the sequence [106] shown in Figure 25.

Drug must be released from the tablet into the gastrointestinal fluids for absorption to occur. The tableting of a medicinal substance allows the introduction of several variables during the manufacture of the dosage form. Process and formulation variables can be adjusted to assure

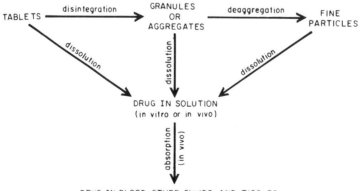

Figure 25   Drug dissolution from a tablet dosage form followed by absorption into the bloodstream. (From Ref. 106.)

bioequivalence of generic dosage forms produced by different manufacturers but may also result in bioinequivalence, and this subject will be addressed later in the chapter. The introduction of direct compression excipients in tablet formulations has circumvented many of the problems of wet granulation associated with the granulating and drying stages. However, drug stability and physical tablet properties, such as color, shape, size, weight, hardness, and dissolution profile, must all be maintained within narrow limits for direct-compressed tablets. In addition to these properties, the characteristics and processing of tablets that influence disintegration and drug release include:

Nature of diluents
Process of mixing
Granule size and distribution
Nature of disintegrant
Nature and concentration of lubricant
Age of finished tablets
Presence or absence of surface-active agent
Physical properties of the drug
Flow of granulation through hopper and into dies
Compressional force in production

It is evident from this list that the formulation of a stable and bioavailable product requires a thorough study of the physicochemical properties of drug and tablet to ensure efficacy.

The search for an apparatus that will afford reliable and reproducible information concerning the dissolution of pharmaceutical dosage forms continues. Unfortunately, there appear to be as many varieties of dissolution apparatus as there are investigators studying dissolution phenomena. The aim is essentially to develop an apparatus that enables correlation between in vitro data and in vivo results. In a comprehensive review [107], Wagner avers that an apparatus cannot be devised to simulate the human intestinal tract because of the complexity of the physiological environment. More will be said about in vitro apparatus and in vitro/in vivo correlation later in this chapter.

B. Dissolution: Theory and Practice

To be absorbed through the gastrointestinal membrane, a drug must first pass into solution. Drugs with poor solufility are absorbed with difficulty, and with such compounds the rate of dissolution in gastrointestinal fluids is generally the rate-controlling step for absorption.

According to Higuchi [108], there are three processes (see Fig. 26) which either alone or in combination describe dissolution-rate mechanisms: the diffusion layer model, the interfacial barrier model, and Danckwert's model. Dissolution by the diffusion layer model (Fig. 26A) is diffusion-limited and consists of two stages: (1) interaction between the solvent with the surface of the drug to form a layer of saturated solution around the drug particle, and (2) the diffusion of drug molecules into the bulk of the system. The diffusion of drug away from the saturated layer is regarded as the rate-determining step. Therefore, this model regards the rate of dissolution as being diffusion-limited. Once the molecules of solute

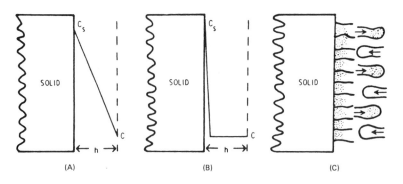

Figure 26   Mechanisms of dissolution. (A) Diffusion layer model, (B) interfacial barrier model, (C) Danckwert's model. (From Ref. 108.)

pass the liquid film/bulk interface, rapid mixing will destroy the concentration gradient. In the interfacial barrier model (Fib. 26B), it is proposed that all collisions of solvent molecules with the solid surface do not result in release of solute molecules because of high free energy of activation requirements. Danckwert's model (Fig. 26C) postulates that removal of solute from the solid is achieved by macroscopic packets of solvent being carried right up to the solid–liquid interface by eddy currents. Goyan [109] used Danckwert's model to study the dissolution of spherical particles.

Noyes and Whitney's Equation

Noyes and Whitney [110] proposed the following relationship, which applies under standard conditions of agitation and temperature to the dissolution rate process for solids:

$$\frac{dw}{dt} = kS(c_s - c_t) \tag{13}$$

The loss of weight of a particle per unit time dw/dt is proportional to the surface area of the solid S and to the difference between the concentration at saturation c_s and the concentration of the solid at a given time, c_t. The rate of dissolution $dw/dt(1/S)$ is the amount dissolved per unit area per unit time and for most solids can be expressed in units of g cm^{-2} sec^{-1}.

When c_t is less than 15% of the saturation solubility c_s, c_t has a negligible influence on the dissolution rate of the solid. Under such circumstances, the dissolution of the solid is said to be occurring under "sink" conditions and Eq. (13) will reduce to

$$\frac{dw}{dt} = kSc_s \tag{14}$$

In general, the surface area S is not constant except when the quality of material present exceeds the saturation solubility, or initially when only small quantities of drug have dissolved. As an example of the Noyes-Whitney equation used under sink conditions, consider a drug weighing 2.5 g and having a total particle surface area of $0.5 \text{ m}^2 \text{ g}^{-1}$. When this drug was added to 2000 ml of water, 600 mg of drug dissolved after 1 min. If the dissolution rate constant k is $7.5 \times 10^{-5} \text{ cm sec}^{-1}$, calculate the saturation solubility c_s and the dissolution rate dw/dt of the drug during the first minute. Is the experiment conducted under sink conditions?

The surface area is $2.5 \times 0.5 \times 10^4 \text{ cm}^2$ (i.e., $1.25 \times 10^4 \text{ cm}^2$. [Note: $1 \text{ m}^2 = (100)^2 \text{ cm}^2 = 10^4 \text{ cm}^2$.] Using Eq. (14) yields

$$\frac{600}{60} = 7.5 \times 10^{-5} \times 1.25 \times 10^4 \times c_s$$

$$c_s = 10.67 \text{ mg cm}^{-3}$$

$$\text{Rate of dissolution} = \frac{dw}{dt} = \frac{600}{60} = 10 \text{ mg sec}^{-1}$$

Now $c_t = 2.5$ g per 2000 cm^3 (i.e., $c_t = 0.3 \text{ mg cm}^{-3}$), so

$$\frac{c_t}{c_s} = \frac{0.3}{10.67}$$

$$= 0.028$$

$$\frac{c_t}{c_s} \times 100 = 2.8\%$$

Therefore, sink conditions are in effect.

Hixon and Crowell's Cube-Root Equation

As a solid dissolves, the surface area S changes with time. The Hixon and Crowell cube-root equation for dissolution kinetics is based on the assumption that:

1. Dissolution occurs normal to the surface of the solute particle.
2. Agitation is uniform over all exposed surfaces and there is no stagnation.
3. The particle of solute retains its geometric shape.

For a monodisperse powder with spherical particles of radius r, the surface area S of N particles at time t is

$$S = N \times 4\pi r^2 \, dr \tag{15}$$

The change in volume of the particle or the volume of particle dissolved over an infinitesimally small time increment dt is

$$dV = -N \times 4\pi r^2 \, dr \tag{16}$$

Since $dw/dt = kSc_s$, according to the Noyes-Whitney equation,

$$dw = \rho \, dV = kSc_s \, dt \tag{17}$$

or

$$-N\rho \times 4\pi r^2 \frac{dr}{dt} = kN \times 4\pi r^2 c_s \tag{18}$$

which reduces to

$$-\rho \frac{dr}{dt} = kc_s \tag{19}$$

Integration gives

$$r = r_0 - \frac{kc_s}{\rho} t \tag{20}$$

or

$$d = d_0 - \frac{2kc_s}{\rho} t \tag{21}$$

where d is the diameter of the particle and d_0 the diameter at $t = $ zero. The weight of a spherical particle is related to its diameter by

$$w = N\rho \frac{\pi}{6} d^3 \tag{22}$$

or

$$w^{1/3} = \left(\frac{N\rho \pi}{6}\right)^{1/3} d \tag{23}$$

The dissolution equation then becomes

$$w_0^{1/3} - w^{1/3} = Kt \tag{24}$$

where

$$K = w_0^{1/3} \frac{2kc_s}{\rho d_0} \tag{25}$$

Equation (24) is the Hixon-Crowell cube-root dissolution law and K is the cube-root dissolution-rate constant.

As an example of the use of the cube-root law, considera a sample of essentially spherical particles of a sulfonamide powder having the initial weight of 500 mg, dissolved in 1000 cm^3 of water. The results obtained

Table 8 Dissolution of a Sulfonamide as a Function of Time

Time (min)	Concentration (mg cc^{-1})	Weight undissolved (g)	$w_0^{1/3} - w^{1/3}$	K
0	0	0.500	0	–
10	0.240	0.260	0.150	0.0150
20	0.392	0.108	0.310	0.0155
30	0.471	0.029	0.487	0.0162
40	0.4940	0.006	0.612	0.0153
50	0.4999	0.0001	0.744	0.0149

$$\Sigma K = 0.0769$$

$$K \text{ (average)} = \frac{\Sigma K}{5} = 0.0153$$

when samples were withdrawn at various times and analyzed for drug content appear in Table 8. From Table 8 the average cube-root dissolution rate constant obtained from these data is 0.0153 where d is the diameter of the particle and d_0 the diameter at t = zero. The weight of a spherical particle is related to its diameter by

$$w = N \rho \frac{\pi}{6} d^3 \tag{22}$$

or

$$w^{1/3} = \left(\frac{N \rho \pi}{6} \right)^{1/3} d \tag{23}$$

The dissolution equation then becomes

$$w_0^{1/3} - w^{1/3} = Kt \tag{24}$$

where

$$K = w_0^{1/3} \frac{2kc_s}{\rho d_0} \tag{25}$$

Equation (24) is the Hixon-Crowell cube-root dissolution law and K is the cube-root dissolution-rate constant.

As an example of the use of the cube-root law, consider a sample of essentially spherical particles of a sulfonamide powder having an initial

weight of 500 mg, dissolved in 1000 cm^3 of water. The results obtained
when samples were withdrawn at various times and analyzed for drug content appear in Table 8. From Table 8 the average cube-root dissolution
rate constant obtained from these data is 0.0153 g$^{1/3}$ min^{-1}.

It will be recalled that Fick's first law [Eq. (1)] involves a diffusion
coefficient D (cm^2 sec^{-1}) and a term h (cm) for the thickness of the
liquid film. These may be combined and expressed as the intrinsic dissolution rate constant, k:

$$k = \frac{D}{h} \times cm \ sec^{-1} \tag{26}$$

In the example above,

$$k = \frac{D}{h} = K \frac{\rho d_0}{2c_s w_0^{1/3}} \tag{27}$$

If the original particle diameter of the drug (assumed spherical) is 32 μm,
the density is 1.33 g cc^{-1}, and solubility 1.0 g liter^{-1}, the intrinsic dissolution rate constant can be calculated as follows:

$$k = 0.0153 \times \frac{(1.33) \ (32 \times 10^{-4})}{2(1 \times 10^{-3}) \ (0.500)^{1/3}}$$

$$= \frac{0.0153 \times 1.33 \times 32 \times 10^{-4}}{2 \times 10^{-3} \times 0.7937}$$

$$= 4.102 \times 10^{-2} \ cm \ sec^{-1}$$

In a well-written and clearly presented monograph on solid dosage
forms, Carstensen [111] differentiated between the dissolution of directly
compressed tablets and those manufactured by the wet granulation process.
Equations and examples are provided here to illustrate these two cases.

Dissolution of Direct-Compressed Tablets

When tablets prepared by direct compression or slugging disintegrate into
the primary particles within a reasonable time period, dissolution follows
the cube-root law (see Fig. 27). The portion AB of the curve can be
represented by the Hixon-Crowell cube-root law:

$$w_0^{1/3} - w^{1/3} = K(t - t_1) \tag{28}$$

where t_1 is the disintegration time and

$$K = \frac{2kc_s}{\rho d_0} w_0^{1/3} \tag{25}$$

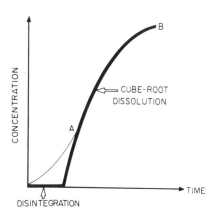

Figure 27 Dissolution-rate curve for a directly compressed or slugged tablet. (From Ref. 111.)

The term c_s is the solubility of the drug in g cm^{-3}, ρ the true density of the drug in g cm^{-3}, k the intrinsic dissolution rate constant in cm sec^{-1}, w_0 the original mass of drugs in the tablet, and d_0 the original diameter of the particles. If the diameters of the particles have increased during compression due to agglomeration, then the size is greater than d_0 of the primary particle. The dissolution process is occurring concomitantly with disintegration, so early in the process that curve does not show a shrap break at t_1 but rather has a smooth curvature AB. A plot of $w_0^{1/3} - w^{1/3}$ versus time is seen in Figure 27, and extrapolation to the horizontal axis will give a good measure of the disintegration time t_1.

As an example of the use of Eq. (28) for the disintegration of tablets into granules and liberation of drug into the bulk liquid, consider an aspirin tablet that disintegrates in 2 min in aqueous medium. If the tablet contains 325 mg of acetylsalicylic acid and 60% of the drug is released in a dissolution test in the first 10 min, what is the time required for 90% of the drug to be released?

Forty percent of 325 mg, or 130 mg, of aspirin remains after 10 min. Equation (28) gives

$$(325)^{1/3} - (130)^{1/3} = K(10 - 2)$$

$$K = 0.226 \text{ mg}^{1/3} \text{ min}^{-1}$$

At the time desired, $t_{10\%}$, w = 32.5 mg, since 90% of the aspirin has dissoolved in the medium.

$$(325)^{1/3} - (32.5)^{1/3} = 0.226(t - 2)$$

$$t_{10\%} = 18.32 \text{ min}$$

Thus, it requires 18.3 min for 90% of the aspirin in this tablet to be released from the granule and pass into the solution.

Dissolution of Wet Granulated Tablets

When tablets are manufactured by wet granulation techniques, they first
distintegrate into various size granules containing drug and excipients,
rather than into primary drug particles, as in the case of directly compressed tablets. Two cases may be considered: tablets can disintegrate
into porous or into relatively nonporous granules.

First, for the disintegration of tablets into porous granules and diffusion of drug from the granules into the bulk solution, Carstensen [111]
gives the equation

$$\ln \frac{W}{V} - C = -k' (t - t_1 - t_2) + \ln \frac{W}{V} \qquad (29)$$

where W is the amount of drug in the dose being dissolved, C the concentration of drug in the solution, t the time, t_1 the disintegration time of the
tablet into granules, t_2 the time required for penetration of liquid into the
porous granule, and t_3 or $(t - t_1 - t_2)$ the time for the drug to diffuse
into the bulk solution (see Fig. 28).

If, in the second case, the granules contain insoluble material and are
relatively nonporous, the time for penetration of the liquid into the granule
may be rate-determining rather than the process of drug diffusion into the
bulk solution.

In this case the drug is released from the granules according to the
equation

$$Q = (K'B \varepsilon t)^{1/2} \qquad (30)$$

where Q is the amount of drug dissolved per unit area of surface, B the
fraction of drug in the tablet or granule, ε the porosity of the granules or
dosage form mass, and t the time. K' is a constant equal to $2DC_s$, where

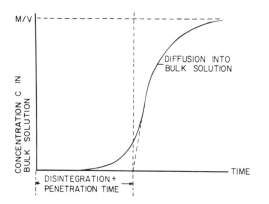

Figure 28   Dissolution-rate curve for a wet granulated tablet. (From
Ref. 111.)

D is the diffusion coefficient of drug in the dissolving medium, and c_s the solubility of drug in the medium. This equation is a form of the Higuchi square-root law [112]. Equation (30) is also applicable to the release of a drug from a capsule containing hydrophobic excipients such as talc and magnesium stearate. The dissolving liquid penetrates this mass only with difficulty, and the time for penetration is therefore the rate-determining step.

The dissolution-rate constant K' is calculated as follows. A tablet of nonporous granules contains 200 mg of drug and 150 mg of excipients, both of density 1.6 g cc^{-1}. The tablet has a surface area of 1.22 cm^2 and a volume of 0.25 cm^3. Calculate the dissolution rate constant K' and obtain Q, the amount of drug dissolved per unit area of tablet surface after 25 min. Experimentally, it is found that 180 mg of the drug has been released from the tablet after 5.0 min.

The total amount of drug and excipient is 0.35 g. The volume taken up by this mass is 0.35 g/1.6 (g/cc^{-1}) or 0.219 cc of drug plus excipient. Since the volume of the tablet is 0.230 cc, the air space in the tablet is 0.230 cc minus 0.219 cc, or 0.011 cc. This amounts to a porosity of 0.011 cc. This amounts to a porosity of 0.011/0.230 = 0.048, or 4.8%.

1. Using Eq. (30), we obtain for Q of 180 mg, at a t of 5 min and B = 200/350, the following:

$$180 \text{ mg cm}^{-2} = \left[K' \frac{200}{350} (0.048) (5.0 \text{ min}) \right]^{1/2}$$

$$K'^{1/2} = \frac{180 \text{ mg}}{0.370} = 486.1$$

$$K' = 236,250 \text{ mg}^2 \text{ cm}^{-4} \text{ min}^{-1}$$

2. After 2 min, the amount of drug dissolved is

$$Q = \left[236,250 \left(\frac{200}{350} \right) (0.048) (25) \right]^{1/2}$$

$$= 403 \text{ mg cm}^{-2}$$

Dissolution of Coated Tablets

Tablets may be film coated to seal the ingredients from moisture and to inhibit photolytic degradation of the active constituents. Tablets and pellets are also coated to produce a sustained release product or provide enteric properties, thus protecting acid-sensitive drugs from decomposition in the gastric fluids. Ideally, a sustained-release preparation should provide part of the drug quickly at the absorption site to achieve sufficient absorption and produce a rapid therapeutic response. The balance of the drug should be provided at a sufficient rate to maintain pharmacological activity over an extended time. In the simplest case (i.e., a one-compartment open model with essentially 100% absorption and total urinary excretion via first-order kinetics), the drug should be provided to the blood at a rate equal to the rate loss from the compartment [113].

As in other cases previously described, liquid must penetrate the film of the tablet or pellet and enter the dosage matrix in order for the drug to be released and diffused into the bulk solution. Barriers such as polymeric coatings and wax matrices, used in timed-release medication, can function to prolong therapeutic activity, however, such dosage forms suffer the inherent problem of possible drug nonavailability and must be carefully formulated so that they provide a uniform drug release over the desired time interval.

El-Fattah and Khalil [114] studied the dissolution rates of 14 batches of sugar-coated chlorpromazine tablets (10, 25, and 100 mg) using the USP XXI method I apparatus. Although all batches of tablets passed the U.S.P. disintegration test in 0.1 N HCl, none passed the U.S.P. dissolution limit (not less than 80% dissolved after 30 min). Poor dissolution rates were ascribed to delayed break-up of the sugar-coat. The dissolution and dialysis rates of tablets for one batch were dependent on the medium composition suggesting a possible drug-excipient interaction.

The dissolution of phenylpropanolamine hydrochloride from a wax matrix timed-release tablet was shown by Goodhart et al. [115] to follow the diffusion equation proposed by Higuchi [112]:

$$Q = \left[\frac{D\varepsilon}{\tau} (2A - \varepsilon c_s) c_s t \right]^{1/2} \tag{31}$$

Here Q is the amount of drug released per unit area of the tablet exposed to the solvent, D the diffusion coefficient of the drug in the permeating fluid, ε the porosity of the matrix, τ the tortuosity of the matrix, A the concentration of solid drug in the matrix, c_s the solubility of drug in the permeating fluid, and t the time. If

$$K'' = \left[\frac{D\varepsilon}{\tau} (2A - \varepsilon c_s) c_s \right]^{1/2} \tag{32}$$

then

$$Q = K'' t^{1/2} \tag{33}$$

For a diffusion-controlled mechanism as postulated in Eq. (31), a plot of the amount released per unit area versus the square root of time should be linear, as predicted by Eq. (33), and the slope of the line would equal K''. Goodhart et al. [115] showed that after 1 hr, a drug release from the tablet matrix followed Higuchi's equation and that different tablet thickness and hardness caused less than 10% variation in drug release at any particular time interval. As seen in Figure 29, wax matrix tablets are slowly permeated by the dissolution media as a function of time.

The percentage volume penetration of dissolution fluid was proportional to $t^{1/2}$. In the earlier time period, drug release lagged about 1 hr behind fluid penetration. This lag time increased at later time periods. The authors found from extrapolation of the curves that 7 hr was required for complete penetration and 11.5 hr for complete drug release.

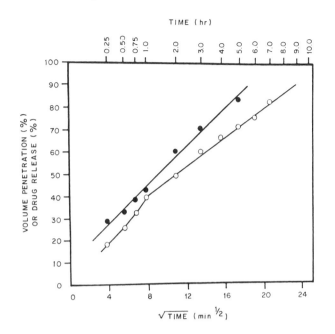

Figure 29 Comparison of fluid penetration and percent drug release from a phenylpropanolamine hydrochloride 150-mg wax matrix tablet. Compression force was 544.3 kg. •, Percent volume penetration of dissolution fluid; ○, percent drug release. (From Ref. 116.)

C. Dissolution Apparatus

Taking into consideration the considerable amount of work done to date on dissolution of tablet dosage forms, it is not surprising that more than 100 different apparatuses have been proposed for the measurement of in vitro drug release from solid dosage forms. Pernarowski [116] cited 100 published methods, and Lettir [117], Hersey [118], and Baun and Walker [119] described the technology in detail. It is not our intention to review the apparatus and methods in detail, but rather to highlight official methods, together with others that have gained popularity.

Swarbrick [120] classified the various techniques of dissolution from a consideration of their associated hydrodynamics. Hersey [118] classified dissolution methods on the basis not only of the type of agitation but also whether the dissolution process occurs under sink or nonsink conditions. Stricker [121] divided the dissolution methods into three groups: closed-compartment systems, open-flow-through chambers, and dialysis and diffusion models. Table 9 illustrates this classification. In diffusion models, dissolved substance passes through a membrane or dividing layer into a second compartment. Closed-compartment systems usually employ large volumes of dissolution solvent. Open flow-through chambers also use

Table 9   In Vitro Methods for the Study of Drug Dissolution

Closed-compartment systems	Open flow-through systems	Dialysis and diffusion models	Other methods
Rotating basket USP XXI	Pernarowski et al. [146]	Marlow and Shangraw [222]	Tape method (Goldberg et al. [225])
Hanging pellet (Nelson [21])	Striker [121]		
Rotating disk (Nelson and Levy [48])			
Rotating bottle (Souder and Ellenbogen [216])	Langenbucher [220]	Barzilay and Hersey [223]	Coulter Counter (Edmundson and Lees [226])
Oscillating tube (Vieit [217])	Marshall and Brook [121]		
Beaker method (Levy and Hayes [137])		Northern et al. [224]	Simultaneous dissolution and partition rates (Niebergall et al. [228])
Static disk (Levy [138])			
Stationary basket (Cook et al. [218])	Shah and Ochs [148]		
Rocking apparatus (MacDonald et al. [23])	Smolen [175]		Methods and Apparatus for Automatic Dissolution Testing of Products (Smolen [175, 176])
Circulating flow-through cell (Baun and Walker [119])			
Paddle method (Poole [145])			
Sintered filter (Cook [219])	Tingstad and Riegelman [227]		
Spin filter (Shah et al. [126, 148])			

large volumes of solvent, but only a small amount, similar to the volume present in the gastrointestinal tract, is actually active in the dissolution process at any point in time.

The types of apparatus, as indicated by Barr [20], differ in a number of respects. These differences involve the type of agitation; the intensity of agitation; the dispersion of the particles; the abrasion of the intact tablet or particles; the volume and rate of exchange of the dissolving medium; the flexibility of the system to vary volumes or agitation intensities; the reproducibility of the system from run to run; the reproducibility of the system in different laboratories, which depends on the availability of standardized components; the container; the stirrer; the volume and rate of exchange of the dissolving fluid relative to the solubility of the drug tested; and experience and documentation available for the method. Excellent reviews of dissolution methodology have recently appeared in the literature [122–124].

Wagner [125] indicated that a dissolution rate apparatus suitable for both research and quality control purposes should meet certain criteria:

1. The apparatus should be economically practical. Ideally, the apparatus should be capable of being fashioned from standard laboratory equipment.
2. The apparatus should be scientifically realistic. The inherent variability in the apparatus should be less than the inherent variability in the products being tested.
3. The apparatus must be flexible in providing an effective degree of agitation. That is, one must be able to alter the effective degree of agitation by altering stirring rate or some similar parameter.

Shah et al. [126] suggested additional criteria:

1. Dissolution rates evaluated by the apparatus under appropriate physiological test conditions should correlate with the in vivo dissolution rate-controlled drug absorption process.
2. The equipment must provide a convenient means for introducing a test sample (tablet, capsule, etc.) into the dissolution medium and holding it at a set position such that the sample is completely immersed in the fluid medium. During the dissolution process, the test sample must be subjected to minimal mechanical impacts, abrasion, and wear in order to retain its microenvironment.
3. The dissolution fluid container must be closed to prevent solvent evaporation, thermostated to regulate fluid temperature, and preferably transparent to permit visual observation of the disintegration characteristics of the test sample and fluid flow conditions during dissolution. It should be possible to maintain solvent sink conditions by employing either a relatively large volume of dissolution fluid or other convenient means, such as continuous flow dilution of the bulk fluid with fresh solvent.
4. Withdrawal of representative fluid sample of the bulk medium for analysis, either by manual or automated methods, must be possible without interrupting solution agitation. As an automated system, it should be possible to conduct continuous filtration of the fluid samples efficiently without encountering operational or analytical problems.

5. The apparatus must be applicable for the evaluation of disintegrating, nondisintegrating, dense, or "floating" tablets and capsules; finely powdered drugs; and all other types of solid drug forms.

USP XXII Apparatus

The apparatus for dissolution testing was described in the USP XXI in detail and the rotating basket and paddle methods are shown in Figures 30 and 31, respectively. The description of the apparatus and method in the USP are as follows:

Apparatus 1. The assembly consists of the following: a covered vessel made of glass or other inert, transparent material (the materials should

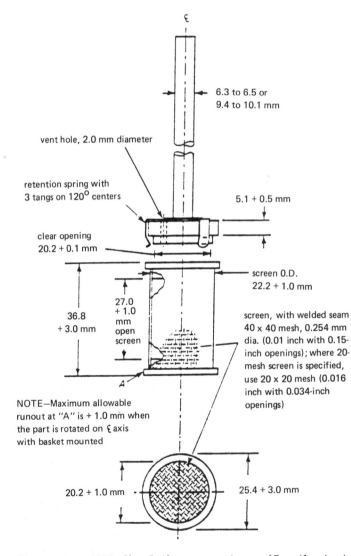

6.3 to 6.5 or
9.4 to 10.1 mm

vent hole, 2.0 mm diameter

retention spring with
3 tangs on 120° centers

5.1 + 0.5 mm

clear opening
20.2 + 0.1 mm

screen O.D.
22.2 + 1.0 mm

27.0
+ 1.0
mm
open
screen

36.8
+ 3.0 mm

screen, with welded seam
40 x 40 mesh, 0.254 mm
dia. (0.01 inch with 0.15-
inch openings); where 20-
mesh screen is specified,
use 20 x 20 mesh (0.016
inch with 0.034-inch
openings)

A

NOTE—Maximum allowable
runout at "A" is + 1.0 mm when
the part is rotated on ₵ axis
with basket mounted

20.2 + 1.0 mm

25.4 + 3.0 mm

Figure 30 USP dissolution apparatus. (See the text for a description.)
(From USP XXII.)

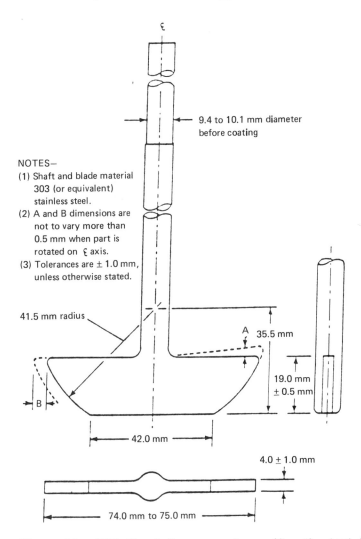

NOTES—
(1) Shaft and blade material 303 (or equivalent) stainless steel.
(2) A and B dimensions are not to vary more than 0.5 mm when part is rotated on ₵ axis.
(3) Tolerances are ± 1.0 mm, unless otherwise stated.

9.4 to 10.1 mm diameter before coating

41.5 mm radius

A 35.5 mm

19.0 mm ± 0.5 mm

42.0 mm

4.0 ± 1.0 mm

74.0 mm to 75.0 mm

Figure 31 USP dissolution apparatus. (See the text for a description.) (From USP XXII.)

not sorb, react, or interfere with the specimen being tested): a motor; a metallic drive shaft; and a cylindrical basket. The vessel is partially immersed in a suitable water bath of any convenient size that permits holding the temperature inside the vessel at 37 ± 0.5° during the test and keeping the batch fluid in constant, smooth motion. No part of the assembly, including the environment in which the assembly is placed, contributes significant motion, agitation, or vibration beyond that due to the smoothly rotating stirring element. Apparatus that permits observation of the specimen and stirring element during the test is preferable. The vessel is cylindrical, with a hemispherical bottom. It is 160 to 175 mm high, its inside diameter is 98 to 106 to 175 mm high, its inside diameter is 98 to 106 mm, and its nominal capacity is 1000. Its sides are flagged at the top.

A fitted cover may be used to retard evaporation. (If a cover is used, it provides sufficient openings to allow ready insertion of the thermometer and withdrawal of specimens.) The shaft is positioned so that its axis is not more than 2 mm at any point from the vertical axis of the vessel and rotates smoothly and without significant wobble. A speed-regulating device is used that allows the shaft rotation speed to be selected and maintained at the rate specified in the individual monograph, within ±4%.

Shaft and basket components of the stirring element are fabricated of stainless steel, type 316 or equivalent, to the specifications shown in Figure 30. Unless otherwise specified in the individual monograph, use 40-mesh cloth. A basket having a gold coating 0.0001 inch (2.5 μm) thick may be used. The dosage unit is placed in a dry basket at the beginning of each test. The distance between the inside bottom of the vessel and the basket is maintained at 25 ± 2 mm during the test.

Apparatus 2. Use the assambly from *Apparatus 1*, except that a paddle formed from a blade and a shaft is used as the stirring element. The shaft is positioned so that its axis is not more than 2 mm at any point from the vertical axis of the vessel, and rotates smoothly without significant wobble. The blade passes through the diameter of the shaft so that bottom of the blade is flush with the bottom of the shaft. The paddle conforms to the specifications shown in Figure 31. The distance of 25 ± 2 mm between the blade and the inside bottom of the vessel is maintained during the test. The metallic blade and shaft comprise a single entity that may be coated with a suitable inert coating. The dosage unit is allowed to sink to the bottom of the vessel before rotation of the blade is started. A small, loose piece of nonreactive material such as not more than a few turns of wire helix may be attached to dosage units that would otherwise float.

Hanson Research Corporation (Northridge, California) offers a multiple-spindle drive apparatus (Model 72) which was redesigned to reduce vibration levels. Preliminary results of their investigations [127] indicate that vibration significantly decreases dissolution times on a linear basis when it is measured at the resin flask and the displacements are in excess of 0.2 ml. Significant changes were noticeable at lower speeds (25 rpm) but were not significant at speeds of 100 rpm or above. The dissolution apparatus previously discussed is based upon the apparatus designed by Gershberg and Stoll [128]. Huber et al. [129], Kaplan [130], Schroeter and Hamlin [131], Schroeter and Wagner [132], and Lazarus et al. [133] have used modifications of the USP-NF tablet disintegration apparatus for drug dissolution studies.

Rotating Flask Dissolution Apparatus

This equipment, as introduced by Gibaldi and Wintraub [26], permitted an absolute quantitative correlation between absorption and in vitro dissolution of aspirin from three dosage forms, as illustrated in Figure 32.

---

*The use of portions of the text of USP XXII is by permission of the USP Convention. The Convention is not responsible for any inaccuracy of quotation or for any false or misleading implication that may arise from separation of excerpts from the original context or by obsolescence resulting from publication of a supplement.

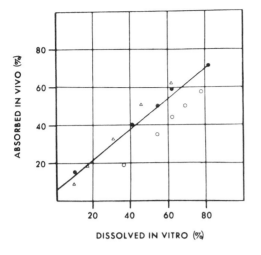

Figure 32   Percent of dose of aspirin absorbed to time T after drug administration versus percent dissolved in vitro at time T.   ○, Conventional tablets; ●, buffered tablets; △, timed-release tablets.   (From Ref. 26.)

Figure 33 shows a schematic diagram of the rotating flask apparatus used by them to determine the rate of release of drug. It consists of a spherical glass flask suspended in a constant-temperature bath. The globe is supported by glass rods, fused to its sides, which form the horizontal axis of the sphere. One support rod is coupled to a constant-speed motor, which provides rotation about the horizontal axis. A sampling port is molded into the sphere to permit introduction of the dosage form and periodic withdrawal of samples. The volume of the dissolution medium (in

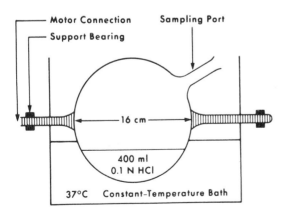

Figure 33   Schematic diagram of rotating flask dissolution apparatus. (From Ref. 26.)

this case, 400 ml) and the position of the sampling port are such that
fluid does not enter the port, regardless of the position of the flask as it
proceeds through a revolution. These measures prevent the accumulation
of undissolved solid in the port. The port is stoppered to prevent loss
of the dissolution medium to the water bath. This method is based on
experience with the apparatus described by Simoons [134]. The hydrodynamics of the two pieces of equipment are similar.

Beaker Methods

Parrott et al. [135] reported the use of a 2-liter, three-neck round-bottom
flask to follow the dissolution of nondisintegrating spherical tablets. They
used a stirring rate of 550 rpm, causing the tablets to rotate freely in the
liquid rather than remaining on the bottom of the flasl. Nelson [136] described a dissolution apparatus in which a nondisintegrating drug pellet
was mounted on a glass slide so that only the upper face was exposed.
The mounted pellet was placed at the bottom of a 600-ml beaker in such a
manner that it could not rotate. The stirring rate was 500 rpm.

    Levy and Hayes [137] were the first to use less intense agitation (80
to 60 rpm); their procedure is one of the simplest yet most widely used
techniques. The dissolution assembly consists of a 400-ml Pyrex Griffin
beaker immersed in a constant-temperature batch adjusted to 37 ± 0.1°C.
A three-blade 5-cm-diameter polyethylene stirrer is attached to an electronically controlled stirring motor affording precision speed control. The
stirrer is immersed in the dissolution medium to a depth of 27 mm and accurately centered by means of a girdle. Stirring rates of 30 to 60 rpm
are usually used. The stirring speed is sufficient to obtain a homogenous
solution for sampling purposes, but at the same time it is low enough so
that the solids of the disintegrated tablet remain at the bottom of the
beakers. Typically, the circular flow of the dissolution medium causes the
powdered drug to aggregate at the center of the bottom of the beaker
within an area of 1 or 2 cm^2.

    This method has been successfully utilized by Levy [22, 138] and by
Levy and Procknal [139]. Modifications to the Levy-Hayes method have
been performed by Campagna et al. [140], Niebergall and Goyan [141],
Gibaldi and Feldman [142], Castello et al. [143], and Paikoff and Drumm
[144].

Paddle Method of Poole [145]

The basic features of this procedure are the use of a three-neck round-
bottom flask as the dissolution vessel and a standard Teflon stirring
paddle located in a standard position relative to the bottom of the flask
and maintained at a constant speed by electronically controlled stirrers.
The dissolution vessel is immersed in a temperature-controlled water bath
maintained constant at 37°C. The solution is pumped from the dissolution
vessel through Tygon tubing to a spectrophotometer by means of a
peristaltic pump. The dissolution vessel is either a 1- or 2-liter three-
neck round-bottom flask. This enables use of from 500 to 2000 ml of solvent media in the test procedure. The stirring paddle is a 7.6-cm-
diameter Teflon paddle and is positioned 2.5 cm from the bottom of the
flask. The stirring rate is maintained at 15 rpm by means of an electronically controlled stirrer. The dosage form is introduced through one
opening of the three-neck flask. In cases where tablets are the dosage

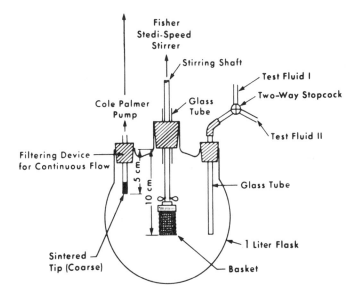

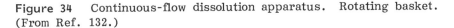

Figure 34   Continuous-flow dissolution apparatus. Rotating basket.
(From Ref. 132.)

form being evaluated, the dosage unit positions itself at the bottom of the
round flask directly under the paddle. In cases where capsules are the
formulation under investigation, a wire spiral around the capsule is
utilized as a sinker and is employed to position the capsule at the bottom
of the flask under the paddle in essentially the same position that the
tablet assumes.

Wagner [125] used this type of dissolution assembly with silicone rubber tubing and directly pumped the solution through a flow cell using a
peristaltic pump. He has obtained a good correlation of in vitro results
with absorption rates.

Hanson Research Corporation (Northridge, California) has modified
this apparatus and offers a vibration-free apparatus with Teflon shafts and
stirrers.

Rotating Basket Method

The NF XIV dissolution method is based on the rotating basket method
introduced by Pernarowski et al. [146]. Figure 34 illustrates the continuous-flow dissolution rotating basket apparatus. The dissolution container
is a 1-liter, three-neck flask. The main neck is 35 mm in diameter; the
secondary necks are 20 mm in diameter. The total volume of the container
is slightly more than 1 liter. If fluid flow or changeover is necessary, the
container is connected (via s suitable filtering device and short lengths of
latex tubing) to a Cole-Parmer series A-76910 or similar pump. Flow rates
of up to 70 ml min^{-1} have been used. Test fluids may be circulated
through a 1-cm flow cell in a spectrophotometer. Dissolution profiles are
graphed externally on a previously calibrated recorder. Figure 35 shows

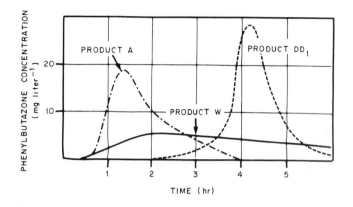

Figure 35 Dissolution profiles for three brands of phenylbutazone tablets. (From Ref. 116.)

the dissolution profile for three brands of phenylbutazone tablets. Figure 36 illustrates an in vivo/in vitro correlation of $t_{90\%}$ dissolution values with in vivo data for seven brands of phenylbutazone tablets using the rotating basket method.

Filter-Stationary Basket Method (Spin Filter) [126]

Essential features of the spin filter apparatus are a stationary sample basket, a large fluid container, and a rotating filter assembly. The

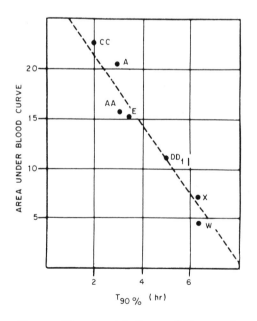

Figure 36 Correlations of $T_{90\%}$ values with in vivo data for seven brands of phenylbutazone tablets. (From Ref. 116.)

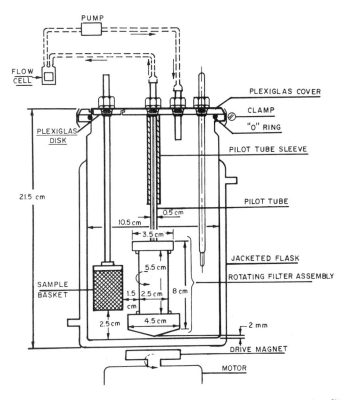

Figure 37 Schematic diagram of the rotating spin filter-stationary basket apparatus. Dashed lines represent the setup for the automated spectrophotometric analysis. (From Ref. 126.)

rotating filter, employed by Himmelfarb in the cultivation of mammalian cells [147] functions as a liquid agitation device as well as an efficient fluid sampling system.

The rotating filter-stationary basket single-test apparatus was constructed by incorporating necessary modifications into a commercially available microbial cell culture cultivation flask (Flasl Model BSC 1000 CA, Virtis Co., Gardiner, N.Y.). Basic features of the apparatus (Fig. 37) are a jacketed dissolution fluid container flask, a stat.onary sample basket, a rotating filter assembly, and an external variable-speed magnetic stirrer (Magnetic Stirrer Model MS-1, Virtis Co., Gardiner, N.Y.). Dashed lines in Figure 37 represent the optional setup for automated dissolution-rate determinations, in which filtered fluid samples are cycled through a spectrophotometer flow cell by means of 2-mm-ID flexible polyethylene tubing and a peristaltic pump (Model 1210, Harvard Apparatus Co., Millis, Massachusetts). The description of individual parts of the apparatus follows.

FLUID CONTAINER FLASK AND COVER. The jacketed glass flask, suitable for holding up to 1.5 liters of dissolution fluid, has a removable Plexiglas cover secured firmly to the neck of the flask by means of an

O-ring and a flexible metal belt. The cover serves as a support for the sample basket and the rotating filter assembly. A rabbeted-edge circular opening in the cover, 3 cm in diameter, provides an entrance pathway for the sample basket. There are three other ports in the cover: one in the center for a glass capillary pilot tube, another for a thermometer, and a third for the return of the dissolution fluid from the spectrophotometer flow cell.

SAMPLE BASKET. The design features of the stationary sample basket are similar to the basket assembly employed in the USP-NF Method I apparatus (NF XII), w.th the exception of using 12-mesh instead of 40-mesh wire cloth screen to facilitate fluid movement through the basket and prevent plugging of the basket screen with solid particles. A rabbeted-edge circular Plexiglas disk is attached to the baslet holding rod with a compression fitting, so that when the basket is introduced into the flask through the cover opening, this disk rests in the corresponding rabbeted-edge opening and holds the basket at a preset level in stationary position. The basket level can be varied by moving the position of the disk along the holding rod. In all experiments the basket was held 2.5 cm from the flask bottom (Fig. 37).

ROTATING FILTER ASSEMBLY. The rotating filter assembly provides a variable intensity of mild laminar liquid agitation and it also functions as an in situ nonclogging filter to permit intermittent or continuous filtration of the dissolution fluid samples efficiently during the dissolution process. The assembly is suspended in the center of the flask on the flared end of a glass capillary pilot tube. Since the pilot tube is secured firmly to the cover with a compression fitting, it remains in a fixed position while the assembly can freely rotate on the flared end of the tube. The assembly rotates by means of a controlled, variable-speed, external magnetic stirrer coupling with a magnetic bar embedded in the bottom part of the assembly. The level of the assembly in the flask can be varied simply by raising or lowering the pilot tube. A stainless steel pilot tube sleeve provides support to the pilot tube and prevents subtle vibration of the assembly. The design features of the assembly (Fig. 38) consist of a filter head, bottom flange, cylindrical filter, two flexible gaskets, and a dynamic seal. The filter head and bottom flange are fabricated from 20% glass-filled Teflon with a magnet embedded in the bottom flange. Cylindrical filters of glass fiber, Teflon, ceramic, or sintered stainless steel are available in the 0.2 to 3 μm porosity range. In assembling these parts, first the filter head is suspended on the flared end of the pilot tube, then the cylindrical filter with one flexible gasket on each end is slipped over the filter head, and finally the bottom flange is screwed into the filter head threads. The spring-action dynamic seal slid over the pilot tube positions into the filter head and prevents passage of liquid through the space between the pilot tube and the filter head. Arrows in the cross-sectional diagram of Figure 38 show the liquid filtration system and flow through the assembly. Dissolution fluid upon filtration through the cylindrical filter flows through a hole in the filter head, channels through a helical path around the pilot tube, and then enters the pilot tube capillary. Fluid samples can be withdrawn continuously or intermittently from the upper end of the pilot tube.

In vivo/in vitro correlations have been obtained using the rotating filter-stationary basket apparatus. Figure 39 illustrates the correlation

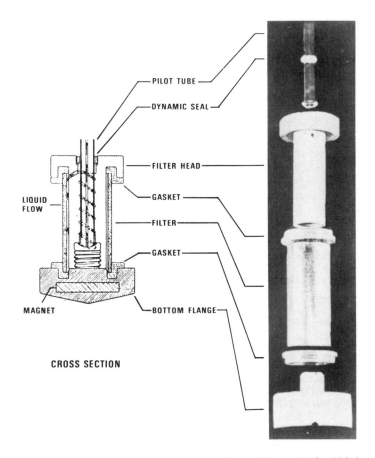

PILOT TUBE
DYNAMIC SEAL
FILTER HEAD
GASKET
FILTER
GASKET
BOTTOM FLANGE
LIQUID FLOW
MAGNET

CROSS SECTION

Figure 38 Rotating filter assembly. (From Ref. 126.)

between in vitro dissolution rates ($t_{50\%}$) and total in vivo response obtained with antidiabetic tablets.

Multiple-Test Apparatus

An automated multiple-test rotating filter-stationary basket apparatus is capable of monitoring up to six dissolution tests simultaneously. The basic design of this apparatus is similar to the single-test unit, with the exception of using a Plexiglas water bath to thermostat all six units and a six-state controlled variable-speed magnetic stirrer operated by a single motor. The upper panel of the stirrer housing is illuminated by a fluorescent light placed underneath the housing, which aids in visual observation of the test environment. Dissolution fluid samples from each flask are continuously cycled by a multichannel pump through one of six flow cells located in the cell compartment of the spectrophotometer. Dissolution rates are monitored by the spectral absorbance recording of the cycling fluid sample.

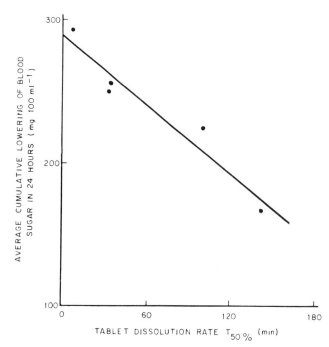

Figure 39 Correlation between the in vitro dissolution rates ($T_{50\%}$) and total in vivo response obtained with antidiabetic tablets. (From Ref. 126.)

Figure 40 shows a comparison of dissolution rates for five antidiabetic tablets obtained by continuous-flow and fixed fluid volume systems. Table 10 shows the correlation between continuous-flow dissolution rates of these antidiabetic tablets and their blood sugar-lowering response in dogs.

Table 10 Correlation Between Continuous-Flow Dissolution Rates of Antidiabetic Tablets and Their Blood Sugar-Lowering Response in Dogs

Sample	Percent dissolved in 60 min	Total blood sugar-lowering response in 24 hr (mg %)
A	92.3	293
B	76.2	256
C	52.5	250
D	35.3	225
E	24.7	167

Source: From Ref. 148.

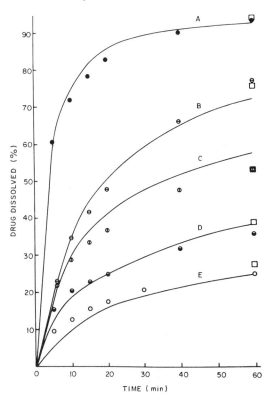

Figure 40   Comparison of dissolution-rate results for tablet samples obtained by continuous-flow and fixed-fluid-volume systems.   Lines represent the results obtained by fixed-fluid-volume experiments and points are the values calculated from continuous-flow experiments.   (From Ref. 148.)

In summary, this apparatus has the following advantages:

1.   Dissolution rates can be determined by either manual or automated methods.
2.   Filtration problems such as clogging of the filter with solid particles is avoided by a dynamic in situ microporous filter element.
3.   It permits the determination of dissolution profiles of tablets, capsules, powdered samples, and bulk drug.
4.   It permits representative sampling of the bulk dissolution medium because of the relatively large filter are extending over the greater portion of the dissolution fluid.
5.   Dissolution-rate determinations can be performed under sink conditions.
6.   Mild agitation conditions can be used.
7.   Retainment of the microenvironment of the test sample and accurate positioning of the sample have been accomplished.   This is a necessary requirement for reliable dissolution studies.
8.   Visual observation of the test sample is possible.

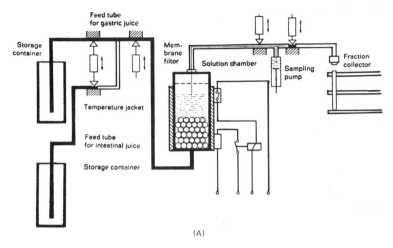

(A)

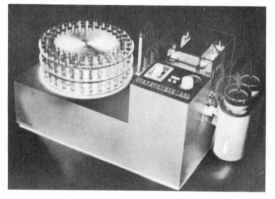

(B)

Figure 41 (A) Schematic diagram of the Sartorius solubility simulator, (B) Photograph. (Courtesy of Knut H. Vogel, Sartorius Filter, Inc., San Francisco.)

One of the disadvantages of the multiple test apparatus is that it is not capable of holding small volumes of fluid in continuous-flow operation.

SARTORIUS SOLUBILITY SIMULATOR. The solubility simulator is used mainly in the development and control of oral pharmaceutical preparations which contain the active ingredient in solid form (tablets, dragees, capsules, powders, suspensions, etc.). Figure 41 shows a schematic diagram and a photograph of the solubility simulator. It consists of two main systems: the solution chamber, which simulates the gastrointestinal tract, and a fraction collector, which represents the biophase. The thermostated (37°C) solution chambers, in which the solid drugs or drug preparations pass into solution, contain a fixed amount of inert filling material in addition to the artificial gastric or intestinal juice. Rotation of the chambers causes a peristaltic movement of the filling material. This both mixes the contents and simulates the mechanical forces in the gastro-intestinal tract. The absorption of dissolved drug is simulated as follows. A sampling pump transports solution (artificial gastric or intestinal juice) discontinuously from the solution chambers, through filtration systems, into the fraction collector tubes. An equal volume of buffer flows simul-taneously into the chambers to replace the sample volume removed. The sampling interval is set on a time-control dial, which automatically puts the fraction collector in motion. When the length of the experiment reaches the average time of stay of a drug in the stomach, the contents of the chamber (artificial gastric juice) are brought to the pH of the natural in-testinal juice. A simple calculation from the analytically determined drug concentration in the individual samples in the fraction collector gives the time dependence of the gastrointestinal dissolution (solubility character-istic) or the resulting rate of absorption (absorption characteristic) for the drug under test.

SARTORIUS ABSORPTION SIMULATOR. The absorption simulator con-sists of a magnetic stirrer peristaltic pump, thermostat, two containers for the artificial gastric or intestinal juice, and a diffusion chamber with an artificial lipid barrier. The lipid barrier consists of an inert membrane, the pores of which are filled with a liquid phase. Two different barriers may be utilized: an artificial stomach-wall barrier and an artificial in-testinal-wall barrier. Both are largely impermeable to hydrogen and hydroxyl ions. Thus, the pH gradient between the aqueous phases can be held constant over long periods of time. Figure 42 shows a schematic diagram and a photograph of this instrument.

Application of the solubility and absorption simulator has been re-ported by Stricker [149, 150], who found close agreement between the ab-sorption characteristics measured with the absorption simulator and ana-logous in vivo studies in humans. Table 11 shows the results obtained

Table 11 Absorption-Rate Constant (k_1) for Acetylsalicylic Acid in the Human Stomach[a]

	$k_1 \times 10^2$ (min^{-1})		
	In vivo		
Test person	Individual values	Mean	In vitro
A. R.	5.5		
H. F.	5.3		
E. S.	5.7		
J. G.	7.6	5.8	5.3 ± 0.5
K. M.	5.3		
I. D.	4.3		
F. H.	7.6		
C. D.	5.0		

[a] In vitro condition: phase I = simulated gastric juice of pH 1.1.
In vivo condition: pH of the orally administered solution was 1.2.

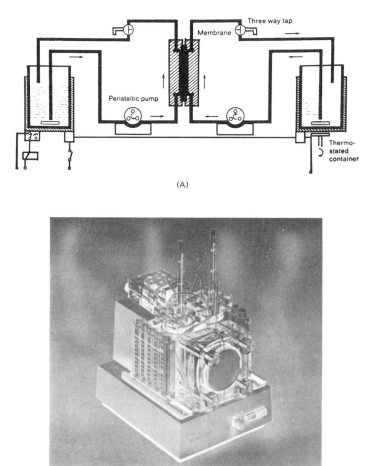

(A)

(B)

Figure 42   (A) Schematic diagram of the Sartorius absorption simulator,
(B) Photograph. (Courtesy of Knut H. Vogel, Sartorius Filter, Inc.,
San Francisco.)

with acetylsalicylic acid.   The absorption-rate constant for acetylsalicylic
acid from the stomach was calculated from blood level measurements following oral administration of dissolved acetylsalicylic acid to a substantial
number of test subjects.   The value of the diffusion-rate constant in vitro
obtained from the absorption simulator is almost identical with the in vivo
average.

Braybrooks et al. [151] examined the effect of mucin on the bioavailability of tetracycline from the gastrointestinal tract using the absorption simulator.   Nozaki et al. [152] studied the absorption rate of
aspirin and phenylbutazone at various pH levels using this apparatus.
The gastric absorption of phenylbutazone decreased in proportion to ele-
vation of pH in the solution.   However, the aspirin absorption rate was
only rarely increased by changes in pH.   Tovaraud [153] investigated

the permeability of phenobarbital with and without the addition of polyethylene glycol (PEG) 6000 by use of the absorption simulator. Results
showed that the rate of permeation was not changed by the addition of
PEG 6000, in agreement with findings of Singh et al. [154] and Solvang
and Finholt [155].

Computer Prediction of Drug Product Bioavailability Data:
Computational and Operational Approaches

In 1982, Smolen discussed the importance of dissolution testing to predict
in vivo bioavailability [156]. Smolen suggested that it is entirely impractical to perform the extensive and expensive human testing of drug
products which is needed to: (a) optimize the bioavailability dynamics
of formulations of new drugs in order to develop products having a maximum therapeutic benefit and attain a desired duration of action, (b) assure the bioequivalency of generic drug products or develop controlled
release drug delivery systems for old drugs, (c) assure bioequivalency
through lot-to-lot reproducibility testing; overly sensitive, in vivo
irrelevant, in vitro tests result in discarding lots whose in vivo performance is satisfactory, and (d) assure satisfactory bioavailability of drug
products through to their expiry dates; the use of in vivo irrelevant tests
can indicate that reductions in bioavailability have occurred through apparent physical instability whereas in fact such changes may be entirely
irrelevant to biological performance; needless product recalls and early
expiry dating can be the result. What is required in every case is an
in vivo-relevant in vitro test that can be rapidly and easily performed
to produce results which are optimally predictive of a drug product's performance in vivo. If the in vitro test is not biologically relevant, then it
may be better not to perform such testing at all than to suffer the fi-
nancial losses which arise from discarding product batches which actually
have a satisfactory in vivo bioavailability. Costly misdirections and delays can also occur in product development programs as a result of using
bio-irrelevant in vitro tests of candidate product formulations to guide
their further development to achieve sought in vivo bioavailability
objectives.

Drugs must be in solution if they are to become available to their sites
of absorption and subsequently become bioavailable to their sites of action.
The rate(s) of a drug's release from dosage forms to become dissolved in
the medium from which it is absorbed into the body becomes the rate-
limiting factor in the drug's bioavailability, especially for controlled release drug delivery systems and determines the quality of a drug product's
therapeutic performance. Therefore, from all the various in vitro physical
and chemical tests which can be performed on a drug product, in vitro
dissolution testing is potentially, the most biologically relevant and useful
tool in predicting in vivo bioavailability.

Smolen points out that in vitro—in vivo correlations reported in the
literature are of the single-point type. These single point type of correlations commonly attempted between amounts dissolved in vitro (or times
to dissolve given amounts) and univariate characteristics of in vivo blood
level versus time profiles (areas under the curve, peaks, times to peak,
etc.) are arbitrary, sometimes irrational and often entirely fortuitous when
observed, as well as not taking advantage of all the data available. The
correlations are also made after-the-fact and the results can be misleading.

For example, it has been shown that digoxin tablets often fractionate
in vitro leading to a rapid initial dissolution rate [157]; however, this
does not necessarily mean that the rest of the tablet releases drug similarly. Therefore, a correlation, such as amount of drug dissolved in
thirty minutes versus peak blood levels, could cause misleading results.

A better approach is to predict the entire time course of a drug
product's in vivo response profile from the results of an in vitro dissolution test. Methods for the computational conversion of dissolution data
into body fluid drug levels over time [158–162] or pharmacological response versus time profiles [163] have been described and implemented
[158–172]. The computational method utilized by the BioConverter program and described in published reports [170, 171] utilizes the mathematical operations of convolution and deconvolution to establish transfer
function (weighting functions in the time domain) relationships between
corresponding sets of in vitro test data and in vivo data obtained on one
or more reference dosage forms. Briefly, as an example of this approach,
the BioConverter program consists of a set of rigorous mathematical algo-
rithms for computationally transforming related sets of experimental data
(e.g., dissolution test results, plasma drug concentration samples, biologic response profiles, etc.) in the complex frequency domain. A
weighted mean system transfer function is identified by deconvoluting
in vitro dissolution test data for one or more reference dosage forms with
their corresponding known in vivo response profiles. Predicted in vivo
response functions for test dosage forms are then obtained by the inverse operation of convolving their in vitro dissolution test results with
the previously determined transfer function. The operations are performed numerically and no a priori assumptions or restrictions are imposed
as to pharmacokinetic or dissolution equation models or the shape of either
the in vitro dissolution versus time profiles or the in vivo bioavailability
response data.

Graphic results produced from the application of the Bio-Converter
program are exemplified in Figures 43 and 44 for nitrofurantoin, where
computationally predicted percentages of the dose of the drug excreted in
the urine over time are compared with temporally corresponding mean values experimentally observed in a panel of human subjects. The weighted
average transfer function utilized to perform the computations shown in
Figures 43 and 44, was constructed from six sets of in vitro and in vivo
data on six different 50 mg nitrofurantoin dosage forms [174].

The computational approach can only be applied when the dissolution
test conditions, as determined by the process variables, are in vivo relevant. For example, agitation rates, dissolution medium composition, and
sink conditions can be chosen to be so harsh as to obscure real in vivo
bioavailability differences between dosage forms; on the other hand,
process variables can be chosen to render a dissolution test too sensitive
in detecting differences which have no in vivo counterpart. These problems are circumvented by implementing the second approach which employs
an apparatus-based operational methodology (BioPredictor) which predicts
the time course of in vivo drug response in the form of a dissolution rate
versus time profile. The dissolution test process variables, such as dissolution medium composition, agitation, or solubility volume (sink conditions), are automatically, continually, and optimally changed by feedback
control throughout the in vitro test process to produce a dissolution rate

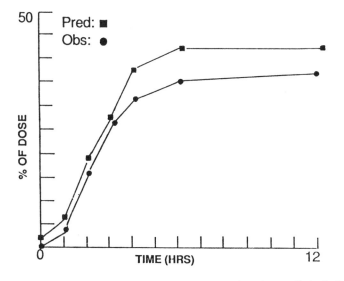

Figure 43   Comparison of computational predicted from in vivo dissolution data, and experimentally observed nitrofurantoin urinary recovery profiles. ■ Predicted, ● observed.

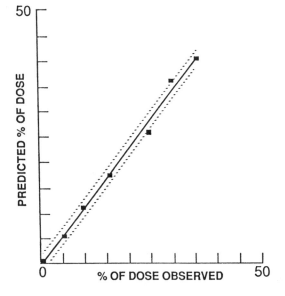

Figure 44   Comparison of computational predicted from in vitro dissolution data, and experimentally observed nitrofurantoin urinary recovery profiles. Top = upper 95%, center = linear reg., bottom = lower 95%, ■ = predicted versus observed.

profile which simulates a time and amplitude scaled in vivo response profile previously determined in humans for a *reference* dosage form undergoing dissolution. The scaled in vivo response profile constitutes the dissolution standard. For a detailed description of the BioPredictor feedback control system, the reader should consult the U.S. patents [175, 176].

D. Dissolution Apparatus Suitability Test

The use of dissolution apparatus calibrators is defined in the USP XXII as an apparatus suitability test. The test involves individually testing one tablet of the USP dissolution calibrator, disintegrating type (available from USP-NF Reference Standards, 23601 Twinbrook Parkway, Rockville, MD 20852) and one tablet of USP dissolution calibrator, nondisintegrating type, according to the operating conditions specified. The apparatus is suitable if the results obtained are within the acceptable range stated in the certificate of that calibrator in the apparatus tested. In 1978, the PMA (Pharmaceutical Manufacturers Association) conducted a collaborative study to determine whether the use of a calibrator was possible and if such a calibrator proved feasible, with the purpose to define its proper use in the standardization of dissolution testing [177].

Each of the collaborating laboratories received bottles with 60 tablets of each of the test samples, which included nondisintegrating 300 mg salicylic acid tablets (USP standard; Hoffmann-La Roche, Inc., Nutley, NJ) as well as disintegrating 50 mg prednisone tablets (research lot 18,747; The Upjohn Co., Kalamazoo, MI) and 2100-mg nitrofurantoin tablets (research lot Rx T11486; Parke, Davis & Co., Detroit, MI). In addition, approximately 1 g of salicylic acid, prednisone, and nitrofurantoin was supplied for use as reference standards.

The collaborators received instructions on the objectives of the study as well as on how to collect and submit data. The instructions were explicit for manual methods for sampling and UV analysis, though automated methods were also permitted. Two dissolution apparatuses were described, neither of which was official at the time the study began late in 1978, but which are now official as USP XXII Apparatus 1 (rotating basket) and USP Apparatus 2 (rotating paddle).

The rotating basket was to be operated at 50, 100, or 150 rpm, the rotating paddle at 50 or 100 rpm. Samples were to be taken at 15, 30, 45, and 60 min after the start of the test. Collaborators were instructed to report results derived with six tablets.

A total of 15 collaborators submitted data. Only data from the 30 min test point was used, a decision consistent with USP's single-point definition of dissolution as a percentage dissolved in a specified time.

Analysis of variance was conducted to calculate laboratory means, within-laboratory variance, and between-laboratory variance. A standard F test demonstrated that for all 30 min data points, the variance between laboratories was significantly greater than the variance within laboratories at the 99.5% confidence level. It was thereby established that the observed variance was not solely attributable to the samples being tested. If the F value had *not* been statistically significant, it would have meant that none of the between-laboratory variation could be attributed to anything other than the test samples, and the samples would therefore not have been acceptable as calibrators. The collaborative study's first objective was

Table 12   Summary of Acceptance Limits[a]

Sample	Apparatus	Speed (rpm)	Acceptance limits	
			$\overline{X}$	Sx
Salicylic acid	Basket	50	13 – 19	2.4
	Basket	100	22 – 30	3.4
	Paddle	50	15 – 23	3.7
	Paddle	100	16 – 34	4.3
Prednisone	Basket	50	21 – 49	6.7
	Basket	100	48 – 80	7.4
	Paddle	50	49 – 75	9.3
	Paddle	100	66 – 83	3.4

[a]Based on percent of nominal label claim dissolved in 30 min.

thus satisfied, and the selected samples were deemed acceptable as calibrators.

The second objective of the PMA study involved defining the use of the calibrators and establishing acceptance limits. Acceptance limits were computed based upon each laboratory's reported mean value for six tablets and the within-laboratory standard deviation. Table 12 presents the computed acceptance limits for the salicylic acid and prednisone tablets, while Table 13 presents the current USP prednisone calibrator tablet acceptance ranges for lot F [177].

The use of calibrators, ultimately defined by USP as an apparatus-suitability test, employs a single-tablet test criterion more in line with USP's general testing policies. Suitability is thus determined individually on each spindle of the dissolution apparatus, rather than by the use of mean values. This procedure obviates the requirement for assessing within-laboratory variance. In order to maintain the approximate 95% confidence limits on single-tablet test results, USP's acceptance ranges are

Table 13   Current USP Prednisone Calibrator Tablet Acceptance Ranges (Lot F)

Apparatus	Percent label dissolved at 30 min	
	50 rpm	100 rpm
Rotating Basket	21 – 49	49 – 81
Rotating paddle	51 – 77	68 – 85

similar, but not identical to the limits described in Table 12 and originally proposed by the PMA committee. The differences, however, are small, as can be seen from Tables 12 and 13.

The PMA Committee believes that careful definition of operating parameters, such as basket or paddle dimensions and limits on rotational speed, along with the use of standard samples as calibrators, will improve the agreement of dissolution data obtained by different laboratories.

E. The Role of Dissolution Testing in Bioavailability and Bioequivalence Testing

The PMA's joint Committee on Bioavailability recently published some of their views regarding dissolution testing and the Drug Price Competition and Patent Restoration Act of 1984 (referenced in text as the Act) [178]. The Act of 1984 provides, in part, for a modification of the drug approval process to facilitate the introduction of pharmaceutical equivalents into the marketplace. Title I of the Act adds a new subsection, 505(j), to the Food, Drug, and Cosmetic Act to permit the filing and approval of abbreviated applications (ANDAs) for duplicate versions of new drugs first marketed after 1962. The abbreviated application must contain information to show the following:

> The indications are the same as one or more of the indications of a previously approved pioneer drug (a *listed drug*)
> The route of administration, dosage form, and strength are the same
> The labeling is the same
> The drug is bioequivalent to the listed drug

The FDA, in response to the question of what type of bioequivalence requirement will be imposed, has stated: "In vivo data will be required for single-source and post-1962 drugs until such time as a correlation between in vivo and in vitro standards can be established for individual drugs." The FDA's position on bioequivalence is both appropriate and timely because dissolution testing has been proposed in some quarters as a single, free-standing test procedure sufficient to demonstrate the pivotal acceptability characteristic of bioequivalence for generic formulations.

The PMA's committee on bioavailability suggests that dissolution testing can be used only as a guide to a formulator in the early stages of drug product design. For some drugs, correlations can be made between in vitro dissolution and in vivo absorption. These correlations, however, can be developed only after biological data have been obtained. Although dissolution testing is one of the critical assessments that must be performed to ensure that a formulation proven safe and effective in the clinic is being manufactured with consistent quality, it is not sufficiently predictive to replace biological testing. Once a drug has been designed and has been shown by in vivo testing to be safe and efficacious, control of the dissolution rate from lot to lot is important for ensuring consistent quality.

Correlations between in vivo bioavailability parameters with in vitro dissolution parameters have shown that it is possible, retrospectively, to develop correlations for immediate-release [179–183] and for controlled-release products [184–186]. However, these correlations apply only to the specific products studied. Thus, a new formulation may not relate to the previously demonstrated correlation.

The PMA Committee suggests that developing and validating an in vitro model that could account for the in vivo complexities of the absorption process (e.g., stomach emptying, intestinal transit, changing pH, and the influence of food on various physiologic components of the G.I. tract) would be a monumental undertaking, applicable only to a single drug of interest. Consequently, the approach of the FDA to request in vivo bioavailability/bioequivalence trials as the definitive evaluative tool appears to be appropriate. However, it should be remembered that in many instances, such as, in the case of anticancer drugs bioequivalence studies in health volunteers could be considered unethical.

Differences in bioequivalence between drug products are not, by themselves, evidence that the use of such products will produce significant problems in the treatment of patients. When bioequivalence may have therapeutic significance that may result in therapeutic failure or hazard to a patient, however, bioequivalence is vitally important.

Examples of bioinequivalence that have been reported in the literature include:

Digoxin [187]
Phenytoin [188–190]
Aminosalicylate [191]
Chloramphenicol [192]
Chloropamide [193]
Diazepam [194]
Levodopa [195]
Nitrofurantoin [196]
Oxytetracycline [197]
Phenylbutazone [198]
Prednisone [199]
Tetracycline [200]
Warfarin [201]

The PMA Committee on bioavailability concluded that dissolution testing should be used as a control device to ensure process and batch-to-batch consistency for a particular formulation of a particular manufacturer and as a screening tool in formulation development. Dissolution testing has failed, thus far, to reliably predict differences among products that are poorly bioavailable, among those that are superbioavailable, and among those that are absorbed to an equivalent degree but whose clinical response is dependent not only on the extent of absorption but on the rate of absorption as well. Unfavorable outcomes of these differences are preventable through appropriate in vivo bioavailability testing.

In the fiscal year 1985, the FDA approved the marketing of 122 generic equivalents of drugs introduced after 1962. In fiscal year 1986, the figure was 398. In fiscal year 1987, from October 1986 through February 1987, 232 new generic equivalents of post-1962 drugs were approved. By contrast, from 1962 through September 1984, a cumulative total of fewer than 75 such generic products had been approved (N.E.J.M.). The FDA has estimated that as a result of the 1984 legislation, manufacturers of generic drugs may realize an increase in revenues of $2 billion a year—i.e., a 50 percent increase over the $4 billion share of the retail prescription drug market that they held in 1984 [202]. Although the large stakes have naturally heightened the controversy over generic equivalence that has gone on for decades, the major clinical and scientific issues underlying the controversy have not been resolved [203, 208–214].

Strom [202] suggested that the FDA's current method of approving new generic products—i.e., on the basis of bioavailability data—seems to be an acceptable interim approach. Clearly, it should be improved as the technology evolves, and attempts are being made to improve it [211].

However, the FDA should encourage the development of clinical data to test the assumptions inherent in the existing approach. Inasmuch as generic products are already on the market, and since studies of the relative effects of two products containing the same drug would require very large sample sizes [211, 212], the most cost-efficient way of collecting these clinical data may be by postmarketing drug surveillance. A number of techniques are not available with which to perform such studies [211, 212]. Yet, postmarketing surveillance has usually been used to study adverse reactions to drugs, instead of their effectiveness, and the most important questions to be addressed in the current context are questions of effectiveness.

It is evident from these discussions that the chapter on bioequivalence has not been completed, and perhaps future work should include bioequivalence studies based on therapeutic response and not only on drug plasma levels. We should keep in mind that in the definition of generic equivalence, both bioequivalence and therapeutic equivalence have equal weight.

F. In Vitro/In Vivo Correlations for Extended-Release Oral Dosage Forms

The USP Subcommittee on Biopharmaceutics [213] defined in vitro/in vivo correlations as follows: the establishment of a relationship between a biological property, or a parameter derived from a biological property produced by a dosage form, and a physicochemical characteristic of the same dosage form.

Historically, in vitro/in vivo correlations have been utilized mostly with immediate-release dosage forms by relating model-independent pharmacokinetic parameters such as AUC, C_{max}, or T_{max} to the percent released in vitro under a given set of conditions. More recently, similar relationships, in addition to some other correlative procedures, have been used for extended-release products.

The USP Subcommittee categorize in order of importance the various correlative methods possible. The correlations were categorized into Levels A, B, C, and D in descending order of quality.

Correlation Level A. This category represents the highest level of correlation. It demonstrates a 1:1 relationship between in vitro and in vivo dissolution. In such a correlation, the in vitro and in vivo dissolution curves are superimposable; the mathematics that describes one, describes the other. Such a procedure is most applicable to extended-release systems that demonstrate an in vitro release rate essentially independent of the dissolution medium. With this correlative procedure, one compares a product's in vitro dissolution curve to the in vivo dissolution curve (i.e., the curve produced by deconvolution of the plasma-level data). This may be done by using the Wagner-Nelson procedure or the Loo-Riegelman method or by direct mathematical deconvolution. Therefore, model-dependent or -independent methods may be used. A modification of the above technique is one that uses the same plasma-level deconvolution procedure but compares the results to the in vitro dissolution data obtained under various conditions, until the dissolution conditions producing a 1:1 correlation are established. The in vitro procedure producing this relationship should be employed for quality control purposes.

The advantages of correlation level A are as follows:

1. One develops a 1:1 in vitro/in vivo correlation that is not found with any other correlative method. A major advantage is that it is developed using every plasma level and dissolution point available; thus, it reflects the complete plasma-level curve shape.
2. A truly meaningful (in vivo indicating) quality control procedure that is predictive of product performance is defined for the product.
3. The extremes of the in vitro quality control standards can be justified by a convolution or a deconvolution procedure.
4. A change in manufacturing site, method of manufacture, raw-material supplies, minor formulation modification, and even in product strength using the same formulation can be justified without the need for additional human studies.

Correlation Level B. Many examples of this type of correlation procedure are found in the literature. This procedure uses the principles of statistical moment analysis. One compares the mean in vitro dissolution time to either the mean residence time of the product in vivo or the mean in vivo dissolution time. This second-level correlation procedure also uses all the in vitro and in vivo data, but is not considered to be a 1:1 correlation since it does not reflect the actual in vivo plasma-level curve; that is, a number of differences in the in vivo curves can produce similar mean residence times. Any data that fit correlation level A will also fit correlation level B, but not necessarily vice versa.

Correlation Level C. This category relates one dissolution time ($t_{50\%}$, $t_{90\%}$, etc.) to one pharmacokinetic parameter, such as AUC, C_{max}, T_{max}. It represents a single point correlation, and does not really reflect the *complete* blood level curve shape, which may be a critical factor for extended-release products.

Correlation Level D. This would include such items as disintegration relationship to in vivo performance or qualitative in vitro/in vivo relationships. We see no real value to such correlations.

Skelly [214, 215] recently reported an innovative method for correlating in vitro dissolution data with in vivo parameters. The method is referred to as a topographical dissolution characterization for controlled release products. Skelly suggests that with most controlled release oral drug dosage forms, dissolution is the rate limiting step in drug release. While in vivo drug absorption and elimination involve a number of complex factors, characterization of in vitro dissolution rate under controlled conditions (pH, solvent, speed, etc.) should be able to provide valuable insights into in vivo drug bioavailability.

Frequently, the analysis of these factors becomes obscured when a variety of data are presented in conventional two-dimensional plots. The choice of approval or disapproval of a new drug product based on such data becomes difficult. We have therefore examined the characteristics of drug product dissolution using a multidimensional technique as a means of more effectively delineating properties of dissolution rate. The results of

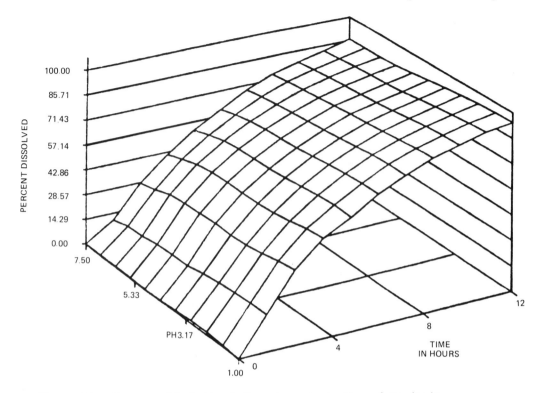

Figure 45   Topographical dissolution characterization of Squibb's Pronestyl-SR controlled release procainamide 500-mg tablets as a function of time and pH.

our studies show that more definitive information can be discerned in a multi-dimensional topographic image which has been shown to be predictive of in vivo drug plasma concentrations.

An example of a multidimensional image generated showing in vitro dissolution rate versus pH is shown in Figure 45. This figure shows a profile of Squibb's Pronestyl-SR procainamide controlled release 500-mg tablets. This dissolution analysis was run at four different pH values over a twelve hour dissolution time span. The profile was performed at a tilt angle of 60° and a rotation angle of 45°. It is readily apparent that the profile over the entire pH range is smooth and unremarkable. Nevertheless, it clearly demonstrates the pH-independent dissolution character of this controlled release formulation which has been shown by studies submitted to the FDA to be fully bioavailable. In situations where a complex relationship exists between in vitro dissolution and in vivo bioavailability, and where dissolution varies as a function of pH, the advantage of topographical analysis is even more obvious.

The use of topographical analysis is a more definitive and predictive method than two-dimensional analysis. This is demonstrated by the effects of pH on dissolution for product formulations of the same drug. The use of the topographical techniques in the selection of an in vitro dissolution medium is illustrated in Figures 46 and 47. The topographical

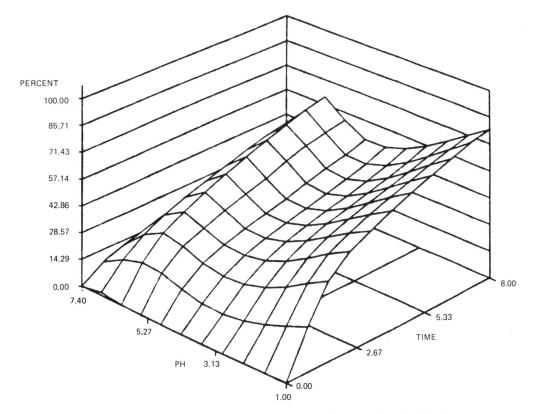

Figure 46 Topographical dissolution characterization of a Product as a function of time and pH. Data from pH 5.4 acetate buffer.

surfaces of the Product in pH 5.4 acetate buffer and the Product in pH 5.4 phosphate buffer clearly demonstrate that the pH 5.4 phosphate buffer is the most discriminating dissolution medium.

The increased complexity of the in vivo/in vitro association for controlled release drug products compared to conventional release is clear. While the conventional release solid oral dosage form in vivo/in vitro relationship is two-dimensional (i.e., the percent dissolved at a time interval versus the amount absorbed), the relationship for controlled release should be viewed as being multi-dimensional with pH being one important factor (in the case of an orally administered drug).

Once the in vivo/in vitro relationship is fully characterized, one should be able to employ dissolution testing in lieu of in vivo data for certain regulatory processes (e.g., minor equipment changes, process or manufacturing changes, site of manufacturing change, etc. An in vivo/in vitro relationship is characterized by the simulation in Figure 48. If one is operating on such a plateau, assurance is provided that minor changes in one parameter will have only a negligible effect on other parameters. If on the other hand, the in vitro dissolution rate over time increases as the pH of the media increases, the extent of absorption will also increase (reflective of the greater amount in solution at higher pH). Such a case may

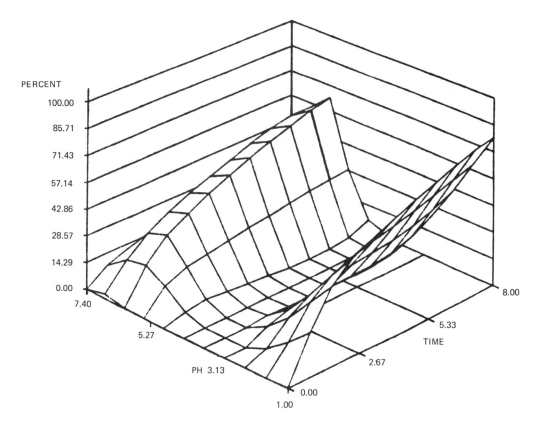

Figure 47   Topographical dissolution characterization of a Product as a function of time and pH.   Data from pH 5.4 phosphate buffer.

be described by the simulation in Figure 49.   Where the slope is steep, a slight change in dissolution could yield quite unexpected in vivo results. If one is operating on such a slope, then duplicative testing of material manufactured at the two different sites of several dissolution media pHs should be sufficient, if the data obtained are the same.   If one has not pertubated their dissolution system so as to ascertain whether the topographic surface is flat or sloping, several tests may be necessary so as to determine the appropriate, sensitive variables.

Figure 50 is an example of a three-dimensional in vivo/in vitro association for an oral controlled release dosage form where the rate of dissolution is independent of the pH of the dissolution media.   In this example, the apparent half-life of absorption is related to the inverse fluctuation of the drug concentration within the therapeutic window.

In summary, Skelly and co-workers feel that the technique of multi-dimensional topographic analysis, which is widely available to the scientific community, lends itself to more accurately predicting the role of in vitro dissolution to in vivo response and should be examined more thoroughly to develop its potential.

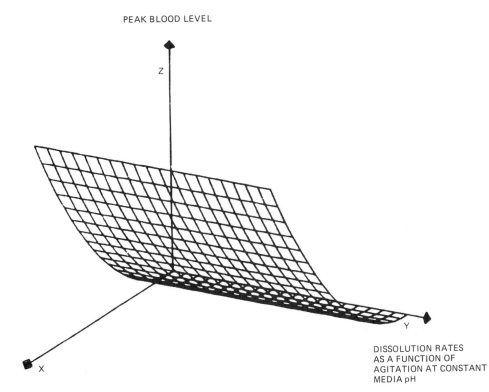

PEAK BLOOD LEVEL

Z

Y

X

DISSOLUTION RATES
AS A FUNCTION OF
AGITATION AT CONSTANT
MEDIA pH

DISSOLUTION DATA AS
A FUNCTION OF MEDIA pH
AT CONSTANT AGITATION

Figure 48 An example of a three dimensional in vivo/in vitro association for an oral controlled release dosage form where the dissolution rate at a particular time interval varies as a function of the pH of the dissolution media. Note that the dissolution rate at that time interval does not vary as a function of the rate of agitation.

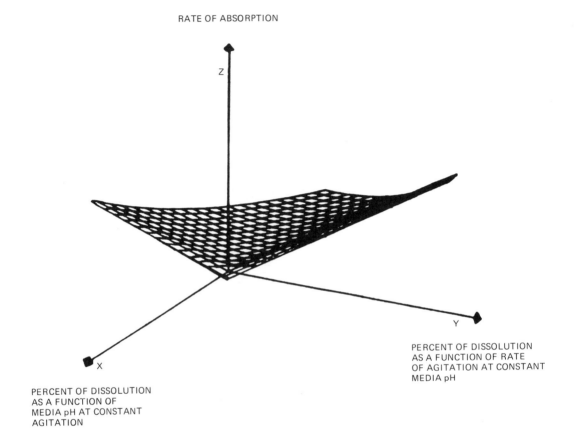

Figure 49   An example of a three-dimensional in vivo/in vitro association for an oral dosage.

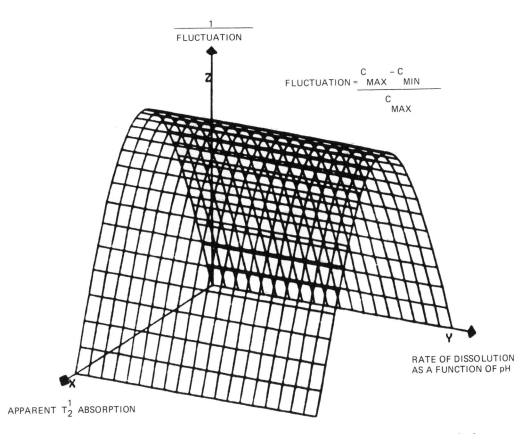

Figure 50 An example of a three-dimensional in vivo/in vitro association for an oral controlled release dosage form where the rate of dissolution is independent of the pH of the dissolution media. Note that the apparent half-life of absorption is related to the inverse of the fluctuation of the drug concentration within the therapeutic window.

G. Dissolution Media

Agitation, composition, pH, ionic strength, viscosity, surface tension, and temperature of the dissolution medium have been exhaustively studied. All of these factors must be considered in order to successfully correlate in vitro data with the situation in vivo.

The relative intensity of agitation is extremely important in dissolution-rate testing. Stirring speeds must be in the correct range to obtain data that will correlate with in vivo results. At a high agitation rate, diffusion control is diminished and there is a tendency for the dissolution rate to be controlled either by the rate of release or by solvation of the molecules from the crystalline matrix [229]. Diffusion control is operative when the rate-determining step is the transport of the solute from the interfacial boundary to the bulk of the surrounding solution. Since diffusion constants are inversely proportional to viscosity, the passage of solute molecules through the interfacial boundary will decrease as viscosity is increased.

Using compressed disks of methyl prednisolone, Hamlin et al. [230] first showed that agitation intensity was of great importance. More dramatically, however, Levy and Hayes [137] and Campagna et al. [140] have shown that agitation intensity is of critical concern. An extremely slow stirring technique was used to correlate the in vitro results with established in vivo differences. Faster stirring rates distinguished the effects of the excipient upon the stirring rate which were not evident with slower stirring [231].

The presence of surface-active agents in the dissolution medium promotes wetting of the solute particles and enhances the dissolution rate, even if the concentration of surfactant is below the critical micelle concentration [229]. This is extremely important for particles of irregular shape with pores and crevices. Owing to occlusion by air, the total surface area of these particles may be incompletely exposed to the solvent. Surface-active agents are discussed in Sec. III.R.

When neutral ionic compounds or unreactive organic additives are added to the dissolution medium, the dissolution rate of a drug in the combined medium that is produced may depend significantly on the drug's solufility in the mixed solvent. Such a dependence was observed for the dissolution rate of benzoic acid in sodium chloride, sodium solfate, and dextrose solutions [135].

H. Tablet Hardness

A decrease in effective surface area of the active ingredients as a result of granulation and compaction of drug particles can seriously affect the dissolution of drug from a tablet, unless the process of compaction is easily reversible when the tablet comes into contact with the dissolution medium.

In pharmacy manufacture, hardness is a measure of resistance of a solid dosage form to mechanical deforming. The assessment of the hardness of tablets is a very useful quality control check in tablet manufacture, and various techniques have been used, including fracture resistance [232], bending strength, tensile strength [233], and crushing strength [234].

Huber and Christenson [235] investigated the influence of tablet hardness and density variation on in vitro dissolution of a dye from controlled-release tablets made with different types and viscosity grades of hydrophilic polymers. Differences in density and porosity could influence the dissolution rate of drug from the tablet by affecting the initial rate of penetration of water at the tablet surface and subsequent disintegration and dissolution. However, these authors reported that for tablets made of varying hardness, markedly different release characteristics were not observed.

Tablet hardness studies [236] with phenobarbital tablets containing lactose and silicon dioxide and/or arabinoglactan as binder showed a slight increase in hardness when the tablets were aged for 16 days at 55°C; however, there was no decrease in dissolution rate.

Stern [237] investigated the effect of five conventional film-coating materials on tablet hardness. The author pointed out that the term "tablet hardness" is widely used in a nonspecific or generic manner as an all-inclusive description of several important tablet parameters, including bending or attrition resistance and impact or crushing strength, the latter being the most widely used to assess tablet integrity. Stern demonstrated that placebos showed linear increases in hardness as coatings were applied. However, the coating process itself did not alter core hardness, since tablets from which the film could be stripped showed original values.

I. Adjuvants

In addition to the compressional force used to manufacture a tablet, the chemical components in the formula have also been shown to prolong disintegration times, which subsequently affect the drug dissolution rate and the bioavailability.

Inert fillers have been found to potentiate the chemical degradation of active ingredients and to cause the disintegration time and the dissolution rate of compressed tablets to change with storage. In addition, adjuvants can influence the therapeutic effectiveness of the medicament in a tablet by modifying its absorption characteristics, cause changes in tablet color, and affect other physical properties such as friability [238].

Alam and Parrott [239] have shown that hydrochlorthiazide tablets granulated with acacia and stored at various temperatures (room temperature to 80°C) increased in hardness with time. The disintegration and dissolution times were also increased. These times were essentially unchanged with tablets granulated with starch and polyvinylpyrrolidone (PVP).

Kornblum and Hirschorn [240] evaluated excipient dilution and compression force effects on the dissolution rate and demonstrated the importance of the excipient/drug ratio to optimize the dissolution rate. The dissolution rate of a quinazolinone compound has been found to increase as the excipient/drug ratio increased. The dissolution data from tablets of 200, 400, and 600 mg, each containing 50 mg of drug, are seen in Figure 51. Changes in compression force were more significant with small tablets, indicating a less pronounced effect as the dilution factor increased. The data supported the conclusion that a larger tablet than necessary for technical reasons could lead to an optimum dissolution rate. The authors also found an increase in the half-lives for dissolution as the compression force increased. The results are seen in Table 14.

Table 14   Half-Lives (min) of Quinazolinone Compound to 100 ml[a]

Tablet weight half-life pressure applied (psi)	200-mg $t_{50\%}$	400-mg $t_{50\%}$	600-mg $t_{50\%}$
12,000	6.8	4.2	2.5
18,000	9.4	6.4	3.4
24,000	14.8	9.4	4.8

[a]Aqueous solution at pH 1.2 for tablets of 200, 400, and 600 mg at various compression forces.
Source: From Ref. 240; reproduced with permission of the copyright owner.

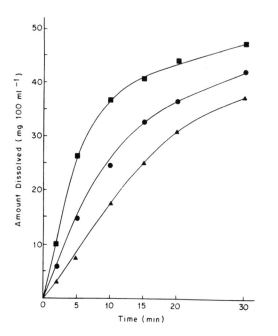

Figure 51   Dissolution of quinazolinone compound in 100 ml of aqueous solution at pH 1.2 from compressed tablets at 24,000 psi. ▲, 200 mg; ●, 400 mg; ■, 600 mg. (From Ref. 240.)

By microscopic examination of disintegrated tablets, Johnsgard and
Wahlgren [241] found that the greater the ratio of excipients to drug, the
less was the tendency for aggregates of the active substance to form.
In vitro studies with tablets prepared by wet granulation showed that much
aggregation caused a marked decrease in the rate of dissolution of slightly
soluble drugs but not of highly soluble substances.

Hydrophilic fillers, such as starch, have been shown to enhance the
dissolution of drugs, particularly when the starch was granulated with the
drug. Marlowe and Shangraw [222] prepared sodium salicylate tablets by
wet granulation techniques, using either lactose or a mixture of lactose and
cornstarch as filler, and found that the presence of starch dramatically increased the dissolution rate. Shotten and Leonard [242] reported that
dividing the disintegrant between the interior of the granules and the
extragranular void pores can accelerate disintegration into fine particles.

A lubricant is a fine material that functions to enhance flowability of
the granulation and decrease die wall friction. Many efficient tablet
lubricants are hydrophobic and may retard disintegration and drug dissolution. Owing to the high pressure involved, lubricants are needed to minimize friction, but, if possible, the lubricant effect should be restricted to
the die wall because interparticula lubrication inhibits bonding. The
type of lubricant, its concentration, and the method of incorporation must
be optimized during formulation development. The efficiency of mixing
magnesium stearate with the tablet granulation can influence the lubricant
effect and drug release from the granules. The method of incorporating
the lubricant [243] can influence penetration into the tablet by the solvent
medium, as seen in Figure 52.

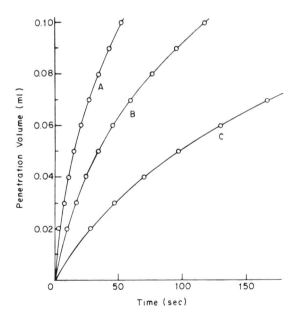

Figure 52 Water penetration into tablets containing lubricant added in
different ways. Key: A, 1% magnesium stearate tumbler-mixed with magnesium carbonate powder; B, 1% shear-mixed with powder; C, 0.5% wet-
mixed during granulation. (From Ref. 243.)

Finholt [244] states that the effect of lubricant on the dissolution rates of drugs from tablets will depend upon the properties of the granules and lubricant and upon the amount of lubricant used. If the granule particles are hydrophilic and fast-disintegrating, a surface-active agent would have little effect. However, when the granules are less hydrophilic and slow to disintegrate, a surface-active lubricant such as magnesium lauryl sulfate may enhance dissolution.

The in vitro dissolution of digoxin tablets was shown by Khalil [245] to be suppressed by a commercial antacid containing aluminum hydroxide and magnesium trisilicate. The significance of this finding was later questioned by Loo et al. [246], who found that with mongrel dogs, the antacids had no significant influence on the blood levels of digoxin.

Microcrystalline cellulose is a widely used tablet excipient and functions both as a diluent and a binder and also aids in disintegration. It is an excellent excipient in the preparation of direct-compressed tablets and is also widely used in tablet formulations prepared by wet granulations procedures. In the past few years several studies have addressed the potential for drug absorption to this excipient. Certain steroids, phenothiazines, antihistamines, and antibiotics have been reported to be absorbed on microcrystalline cellulose from aqueous solutions, and several adsorption mechanisms have been proposed. Contradictory results were obtained by Nyqvist and co-workers [247] and Frantz and Peck [248] concerning the effect of pH on adsorption and desorption of phenothiazines by microcrystalline cellulose. In a recent study by Okada and co-workers [249], the adsorption of diphenhydramine, chlorphenirimine, isoniazid, and *p*-aminobenzoic acid was very slight or negligible, whereas the adsorption of four phenothiazine derivatives was considerable. The adsorption of acrinol was due to an ion exchange mechanism and to nonelectrostatic forces. Marked adsorption of acrinol onto microcrystalline cellulose was interpreted in terms of the presence of polar groups capable of hydrogen-bond formation and the coplanar arrangement of the acridine ring [249].

Khalil and co-workers [250] reported that in human volunteers, both the rate and extent of urinary excretion of riboflavin were significantly reduced (p < 0.05) when attapulgite was coadministered with the drug. About 50% reduction occurred in the cumulative amount excreted following the concurrent administration of 10 mg riboflavine in a solution form and 2 g of regular attapulgite. The coadministration of the drug with a 30 ml dose of a commercial antidiarrheal suspension containing 10% activated attapulgite and 3% colloidal attapulgite produced a relatively lesser effect the reduction in extent of absorption being 40%). No statistically-significant effect was found when the adsorbent was ingested 2 hours prior to the drug. The observed reduction in drug bioavailability in the presence of attapulgite was attributed to the significant uptake of the drug by the adsorbent.

Singh and Gupta studied the adsorption of norfloxacin to several pharmaceutical adjuvants [251]. Their studies indicated that the maximal adsorption was found with activated charcoal and bentonite. It was proposed that the adsorption onto the clay was due to the residual valences on the edges, corners, and cracks present on the surface of the clay. These surface defects, plus the higher surface area and exchange capacity of bentonite, were the principle factors involved in the adsorption process. Activated charcoal has been studied by several investigators for its adsorption properties, and Singh and Gupta concluded that the maximum capacity of the charcoal was due to a particle size phenomenon. They also suggested that the administration of activated charcoal would be a suitable antidote in overdosing cases, due to the high binding capacity for norfloxacin.

J. Salts and pH Effects

The equilibrium solubility and dissolution rate of a drug are important properties governing the effective concentration that a drug, particularly a relatively insoluble one, achieves at the absorption site in the gastrointestinal tract. The factors that govern solubility of drugs are temperature, particle size, crystalline state, complexation, and variations in pH and salt concentration.

Dissolution is the sum total of various factors involved in the transference of a solute molecule from the solid to the solution phase [252]. Attempts to increase solubility can often be achieved by judicious selection of a suitable excipient or by using a more soluble drivative of the drug.

The dissolution rate of drugs may be increased by adjusting the pH of the microenvironment surrounding the drug particle. The resulting increase in solubility in the diffusion layer in these cases is nearly always due to salt formation following an acid-base reaction.

The solution of a relatively insoluble organic acid in water can be represented by the equilibrium equations

$$[HA] \text{ (solid phase)} \xrightarrow{K_s} [HA] \text{ (solution phase)} \xrightarrow{K_a} [H^+] + [A^-] \quad (34)$$

The equilibrium constant K_s of the first reaction above corresponds to the concentration of the undissociated acid in equilibrium with the solid phase. The equilibrium constant K_a of the second reaction is merely the dissociation constant of the acid,

$$K_a = \frac{[H^+][A^-]}{[HA]} \quad (35)$$

Since the total concentration of the compound in solution c_s would be the sum of the ionized and nonionized form, one can write

$$c_s = [HA[+ [A^-] = [HA] + K_a \frac{[HA]}{[H^+]} \quad (36)$$

But since $K_s = [HA]$,

$$c_s = K_s + K_s \frac{K_a}{[H^+]} = K_s \left(1 + \frac{K_a}{[H^+]} \right) \quad (37)$$

When $[H^+] \ll K_a$, $K_a/[H^+]$ is much larger than K_s, and

$$c_s = \frac{K_s K_a}{[H^+]} \quad (38)$$

Expressed in logarithmic form, Eq. (38) becomes

$$\log c_s = \log K_s + \log K_a - \log [H^+] \qquad (39)$$

or

$$\log c_s = \log K_s + pH - pK_a \qquad (40)$$

The solubility c_s of a weak acid actually represents the concentration of the drug in the diffusion layer and [from Eq. (40)] would increase with an increase in pH.

Equivalently, the dissolution of a relatively insoluble organic base can be written as

$$low \ c_s = pK_w - pH - pK_b + \log K_s \qquad (41)$$

where K_w is the dissociation constant of water and K_b the dissociation constant of the base.

The solution rate of a weak acid (or base) is not dependent directly on its intrinsic solubility in the medium, but on the solubility that exists in the diffusion layer. The pH of this thin layer for an acidic drug may be increased by including in the formulation agents such as sodium citrate, sodium bicarbonate, and magnesium carbonate. The dissolution rate and the absorption rate of aspirin are increased in buffered tablets as compared to plain aspirin [253]. The pH of the stomach content is significantly altered in the presence of the buffering agent and when the microenvironmental pH is raised sufficiently high to increase the rates of dissolution and absorption.

Techniques for forming sodium, potassium, and other water-soluble salts, such as hydrochloride, have long been used to improve the bioavailability of poorly soluble drugs. Generally, the salt will show higher dissolution rates than the corresponding nonionic drugs at the same pH, even though the final equilibrium solubility of the drug and its salt are alike [254]. Higuchi et al. [254] have shown that under physiological conditions of pH favoring conversion of the salt to a nonelectrolyte, the salt dissolves rapidly, and the nonelectrolyte formed then precipitates as fine particles having desirable characteristics for proper redissolution and bioabsorption.

Anderson and Sneddon [255] did not find this explanation applicable when comparing the dissolution rates in 0.1 N aqueous hydrochloric acid solutions of phenobarbital and sodium phenobarbital tablets produced by the same manufacturer, as displayed in Figure 53. Dissolution of the parent acid compound in both water and acid was very similar. The sodium phenobarbital tablets dissolve rapidly in water; however, dissolution was greatly retarded in acidic media, which, like gastric acid, had a pH of about 1.5. Although 0.1 N hydrochloric acid with or without pepsin is often used as simulated gastric juice for in vitro experiments, Finholt and Solvang [256] discovered that inclusion of a low concentration of a surface-active agent such as polysorbate 80 in the dissolution medium reproduced more closely the conditions in the stomach. The results from the investigation of Anderson and Sneddon found in Table 15 demonstrate that the surfactant had little effect on the formulations tested.

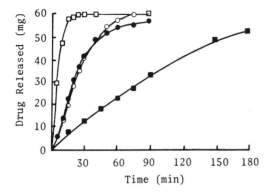

Figure 53   Release of barbiturate from sodium phenobarbital and phenobarbital tablets in water and acid, as a function of time.   □, Sodium
phenobaribtal in water; ○, phenobaribtal in water; ■, sodium phenobarbital in 0.1 N HCl, ●, phenobarbitol in 0.1 N HCl.   (From Ref. 255.)

The results of this study [255] are in conflict with an earlier study
by Nelson [21], who demonstrated that compressed pellets of phenobarbital dissolved much more slowly than similar pellets of sodium phenobarbital and that this held for acidic, neutral, and alkaline conditions
(see Table 16).

Table 15   Times for Dissolution (as $T_{50\%}$ Values) of Barbiturate
Tablets in Various Media at 37°C

Tablet	Medium	$T_{50\%}$ (min)	Average $T_{50\%}$
Phenobaribtal (60 mg)	Water	18, 22, 24	21
	0.1 N hydrochloric acid	19, 20	20
	0.1 N hydrochloric acid with 0.01% polysorbate 80	12, 12	12
	0.1 N hydrochloric acid with 0.05% polysorbate 80	10	10
Phenobarbital sodium (60 mg)	Water	4, 5, 6	5
	0.1 N hydrochloric acid	80, 86	83
	0.1 N hydrochloric acid with 0.01% polysorbate 80	82	82
	0.1 N hydrochloric acid with 0.05% polysorbate 80	75, 84	80

Source: From Ref. 255.

Table 16   Dissolution Rate of Weak Acids and Their Sodium Salts

Compound	pK_a	Dissolution rate ($mg/100\ min/cm^2$)		
		0.1 N HCl, pH 1.5	0.1 M phosphate, pH 6.8	0.1 M borate, pH 9.0
Benzoic acid	4.2	2.1	14	28
Sodium salt		980	1170	1600
Phenobarbital	7.4	0.24	1.2	22
Sodium salt		∿200	820	1430
Salicylic acid	3.0	1.7	27	53
Sodium salt		1870	2500	2420
Sulfathiazole	7.3	<0.1	∿0.5	8.5
Sodium salt		550	810	1300

Source: From Ref. 21.

The tremendous differences seen in Table 14 for the acid and the salt compound suggest that the tablet formulations and physical properties of the dosage forms (Fig. 53) may exert more influence on drug release than that exerted by the nature of the active ingredient.

Vivino [257] compared the blood levels of theophylline following the administration of theophylline isopropanolamine and theophylline ethylenediamine to humans. He found that the isopropanolamine salt gave a more rapid rise in blood levels and higher and more prolonged blood levels. In an earlier study, Gagliani et al. [258] showed that choline theorphyllinate also gave earlier and higher levels of theophylline in the blood than did theophylline ethylenediamine. These results may be related to the dissolution rates, which appear in Figures 54 and 55. The choline and isopropanolamine salts dissolve between two and three times as fast as the ethylenediamine salt, depending on the media used [136].

Later work by Nelson [259] correlated the excretion rates of tetracycline and its various salts with the dissolution rates as seen in Figure 56.

Correlations between dissolution rates and blood levels in humans have been made with penicillin V and its salts [260]. The rates of solution at pH 2 and 8 occur in the order: potassium salt > calcium salt > free acid > benzathine salt. Studies in human subjects showed that blood levels followed the same sequence, indicating a strong correlation and dependence on the solution rates of the salts.

Salt formation does not result in all cases in faster dissolution rates of weak electrolytes in media of various pH. The conversion of a weak acid on the surface of a tablet may form a film that is insoluble in acid media,

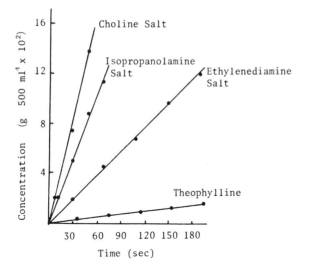

Figure 54 Solution rate of theophylline and salts in 0.1 N hydrochloric acid. (From Ref. 136.)

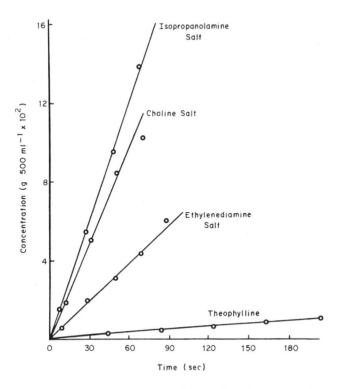

Figure 55 Solution rate of theophylline and salts in 0.1 M phosphate buffer. (From Ref. 136.)

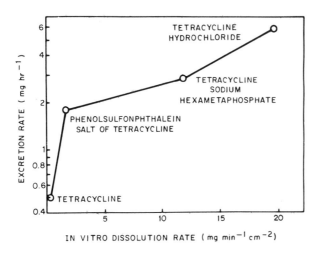

Figure 56   Correlation between excretion rate at 1 hr and in vitro dissolution rate when various tetracyclines are taken in the form of pellets. (From Ref. 259.)

and this film can prevent penetration of the liquid into the tablet, inhibiting disintegration and dissolution.   The precipitation of insoluble alginic acid and carboxymethylcellulose from water-soluble salts of these gums may have a similar effect.   Studies with aluminum acetylsalicylate [261], warfarin sodium [262], and benzphetamine pamoate [263] showed that administration of the salt slowed dissolution and subsequent absorption of the drug compared to the nonionized form.   This decrease appeared to be a result of precipitation of an insoluble particle or film on the tablet surface.

The formation of salts and esters of drugs has helped to stabilize the active moiety against degradation in the acidic medium of the stomach. Blood levels with erythromycin estolate, an ester, were demonstrated to be several times higher than those obtained with erythromycin base or the stearate salt [264–266].   These differences were found in both fasting and nonfasting subjects, suggesting that food exerted little influence on absorption of erythromycin estolate.   This phenomenon is probably due to the high acid stability of the estolate derivative compared to the base and stearate salt.   Unfortunately, erythromycin estolate is highly bound to proteins in the blood, and the concentration that is free for antibacterial action in the body is essentially no greater than erythromycin from the salt or base.   Furthermore, the estolate is known to cause reversible hepatotoxicity in a small number of cases and must be used with some caution.

The bioavailability of aminosalicylic acid and its sodium, calcium, and potassium salts in tablet form has been examined by Wan et al. [267].   In tests on 12 volunteers, doses of 4 g of the free acid, and 2.8 g and 2.6 g of the sodium, potassium, and calcium salts, were given orally.   The absorption from the salts was complete and rapid, but only 77% of the free acid was absorbed, the dissolution rate of this relatively insoluble substance being the rate-limiting factor.   The salts gave a greater area under the plasma concentration curve than did the unmetabolized drug, although

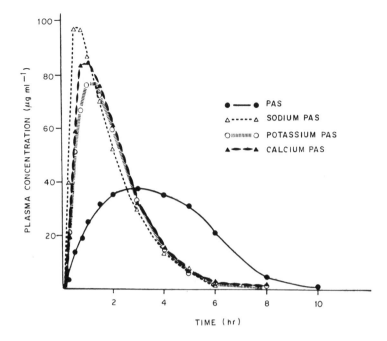

Figure 57 Mean plasma concentrations of unchanged drug from 12 subjects following administration of four different preparations of aminosalicylic acid (PAS). Data were corrected to 70-kg body weight. (From Ref. 267.)

the absolute amount of free acid absorbed was higher. The authors attribute this phenomenon to the limited capacity of humans to acetylate the drug, especially during the first pass in the gastrointestinal and liver tissues (see Fig. 57).

Berge and co-workers [268] have reviewed pharmaceutical salts and discussed the physicochemical properties, bioavailability, and toxicological considerations that must be considered in selecting the most useful salt form of a drug. This article, published in 1977, contained 294 references. In 1981, Miyazaki and co-workers [269] cautioned against the use of hydrochloride salts in pharmaceutical formulations. These authors recognized that salt formation was one of the first approaches to modify drug solubility in dissolution rates. Berge and co-workers [268] reported that due to the simple availability and physiology, the monochloride salts had been the most frequent choice of the available salts of basic drugs. However, reports in the literature have shown that hydrochloride salt formation does not necessarily enhance solufility and bioavailability in all cases. This finding is based on the common ion effect of chloride on the solubility product equilibrium of hydrochloride salts, which is often overlooked [270]. Hydrochloride salts of drugs frequently exhibit less than desirable solubility in gastric fluid because of the abundance of chloride ion. Miyazaki and co-workers studied the relationship between solubility in water and the extent of the common ion effect, and a high correlation was found, suggesting that hydrochlorides possessing a solubility in water at least of the order observed for papaverine and demeclocyline hydrochlorides (approximately 32 mg/ml at 25°C and 42 mg/ml at 37°C), are less soluble than the corresponding free base in gastric pH [269].

Miyazaki and co-workers [271] investigated the dissolution properties of the hydrochloride, sulfate, and iodide salts of berberine. They also investigated a common ion effect on the solubility of berberine hydrochloride. Sodium chloride showed a salting out effect in the hydrochloride salt solution, indicating the existence of a significant common ion effect owing to the addition of excess chloride. The chloride ion significantly reduced the dissociation of the hydrochloride salt and reduced its solubility. A similar salting out effect was noted with potassium chloride. Since the data for the two salts were similar, significant effects due to the cation are considered to be negligible. The presence of sodium sulfate on the other hand, appeared to have little influence on the solubility of berberine hydrochloride. In addition, the solubility of the sulfate salt was only slightly effected by the addition of sodium chloride, as shown in Table 17, which summarizes the salting out constants. These results indicate that the solubility of berberine hydrochloride decreased considerably with an increase in chloride-ion concentration. The dissolution behavior of the two salt forms in pH 7.4 isotonic phosphate buffer is shown in Figure 58. The differences were similar to those in hydrochloric acid solutions, with the sulfate salt passing into solution more rapidly and after 30 min having significantly more drug in solution than the hydrochloride salt. The results of the study by Miyazaki and co-workers indicate that the apparent solubility and dissolution rate of the hydrochloride salt of berberine were considerably less than those of the sulfate salt in chloride containing media, which could result in complete dissolution of the hydrochloride salt in the gastrointestinal tract. In such cases, the use of an alternative salt form, for example the sulfate salt, may improve the dissolution and bioavailability of the drug.

In an effort to protect xilobam from the effects of high temperatures and high humidities adversely influencing its dissolution from tablets, three arylsulfonic acid salts and a saccharin salt were prepared and characterized by Walkling and co-workers [272]. All of the salts were determined to be more stable at 74% relative humidity and 70°C than the free base. In spite of the large differences between the effect of high humidity at a high temperature on the salts versus the free base, the dissolution of the

Table 17   Salting-Out Constants of Salt
Forms of Berberine at 37°

Salt form	Salt	Salting-out constant, k
Hydrochloride	NaCl	36.67
Hydrochloride	KCl	35.00
Hydrochloride	Na_2SO_4	3.75
Sulfate	NaCl	1.67

Source: From Ref. 271.

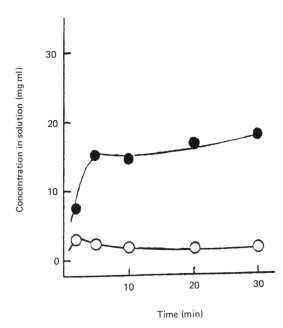

Time (min)

Figure 58   Dissolution curves of hydrochloride (○) and sulfate (●) salts of berberine in pH 7.4 isotonic phosphate buffer at 37°.

most stable salt (1-napsylate) was essentially equivalent to the dissolution of the free base when both were prepared as formulated tablets. The results reported in Table 18 show that all of the salts tested were more stable than the free base, especially after seven days. This data also indicated that the 1-napsylate was the most stable form. The authors also reported that a tablet formulation containing the 1-napsylate salt, actually released the xilobam at a faster rate than the free base as shown in Figure 59. Thus, it was demonstrated that a strong acid with an aryl group could protect a base that is easily hydrolysed, from the adverse effects of high humidity at a high temperature under non-sink conditions. At the same time, dissociation from that base under appropriate sink conditions, as in a dissolution test, will permit rapid bioavailability of the base, in vivo [272].

Benjamin and Lin [273] prepared the hydrochloride, acetate, tartrate, sulfate, p-hydroxybenzoate, ebonate, napsylate, 3-hydroxynapthoate, and methacrylic acid-methacrylate copolymer salts of 9-[2-(indol-3-yl)ethyl]-1-oxa-3-oxo-4, 9-diazaspira[5,5] udecane. In vitro dissolution rates for the pure salts were determined using the rotating disk method in 0.1 N HCl, water, and 0.05 M phosphate buffer pH 7.5. The intrinsic dissolution rates in all media showed dramatic differences among various salts corresponding to the differences in their solubilities in water. The in vitro dissolution rates in phosphate buffer and water showed marked differences among salts. However, there were no significant differences in dissolution rates when 0.1 N HCl was used as the medium. The data also indicated

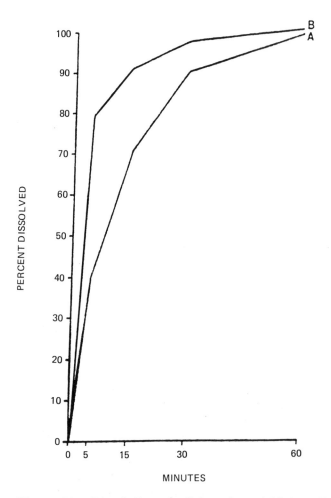

Figure 59   Dissolution of xilobam from tablets: Key: A, free base; B, 1-napsylate. (From Ref. 00.)

Table 18 Solid-State Stability at 70° and 74% Relative Humidity

Days	Percent intact xilobam				
	Free base	Tosylate	Saccharinate	2-Napsylate	1-Napsylate
5	93.6	97.9	99.7	98.0	100.1
	93.0	98.1	99.0	98.7	99.7
	93.8	97.8	98.4	99.4	100.8
	$\overline{X} = 93.5$	$\overline{X} = 97.9$	$\overline{X} = 99.0$	$\overline{X} = 98.7$	$\overline{X} = 100.2$
7	15.6	88.1	78.7	83.4	100.0
	24.6	79.7	82.5	72.9	99.4
	13.8	76.6	82.2	76.8	99.4
	$\overline{X} = 18.0$	$\overline{X} = 82.5$	$\overline{X} = 81.1$	$\overline{X} = 77.4$	$\overline{X} = 99.6$

$\overline{X}$ = mean.
Source: From Ref. 272.

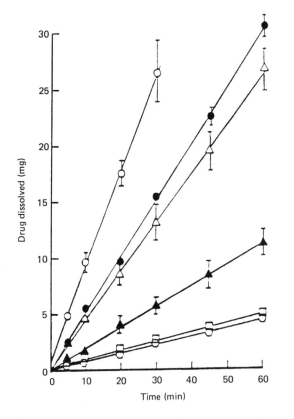

Figure 60   Common-ion effect on the dissolution profiles of the sodium salt of REV 3164 in water from a surface area of 0.95 cm^2 at 25°C. Sodium chloride solutions in water only ($\circ$), 0.01 ($\bullet$), 0.02 ($\triangle$), 0.5 ($\blacktriangle$), and 0.10 M ($\square$) concentrations, and 0.10 M sodium carbonate-bicarbonate buffer (pH 10) ($\circ$) were used. Each datum point represents the average $^\circ$ s.d. of three determinations.

that the ebonate, 3-hydroxynaphtoate, and napsylate salts, when formulated in an enteric coated dosage form, would provide a slow release of the drug.

The solubility and the dissolution rate of the sodium salt of an acidic drug (REV 3164; 7-chloro-5-propyl-$1H$,$4H$-[1,2,4]triazolo[4,3-a]-quinoxaline-1,4-dione) decreased by the effect of a common ion present in aqueous media [274]. The solubility of the sodium salt of REV 3164 in a buffered medium was much lower than that in an unbuffered medium. Also, the presence of NaCl decreased its solubility in water, as seen in Figure 60. The apparent solubility product (K'_{sp}) of the salt, however, did not remain constant when the concentration of NaCl was changed. A decrease in K'_{sp} value with the increase in NaCl concentration was observed; for example, the K'_{sp} values at 0 and 1 M NaCl were 7.84×10^{-4} and 3.94×10^{-4} M^2, respectively. Even when corrected for the effect of ionic strength, the solubility product decreased. This decrease in the solubility product in the presence of NaCl indicated a decrease in the degree of self-association (increase in activity coefficient) of the drug in aqueous media.

K. Particle Size

As stated earlier, drugs administered orally in a solid dosage form must first dissolve in gastrointestinal fluids before they are absorbed. Since dissolution rate is directly proportional to surface area [see Eq. (13)], a decrease in size of the primary particles of the drug will create a greater surface area in contact with the dissolution medium, resulting in a faster rate of solution. This becomes important where the absorption is rate-limited by the dissolution process. Particle size is generally important for poorly or slowly soluble drugs. The dissolution of drugs from granules prepared by wet and dry granulating techniques was discussed earlier in the chapter.

The classic works of Bedford and co-workers [275, 276], which showed how griseofulvin blood levels were markedly affected by particle size, are often quoted. Extensive studies on the influence of particle size on the bioavailability of digoxin was recently reported by Shaw and Carless [277] (see Figs. 61 and 62) and by Jounela et al. [278].

Although the reduction in particle size remains an accepted method for increasing dissolution rates, it must not be assumed that finer particles will always exhibit faster dissolution rates than coarser drug particles. Aggregation may reduce the effective surface area in contact with the dissolution medium. During tablet compression, the particular shape [279] and particle size [280] may change.

Solvang and Finholt [155] illustrate the complexities of particle size effect in solid dosage forms. They showed that phenacetin was released faster from granules than from tablets, whereas the reverse was true for prednisone and phenobarbital. These results could be due to a wetting phenomenon, yet other factors besides particle size appear to exert an

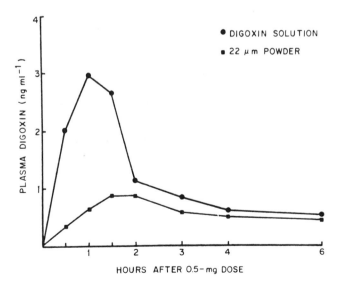

Figure 61 Mean plasma digoxin levels recorded in four healthy volunteers after 0.5-mg doses of (1) digoxin powder of 22-μm mean particle diameter and (2) digoxin in solution. (From Ref. 277.)

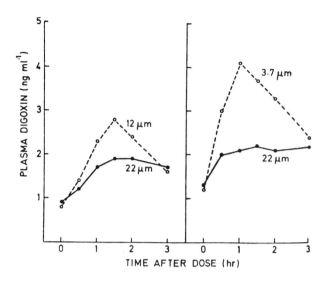

Figure 62   Mean plasma digoxin levels recorded in fasting patients on maintenance dixogin therapy before (●) and after (○) 0.5 mg of digoxin powder of mean particle size 22 μm (four patients) and 12 μm and 3.7 μm (four patients). (From Ref. 277.)

influence on drug dissolution. Kornblum and Hirschorn [281] compared the dissolution rates of powders and tablets of a quinazolinone drug that had been spray dried and air attrited. The drug that was micronized by air attrition had the smaller particle size but formed aggregates in solution; thus, faster dissolution rates were observed for the spray dried material. The reverse was true when the drug was incorporated into tablets containing microcrystalline cellulose and lactose as filters. The addition of hydrophilic diluents to the hydrophobic drug imparted hydrophilic properties to the tablets, and particle aggregates experienced with the attrited powder did not form.

In addition to compaction during manufacture, other factors, such as adsorption of air on the particle surface, static surface charge, hydrophobicity imparted by adsorption of tablet lubricants, and improper choice of tablet excipients, may cause fine particles to dissolve more slowly than larger particles. In those instances where particle size is important, care must be exercised during moist granulating to prevent crystal growth or condensation into aggregates. These effects must therefore be identified and treated appropriately in the course of good formulation practices.

A reduction in particle size is not desirable in all cases. For example, a particle size reduction of nitrofurantoin will increase dissolution rate (see Fig. 63) and blood levels; however, smaller size particles will also increase gastrointestinal irritation, which explains why a macrocrystalline rather than an amorphous form of nitrofurantoin appears in the marketed product.

Monkhouse and Lach [283] have increased the dissolution rates of various poorly soluble drugs by adsorbing the drug onto an adsorbent and

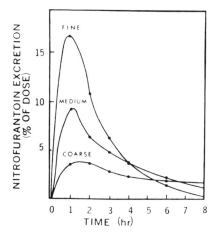

Figure 63 Effect of crystal size of orally administered nitrofurantoin on urinary recovery rate in the rat. Coarse, 50−80 mesh (300−800 μm); medium, 80−200 mesh (180−75 μm); fine, 200 mesh to micronized (75−10 μm or less). (From Ref. 282.)

increasing the surface area of the drug in contact with dissolution media. This was accomplished by equilibrating the drug in an organic solvent with an insoluble excipient having an extensive surface (e.g., fumed silicon dioxide), and evaporating the mixture to dryness. The dissolution data for indomethacin are seen in Figure 64. An increased rate of release from the miniscular drug delivery system, as Monkhouse and Lach called their dosage form, was observed with all drugs studies.

Studies by Abdallah and co-workers [284] with griseofulvin-silicon dioxide adsorbates prepared from solvent deposition studies, demonstrated that the drug particle size increased in griseofulvin-rich samples and incomplete drug recovery was experienced from samples containing high levels of the insoluble carrier. The authors noted that these were two drawbacks that should be considered in solvent deposition systems. Other investigators have reported poor dissolution from solvent deposited drugs on insoluble carriers in spite of a low drug-carrier ratio [285]. Factors such as drug instability, solvent migration, and drug entrapment should be considered in all of these systems.

McGinity and Harris investigated the adsorption of griseofulvin, indomethacin, and prednisone to colloidal magnesium aluminum silicate and demonstrated that this process markedly improved the dissolution rates of these hydrophobic and poorly soluble drugs [286]. The rapid release of drug from the surface of the clay was due to the weak physical bonding between the two materials and to the swelling of the clay in aqueous media. The hydrophilic and swelling properties of the montmorillonite clay in aqueous media also helped to facilitate the wetting of the hydrophobic drug substances. The dissolution profiles of the indomethacin-montmorillonite adsorbates in aqueous media containing polysorbate 80 (0.02%) are shown in Figure 65.

Eckert-Lill and co-workers [287] studied the chemiadsorption of drug molecules with reactive hydroxyl groups onto porous silica supports having

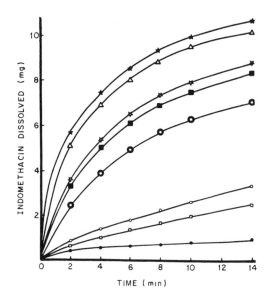

Figure 64   Dissolution profiles of miniscular indomethacin in water at 240 rpm. ★, 20% fumed silicon dioxide EHS; △, 10% fumed silicon dioxide EHS; ✶, 20% fumed silicon dioxide M7; ■, 10% fumed silicon dioxide M7; o, 20% silicic acid; ○, 5% fumed silicon dioxide EHS; □, 10% silicic acid; ●, indomethacin powder only. (From Ref. 283.)

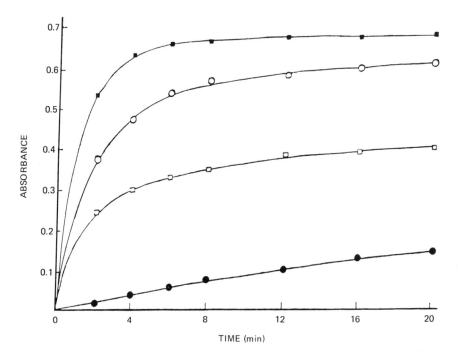

Figure 65   Dissolution profiles of indomethacin: montmorillonite adsorbates (equilibrated in acetone) in aqueous polysorbate 80 solution 0.02%, at 37°. Key: ● pure drug; □ 1:1 adsorbate; ○ 1:4 adsorbate; ■ 1:9 adsorbate.

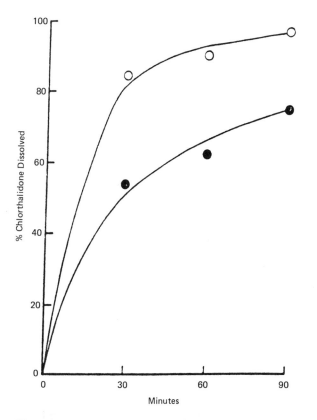

Figure 66 Dissolution profiles of chlorthalidone from chlorthalidone/ propranolol hydrochloride tablets. Key: micronized chlorthalidone ○; Fitmilled chlorthalidone ●.

a mean pore size of 10 nm. This adsorption occurred for a great number of alcohols and phenols with a variety of different structures, including codeine and p-hydroxybenzoic acid esters. The strong pH dependence of the hydrolytic cleavage of drug chemiadsorbates from the silica resulted in an almost constant drug release rate, provided that the dissolution test was performed under the so-called half-change conditions [288]. Increasing rates of cleavage with an increasing pH of the dissolution fluid compensated for the typical matrix liberation effects of the porous silica support.

The particle size reduction of chlorthalidone by fluid energy milling, Alpine milling, and Fitzpatricl milling were evaluated by Narurkar and co-workers [289]. The desired particle size was achieved by both the fluid energy milling and Alpine milling processes. Alpine milling, being a more complex process, is susceptible to product decomposition, whereas fluid energy milling is a simple and efficient process without any risk of product decomposition. The desired particle size could be achieved by Fitzmilling because of the low probability of impaction force on particles.

The dissolution rate of the chlorthalidone from chlorthalidone/propranolol hydrochloride tablets (25/80 mg) prepared with fluid energy milled chlorthalidone was significantly better than the tablets prepared with Fitzpatrick-milled chlorthalidone, as shown in Figure 66. The minimum effective specific surface area of chlorthalidone needed for maximum dissolution in water was found to be approximately 3.5 m^2/g.

L. Prodrug Approach

A prodrug results from a chemical modification of a biologically active substance to form a new compound, which upon in vivo enzymatic attack will liberate the parent compound [290]. This definition has been extended by Kupchan and Isenberg [291] to include nonenzymatic as well as enzymatic release. Higuchi [292] has outlined the various mechanisms that can be employed to release the agent from the inactive form in the body. These include simple dissolution, dilution, pH changes, action of endogenous esterases, dealkylation, decarboxylation, deamination, oxidation, and reduction.

Stella [293] reported the following applications for prodrugs. They:

1. Facilitate passage through lipid membranes for drugs with poor lipid solubility
2. Eliminate problems associated with drug odor and taste
3. Prolong drug activity in the body by decreasing the absorption rate of the drug
4. Increase water solubility of the drug to allow for direct i.v. injection
5. Simulate natural body transport and storage to lower the toxicity of i.m. injections
6. Increase the stability of compounds that undergo rapid degradation
7. Increase the bioavailability of drugs

The alteration in physical properties and/or modification of the chemistry of active drug substances can in certain instances lead to easier pharmaceutical processing. Candidates with desired melting point, solubility, dissolution, stability, and permeability can be synthesized to allow the dosage-form developer to select, more or less at will, the optimum characteristics desired for the purpose [292].

A wide variety of prodrug chemical linkages are known to be enzymatically hydrolyzed [294]. In many cases, the host tissue in which hydrolysis occurs is also known. Thus, prodrugs administered orally are dependent on enzymes present in the gastrointestinal tract, blood, and liver to regenerate the parent drug. Parenterally administered prodrugs are hydrolyzed by enzymes localized in the circulation and in the liver; whereas site-activated prodrugs are hydrolyzed by enzymes found in specific tissues.

The bioavailability of ampicillin has been improved by the preparation of prodrugs. Pivampicillin was synthesized by Daehne et al. [295] as a prodrug of ampicillin and, as shown in Figure 67, it produced higher blood levels of ampicillin after oral dosing than did ampicillin itself. Pivampicillin is a much more lipophilic derivative of ampicillin; in solution, ampicillin exists as a very nonlipophilic ion.

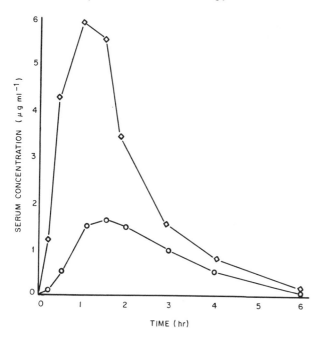

Figure 67 Mean serum levels of ampicillin in normal volunteers following oral administration of 250 mg of ampicillin (○) and 358 mg of pivampicillin HCl (∿250 mg of ampicillin) (◊) on an empty stomach. [From Daehne, W. V., Fredericksen, E., Gundersen, E., Lund, F., Morch, P., Peterson, H. J., Roholt, K., Tybring, L., and Godtfredsen, W. O., *J. Med. Chem.*, *13*:607 (1970).]

Hetacillin is also a prodrug of ampicillin and may be considered as a condensation product of acetone and ampicillin. Schwartz and Hayton [296] have shown concentrated solutions of hetacillin to be more stable. Prodrugs of carbenicillin [297], lincomycin, and clindamycin [298] have also been made.

Erythromycin 2'-N-alkylsuccinamate and 2'-N-alkylglutaramate prodrugs afford tasteless derivatives and display blood levels equivalent to or greater than those of erythromycin base. The erythromycin 2'alkylthio-succinate and thioglutarate prodrugs were reported to be virtually taste-less and extremely stable in a suspension formulation [299].

In a multi-authored text edited by Bundgaard [300], the properties and applications of prodrugs proposed earlier by Stella [293] have been expanded. The various authors in this text have utilized prodrugs to sustain drug action, improve formulation properties, promote skin absorp-tion, and for cancer chemotherapy and site-specific drug delivery.

M. Molecular Dispersion Principles

The dispersion of a drug within a water-soluble carrier effectively causes a reduction in particle size of the dispersed drug. Enhancement of rate of dissolution by this method and thus a possible absorption rate increase has generated considerable interest [301–317].

The unique approach of solid dispersions to reduce the particle size of drugs and increase rates of dissolution and absorption was first demonstrated in 1961 by Sekiguchi and Obi [301]. They prepared a eutectic mixture of the drug sulfathiazole and the carrier urea, followed by rapid solidification. The crushed dispersions were expected to release drug faster in aquous fluids because of the fine dispersion of the sulfathiazole in the matrix and the rapid dissolution of the urea.

Among the several carriers employed by workers to prepare solid dispersions, the most successful include polyethylene glycol 4000 and 6000, urea, dextrose, citric acid, succinic acid, and PVP.

In addition to the fusion or melt method used by Sekiguchi and Obi, another commonly used technique for the preparation of solid dispersion is the solvent method. A physical mixture of drug and carrier is dissolved in a common solvent, and upon evaporation of the solvent, the dissolved substances are coprecipitated from solution. The obvious advantage to the solvent method is its usefulness for drugs that thermally decompose at relatively low temperatures.

Several factors, including the cooling rate of the melt, choice of solvent, and evaporation rate of the solvent, may contribute to solid dispersions of varying physical characteristics and drug dissolution rates. McGinity et al. [312] prepared melt and coprecipitates of sulfabenzamide using six carrier systems; a comparison of the dissolution rates indicated that the method of preparation influenced the rate of solution of the sulfabenzamide.

Although the technology of solid dispersion has advanced during the past 25 years, most pharmaceutical studies are restricted to powdered dispersions rather than tablets. The formulation of tablets from solid dispersions provides a real challenge to the formulator. Storage at elevated temperatures for long periods of time may induce changes in crystal shape and size and other physical alterations in the dispersed drug, which in turn may influence bioavailability.

Several authors have correlated in vitro dissolution data with pharmacological response and have demonstrated a significant increase in drug activity from the solid dispersion system [313–315]. Svoboda et al. [312] compared the LD_{50} of the experimental antitumor agent acronycine with an acronycin-PVP coprecipitate and demonstrated a significant decrease in LD_{50} for the coprecipitate over the pure drug.

Stupack and Bates [316] reported that the dissolution rate of reserpine from PVP coprecipitates was significantly faster than from a PVP physical mix with micronized reserpine, as seen in Figure 68. Stoll et al. [314, 315] also showed that PVP coprecipitates of reserpine gave a superior pharmacological response over the pure drug.

In more recent years, research on molecular dispersions has addressed problems related to mechanisms of drug release from solid dispersions and the characterization of the drug molecules in these systems [318]. The physical and chemical stability of these dispersions has also received considerable attention. In a report by Ford [319], differential thermal analysis was utilized to study the properties of solid dispersions. McGinity and co-workers [320] used X-ray diffraction and scanning electron microscopy to study the influence of cooling rate on the properties of solid dispersions prepared by the melt-method. Tolbutamide was the model drug

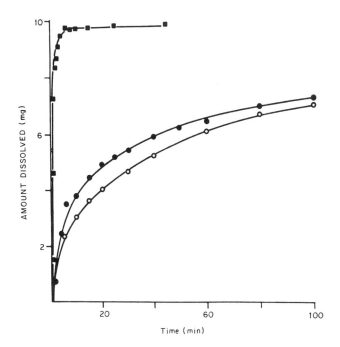

Figure 68 Dissolution rate of reserpine. ○, Reserpine crystals (6–30 μm); ●, 1:5 physical mixture with polyvinylpyroolidone; ■, 1:5 co-precipitate with polyvinylpyrrolidone. (From Ref. 316.)

investigated and the carriers included urea and polyethylene glycol 6000. Slow cooled urea dispersions of tolbutamide demonstrated a complete lack of crystallinity, suggesting formation of an amorphous material. A rapidly cooled dispersion showed peaks for urea and an absence of drug in the X-ray pattern, suggested that a true molecular dispersion was formed. The X-ray patterns of rapid and slow cooled dispersions of tolbutamide and polyethylene glycol 6000 demonstrated that a physical mixture of the drug and carrier resulted from both methods of dispersion preparation.

The stability and dissolution rates of corticosteroids in polyethylene glycol solid dispersions were investigated by Khalil and co-workers [321]. The dissolution rates of the steroids were relatively fast from the solid dispersions and showed no significant changes upon storage. However, of the five PEG samples used, three increased the chemical instability of the steroids, and oxidation was presumably accelerated by a perixide impurity in the PEG samples. Polyethylene glycols are polyethers and the presence of peroxides as impurities has been reported [322]. The instability of drugs including penicillin and bacitracin [323], chloramphenicol [324], and an experimental topical corticosteroid [325] was attributed to the presence of peroxides in PEG samples containing these drugs. McGinity and co-workers reported that in some cases the level of peroxide in the glycol sample can increase with aging [325]. Deshpande and Agrawal [326] studied the dissolution and stability of benzothiadiazine derivatives in polyethylene glycol 6000 dispersions prepared by the melt

and solvent evaporation methods. The dissolution rates of four water insoluble drugs were found to markedly increase when dispersed in polyethylene glycol 6000. The stability of bendroflumethiazide and methyclo-
thiazide was decreased in dispersions prepared by either method.

The stability of nifedipine in coprecipitates utilizing urea, PVP K-25,
K-30, K-90 and PEG 4000, 6000, 10,000 as the carrying materials was
studied by Sumnu [327]. It was found that Nifedipine in the urea
containing coprecipitates was chemically unstable. The storage of co-
precipitate systems of the drug with the PVPs under humid conditions
was found to influence both dissolution and bioavailability. It was suggested by the author that reduced dissolution and bioavailability of the
drug in the PVP systems resulted from partial crystallization of amorphous
nifedipine in the PVP matrix. The coprecipitates of nifedipine with PEG
were found to be physicochemically stable to humidity, and it was concluded
that the glycols were the carrier materials of choice for nifedipine coprecipitates.

N. Polymorphism (and Crystal Form)

Many organic medicinal compounds are capable of existing in two or more
crystalline forms with different arrangements of the molecules in the
crystal lattice, and these are referred to as polymorphs. Two polymorphs
of a given compound may be as different in structure and properties as
the crystals of different compounds. The X-ray diffraction patterns,
densities, melting points, solubilities, crystal shape, and electrical properties vary with the polymorphic form. However, in the liquid or vapor
state, no difference in properties is discernible.

At room temperature and pressure, one polymorph may be thermodynamically more stable than the other forms in the solid state, as explained by Carstensen [111]. The metastable polymorph possesses a higher
solubility and dissolution rate than does the stable form, and this phenomenon may be used to advantage in biopharmaceutics. The appropriate
selection and preparation of the most suitable polymorph can often significantly increase the absorption and medicinal value of drugs, particularly those with low solubilities. With poorly soluble drugs it is possible to
increase the solubility simply by modifying their crystalline nature [317,
328]. However, metastable crystalline forms may not be stable and may
revert on standing to the stable polymorph; such stability problems must
be taken into consideration. When incorporated into the final tablet dosage
form it is, of course, necessary to ensure against transformation to a more
stable and less soluble crystalline state.

The polymorphism of succinylsulfathiazole has been examined by several
investigators [329-334]. Literature reports on this drug suggest a degree
of uncertainty concerning the number of crystal forms and the lack of reproducibility in preparation and characterization. Recent studies on this
drug by Moustafa et al. [332] showed that physical instability was exhibited by some aqueous suspensions of succinylsulfathiazole. Some of the
problems encountered were crystal growth, formation of cementlike precipitates, and difficult resuspendability. These workers isolated six
crystal forms and one amorphous form of succinylsulfathiazole. Suspension
of all forms in water resulted in a transformation to the more stable form II.
The transformation of form I to form II in aqueous suspensions is seen in
Figure 69.

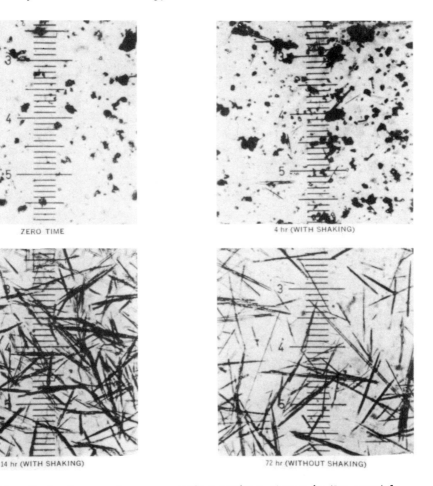

ZERO TIME   4 hr (WITH SHAKING)

14 hr (WITH SHAKING)   72 hr (WITHOUT SHAKING)

Figure 69   Photomicrographs representing various stages in the crystal growth accompanying the transformation of succinylsulfathiazole Form I to Form II in aqueous suspension (1 small micrometer division = 100 μm). (From Ref. 332.)

    The formation of polymorphs of a potential tricyclic antidepressant drug was demonstrated by Gibbs et al. [335] to dratmatically improve the bioavailability of the drug, as seen in Figure 70. Formulation 1 contained untreated drug and excipient. Drug in formulation 2 was micronized, resulting in a twofold increase in the area under the curve. Drug in formulation 3 was present as a 1:1 (w/w) lyophilized combination of active moiety and poloxamer 407 (Pluronic F-127). The X-ray diffraction, differential thermograms, and infrared analyses confirmed the formation of a more rapidly soluble polymorph in the lyophilized sample. The dissolution profiles of the three formulas appear in Figure 71.

    Theoretical considerations predict that amorphous solids will, in general, be better absorbed than will crystalline ones. These considerations are based on the relative energies involved in the dissolution phenomena.

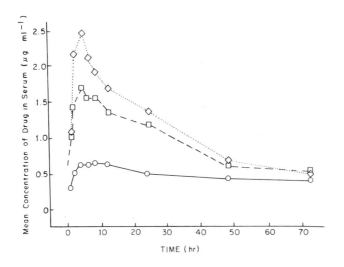

Figure 70 Mean concentrations of unchanged drug in the serum of six healthy male volunteers after oral administration of 200-mg doses of three different capsule formulations of an experimental tricyclic antidepressant drug in a three-way crossover design study. $\circ$, Drug plus excipients (AUC = 43.6 μg ml^{-1} hr^{-1}); $\square$, micronized drug plus excipients (AUC = 68.2 μg ml^{-1} hr^{-1}); $\diamond$, lyophilized drug-poloxamer 407 combination plus excipients (AUC = 81.2 μg ml^{-1} hr^{-1}). (From Ref. 335.)

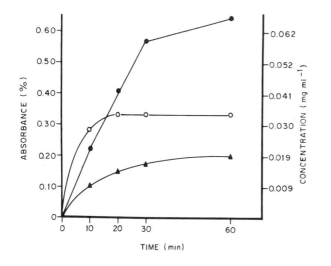

Figure 71 Dissolution profiles in 0.1 N hydrochloric acid (absorbance and concentration versus time) for three capsule formulations of an experimental tricyclic antidepressant drug. $\blacktriangle$, Drug plus excipients; $\circ$, micronized drug plus excipients; $\bullet$, lyophilized drug-poloxamer 407 combination plus excipients. (From Ref. 335.)

An amorphous solid lacks strong cohesive bonds between the molecules. The molecules are randomly arranged, and less energy iss required to separate the molecules of the amorphous material and dissolve the solid in contrast to a crystalline material. Techniques commonly used in preparing drugs in the amorphous state generally reduce the particle size of the drug and result in a faster rate of dissolution than occurs with a crystalline form. Since the amorphous state is predictably unstable, there is a strong tendency to transform to the crystalline state. Macek [336] reported that amorphous forms of the sodium and potassium salts of penicillin G obtained by evaporation from solution are less stable chemically than are their crystalline counterparts. Crystalline potassium penicillin can withstand dry heat for several hours without significant decomposition. Under similar conditions, the amorphous forms lose considerable activity. The amorphous form of novobiocin is 10 times more soluble but less stable than the crystalline form of the drug. Sokoloski [337] utilized methylcellulose to block this transformation from amorphous back to crystalline.

Ueda and co-workers have studied the dissolution properties of polymorphic forms of tolbutamide [338] and chlorpropamide [339]. Two polymorphs of the tolbutamide were characterized and eight polymorphs of the chlorpropamide were isolated. Dissolution studies with six forms of the drug indicated that two polymorphs demonstrated an initial two and three fold increase in solubility in pH 2.0 buffer media, over the remaining polymorphs.

More recent studies have placed an emphasis on the characterization of polymorphic changes that occur during processing and other mechanical treatments of drug substances. Takahashi and co-workers characterized two crystal forms of fostedil using X-ray diffraction and infrared spectra [340]. Solubility studies demonstrated that Form 2 was slightly more soluble than the Form 1 polymorph. Compression of Form 2 at a compression force of $500-1000$ kg/cm^2 induced polymorphic changes in the crystal. Similar changes were produced through grinding, as shown in Figure 72. Microcrystalline cellulose and cornstarch were ground with the Form 2 polymorph and were shown to accelerate the polymorphic transformation to Form 1. The authors concluded that Form 1 was the more suitable form for development due to polymorphic transitions of fostedil during grinding and compression. Similar polymorphic transitions were experienced by Lefebvre and co-workers [341] for carbamazepine during grinding and compression. Narurkar and co-workers [342] found that two polymorphs of celiprolol hydrochloride demonstrated a difference in hygroscopicity. They demonstrated that the high melting Form 1, which was the less hygroscopic of the two forms, underwent a transition to a low melting Form 2 at higher relative humidity.

O. Solvates and Hydrates

As a corollary to the importance of polymorphic forms on drug availability, hydrates and solvates of poorly soluble drugs should be considered. Solvates are different from polymorphs; they are the crystalline forms of drugs that associate with solvent molecules. When water is the solvent, the solvate formed is called a hydrate.

A comparative study [330] on the dissolution behavior of hydrated and nonsolvated forms of cholesterol, theophylline, caffeine, glutathimide, and

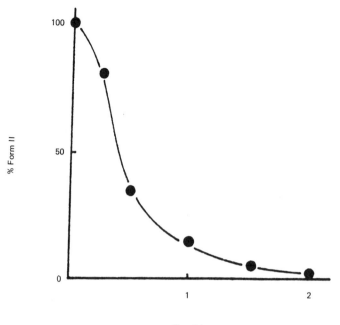

Figure 72   Effect of grinding on the polymorphic transformation of Form II of Fostedil.

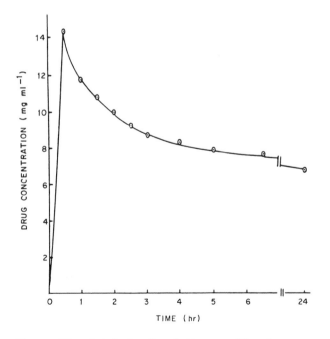

Figure 73   Intrinsic dissolution profile of a new antihypertensive drug in 0.1 N hydrochloric acid at 500 rpm.   (From Ref. 344.)

succinylsulfathiazole, showed that the anhydrous forms dissolved more rapidly in water and in all cases yielded drug concentrations in solution sub-
stantially higher than the hydrated states. Conversely, Shefter and
Higuchi [330] showed that the solvated forms of fluorocortisone with
n-pentanol or ethyl acetate and of succinylsulfathiazole with *n*-pentanol dissolved much more rapidly than did nonsolvated forms of the drugs.

Ballard and Biles [343] studied the in vitro absorption rates of hydro-
cortisone tert-butyl acetate and prednisolone tert-butyl acetate and their
solvates, by a pellet-implantation technique. Their results indicated that
drug solvates may exhibit dimorphism (two polymorphic forms) and each
form may exhibit different in vivo absorption rates.

Lin and Lachman [343] employed photomicrographic and dissolution
methods to study the in situ crystalline transformation of a new antihypertensive drug. The intrinsic dissolution profile of this drug, as seen in
Figure 73, shows an apparent rapid dissolution and attainment of a peak
concentration of drug in solution. Following this peak, there is a pronounced decline of drug in solution with time, which was attributed to the
formation of a less soluble species, such as a hydrate of the drug.

The dissolution properties and physical characterizations of erythromycin dihydrate, anhydrate, and amorphous forms were reported by
Fukumori and co-workers [345]. Erythromycin also forms solvates with
acetone, chloroform, *n*-butanol, and isopropanol. Many kinds of solvates
can easily be desolvated by mild heat treatment or even by exposure at
room temperature [346,347]. Fukomori and co-workers [345] demonstrated
that the temperature dependence of solubility for each form was such that
the solubility increased with a decrease in temperature. The dissolution
profiles for the amorphous form of erythromycin in distilled water as a
function of temperature are displayed in Figure 74. The heats of solution
increased with temperature and the plots against temperature for the three
forms could be fitted to a straight line, as seen in Figure 75. The slope
of the plot appeared to be identical for the three forms suggesting that
the peculiar temperature dependence of solubility might result from some
intermolecular interaction in the aqueous solution.

P. Complexation

The formation of molecular complexes can either increase or decrease the
apparent solubility of many pharmaceuticals. Higuchi and Lach [348] reported the use of xanthine to increase the solubility of drugs. The delayed
onset of action of drugs in tablets containing agents for the relief of
asthma was due to the formation of an insoluble complex. The dissolution
of theophylline from various generic tablets is seen in Figure 76. In Figure 77 the bioavailability of theophylline complexed with penobarbital is
compared with blood levels of theophylline alone and a physical mix of the
two drugs. The complexation of theophylline to the barbiturate resulted
in a significant decrease in theophylline blood levels after 0.5- and 1-hr
periods.

In studies with the benzocaine-caffeine complex, Higuchi et al. [350]
observed that the fastest rate of dissolution for either compound occurred
when the molar ratio was 1:1. Zoglio et al. [351] later showed that caffeine forms soluble complexes with the ergot alkaloids.

Higuchi and Ikeda [352] prepared a rapidly dissolving form of digoxin
by complexing the drug with hydroquinone. The dissolution profiles

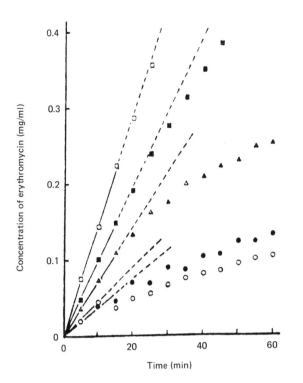

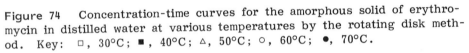

Figure 74 Concentration-time curves for the amorphous solid of erythromycin in distilled water at various temperatures by the rotating disk method. Key: □, 30°C; ■, 40°C; △, 50°C; ○, 60°C; ●, 70°C.

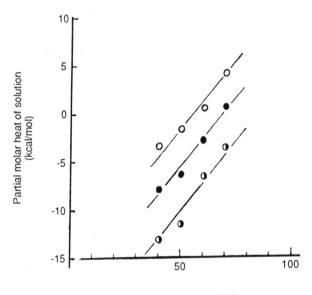

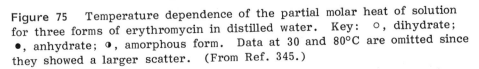

Figure 75 Temperature dependence of the partial molar heat of solution for three forms of erythromycin in distilled water. Key: ○, dihydrate; ●, anhydrate; ◑, amorphous form. Data at 30 and 80°C are omitted since they showed a larger scatter. (From Ref. 345.)

468

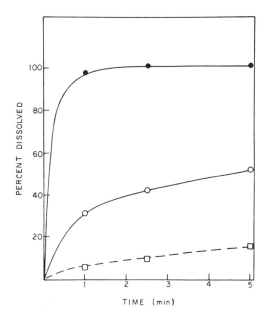

Figure 76   Dissolution profiles of theophylline in simulated gastric fluid at 37°C from theophylline, ephedrine hydrochloride, and phenobarbital tablets.   ●, Brand name; ○, generic B; □, generic A.   (From Ref. 349.)

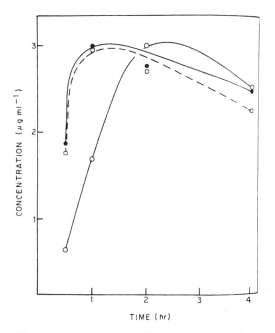

Figure 77   Theophylline serum levels, subject JWB, following a single 100-mg oral dose of theophylline.   (1) Physically mixed with phenobarbital, (2) complexed with phenobarbital.   ●, Free; ○, complex; □physical mixture.   (From Ref. 349.)

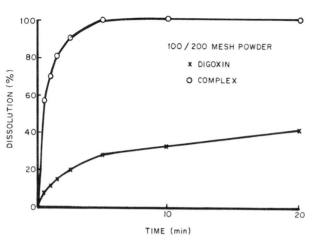

Figure 78   Dissolution-rate profiles obtained for the hydroquinone-digoxin complex and for digoxin itself under comparable conditions. (From Ref. 352.)

appear in Figure 78. It was suggested that the formation of a complex may overcome the processing problems associated with digoxin solid dosage forms because the complex completely dissociates when dissolved.

N-Methylglucamine, a basic compound with a pK_a of 9.3 and aqueous solubility of 1 g ml^{-1}, has been successfully employed as a complexing agent to enhance the absorption of Coumermycin A_1 [353]. When the drug

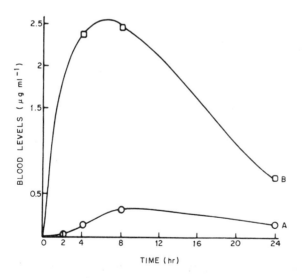

Figure 79   Mean coumermycin blood levels in humans following a single oral dose. A, alone; B, in combination with four parts of N-methylglucamine. (From Ref. 353.)

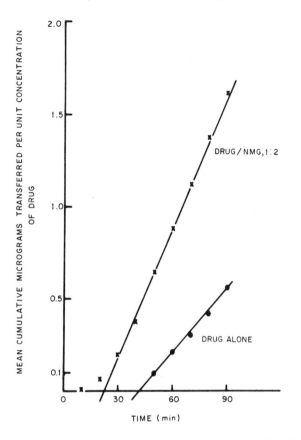

Figure 80   Everted intestinal sac data of a drug exhibiting poor in vitro permeability characteristics with and without the addition of 2 parts N-methylglucamine.   (From Ref. 353.)

was admixed with four parts of the complexing agent and administered to humans, the blood levels of the drug increased significantly, as seen in Figure 79.   The in vitro everted intestinal sac preparation was used with this drug, plus two parts of the N-methylglucamine, and compared with the diffusion of the drug alone.   The data in Figure 80 suggest that the permeability of drug from solutions was enhanced by the addition of the complexing agent.   Overall, it appears that the complexing agent altered both the dissolution and permeability characteristics of Coumermycin A$_1$, to allow for a more prolonged absorption of an otherwise negligibly absorbed drug.

In a recent review by Duchene and co-workers [354], the properties of inclusion complexes of drugs with cyclodextrins were discussed.   The more rapid dissolution of drug from these compounds resulted in higher blood concentrations, earlier peak times, and larger areas under the blood level curves for drug present in inclusion compounds, compared with pure drug alone.   In 1987, Szeman and co-workers [355] complexed several drugs with water soluble cyclodextrin polymers to improve the solubility and dissolution rates of the drugs.   The inclusion complexes with cyclodextrin often resulted in improved stability of the guest molecules. Greater stability may also be shown towards high temperature, resulting in lower volatility or higher thermal resistance. Higher stability against oxidation and hydrolysis have also been reported.

Q. Drug-Excipient Interactions

It is well known that the preparation of tablets involves the use of so-called "inert" ingredients. Excipient or adjuvant materials are added as binding agents, lubricants, disintegrants, diluent, or coating materials and are necessary for the preparation of a good-quality drug product. Since these ingredients often constitute a considerable portion of the tablet, the possibility exists for drug-excipient interactions to influence drug stability, dissolution rate, and drug absorption; but a physical or chemical interaction between the drug and adjuvant may result in the modification of the physical state, particle size, and/or surface area of the drug available to the absorption site. In addition, the formation of a surface complex or changes in chemical stability of the active constituent may result in toxic manifestations. Drugs bound by physical forces to excipients in the solid state generally separate rapidly from the excipient in aqueous solution. However, drugs bound via chemisorption are strongly attached to the excipient, which may result in incomplete absorption through the gastrointestinal membrane.

Several literature reports have appeared over the past decade describing drug-excipient interactions and the influence such interactions may have on drug bioavailability. An intensive review on this subject was conducted by Monkhouse and Lach [106], who stressed that drug products resulting from a generic or trade name manufacturer should be equally efficacious if proper care is taken during the formulation and manufacture of the dosage form to ensure optimum absorption. Space does not allow discussion of the paper by Monkhouse and Lach; however, important excipient studies referred to by them and published in the past few years should be mentioned. The interaction of dicumarol with several excipients was extensively studied by Akers and co-workers [356,357]. Dicumarol administered with talc, Veegum, aluminum hydroxide, and starch resulted in lower plasma levels of the drug in dogs when compared to the drug alone (see Figs. 81 to 83). Significantly higher plasma levels (up to 180% of control values) were observed when dicumarol was administered with magnesium oxide or hydroxide, and this was thought to be due to the formation of a magnesium chelate. The chelate was later isolated and characterized by Spivey [358]. Studies in vivo with dogs confirmed that the dicumarol from the magnesium chelate was more bioavailable than was the dicumarol itself. This effect is very interesting since, to the contrary, chelation has been reported to lower blood levels of drugs (e.g., tetracycline complexes with calcium and iron). Dissolution studies with three commercial dicumarol tablets (see Fig. 84) and in vivo evaluation of these tablets in dogs [357] verified that drug excipient interactions with this drug can be of serious proportions.

In other studies with colloidal magnesium aluminum silicate, cationic drugs were found to bind strongly to the clay [359]. Urinary recovery studies with amphetamine sulfate [360], however, indicated that although absorption was delayed, bioavailability from the amphetamine-clay absorbate was not significantly different from that with the pure drug.

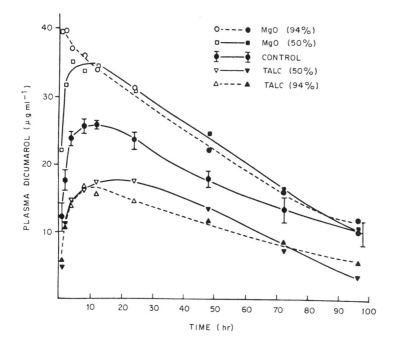

Figure 81 Plasma concentration of dicumarol after single oral doses of the drug given alone (control) or with various excipient materials. The values shown are the mean of four animals. Open data points indicate significant differences from control. Variations about the mean values was not statistically different from that of the control values shown with SEM. (From Ref. 356.)

Sorby [361] studied the influence of attapulgite and activated charcoal on the absorption of promazine and found that charcoal decreased both the rate and extent of absorption. Although attapulgite decreased the initial rate of drug absorption, there was no significant effect on total availability, since the drug was weakly bound to the clay. Later studies by Tsuchiya and Levy [362] suggested that it was possible to make reasonable predictions concerning the relative antidotal effectiveness of activated charcoal in humans on the basis of appropriate in vitro adsorption studies.

In a recent series of publications by Chowhan and Chi, drug and excipients in the powdered state were shown to interact with each other during powder mixing [363-365]. The interaction with disintegrants, lubricants, and fillers in a solid state was shown to effect the dissolution properties of the active ingredient. Chowan and Chi stated that such interactions can occur during any unit operation, including mixing, granulating, drying, and blending. During the initial phases of dosage form development it is essential that the formulators have a thorough understanding of these interactions such that the most appropriate excipients are selected to enable the formulation to perform optimally. Signoretti and co-workers [366] determined the physicochemical compatibility of clenbuterol with various commonly used tablet excipients by using differential scanning calorimetry. Using this technique, clenbuterol was found to be

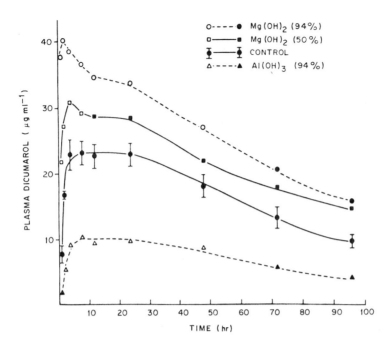

Figure 82　Plasma concentration of dicumarol after single oral doses of the drug given alone (control) or with various excipient materials.　The values shown are the mean of four animals.　Open data points indicate significant differences from control.　Variations about the mean values was not statistically different from that of the control values shown with SEM.　(From Ref. 356.)

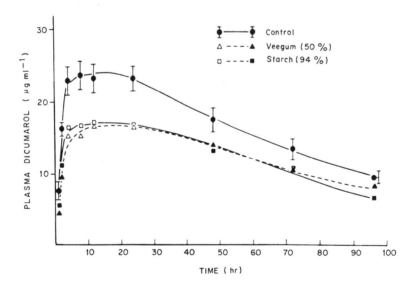

Figure 83　Plasma concentration of dicumarol after single oral doses of the drug given alone (control) or with various excipient materials.　The values shown are the mean of four animals.　Open data points indicate significant differences from control.　Variations about the mean values was not statistically different from that of the control values shown with SEM.　(From Ref. 356.)

474

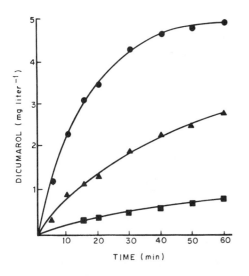

TIME (min)

Figure 84   Dissolution rate of dicumarol from three commercial tablets.
▲, Product A; ●, product B; ■, product C.   (From Ref. 357.)

compatible with talc, stearic acid, magnesium stearate, and titanium dioxide, whereas an incompatibility was shown with maize starch, pre-
gelatinized starch, cornstarch, sodium starch glycollate, polyvinyl
pyrrolidone, Avicel PH 101, and lactose.

    Chrzanowsky and co-workers compared differential scanning calorimetry
to an isothermal stress method for excipient compatibility testing [367].
They found the differential scanning calorimetry method to be an unreliable
compatibility predictor for fenretinide and could not be used with one of
the three mefenidil salts investigated.   Conversely the isothermal stress
method was an accurate compatibility predictor.   The authors stated that
the conditions of the test must be based upon the physical−chemical
properties of the compound and excipient.

    In 1985, Jacobs [368] described a drug-excipient program under ac-
celerated conditions to determine the influence of excipients on the chemical stability of the active ingredient.   Jacobs described the preparation
and testing of binary mixtures of drug substances and excipients stored
at elevated temperature, with and without added moisture.   The author
followed the compatibility of a drug with an excipient using thin layer
chromatography and high-performance liquid chromatography.

    The bioavailability of phenylpropanolamine hydrochloride from tablets
containing croscarmellose sodium was reported by Hollenbacl [369].   The
drug-excipient interaction involving weakly basic drugs and croscarmellose
sodium in aqueous dispersion had been previously well documented [370,
371].   The interaction occurs in vitro under conditions where the cationic
form of the drug exists and can exchange with sodium ions associated
with insoluble dispersed croscarmellose (cross-linked sodium carboxy-
methyl cellulose).   The significance of this interaction was studied by
Hollenbeck in six healthy subjects in a cross-over study to investigate
the physiological significance of the in vitro drug-excipient interaction

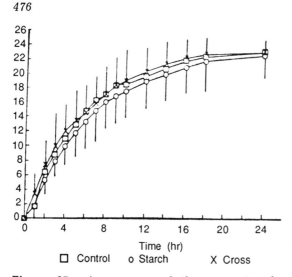

Time (hr)

□ Control   o Starch   X Cross

Figure 85 Average cumulative amounts of phenylpropanolamine excreted in the urine for control (CONTROL), starch-containing (STARCH), and croscarmellose sodium-containing (CROS) dosage forms in all subjects. (Error bars included for the STARCH and CROS treatments represent ±2 S.D. from the mean.) (From Ref. 369.)

[369]. Although a significant interaction between the drug and the excipient was found in vitro in distilled water, this interaction did not adversely influence the bioavailability of phenylpropanolamine hydrochloride from a solid dosage form containing the excipient as a disintegrant, as shown in Figure 85. Since the drug-excipient interaction is based on a nonspecific ion exchange mechanism, it is reasonable to expect these results are not specific for phenylpropanolamine hydrochloride. Hollenbeck concluded that a dissolution medium with ionic strength similar to physiological fluids would therefore seem more appropriate for the testing of dosage forms containing croscarmellose and weakly basic drugs.

R. Surface-Active Agents

The improved oral absorption of drugs when administered with surface-active agents has been attributed to the improved solubility and dissolution rates due to solubilization and/or wetting effects of the surfactants. However, in evaluating the effect of surface-active agents on the absorption rate of a drug, it is essential to establish whether this effect is mediated by an alteration of the absorbing membrane, an interaction with the drug, or by a modification of the physical properties of the dosage form. According to Nogami et al. [75,372,373], the rate-determining step in tablet disintegration is the penetration of media through the pores in the tablet. An equation was derived (42) which was found applicable to tablets:

$$L^2 = \frac{r\gamma\cos\theta}{2\eta} \, t = kt \tag{42}$$

where L is the length penetrated at time t, k the coefficient of penetration, r the average radius of the void space, θ the contact angle, and γ and η the surface tension and viscosity, respectively.

Equation (42) indicates that a surfactant has two effects on penetration of a liquid into the tablet. The addition of a surfactant lowers the surface tension and decreases the contact angle. Thus, the overall coefficient of penetration of a liquid into the tablet rises in the presence of surfactants, and increased penetration generally enhances disintegration. Ganderton [374] examined the effect of including a surfactant such as sodium lauryl sulfate on the breakup and dissolution of phenindione tablets and showed that the surfactant greatly assisted these effects over a wide range of pressures.

The surfactants dioctyl sodium sulfosuccinate and poloxamer 188, which are used internally as fecal softeners, have ben shown to improve the dissolution rates and absorption characteristics of various sulfonamides [375-377].

The presence of a surface-active agent in the dissolution medium has also been investigated. At levels of surfactant below the critical micelle concentration (CMC), the principal effect involved would be a wetting phenomenon rather than solubilization, according to Finholt and Solvang [256]. These workers used phenacetin as the model hydrophobic drug and studied the dissolution rate of phenacetin in 0.1 N aqueous hydrochloric acid containing different amounts of polysorbate 80. The data in Figure 86 show the times for 100 mg of drug to dissolve as a function of the surface tension. Other investigators [378,379] have shown improved dissolution rates at levels of surfactant below the CMC. Recently, Lim and Chen [380] reported that at pH 2.4 and 37°C, the apparent solubility of aspirin increased 17% in solutions of cetylpyridinium chloride above its CMC (0.2%).

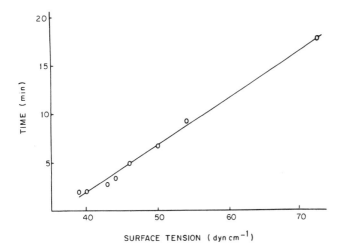

Figure 86   Relationship between the surface tension of the dissolution medium and the time necessary for dissolution of 100 mg of phenacetin (0.21-0.31 mm). Dissolution media: 0.1 N HCl containing different amounts of polysorbate 80. (From Ref. 256.)

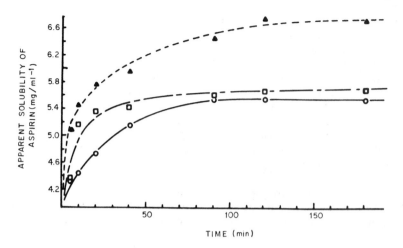

Figure 87   Effect of cetylpyridinium chloride on the apparent solubility of aspirin as a function of time at 37°C in pH 2.4 buffer. ▲, Above CMC; ○, below CMC; □, buffer control. (From Ref. 380.)

However, at concentrations below the CMC, dissolution rate and apparent solubility of aspirin decreased (see Fig. 87). Chiou et al. [381] enhanced the dissolution rates of sulfathiazole, prednisone, and chloramphenicol by recrystallization of the drugs in aqueous polysorbate 80 solutions.

Parrott and others [382,383] have studied the effects of high concentrations of surfactants on the dissolution of benzoic acid. Using concentrations of surfactant exceeding the critical micelle concentration, the dissolution rate rose to a peak and then declined with increase in surfactant concentration, as seen in Figure 88. The total solubility of benzoic acid increased linearly as the concentration of the surfactant increased.

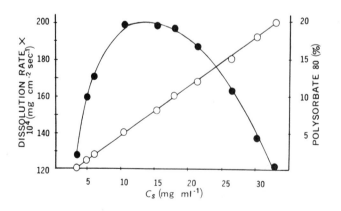

Figure 88   Relationship of total solubility C_S of benzoic acid at 25°C to dissolution rate and concentration of polysorbate 80. ●, Rate; ○, concentration. (From Ref. 383.)

Elworthy and Lipscomb [384] substantiated these results by reporting that at high concentrations of surfactant, the viscosities of dissolution media were enhanced markedly, slowing the dissolution rate of griseofulvin.

The FDA's handbook of drug dissolution standards recommends the use of 0.56% sodium lauryl sulfate in water as the dissolution medium for medroxyprogesterone acetate tablets to meet the recommended dissolution tolerance limits of not less than 85% in 45 min. Fatmi and co-workers [385] demonstrated that these tolerance limits can be achieved by using smaller quantities of the surfactant (0.1%) in 0.1 N hydrochloric acid as the dissolution medium. Both the generic and inventor's products resulted in comparable and acceptable results in both media. The authors recommended that by decreasing the quality of surfactant in the medium, a more discriminating test would result as well as easier handling of the surfactant.

Pandit and co-workers [386] proposed the use of surfactant solutions as media for the dissolution testing of a poorly water-soluble drug. The solubility of 4-(4-biphenylyl)-butanol was dramatically enhanced in the presence of anionic, cationic, and nonionic surfactants. Since no bioavailability problems were experienced following oral administration of the drug, it was concluded that physiological surfactants could be involved in the solubilization of the drug, in vivo. Intrinsic dissolution studies were conducted in water, sodium dodecyl sulfate, and polyoxyethylene lauryl ether solutions and the later surfactant solution was selected as the medium of choice.

Itai and co-workers [387] studied the effect of surfactants, particle size, and additives on the dissolution rate of flufenamic acid. They suggested that extensive micronization may result in a considerable increase in hydrophobicity of the active ingredient and a decrease in the available surface area. Although the influence of surfactants on drug dissolution has been extensively investigated, few reports have dealt with the dissolution behavior of powdered drugs having controlled particle sizes, in surfactant solutions. Using several probability parameters obtained from linear regression of the dissolution data, Itai and co-workers evaluated quantitatively, the effect of varying the amounts os surfactant, particle size, and additives on the time course of the available surface area of flufenamic acid during the dissolution process.

Although surfactants generally increase drug solubility and/or dissolution rate, Feely and Davis [388] demonstrated that the inclusion of sodium dodecylsulphate into a matrix tablet containing hydroxypropyl methylcellulose (HPMC) and the cationic drug, chlorpheniramine maleate, resulted in a decrease in release rates as shown in Figure 89. The release rate constant (k) was calculated from the linear, percentage rebound versus root time curve for each formulation containing the various levels of surfactant. A linear relationship, as shown in Figure 90, was found when k was plotted as a function of the percentage of surfactant.

Daley and co-workers [389] had made a similar observation to Feely and Davis concerning the effect of the surfactant in the HPMC matrix tablet containing chlorpheniramine maleate. They attributed this effect to the binding of the surfactant to the polymer, thereby causing an increase in gel viscosity. Feely and Davis reported that the retardation was due to an ionic interaction between the drug and the surfactant and was dependent upon the number of surfactant molecules present.

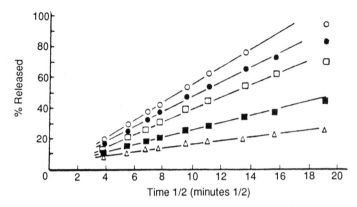

Figure 89   Effect of sodium dodecylsulfate (SDDS) concentration on chlorpheniramine release from Methocel K100M matrices (pH 7). Key: ○, 0% w/w; ●, 2% w/w; □, 5% w/w; ■, 10% w/w; △, 15% w/w. (From Ref. 388.)

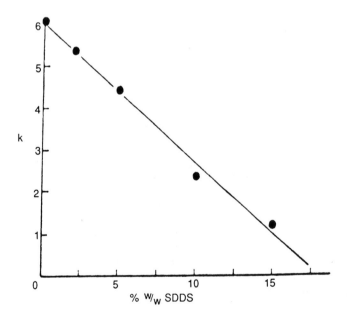

Figure 90   Plot of k vs % w/w sodium dodecylsulfate (SDDS) for chlorpheniramine release from Methocel K100M matrices (pH 7). Slope = -0.33 min$^{-1/2}$, intercept = 6.01 min$^{-1/2}$, correlation coefficient = 0.995. (From Ref. 388.)

IV. PHARMACOKINETIC MODELS AND METHODS

A basic understanding of pharmacokinetics —the quantitative description of the time course of drugs and metabolities in the body —is essential to the intelligent use of biopharmaceutics in tablet development. So far we have attempted to show that dosage formulation variables affect bioavailability and as a consequence alter clinical efficacy of medicinal agents in a significant way.

In the research laboratories and manufacturing plants of modern drug companies it is not enough to know that complex forces are at play. The scientific foundations of physical pharmacy, biopharmaceutics and pharmacokinetics, have advanced to a point where the pharmaceutical scientist is expected to apply current knowledge to the design of a tablet, suppository, suspension, or microcapsule with release properties and stability characteristics that result in maximum efficacy, safety, and therapeutic control.

These demands on the drug scientist require that he or she have at least an acquaintance with the quantitative aspects of pharmacokinetics and biopharmaceutics.

In order to follow the processes of absorption, distribution, metabolism, and elimination of drugs in the body and to relate these events to pharmacological action and therapeutic response, it is convenient to use models, that is, to represent the body as a system of compartments with the drug entering and leaving the compartments according to a postulated kinetic scheme. Modeling employs techniques of statistics, kinetics, and the devising of mathematical constructs in order to cast the observed data, such as blood levels and cumulative urinary excretion, into an organized sequence of steps which make up the model. The model is a hypothetical scheme, and the simplest mathematical construct that corresponds with the observed facts should be used. If it serves to explain the observed phenomena and allows predictions of results not yet obtained, it should be considered adequate even though it proves to be an oversimplification of the real situation. Only when results obtained from the use of a model fail to correspond to observed pharmacokinetic data should more elaborate compartmental models be sought.

Some of the models that have been used with success in pharmacokinetics and biopharmaceutics are described in the following paragraphs.

A. One-Compartment Model: Single Dosing

The one-compartment model, represented by the following scheme, considers the body as a homogeneous unit with an input and an output rate process

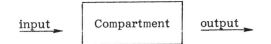

This model does not suggest that the concentration of drug in the blood plasma is equal to the concentration of drug in all tissues or fluids at any one time. The model implies, however, that whatever occurs regarding the drug concentration in the blood plasma is mirrored by changes in

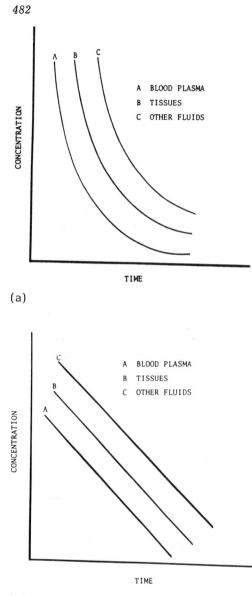

(a)

(b)

Figure 91   (a) Time course of drug in body fluids and tissues (b) in a semilog-arithmic plot of the data in (a).

other tissues and fluids. Hence, if one could follow the time course of drug concentration in tissues and blood plasma, all levels should decline in a parallel fashion. This is illustrated in Figure 91a and b, where Figure 91b is a semilogarithmic plot of the data in Figure 91a. The ratio of the concentration of drug in blood plasma to the concentration of drug in the tissue at any given point in time is constant.

A convenience in utilizing the one-compartment model is that the output of drug from the body is frequently a first-order process. This means that the elimination of drug from the body is proportional to the amount of drug in the body at that time. The proportionality constant K is the apparent elimination-rate constant, drug elimination taking place by several physiological processes. The apparent first-order elimination-rate constant K is the sum of the individual rate constants for different elimination processes:

$$K = k_e + k_b + k_m + k_s + \cdots \tag{43}$$

where k_e and k_b are apparent first-order elimination-rate constants for renal and biliary excretion, respectively, and k_m and k_s are apparent first-order constants for metabolic and salivary processes.

Let us now turn our attention to the analysis of a one-compartment model after single-dose intravenous administration.

Intravenous Injection

PLASMA LEVELS. After intravenous injection of a single dose, the drug is distributed throughout the body by means of the vascular network. When the drug is injected rapidly into the bloodstream, it initially mixes with a small volume of blood, forming a bolus or mass of the administered dose. However, as it passes through the various capillary beds, beds, filtration and diffusion effects cause some of the molecules to diffuse into the surrounding tissues. The rate of uptake of a compound into tissues is controlled by several factors, including the rate of blood flow to the tissue, permeability of the compound across tissue membranes, the mass of tissue, and partition characteristics of the compound between plasma and tissues. Partitioning, in turn, is affected by the pH of the medium, complexation, and plasma protein binding. In addition to distribution processes, drugs are metabolized or excreted unchanged in urine, bile, saliva, and other body fluids. In each of these systems the intact drug may undergo recycling into the body rather than direct elimination. If the drug is distributed and eliminated according to a one-compartment model, the rate of loss of drug from the body is given by the first-order expression,

$$\frac{dA}{dt} = -KA \tag{44}$$

where A is the amount of drug at time t after injection, dA/dt the change of the amount of drug dA in the single compartment representing the body with respect to the infinitesimal duration of time, dt and K, as illustrated in Eq. (43), is the overall elimination-rate constant. The negative sign in Eq. (43) indicates that the amount of drug in the body is decreasing with time.

Equation (44) is a first-order linear differential equation, and integration of this equation according to elementary principles of calculus or by use of Laplace transforms [390–392] results in

$$A = A_0 e^{-Kt} \qquad (45)$$

The initial condition for the integration is that $A = A_0$ = initial intravenous (i.v.) dose. Conversion of Eq. (45) to Briggsian logarithms leads to

$$\log A = \log A_0 - \frac{Kt}{2.303} \qquad (46)$$

It should be understood that owing to the process of distribution, the body cannot be truly considered a homogenous unit, the drug concentration in blood plasma differing from drug concentration in tissues. However, the ratio of blood plasma drug concentration to tissue drug concentration will be constant at any point in time, and a constant relationship exists between the drug concentration C in the plasma and the amount A of drug in the body:

$$A = V_d D \qquad (47)$$

where V_d is a proportionality constant termed "apparent volume of distribution"; the units of V_d are volume units. If A is expressed as milligrams of drug per kilogram of body weight and plasma concentration as mg liter^{-1}, V_d has the units liter kg^{-1}. No physiological meaning should be attached to this constant; rather, it should be considered simply as a proportionality term which allows one to relate amount A in the body to concentration C.

Equation (5) enables the conversion of Eq. (46) to be expressed in concentration terms:

$$\log C = \log C_0 - \frac{Kt}{2.303} \qquad (48)$$

Equation (48) yields a straight line and extrapolation to time zero gives C_0, the plasma concentration at initial injection. The value of the apparent first-order elimination-rate constant K can be obtained from the slope of the line. C_0 may be used to calculate the value of the apparent distribution V_d using the relationship

$$V_d = \frac{A_0}{C_0} \qquad (49)$$

where A_0 is the i.v. dose.

The graphical representation of Eq. (48) is illustrated in Figure 92. The biological or elimination half-life $t_{1/2}$ is defined as the time required for the drug concentration at any point on the straight line to decrease to one-half of the original value. The half-life can be obtained either graphically as illustrated in Figure 92, or by use of the following relationship:

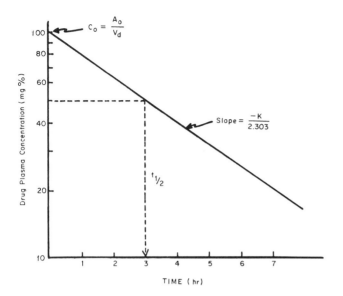

Figure 92 Semilogarithmic plot of the concentration of drug in the blood plasma as a function of time after single intravenous administration.

$$t_{1/2} = \frac{0.693}{K} \tag{50}$$

The best values for K, $t_{1/2}$, and C_0 are obtained by least-squares regression analysis of the data.

Example 1 Sample Calculation of Pharmacokinetic Parameters Using Plasma Concentration-Time Data Following I.V. Administration of a Drug That is Represented by a One-Compartment Model

A subject received an i.v. dose of 100 mg of a drug, and plasma concentrations of drug were determined as a function of time. The results are illustrated in Table 19. Calculate (a) the overall elimination-rate constant K, (b) the volume of distribution V_d, (c) the elimination half-life $t_{1/2}$, and (d) C_0. Assume that the drug is eliminated by an apparent first-order process.

Solution:

Step 1. To solve this problem, start by using Eq. (48), which shows that a plot of the logarithm of the drug plasma concentration versus time is linear. The result of plotting the data is illustrated in Figure 93.

Step 2. Calculate the slope of the line. An equation for obtaining slope is

Table 19   Plasma Concentration
of a Drug After Intravenous
Administration of 100 mg

Time (hr)	Plasma concentration ($\mu g\ ml^{-1}$)
1	60.65
2	36.79
3	22.31
4	13.53
5	8.21
6	4.98
7	3.02

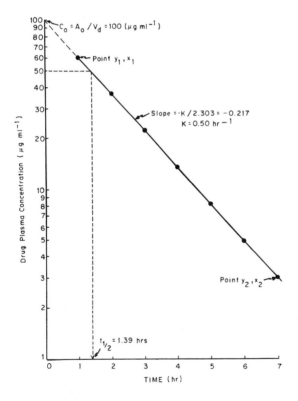

Figure 93   Semilogarithmic plot of the concentration of drug in the blood plasma following intravenous administration of a drug represented by a one-compartment model.

$$S = \frac{\log y_1 - \log y_2}{x_1 - x_2}$$

Using the points $y_1 = 60.65$, $x_1 = 1$ hr and $y_2 = 3.02$, $x_2 = 7$ hr from Figure 93 we get

$$S = \frac{1.78 - 0.48}{1 - 7} = -0.217$$

The slope is equal to -0.217. According to Eq. (48), the slope is equal to $-K/2.303$. Thus,

$$-K = \text{slope} \times 2.303$$

$$K = -(0.217 \times 2.303) = 0.5$$

Step 3. Extrapolate the line to time zero to obtain C_0. In this particular example, C_0 is equal to 100 $\mu g/ml^{-1}$ (see Fig. 93.)

Step 4. Knowledge of C_0 and the intravenous dose enables one to calculate the volume of distribution V_d by means of Eq. (49).

$$V_d = \frac{100,000}{100} = 1000 \text{ ml} = 1 \text{ liter}$$

Step 5. Calculation of the elimination half-life is accomplished using Eq. (50). Thus,

$$t_{1/2} = \frac{0.693}{0.500} = 1.39 \text{ hr}$$

Another method to calculate the half-life is graphical representation of the data. At time $t = 0$, the drug plasma concentration is 100 $\mu g/ml^{-1}$. Using the definition of half-life at drug plasma concentration of 50 $\mu g/ml^{-1}$, or one-half the original value, the half-life is read from the horizontal axis as roughly 1.4 hr (see Fig. 93).

URINARY EXCRETION. K, $t_{1/2}$, and C_0 can also be obtained using urinary excretion data, since the amount of unchanged drug in the urine is proportional to the amount of drug in the body. The excretion rate dA_u/dt can be expressed in terms of first-order kinetics as

$$\frac{dA_u}{dt} = k_e A \tag{51}$$

It is important to recognize that k_e is the apparent first-order elimination-rate constant for unchanged drug. The overall elimination constant K does not appear in this equation, since it is the summation of k_e together with other elimination-rate constants.

Substitution of Eq. (45) into Eq. (51) leads to

dA_u/dt can be approximated by $\Delta A_u/\Delta_t$; therefore,

$$\frac{\Delta A_u}{\Delta t} = k_e A_0 e^{-Kt} \tag{53}$$

Taking the logarithm of this equation results in

$$\log \frac{\Delta A_u}{\Delta t} = \log k_e A_0 - \frac{Kt}{2.303} \tag{54}$$

Equation (54) is a straight line when the excretion rate of unchanged drug in the urine $\Delta A_u/\Delta t$, in mg/hr^{-1}, is plotted versus time; it provides a technique called the "elimination-rate method." The slope of the line is $-K/2.303$. Thus, the overall elimination rate constant K can be obtained from this relationship, and the elimination half-life is calculated using Eq. (50).

It is important to consider that dA_u/dt is not an instantaneous rate but rather an average rate $\Delta A_u/\Delta t$ obtained over the finite time period Δt. Consequently, when constructing the graph, average excretion rates should be plotted versus the midpoint of a short urine-collection-time interval. At the midpoint of each Δt, the average excretion rate will approximate the instantaneous excretion rate.

Other methods exist to analyze urinary excretion data. Swintosky [393] introduced a technique that can be used when drug elimination continues over long periods of time. This method is also employed when the rate of excretion of drug and metabolite are maximum.

SIGMA-MINUS METHOD. Another useful analysis of urinary excretion data can be obtained through the sigma-minus method, a procedure introduced by Martin [394]. This method requires accurate assessment of the total amount of drug or metabolite excreted in the urine. The method becomes impractical when drug elimination is slow or when the data relate to multiple-dose therapy. The sigma-minus method is not applicable when drug elimination is a zero-order process. However, this approach overcomes the problem of fluctuations in the rate of drug elimination which one obtains when using the excretion-rate plot based on Eq. (54). Figure 94 illustrates that fluctuations in the rate of drug elimination are reflected to a much greater extent in the excretion-rate method than in the sigma-minus method.

The following mathematical treatment leads to the equation utilized in the sigma-minus method. Integration of Eq. (52), assuming that $A_u = 0$ at $t = 0$, yields

$$A_u = \frac{k_e A_0}{K} (1 - e^{-Kt}) \tag{55}$$

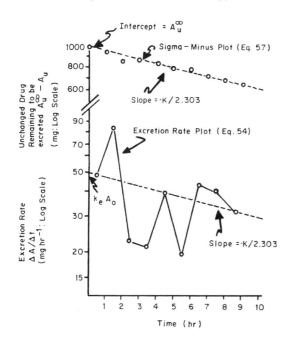

Figure 94   Log sigma-minus plot and corresponding log rate plot relating to data for the excretion of drug in urine. The dashed lines represents a theoretical decline corresponding to K = 0.05 hr^{-1}. Fluctuations in the rate of drug elimination are reflected to a much greater extent in the rate plot. (From Ref. 394.)

where A_u is the cumulative amount of unchanged drug excreted to time t. At time t = ∞, Eq. (55) reduces to

$$A_u^\infty = \frac{K_e A_0}{K} \tag{56}$$

where A_u^∞ is the total amount of unchanged drug eliminated in the urine. Substitution of A_u^∞ for $k_e A_0/K$ in Eq. (55) gives

$$\log (A_u^\infty - A_u) = \log A_u^\infty - \frac{Kt}{2.303} \tag{57}$$

Equation (58) is a straight line with a slope of $-K/2.303$; consequently, K can be determined using urinary excretion data. If the drug is eliminated unchanged in the urine and is not eliminated by other routes, k_e becomes equal to K, and from Eq. (56) it can be seen that A_u^∞ becomes A_0, which is the initial i.v. dose.

   Several practical applications of these methods have been reported in the literature [395 – 397].

Example 2   Sample Calculation of Pharmacokinetic Parameters Following
Intravenous Bolus Injection of a Drug That Is Represented by a One-
Compartment Model Using Urinary Excretion Data

A 100-mg dose of a drug was administered i.v. to a subject and the cumulative amount of drug in the urine was obtained as a function of time.
The results are illustrated in Table 20. Using the sigma-minus method
and the excretion-rate method, estimate (a) the half-life of the drug,
(b) the overall elimination-rate constant K, (c) the rate constant for elimination of unchanged drug, and (d) the cumulative amount of drug excreted unchanged at 4.5 hr.

Solution:

Step 1.   Eq. (54) shows that a plot If log $\Delta A_u / \Delta t$ versus ti will result in
a straight line. The slope is equal to $-K/2.303$ and the intercept $k_e A_0$.
The use of this equation requires that log $\Delta A_u / \Delta t$ be plotted against the
midpoint of a short urine-collection interval (see Table 20). According to
Figure 95, the slope and the intercept of the line are -30 and 20.0 mg,
respectively. Thus,

$$K = -\text{slope} \times 2.303 = -(-0.30 \times 3.303) = 0.691 \text{ hr}^{-1}$$

$$k_e = \frac{\text{intercept}}{A_0} = \frac{20}{100} = 0.20 \text{ hr}^{-1}$$

Step 2.   Eq. (58) shows that a plot of log $(A_u^\infty - A_u)$ versus time will
result in a straight line with a slope equal to $-K/2.303$. According to
Figure 95, the slope is equal to -0.30. Thus,

$$K = -\text{slope} \times 2.303 = -(-0.30 \times 2.303) = 0.691 \text{ hr}^{-1}$$

This is the same value obtained in step 1 for K, as would be expected.

Step 3.   Another way to calculate k_e is given by Eq. (56).

$$k_e = \frac{K A_u^\infty}{A_0} = \frac{0.691 \times 28.85}{100} = 0.20 \text{ hr}^{-1}$$

Step 4.   The cumulative amount excreted unchanged up to 4.5 hr can be
estimated by means of Eq. (55). Thus,

$$A_{u(4.5 \text{ hr})} = \frac{0.20 \times 100}{0.691} (1 - e^{-0.691 \times 4.5}) = 27.61 \text{ mg}$$

Table 20 Cumulative Amount Excreted Unchanged After Intravenous Administration of 100 mg of a Drug

Time, t (hr)	Cumulative amount A_u (mg)	$t_{midpoint}$	Δt	ΔA_u	$\frac{\Delta A_u}{\Delta t}$	$A_u^\infty - A_u$
0	0	–	–	–	–	28.85
0.5	8.45	0.25	0.5	8.45	16.90	20.40
1.0	14.43	0.75	0.5	5.98	11.96	14.42
1.5	18.65	1.25	0.5	4.22	8.44	10.20
2.0	21.64	1.75	0.5	2.99	5.98	7.21
2.5	23.76	2.25	0.5	2.12	4.24	5.09
3.0	25.25	2.75	0.5	1.49	2.98	3.60
3.5	26.31	3.25	0.5	1.06	2.12	2.54
4.0	27.06	3.75	0.5	0.75	1.50	1.79
5.0	27.96	4.5	1.0	0.90	0.9	0.89
6.0	28.41	5.5	1.0	0.45	0.45	0.44
7.0	28.63	6.5	1.0	0.22	0.22	0.22
8.0	28.75	7.5	1.0	0.12	0.12	0.10
∞	$A_u^\infty = 28.85$	–	–	–	–	0.0

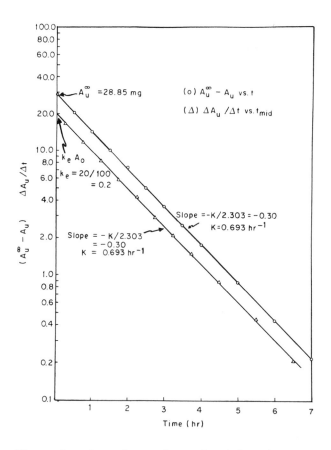

Figure 95 Log sigma-minus plot (○) and corresponding log rate plot (△) relating to data for the urinary excretion of a drug following intravenous bolus injection. The drug is represented by a one-compartment model.

Oral Absorption

The treatment here follows the excellent description of Gibaldi and Perrier [398]. The reader should also refer to Wagner's explanation of dosage regimen and its calculations; he introduced a number of dose regimen equations [399]. Equation (58) represents the pharmacokinetic model of a drug entering the body by an apparent first-order rate process, as is customarily found for oral, rectal, and intra-muscular administration. The drug, administered as a single dose, is absorbed and eliminated from the body by apparent first-order processes. One-compartment characteristics are observed in this case.

$$G \xrightarrow{\ k_a\ } A \xrightarrow{\ K\ } U \tag{58}$$

G is the amount of drug at the absorption site, A the amount in the body, and U the amount eliminated unchanged in the urine.

The differential equation describing the change in A is given by

$$\frac{dA}{dt} = k_a G - KA \tag{59}$$

The term k_a is the apparent first-order absorption-rate constant, and K is the apparent first-order overall elimination-rate constant. The rate of loss at the absorption site is given by

$$\frac{dG}{dt} = -k_a G \tag{60}$$

Integration of Eq. (60), assuming that G is the dose at $t = 0$, leads to

$$G = G_0 e^{-k_a t} \tag{61}$$

However, it should be remembered that in most cases only a fraction of the dose is absorbed. Thus,

$$G = FG_0 e^{-k_a t} \tag{62}$$

where F is the fraction of the administered dose G_0 that is absorbed following oral administration. Substituting Eq. (62) into Eq. (59) and integrating assuming that $A = A_0 = 0$ at $t = 0$ leads to

$$A = \frac{k_a FG_0}{k_a - K} (e^{-Kt} - e^{-k_a t}) \tag{63}$$

which is expressed in terms of concentration as

$$C = \frac{k_a FG_0}{(k_a - K)V_d} (e^{-Kt} - e^{-k_a t}) \tag{64}$$

where V_d is the apparent volume of distribution. It is helpful to consider two situations: the usual case, where absorption is rapid and then subsides to insignificance while elimination continues at a finite rate ($k_a \gg K$); and a second instance, in which K is large relative to k_a (that is, $k_a \ll K$), owing to rapid drug elimination or slow release of the drug from its dosage form. In the first case k_a is appreciably greater than K—say, 10 to 100 times as large—then $e^{-k_a t}$ will become quite small as time proceeds, whereas e^{-Kt} remains significant. Equation (64) then reduces to

$$C = \frac{k_a FG_0}{(k_a - K)V_d} e^{-Kt} \tag{65}$$

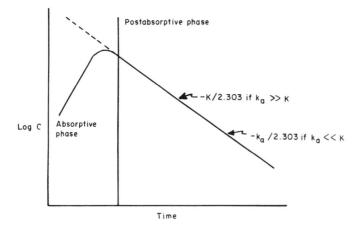

Figure 96   Semilogarithmic plot of drug levels in plasma after oral administration of a single dose of a drug.   The slope values are explained in
the text.

This case is the one more frequently encountered after oral administration
of drugs.   Equation (65) describes the concentration of drug in the body
after absorption has ceased (i.e., during the postabsorptive period).
    The logarithm of Eq. (65) is

$$\log C = \log \frac{k_a F G_0}{(k_a - K)V_d} - \frac{Kt}{2.303} \tag{66}$$

Log C may be plotted on the vertical axis of a graph versus time on the
horizontal axis to yield a curve as shown in Figure 96.   The terminal portion or postabsorptive phase is essentially linear with a slope of $-K/2.303$,
following Eq. (66).   Employing Eq. (50), the half-life for elimination can
also be calculated.
    In the reverse case where K is significantly greater than k_a, the slope
of the line in the terminal phase will now be equal to $-k_a/2.303$.   The flip
in slope from $-K/2.303$ to $-k_a/2.303$ is called a "flip-flop" model and is
usually observed when drugs are rapidly eliminated (K large).   An example of this phenomenon is provided by ampicillin kinetics, as reported by
Doluisio et al. [400].   The value for the rate constant of absorption k_a
may be calculated as follows.   The "method of residuals" (also called
feathering or stripping) is used to obtain a residual line, and the slope
of this line for the usual case where $k_a > K$ is $-k_a/2.303$.   This is illustrated in Figure 97.
    According to Eq. (66), the terminal linear portion of the curve with
slope $-K/2.303$ may be extrapolated to t = 0 to provide an intercept
value, I:

$$I = \log \frac{k_a F G_0}{(k_a - K)V_d} \tag{67}$$

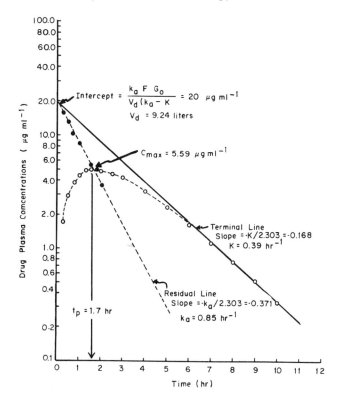

Figure 97 Semilogarithmic plot of the concentration of drug in the blood plasma following single oral administration of a drug represented by a one-compartment model.

The actual plasma levels of the early portion of the curve are then subtracted from the extrapolated line. This procedure produces a series of "residual" concentrations, Cr, as found in Table 20. These residuals are equivalent to the difference between Eq. (64) and Eq. (65):

$$Cr = \frac{k_a FG_9}{(k_a - K)V_d} e^{-k_a t} \tag{68}$$

A plot of Cr on a logarithmic scale versus time

$$\log Cr = \log \frac{k_a FG_0}{(k_a - K)V_d} - \frac{k_a t}{2.303} \tag{69}$$

yields a straight line [Eq. (69)] with a slope of $-k_a/2.303$ and an intercept I as given by Eq. (67).

By such a method of residuals it is possible to resolve the original curve into its component parameters, particularly the absorption constant

k_a and the elimination constant K. The apparent volume of distribution can be calculated from the y intercept if k_a and K are known:

$$V_d = \frac{k_a FG_0}{(k_a - K)I} \tag{70}$$

A better estimate of the volume of distribution can be obtained by integrating Eq. (64) from zero to infinity. This leads to

$$\int_0^\infty C \, dt = \frac{FG_0}{V_d K} \tag{71}$$

where the left term of the equation is the area under the plasma concentration-time curve. Rearrangement of Eq. (71) gives

$$V_d = \frac{FG_0}{K \int_0^\infty C \, dt} \tag{72}$$

If the total dose administered is absorbed, then F is equal to 1.

CALCULATING THE TIME AT PEAK CONCENTRATION t_p. Two quantities are of particular importance in studying the biopharmaceutics of rival products either during the formulation stage or during evaluation of competitive marketed forms of a generic drug. These are the peak or maximum bioconcentration C_{max} attained with a particular dose of the drug, and the time t_p following administration that the blood level reaches its maximum value.

Differentiation of Eq. (64) with respect to time and assuming that at peak concentration in the plasma concentration-time curve dc/dt = 0 results in the expression

$$\frac{k_a}{K} = \frac{e^{-kt_p}}{e^{-k_a t_p}} \tag{73}$$

where t_p is the time to peak.

Further simplification of Eq. (73) leads to a solution for the time to peak t_p:

$$t_p = \frac{2.303}{k_a - K} \log \frac{k_a}{K} \tag{74}$$

It will be observed from Eq. (74) that as the absorption rate increases, the time to peak decreases. This is illustrated in Figure 98.

Maximum plasma concentration C_{max} is easily estimated by substituting t_p for t in Eq. (64), yielding

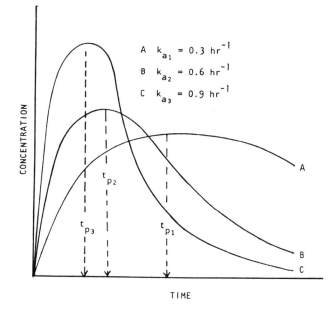

Figure 98 Effect of the absorption rate k_a on the time to peak t_p. As k_a increases, t_p decreases.

$$C_{max} = \frac{k_a FG_0}{V_d(k_a - K)} \; (e^{-Kt_p} - e^{-k_a t_p}) \tag{75}$$

Combining Eqs. (74) and (75) leads to a simple equation for estimating the peak blood level C_{max}:

$$C_{max} = \frac{FG_0}{V_d} e^{-Kt_p} \tag{76}$$

Now that we have presented the equations as derived by Gibaldi and Perrier [398], let us apply them to the oral administration of a drug product.

Example 3   Sample Calculation of Pharmacokinetic Parameters Using Plasma Concentration-Time Data Following Oral Administration of a Drug That Is Represented by a One-Compartment Model

A subject received a single oral dose of 100 mg in a tablet dosage form, and the drug plasma concentration was obtained as a function of time. The results are illustrated in Table 21. Calculate (a) the absorption-rate constant k_a, (b) the elimination-rate constant K, (c) the volume of distribution V_d, (d) time to peak t_p, and (e) the maximum drug concentration C_{max}. Assume that the fraction of the dose absorbed F is equal to 1.0.

Table 21   Concentration Time Data Obtained Following Oral Administration
of a Drug

Time (hr)	Drug concentration ($\mu g \ ml^{-1}$)	Time (hr)	Drug concentration ($\mu g \ ml^{-1}$)
0	0	3.0	4.21
0.25	1.72	4.0	3.22
0.5	2.97	5.0	2.34
0.75	3.84	6.0	1.65
1.0	4.42	7.0	1.14
1.5	4.95	8.0	0.78
1.75	5.0	9.0	0.53
2.0	4.95	10.0	0.36
2.5	4.65		

Solution:

Step 1. Plot the values from Table 21 on semilogarithmic paper. Figure
97 provides a graphical representation of the data (open circles).

Step 2. Extrapolate the terminal linear phase to time zero, where one observes the intercept to be 20.0 $\mu g \ ml^{-1}$.

Step 3. Calculate the slope of the terminal linear phase. According to
Eq. (66), the slope of the line should be equal to $-K/2.303$. Thus,

$$-K = slope \times 2.303$$

$$= -(0.168 \times 2.303) = 0.39 \ hr^{-1}$$

Step 4. Using the method of residuals ("feathering"), calculate the residual concentration values. These values are obtained by subtracting the
true plasma drug concentration values in the absorptive phase from the
corresponding drug concentration values on the extrapolated linear portion
of the line. Table 22 illustrates the results.

Step 5. On the same graph, plot the residual values of column 4,
Table 22 (see Fig. 97). Calculate the slope of this line using the two-
point formula or a desk calculator. The result is -0.371. The slope is
equal to $-k_a/2.303$; therefore,

$$k_a = -(-0.371 \times 2.303) = 0.85 \ hr^{-1}$$

Step 6. Equation (66) indicates that the intercept at time zero is equal to
$k_a F G_0/(k_a - K)V_d$. This allows us to calculate the volume of distribution.
From Figure 97 we see that the intercept I is equal to 20 $\mu g \ ml^{-1}$. Thus,

Table 22 Residual Values: Plasma Concentration-Time Data
Following Oral Administration of a Drug

Time (hr)	Drug concentration ($\mu g \ ml^{-1}$)	Extrapolated concentration ($\mu g \ ml^{-1}$)	Residual concentration ($\mu g \ ml^{-1}$)
0.25	1.72	17.5	15.78
0.5	2.97	16.0	13.03
0.75	3.84	14.0	10.16
1.0	4.42	13.0	8.58
1.5	4.95	10.5	5.55
1.75	5.0	10.0	5.0
2.0	4.95	8.6	3.65

$$V_d = \frac{k_a F G_0}{(k_a - K)(I)}$$

$$= \frac{0.85 \times 1.0 \times 100}{(0.85 - 0.39)20} = 9.24 \text{ liters}$$

A second method to calculate the volume of distribution is given by
Eq. (72). This requires the estimate of the area under the plasma concentration-time curve from time zero to infinity. In this particular case,
the area is approximately equal to 27.75 $\mu g \ ml^{-1} \ hr^{-1}$. The area under
the curve may be calculated using the trapezoidal rule or more elaborate
methods, such as Simpson's rule.

$$V_d = \frac{F G_0}{K \int_0^\infty C \ dt} = \frac{1.0 \times 100}{0.39 \times 27.75} = 9.24 \text{ liters}$$

Step 7. Equation (74) allows calculation of time to peak t_p:

$$t_p = \frac{2.303}{0.85 - 0.39} \log \frac{0.85}{0.39} = 1.7 \text{ hr}$$

See Figure 97 for a visual estimation of t_p in comparison with the calculated value, 1.7 hr.

Step 8. Equation (75) provides an expression for calculating maximum
plasma concentration on the time curve:

$$C_{max} = \frac{0.85 \times 1 \times 100}{9.24 \ (0.85 - 0.39)} (e^{-0.39 \times 1.8} - e^{-0.85 \times 1.7})$$

$$= 5.59 \ \mu g \ ml^{-1}$$

B. One-Compartment Model: Multiple Dosing

The implications and mathematical analysis of multiple-dosing pharmacokinetics on dosage form design have been extensively reviewed by Krüger-
Thiemer and others [401–406]. Both Wagner [407,408] and Gibaldi and
Perrier [409] describe multiple dosing in some detail, and readers will
profit by familiarizing themselves with these sources and the original literature that is referred to in these books. The treatment of this section
on multiple dosing follows the outline of Gibaldi and Perrier [409], and
ends with sample calculations that hopefully provide the reader with a
better understanding of the somewhat complex equations used to describe
multiple dosing. Although the discussion of pharmacokinetics up to this
point has centered on the administration of a single dose of drug, the most
common therapy involves a practice of multiple dosing with the purpose of
reaching and maintaining a desired therapeutic blood concentration over an
extended period of time.

In treating an acute headache, a single dose of aspirin may be given.
For producing sleep, a single dose of sedative is usually effective. But
for mild arthritis, aspirin tablets may be given every 4 hr over a period
of days. For effective antibacterial action, antibotics are ordinarily taken
according to a prescribed dosage regimen for perhaps 10 days or longer.
In the case of onycomycosis, griseofulvin is recommended to be taken for
as long as 6 months to a year, until the infected toe or fingernail shows
no more presence of the infecting organism.

Figures 93 and 97 show the rise and fall in drug blood level curves
for single dosing from time of administration until the concentration of
drug in the body can no longer be determined. As previously indicated,
the area under the concentration-time curve provides an important means
for estimating the relative bioavailability of a drug administered in various
drug delivery systems.

When a dose of drug is repeated at definite time intervals, the therapeutic regimen is referred to as multiple dosing. Such a sequence of
dosing is shown in Figures 99 and 100. It is observed that following the
first dose, the blood level of the second dose adds on to the blood level
remaining from the first dose. Each new dose elevates the blood level
more because it is added to drug concentration remaining from previous
doses. The succession of blood level curves have the shape of the single-
dose curves. Each curve begins at the time a new dose is administered,
rises to a maximum or peak value C_{max}, and then falls as drug is excreted and each dose is exhausted. In the meantime, at a definite dosing
time interval τ, a new dose is administered and another concentration-time
curve rises through a peak value and falls to zero.

As observed in Figures 99 and 100, a program of multiple dosing results in both a C_{max} and a C_{min}, and eventually a steady-state plateau is
reached where C_{max} and C_{min} no longer change in value with the administration of successive doses. By following the increases in blood level
as each new dose is added to the figures, readers can satisfy themselves
that the plateau is reached when the first dose is essentially eliminated
from the body. Actually, the single-dose value approaches zero asymptot-
ically, and complete elimination is never reached. However, 97% of the
plateau value is attained in a period of five half-lives, and 99% is attained
after seven half-lives. For a drug with $t_{1/2}$ = 5 hr, the plateau is therefore reached in 25 to 35 hr.

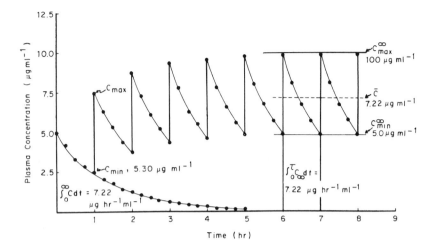

Figure 99 One-compartment model of multiple-dose intravenous administration of equal doses of a drug at a uniform time interval τ.

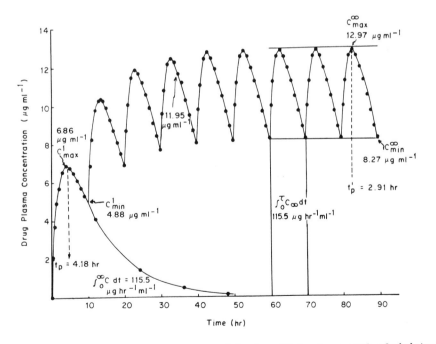

Figure 100 One-compartment model of multiple-dose oral administration of equal doses of a drug at a uniform time interval τ.

Multiple Dosing by Intravenous Administration

Benet introduced a method by which multiple-dose equations can be readily obtained [392]. He has shown that any equation describing the time course of a drug leaving a compartment after a single dose may be changed into a multiple-dose equation by multiplying each exponential term containing t (time)(i.e., $e^{-k_i t}$) by the function

$$\frac{e^{(n-1)k_i \tau} - e^{-k_i \tau}}{1 - e^{k_i \tau}} \tag{77}$$

where τ is the dosing interval, k_i the apparent first-order rate constant in each exponential term, and n is equal to the number of doses.

Based on these considerations, Eq. (45) can be converted to the following multiple-dose equation:

$$A \left(\frac{1 - e^{-nK\tau}}{1 - e^{-K\tau}} \right) = A_0 \left(\frac{1 - e^{-nK\tau}}{1 - e^{-K\tau}} \right) e^{-Kt} = A_n \tag{78}$$

which in concentration terms becomes

$$C_n = \frac{A_0}{V_d} \left(\frac{1 - e^{-nK\tau}}{1 - e^{-K\tau}} \right) e^{-Kt} \tag{79}$$

where t is the time elapsed since dose n was administered. Equation (79) allows the calculation of the drug plasma concentration at any point in time during a dosing interval. It can be seen from this equation that the plasma concentration increases with time and approaches a steady-state level. After multiple dosing for a time equal to seven half-lives, the plasma concentration is within 1% of the steady-state level or plateau level.

To obtain the plasma concentration at steady state, Eq. (79) can be used. By setting n to infinity we obtained C_∞, which is the plasma concentration as a function of time at steady state.

$$C_\infty = \frac{A_0}{V_d} \left(\frac{1}{1 - e^{-K\tau}} \right) e^{-Kt} \tag{80}$$

Similarly, the minimum plasma concentration C_{min} at steady state can be expressed as

$$C_{min}^\infty = \frac{A_0}{V_d} \left(\frac{1}{1 - e^{-K\tau}} \right) e^{-K\tau} \tag{81}$$

and the maximum plasma concentration at steady state becomes

$$C_{max}^\infty = \frac{A_0}{V_d} \left(\frac{1}{1 - e^{-K\tau}} \right) \tag{82}$$

The "average" concentration of drug at steady state $\overline{C}_\infty$ is frequently referred to in the literature of multiple dosing:

$$\overline{C}_\infty = \frac{\int_0^\tau C_\infty \, dt}{\tau} \qquad (83)$$

In Eq. (83), $\int_0^\tau C_\infty \, dt$ is the area under the curve at steady state during a dosing interval (see Fig. 99 for a graphical depiction of this area) and is not a true average value of C_{max}^∞ and C_{min}^∞. The area under the curve may be obtained from the Simpson or trapezoidal rule or calculated from the expression

$$\int_0^\tau C_\infty \, dt = \frac{A_0}{V_d K} \qquad (84)$$

Substituting Eq. (84) into (83) yields

$$\overline{C}_\infty = \frac{A_0}{V_d K} \frac{1}{\tau} \qquad (85)$$

Krüger-Thiemer and Bunger [403] have extensively discussed the concept of loading dose when drugs are administered repetitively. If a drug has a long half-life, considerable time may be required before the plateau blood level is reached. This delay may be circumvented by use of a loading dose. The loading dose A_0^* is estimated using the equation

$$A_0^* = A_0 \left(\frac{1}{1 - e^{-K\tau}} \right) \qquad (86)$$

where A_0 is the maintenance dose. This equation applies when the drug is administered intravenously and confers one-compartment model characteristics on the body. A practical example of this equation has been illustrated by Krüger-Thiemer et al. [410].

It is interesting to note that if the half-life ($0.693/K$) of the drug is equal to the dosing interval τ, then Eq. (86) becomes

$$A_0^* = 2A_0 \qquad (87)$$

which indicates that the loading dose is twice the maintenance dose.

Example 4   Sample Calculation of Pharmacokinetic Parameters Following Multiple Intravenous Administration of a Drug That Is Represented by a One-Compartment Model

---

A subject was administered 50 mg of a drug solution intravenously every hour for a period of 9 hr and plasma concentrations of drug were obtained as a function of time. The results are illustrated in Figure 99. Two weeks prior to this treatment the subject received a single intravenous dose of 50 mg of the drug solution. The elimination half-life of the drug, the area under the plasma concentration-time curve, and the volume of distribution were found from the single-dose study to be 1 hr, 7.22 µg hr^{-1} ml^{-1}, and 10 liters, respectively. Assuming that there was no change in renal and metabolic function of the subject, when multiple dosing was conducted, calculate (a) the elimination rate constant K, (b) the plasma concentration of drug 0.5 hr after the second dose, (c) the minimum, C_{min}^{∞} and maximum, C_{max}^{∞} concentration of drug at steady state, (d) the average concentration of drug at steady state $\overline{C}$, and (e) the loading dose required to produce an immediate steady-state plasma level of the drug. The area under the plasma concentration-time curve during the 6- to 7-hr dosing interval was found to be 7.22 µg ml^{-1} hr^{-1}. Assume the steady state was achieved after seven doses.

Solution:

Step 1. The elimination-rate constant can be calculated by using Eq. (83). Thus,

$$K = \frac{0.693}{t_{1/2}} = \frac{0.693}{1.0} = 0.693 \text{ hr}^{-1}$$

Step 2. The plasma concentration of drug 0.5 hr after the second dose can be calculated using Eq. (79). In this case, τ, the dosing interval, is equal to 1 hr. Thus,

$$C = \frac{50}{10} \left(\frac{1 - e^{-2 \times 0.693 \times 1.0}}{1 - e^{-0.693 \times 1.0}} \right) e^{-0.693 \times 0.5}$$

$$= 5.30 \text{ µg ml}^{-1}$$

Compare with Figure 99 at 1.5 hr.

Step 3. The minimum C_{min} and maximum C_{max} drug plasma concentrations at steady state can be calculated from Eqs. (81) and (82), respectively. Thus

$$C_{min}^{\infty} = \frac{50}{10} \left(\frac{1}{1 - e^{-0.693 \times 1.0}} \right) e^{-0.693 \times 1.0} = 5.0 \text{ µg ml}^{-1}$$

and

$$C_{max}^{\infty} = \frac{50}{10} \left(\frac{1}{1 - e^{-0.693 \times 1.0}} \right) = 10.0 \text{ µg ml}^{-1}$$

Compare with Figure 99.

Step 4. The average concentration of drug at steady state $\overline{C}$ can be calculated from Eq. (83) or (85). Thus,

$$\overline{C} = \frac{7.22}{1.0} = 7.22 \ \mu g \ ml^{-1}$$

or

$$\overline{C} = \frac{1}{10 \times 0.693 \times 1.0} = 7.22 \ \mu^{-1}$$

Compare with Figure 99.

Step 5. Equation (86) allows the calculation of the loading dose. Thus,

$$A_0^* = 50 \ \frac{1}{1 - e^{-0.693 \times 1.0}} = 100 \ mg$$

In this particular case, $t_{1/2}$ is equal to τ. Thus, Eq. (87) can be employed and the result is

$$A_0^* = 2 \times 50 = 100 \ mg$$

Multiple Dosing with First-Order Absorption
(Oral Dosing)

The scheme in Sec. IV.A may be used to estimate drug plasma levels following multiple oral dosing (usually representing first-order absorption) and assuming a one-compartment model. Applying the method developed by Benet [392], it can be shown that the result of multiplying each exponential term in Eq. (64) containing t (time) (that is, $e^{-k_i t}$ 0 by the function given in Eq. (8) will yield an equation for calculating multiple oral dosing.

$$C_n = \frac{k_a F G_0}{V_d(k_a - K)} \left[\left(\frac{1 - e^{-nK\tau}}{1 - e^{-K\tau}} \right) e^{-Kt} - \left(\frac{1 - e^{-nk_a\tau}}{1 - e^{-k_a\tau}} \right) e^{-k_a t} \right] \tag{88}$$

Equation (92) is employed to predict the drug plasma concentration at any time during a dosing interval (e.g., the concentration C_3 following the third dose of a drug). The terms of Eq. (92) have the same meaning here as in earlier equations in this section.

The terms $e^{-nk_a\tau}$ and $e^{-nK\tau}$ will tend to zero as the number of doses increase. This leads to Eq. (93), which describes the drug plasma concentration C_∞ as a function of time at steady state:

$$C_\infty = \frac{k_a F G_0}{V_d(k_a - K)} \left[\left(\frac{1}{1 - e^{-K\tau}} \right) e^{-Kt} - \left(\frac{1}{1 - e^{-k_a\tau}} \right) e^{-k_a t} \right] \tag{89}$$

The average plasma concentration at steady state $\overline{C}_\infty$ is given by an equation analogous to that for intravenous multiple dosing. It can be seen from Eq. (90) that $\overline{C}_\infty$ depends on the fraction of the dose absorbed, the magnitude of the dose given, the volume of distribution, the elimination-rate constant, and the dosing interval:

$$\overline{C}_\infty = \frac{FG_0}{V_d K \tau} \tag{90}$$

The area under the plasma concentration-time curve for time zero to infinity following single oral administration is equal to the area under the curve during a dosing interval at steady state. Consequently,

$$\int_0^\infty D \ dt = \int_0^\infty C_\infty \ dt \tag{91}$$

Now, integration of Eq. (89) from 0 to τ yields the expression

$$\int_0^\tau C \ dt = \frac{FG_0}{V_d K} \tag{92}$$

Combining Eqs. (90) and (92), we obtain

$$\overline{C}_\infty = \frac{\int_0^\tau C \ dt}{\tau} \tag{93}$$

Equation (93) allows the calculation of the average plasma concentration of drug at steady state. This equation is useful because it does not require knowledge of the volume of distribution, V_d, or the fraction, F, of the dose absorbed.

Time for Maximum Drug Plasma Concentration

Assuming that F remains constant during the multiple-dosing regimen, the time t_p', at which the maximum drug plasma concentration at steady state occurs, can be expressed by

$$t_p' = \frac{1}{(k_a - K)} \ln \frac{k_a(1 - e^{-K\tau})}{k(1 - e^{-k_a \tau})} \tag{94}$$

The knowledge of t_p' allows the calculation of the maximum plasma concentration at steady state C_{max}. It is shown by Gibaldi and Perrier [409] that

$$C_{max}^\infty = \frac{FG_0}{V_d} \left(\frac{1}{1 - e^{-K\tau}} \right) e^{-Kt_p'} \tag{95}$$

Similarly, by setting t equal to τ in Eq. (89), the following equation for the minimum plasma concentration C_{min} at steady state results:

$$C_{min}^{\infty} = \frac{k_a FG_0}{V_d(k_a - K)} \left[\left(\frac{1}{1 - e^{-K\tau}}\right) e^{-K\tau} - \left(\frac{1}{1 - e^{-k_a\tau}}\right) e^{-k_a\tau} \right] \qquad (96)$$

The maximum drug plasma concentration after the first dose is given by the equation

$$C_{max}^{1} = \frac{FG_0}{V_d} e^{-Kt_p} \qquad (97)$$

where t_p is the time for appearance of maximum plasma concentration of drug after the first dose. The time t_p is given by the expression

$$t_p = \frac{1}{k_a - K} \ln \frac{k_a}{K} \qquad (98)$$

Similarly, the minimum plasma drug concentration after the first dose is given by

$$C_{min}^{1} = \frac{k_a FG_0}{V_d(k_a - K)} (e^{-K\tau} - e^{-k_a\tau}) \qquad (99)$$

The loading dose, A_0^*, following first-order input (oral or intramuscular dosing, for example) is calculated using the expression

$$A_0^* = A_0 \frac{1}{1 - e^{-K\tau}} \qquad (100)$$

which is identical to Eq. (86) for intravenous administration if the maintenance dose A_0 is administered in the postabsorptive period.

Example 5   Sample Calculation of Pharmacokinetic Parameters Following Multiple Oral Administration of a Drug That Is Represented by a One-Compartment Model

A subject was administered a tablet dosage form containing 100 mg of a drug every 10 hr for a period of 100 hr. Plasma concentration of drug was obtained as a function of time. The results are illustrated in Figure 100. Two weeks prior to this treatment the subject received a single oral dosage of the dosage form, and after performing a Wagner–Nelson calculation, the absorption-rate constant k_a, the elimination half-life of the drug, the area under the curve from time zero to infinity, and the volume of distributioo were found to be 0.5 hr^{-1}, 7.7 hr, 115.5 μg ml^{-1} hr^{-1}, and 10 liters, respectively. Calculate (a) the elimination-rate constant K, (b) the plasma concentration of drug 5 hr after the fourth dose, (c) the minimum C_{min}^1, and maximum C_{max}^1 drug plasma concentration after the first dose, (d) the minimum C_{max}^∞ drug plasma concentration at steady state, (e) the average drug concentration of steady state, and (f) an estimation of a loading dose assuming that the maintenance dose is equal to 100 mg and is administered in the postabsorptive phase. Assume that the fraction of drug absorbed F is equal to 1.0.

Solution:

Step 1. The elimination-rate constant can be calculated by using Eq. (41). Thus,

$$K = \frac{0.693}{t_{1/2}} = \frac{0.693}{7.7} = 0.09 \text{ hr}^{-1}$$

Step 2. The plasma concentration of drug 5 hr after the fourth dose can be calculated using Eq. (88). In this case, τ, the dosing interval, is 10 hr. Thus,

$$C = \frac{0.5 \times 1 \times 100}{10(0.5 - 0.09)} \left[\left(\frac{1 - e^{-4 \times 0.09 \times 10}}{1 - e^{-0.09 \times 10}} \right) e^{-0.09 \times 5} \right.$$

$$\left. - \left(\frac{1 - e^{-4 \times 0.5 \times 10}}{1 - e^{-0.5 \times 10}} \right) e^{-0.5 \times 5} \right] = 11.95 \text{ µg ml}^{-1}$$

See Figure 100 for comparison of the results.

Step 3. The minimum concentration of drug C_{min}^1 after the first dose can be calculated using Eq. (99). Thus,

$$C_{min}^1 = \frac{0.5 \times 1 \times 100}{10(0.5 - 0.09)} (e^{-0.09 \times 10} - e^{-0.5 \times 10})$$

$$= 4.88 \text{ µg ml}^{-1}$$

The maximum drug plasma concentration C_{max}^1 is given by Eq. (97). However, if it is necessary to calculate the time to peak t_p after the first dose, t_p is given by Eq. (98). Consequently,

$$t_p = \frac{1}{0.5 - 0.09} \ln \frac{0.5}{0.09} = 4.18 \text{ hr}$$

and

$$C_{max}^1 = \frac{1 \times 100}{10} e^{-0.09 \times 4.18} = 6.86 \text{ µg ml}^{-1}$$

See Figure 100 for comparison of results.

Step 4. The minimum drug plasma concentration C_{min}^{∞} at steady state can be calculated using Eq. (95). Thus,

$$C_{min}^{\infty} = \frac{0.5 \times 1 \times 100}{10(0\cancel{\times}5 - 0.09)} \left[\left(\frac{1}{1 - e^{-0.09 \times 10}} \right) e^{-0.09 \times 10} \right.$$

$$\left. - \left(\frac{1}{1 - e^{-0.5 \times 10}} \right) e^{-0.5 \times 10} \right] = 8.27 \ \mu g \ ml^{-1}$$

See Figure 100 for comparison of results.

The maximum drug concentration C_{max}^{∞} at steady state can be calculated using Eq. (95). However, use of this equation requires knowledge of the time to peak t_p', which is given by Eq. (94). Thus,

$$t_p' = \frac{1}{0.5 - 0.09} \ln \frac{0.5(1 - e^{-0.09 \times 10})}{0.09(1 - e^{-0.5 \times 10})} = 2.91 \ hr$$

Consequently,

$$C_{max}^{\infty} = \frac{1 \times 100}{10} \left(\frac{1}{1 - e^{-0.09 \times 10}} \right) e^{-0.09 \times 2.91} = 12.97 \ \mu g \ ml^{-1}$$

See Figure 100 for comparison of results.

Step 5. An estimate of a loading dose can be obtained using Eq. (100). Thus,

$$A_0^* = 100 \times \frac{1}{1 - e^{-0.09 \times 10}} = 169 \ mg$$

C. Two-Compartment Model: Single Dosing

In the beginning of Sec. IV it was observed that drugs distribute throughout the body, and this fact prompted investigators to develop a more complex mathematical model, including a central and at least one peripheral compartment. The two-compartment model is sufficiently realistic when viewed on a physiological basis, and it is perhaps mathematically more acceptable than a one-compartment model. However, when calculations using a one-compartment model yield results that correspond satisfactorily with the experimental data, the more complex two-compartment model need not be employed.

Intravenous Injection (Single Dose)

The two-compartment model, with bolus intravenous injection and with elimination occurring from the central compartment, can be represented by the scheme, where k_{12} is the first-order rate constant for transfer of drug from compartment 1 to compartment 2, k_{21} the first-order rate constant for

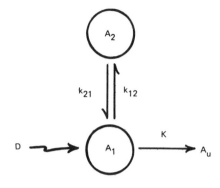

transfer of drug from compartment 2 to compartment 1, K the overall
first-order rate constant for elimination of drug by all processes from compartment 1, A_1 the amount of drug in compartment 1 at time t, and A_2 the
amount of drug in compartment 2 at time t. D is the amount of drug representing the intravenous dose, and A_u is the amount of drug in the
urine. The rate of change in amount of drug in compartment 1 can be
described by the following differential equation:

$$\frac{dA_1}{dt} = k_{21}A_2 - k_{12}A_1 - KA_1 \tag{101}$$

A second equation may be written to describe the rate of change of the
amount of drug in the second compartment:

$$\frac{dA_2}{dt} = k_{12}A_1 - k_{21}A_2 \tag{102}$$

Integration of Eqs. (101) and (102) leads to

$$A_1 = \frac{D(\alpha - k_{21})}{\alpha - \beta} e^{-\alpha t} + \frac{D(k_{21} - \beta)}{\alpha - \beta} e^{-\beta t} \tag{103}$$

which is referred to as a biexponential equation because of the two terms
containing exponents. Equation (103) describes the amount of drug in
compartment 1 as a function of time. In this equation, D is the intravenous dose and thus the amount of drug in compartment 1 at t equals
zero; the quantities α and β are hybrid rate constants:

$$\alpha = \frac{1}{2}\left[(k_{12} + k_{21} + K) + \sqrt{(k_{12} + K_{21} + K)^2 - 4k_{21}K} \right] \tag{104}$$

$$\beta = \frac{1}{2}\left[(k_{12} + k_{21} + K) - \sqrt{(k_{12} + k_{21} + K)^2 - 4k_{21}K} \right]$$

and

$$\alpha \cdot \beta = k_{21}K \tag{105}$$

$$\alpha \cdot \beta = k_{12} + k_{21} + K \tag{106}$$

The integrated equation describing the amount of drug A_2 in compartment 2 as a function of time can be described by

$$A_2 = \frac{k_{12}De^{-\beta t}}{\alpha - \beta} - \frac{k_{21}De^{-\alpha t}}{\alpha - \beta} \tag{107}$$

or

$$A_2 = \frac{k_{12}D}{\alpha - \beta} - (e^{-\beta} - e^{-\alpha t})$$

A linear relationship exists between the drug concentration in the plasma C and the amount of drug in compartment 1; that is,

$$A_1 = V_1C \tag{108}$$

where V_1 is the apparent volume of compartment 1. Equation (108) enables the conversion of Eq. (103) from amount to concentration,

$$C = \frac{D(\alpha - k_{21})}{V_1(\alpha - \beta)} e^{-\alpha t} + \frac{D(k_{21} - \beta)}{V_1(\alpha - \beta)} e^{-\beta t} \tag{109}$$

and

$$C = Pe^{-\alpha t} + Qe^{-\beta t} \tag{110}$$

where the coefficients P and Q of these biexponential equations are defined by the expressions

$$P = \frac{D(\alpha - k_{21})}{(\alpha - \beta)V_1} \tag{111}$$

and

$$Q = \frac{D(k_{21} - \beta)}{(\alpha - \beta)V_1} \tag{112}$$

If the logarithm of plasma concentration of drug is plotted against the time t, following Eq. (110), a biexponential curve is obtained (see Fig. 101). The curve is referred to as biexponential because it can be factored into two curves by a technique called "feathering" or "stripping." The terminal linear segment of the biexponential curve is extrapolated to time t = 0, and is shown in Figure 101 as a dashed line. The data are feathered or stripped by subtracting each drug concentration value on the extrapolated dashed portion of the biexponential curve from the

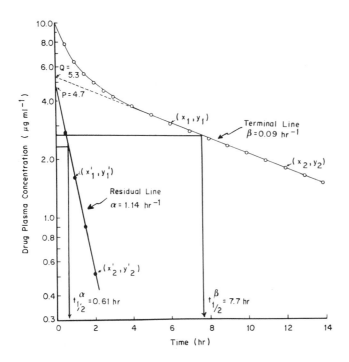

Figure 101 Semilogarithmic plot of the concentration of drug in the blood plasma following single intravenous administration of a drug represented by a two-compartment model.

experimental points above it on the curved part of the biexponential line at the particular time (see Example 6). As observed in Figure 101, the $Pe^{-\alpha t}$ curve will approach zero and $Qe^{-\beta t}$ will retain a finite value. When $e^{-\alpha t}$ has approached closely to zero, this period is referred to as the postdistributive phase. At this point Eq. (110) reduces to

$$P = Qe^{-\beta t} \qquad\qquad (113)$$

or in logarithmic form,

$$\log P = \log Q - \frac{\beta t}{2.303} \qquad\qquad (114)$$

To summarize, one begins the analysis in the case of a two-compartment model by plotting the results on semilogarithmic graph paper, feathering the data so as to obtain two curves, then calculating β using Eq. (114), corresponding to the terminal part of the biexponential curve. Q, the coefficient for the β exponential term of Eq. (113), is obtained from the extrapolation value [see Eq. (114)], where the dashed line crosses the vertical axis at t = 0. The value of α is obtained from the slope of the linear segment resulting from a plot of the residuals, and the P value is found where this line crosses the vertical axis at zero time.

The half-lives for the α and β phases are obtained in the ordinary manner, employing the equations

$$t^{\alpha}_{1/2} = \frac{0.693}{\alpha} \tag{115}$$

$$t^{\beta}_{1/2} = \frac{0.693}{\beta} \tag{116}$$

It should be noted that β is not an elimination-rate constant, but rather depends both on elimination and distribution of the drug according to the expression

$$\beta = fK \tag{117}$$

where f, the fraction of drug in the central compartment in the postdistributive phase, is

$$f = \frac{k_{21} - \beta}{k_{21} + k_{21} - \beta} \tag{118}$$

Thus, β is smaller than the elimination-rate constant K, being K multiplied by a fractional quantity f. The quantity K is the rate constant for elimination from the central compartment and β is the elimination constant for the body. The quantity $t^{\beta}_{1/2}$ gives the biological half-life.

If f is unity or near to a value of 1.0, the drug is present almost totally in the central compartment, and a one-compartment model will describe its kinetics. In this case, β simply becomes the elimination-rate constant K. Currently, computer programs are available to fit and feather the data shown in Figure 101 and to give the constants α , β, P, and Q and the half-lives. The computer can also be programmed to calculate and print the values for k_{12}, k_{21}, and K, as well as V_1, the apparent volume of the central compartment.

Example 6   Sample Calculation of Pharmacokinetic Parameters Following Single Intravenous Administration of a Drug Represented by a Two-Compartment Model

---

A subject received a single intravenous dose of a drug solution containing 100 mg of drug. The drug plasma concentration was obtained as a function of time. The results are illustrated in Table 23. Calculate (a) the values for α and β, and (b) the half-life for the distributive phase α and the elimination phase β. (c) Write an equation that will give the concentration of drug C as a function of time and calculate the concentration of drug 9.5 hr after administration. Calculate (d) the volume of distribution of the central compartment V_1; (e) the fraction of drug in the central compartment in the postdistributive phase; (f) the values of k_{12}, k_{21}, and K; and (g) the area under the plasma concentration-time curve. Assume that the drug plasma levels are represented by a two-compartment model.

Table 23   Time Data Obtained
Following Intravenous Administration
of a Drug

Time (hr)	Drug plasma concentration ($\mu g\ ml^{-1}$)
0.5	7.78
1.0	6.40
1.5	5.51
2.0	4.91
2.5	4.89
3.0	4.17
4.0	3.70
5.0	3.35
6.0	3.05
8.0	2.54
10.0	2.12
12.0	1.77
14.0	1.48

Solution:

Step 1.   Plot the data in semilogarithmic graph paper.   Figure 101 illustrates the graphical representation of the data (open circles).

Step 2.   To calculate the value for the elimination phase β, extrapolate the terminal linear segment of the biexponential to time zero.   According to Eq. (114), the slope of this line is equal to $-\beta 2.303$.   For practical purposes, the points (x_1, y_1) and (x_2, y_2) in the graph will be used to estimate the slope.   However, it should be noted that the best way to obtain the slope is by using linear regression analysis.

$$\text{Slope} = \frac{\log y_2 - \log y_1}{x_2 - x_1} = \frac{\log 3.05 - \log 1.77}{6 - 12} = 0.0394$$

Thus,

$$\beta = -(-0.0394 \times 2.303) = 0.09\ hr^{-1}$$

In order to calculate the value for the distributive phase α, the method of residuals is employed.   The residual values are obtained by subtracting from the true plasma concentration values in the distributive phase the corresponding drug concentration values on the extrapolated line (dashed

Table 24 Residual Values Plasma Concentration-Time Data
Following Single Intravenous Administration

Time (hr)	Drug concentration ($\mu g \ ml^{-1}$)	Extrapolated concentration ($\mu g \ ml^{-1}$)	Residual concentration ($\mu g \ ml^{-1}$)
0.5	7.18	5.01	2.77
1.0	6.40	4.80	1.60
1.5	5.51	4.61	0.90
2.0	4.91	4.40	0.51

line, see Fig. 101). Table 24 illustrates the results. On the same sheet of graph paper, plot the residual values (solid circles, Fig. 101). Calculate the slope of this line using the points (x_1', x_1') and (x_2', x_2').

$$\text{Slope} = \frac{\log y_2' - \log y_2'}{x_2' - x_1'} = \frac{\log 0.51 - \log 1.60}{2 - 1} = -0.497$$

Thus,

$$\alpha = -(\text{slope} \times 2.303) = -(-0.497 \times 2.303) = 1.14 \ hr^{-1}$$

Step 3. To calculate the half-life for the α phase $t_{1/2}^{\alpha}$ and the half-life for the β phase, $t_{1/2}^{\beta}$, Eqs. (115) and (116) are used. Thus,

$$t_{1/2}^{\alpha} = \frac{0.693}{1.14} = 0.61 \ hr$$

and

$$t_{1/2}^{\beta} = \frac{0.693}{0.09} = 7.70 \ hr$$

The half-lives can also be obtained from the graphical representation of the data. The extrapolated line (dashed line, Fig. 101) crosses the y axis at time zero at 5.3 $\mu g \ ml^{-1}$ (Q), and the residual line at 4.7 $\mu g \ ml^{-1}$ (P). Using the half-life definition, at a drug concentration of 5.3/2, the half-life for the β phase is 7.7 hr, and at a drug concentration .47/2, the half-life for the α phase is approximately 0.6 hr.

Step 4. The equation describing the plasma concentration of drug as a function of time is given by

$$C = Pe^{-\alpha t} + Qe^{-\beta t}$$

The values for α and β have been calculated in steps 2 and 3. P and Q are the y intercepts of the residual line and terminal line at $t = 0$, respectively (see Fig. 101). Thus,

$$C = 4.7e^{-1.14t} + 5.3e^{-0.09t}$$

Therefore, the concentration of drug 9.5 hr postadministration will be

$$C = 4.7e^{-1.14 \times 9.5} + 5.3e^{-0.09 \times 9.5} = 2.25 \; \mu g \; ml^{-1}$$

See Figure 101 for comparison of the calculated result 2.25 $\mu g \; ml^{-1}$ with that read from the graph.

Step 5. The value of the central compartment V_1 can be estimated from Eq. (110). At time $t = 0$, Eq. (110) reduces to

$$C_0 = P + Q = 4.7 + 5.3 = 10.0$$

and

$$V_1 = \frac{dose}{C_0} = \frac{100,000 \; g \; ml^{-1}}{10 \; g \; ml^{-1}} = 10,000 \; ml \qquad or \qquad 10 \; liters$$

Step 6. To calculate k_{12}, k_{21}, and K, start by calculating k_{21} from Eq. (111) or (112). Thus,

$$k_{21} = \alpha - \frac{P(\alpha - \beta)V_1}{D}$$

$$= 1.14 - \frac{4.7(1.14 - 0.09)10,000}{100,000} = 0.6 \; hr^{-1}$$

or

$$k_{21} = \frac{Q(\alpha - \beta)V_1}{D} + \beta$$

$$= \frac{5.3(1.14 - 0.09)10,000}{100,000} + 0.09 = 0.6 \; hr^{-1}$$

To calculate the elimination-rate constant K, Eq. (105) is used. Thus

$$K = \frac{\alpha \cdot \beta}{k_{21}} = \frac{1.14 \times 0.09}{0.65} = 0.16 \; hr^{-1}$$

And finally, k_{12} can be calculated using Eq. (106). Thus

$$k_{12} = 0.09 + 1.14 - 0.16 - 0.6 = 0.4 \; hr^{-1}$$

Step 7. The fraction of drug in the central compartment in the post-distributive phase can be obtained using Eq. (117) or (118):

$$f - \frac{\beta}{K} = \frac{0.09}{0.16} = 0.56$$

or

$$f = \frac{0.6 - 0.09}{0.6 + 0.4 - 0.09} = 0.56$$

In this case f_1 is not unity, and consequently the data cannot be described by a one-compartment model. In addition, it should be remembered that β is smaller than K, and consequently the biological half-life is given by β while the elimination of drug from the central compartment is given by K.

Step 8. The area under the plasma concentration-time curve can be obtained by integrating Eq. (110) from time zero to infinity. Thus,

$$\text{area} = \int_0^\infty C \, dt = \frac{P}{\alpha} + \frac{Q}{\beta} = \frac{4.7}{1.14} + \frac{5.3}{0.09} = 63.0 \ \mu g \ ml^{-1} \ hr^{-1}$$

Urinary Excretion

A drug following the two-compartment model may be subjected to urinary excretion analysis in order to obtain the pharmacokinetic parameters that were described in Sec. IV.C.

According to the following scheme

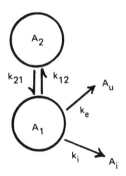

where A_u is the unchanged drug amount eliminated in the urine; A_i the amount of drug in its various forms eliminated by other excretion pathways, such as salivary and biliary; and k_e and k_i are the respective first-order elimination-rate constants. Thus,

$$K = k_e + k_i \tag{119}$$

The rate of excretion of unchanged drug according to the foregoing scheme is given by

$$\frac{dA_u}{dt} = k_e A_1 \tag{120}$$

where A_1, the amount of drug in the central compartment, is given by Eq. (103). Substitution of this equation into Eq. (121) leads to

$$\frac{dA_u}{dt} = \frac{k_e D(\alpha - k_{21})}{(\alpha - \beta)} e^{-\alpha t} + \frac{k_e D(k_{21} - \beta)}{(\alpha - \beta)} e^{-\beta t} \tag{121}$$

which can be simplified to

$$\frac{dA_u}{dt} = P'e^{-\alpha t} + Q'e^{-\beta t} \tag{122}$$

where

$$P' = \frac{k_e D(\alpha - k_{21})}{(\alpha - \beta)} \tag{123}$$

and

$$Q' = \frac{k_e D(k_{21} - \beta)}{(\alpha - \beta)} \tag{124}$$

If the logarithm of the excretion rate dA_u/dt is plotted versus time, a biexponential curve will result. This is illustrated in Figure 102. Using the "method of residuals" or "feathering," the biexponential curve can be broken into two lines. The slope of the terminal line is equal to $-\beta/2.303$ and the slope of the residual line is equal to $-\alpha/2.303$. The respective y intercept at time $t = 0$ are P' and Q'. Gibaldi and Perrier [411] have shown that the elimination-rate constant, k_e, can be calculated using the expression

$$k_e = \frac{P' + Q'}{D} \tag{125}$$

Similarly,

$$k_{21} = \frac{P'\beta + Q'\alpha}{P' + Q'} \tag{126}$$

K and K_{12} can be calculated from Eqs. (105) and (106).

Another approach to calculate the pharmacokinetic parameters from urinary excretion data is the sigma-minus method. This method requires knowledge of the total amount of unchanged drug excreted to time infinity (see Sec. IV.I).

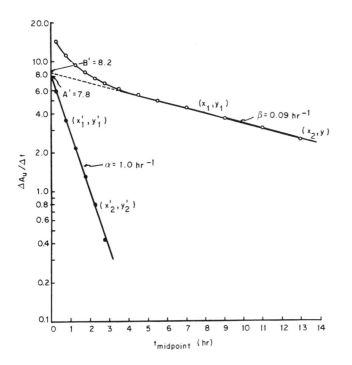

Figure 102 Log rate plot relating to data for the urinary excretion of a drug following intravenous bolus injection. The drug is represented by a two-compartment model.

Example 7 Sample Calculation of Pharmacokinetic Parameters Following Intravenous Bolus Injection of a Drug Represented by a Two-Compartment Model Using Urinary Excretion Data

A subject received an i.v. bolus injection of a solution containing 100 mg of a drug. The cumulative amount of drug in the urine was obtained as a function of time. The results are illustrated in Table 25. Assume that the drug is represented by a two-compartment model. Calculate (1) α, β, P', and Q'; (2) the rate constant k_e for elimination of unchanged drug in the urine; (3) the intercompartmental first-order rate constant k_{21}; and (4) the fraction of unchanged drug excreted in the urine.

Solution:

Step 1. Equation (122) shows that a plot of log $\Delta A_u / \Delta t$ versus t will result in a biexponential curve. The use of this equation requires that log $\Delta A_u / \Delta t$ be plotted against the midpoint of a short urine interval (see Table 25). Figure 102 illustrated the graphical representation of the data (open circles).

Step 2. Extrapolate the terminal linear phase to time zero, where one observes the intercept to be 8.2 mg hr^{-1}. Thus,

$$Q' = \text{intercept} = 8.2 \text{ mg hr}^{-1}$$

Table 25   Urinary Excretion Data After Intravenous Administration of 100 mg of a Drug Solution

Time (hr)	Cumulative amount of drug excreted unchanged (mg)	ΔA_u	Δt	$\Delta A_u / \Delta t$	$t_{midpoint}$
0	0				
0.5	7.04	7.04	0.5	14.08	0.25
1.0	12.68	5.64	0.5	11.28	0.75
1.5	17.42	4.74	0.5	9.48	1.25
2.0	21.57	4.15	0.5	8.30	1.75
2.5	25.32	2.74	0.4	7.50	2.25
3.0	28.78	3.46	0.5	6.92	2.75
4.0	35.06	6.28	1.0	6.28	3.5
5.0	40.68	5.62	1.0	5.62	4.5
6.0	45.79	5.11	1.0	5.11	5.5
8.0	54.70	8.91	2.0	4.46	7.0
10.0	62.14	7.44	2.0	3.72	9.0
12.0	68.36	6.22	2.0	3.11	11.0
14.0	73.56	5.20	2.0	2.60	13.0

Step 3.   Calculate the slope of the terminal linear phase.   The slope of the line is equal to $-\beta/2.303$.   Thus,

$$\text{Slope} = \frac{\log y_2 - \log y_1}{x_2 - x_1} = \frac{\log 2.6 - \log 4.46}{13 - 7} = -0.039$$

$$\beta = -(-0.039 \times 2.303) = 0.09 \text{ hr}^{-1}$$

Step 4.   Using the method of residuals as previously discussed, calculate the residual amounts.   Table 26 illustrates the results.

Step 5.   On the same sheet of graph paper, plot the residual values of column 4, Table 23 (see Fig. 102).   Calculate the slope of this line, which is equal to $-\alpha/2.303$.   It is also observed that the intercept of this line at time zero is 7.8 mg hr^{-1}.   Thus,

$$\text{Slope} = \frac{\log y_2' - \log y_1'}{x_2' - x_1'} = \frac{\log 0.8 - \log 3.58}{2.25 - 0.75} = -0.43$$

$$\alpha = -(-0.43 \times 2.303) = 1.0 \text{ hr}^{-1}$$

Table 26 Residual Values: Unrinary Excretion Following Intravenous Dosing

Time (hr)	$\Delta A_u/\Delta t$ (mg hr^{-1})	Extrapolated $\Delta A_u/\Delta t$	Residual value
0.25	14.08	8.1	5.98
0.75	11.24	7.7	3.58
1.25	9.48	7.3	2.18
1.75	8.30	7.0	1.30
2.25	7.50	6.7	0.80
2.75	6.92	6.5	0.42

and

$$P' = \text{intercept} = 7.8 \text{ mg hr}^{-1}$$

Step 6. The first-order elimination-rate constant for unchanged drug in the urine k_e can be calculated using Eq. (125). Thus,

$$k_e = \frac{7.8 + 8.2}{100 \text{ mg}} = 0.16 \text{ hr}^{-1}$$

Step 7. The intercompartmental rate constant k_{21} can be calculated from Eq. (126). Thus,

$$k_{12} = \alpha + \beta - k_{21} - K = 0.09 + 1.0 - 0.56 - 0.16 = 0.37 \text{ hr}^{-1}$$

Step 8. The fraction of drug excreted unchanged f, is given by the ratio of k_e/K. Thus,

$$f = \frac{k_e}{k} = \frac{0.16}{0.16} = 1.0$$

This indicates that 100% of the administered drug was excreted unchanged and that no metabolism took place.

Oral Dosing (Two-Compartment Model)
with First-Order Absorption

The most practical modality for drug administration is the oral route. A drug is represented by a two-compartment model after oral (assumed to be first-order) absorption is shown in the scheme where k_a is the first-order absorption-rate constant. The terms k_{12}, k_{21}, K, A_1, and A_u have been previously defined. The amount of drug A_1 as a function of time is given by Eq. (127):

$$A_2$$

$$K_{21} \Big\Uparrow K_{12}$$

$$G \xrightarrow{K_a} A_1 \xrightarrow{K} A_u$$

$$A_1 = \frac{k_a F G_0 (k_{21} - k_a)}{(\alpha - k_a)(\beta - k_a)} e^{-k_a t} + \frac{k_a F G_0 (k_{21} - \alpha)}{(k_a - \alpha)(\beta - \alpha)} e^{-\alpha t}$$

$$+ \frac{k_a F G_0 (k_{21} - \beta)}{(k_a - \beta)(\alpha - \beta)} e^{-\beta t} \tag{127}$$

where F is the fraction of the dose G_0 absorbed. The quantities α and β have been previously defined. Equation (127) can be converted to concentration terms using the relationship $A_1 = V_c C$. Thus,

$$C = \frac{k_a F G_0 (k_{21} - k_a)}{V_c (\alpha - k_a)(\beta - k_a)} e^{-k_a t} + \frac{k_a F G_0 (k_{21} - \alpha)}{V_c (k_a - \alpha)(\beta - \alpha)} e^{-\alpha t}$$

$$+ \frac{k_a F G_0 (k_{21} - \beta)}{V_c (k_a - \beta)(\alpha - \beta)} e^{-\beta t} \tag{128}$$

where V_c is the volume of the central compartment. Equation (128) can be replaced to

$$C = n e^{-K_a t} + L e^{-\alpha t} + M e^{-\beta t} \tag{129}$$

where

$$N = \frac{k_a F G_0 (k_{21} - k_a)}{V_c (\alpha - k_a)(\beta - k_a)} \tag{130}$$

$$L = \frac{k_a F G_0 (k_{21} - \alpha)}{V_c (k_a - \alpha)(\beta - \alpha)} \tag{131}$$

$$M = \frac{k_a F G_0 (k_{21} - \beta)}{V_c (k_a - \beta)(\alpha - \beta)} \tag{132}$$

The typical kinetic behavior of a drug represented by a two-compartment model indicates that the terms $e^{-k_a t}$ and $e^{-\alpha t}$ in Eq. (129) tend to zero as time proceeds. Thus, Eq. (129) reduces to

$$C = Me^{-\beta t} \tag{133}$$

or in logarithmic form

$$\log C = \log M - \frac{\beta t}{2.303} \tag{134}$$

According to Eq. (129), a plot of the logarithm of the drug plasma concentration C versus time will result in a triexponential curve, and according to Eq. (134), the terminal linear segment of the line has a slope equal to $-\beta/2.303$. To obtain α and k_a, the method of residuals is used. In this case two residual lines are obtained. The terminal linear segment of the first residual line has a slope equal to $-\alpha/2.303$, and the second residual line has a slope equal to $-k_a/2.303$. In most instances, it is very difficult to obtain α and k_a from the residual lines, and it is advisable that intravenous data be obtained to gain insight into the values of α, β, k_{12}, k_{21}, and K. When α and k_a have values which are close, the triexponential curve will appear more like a biexponential curve, such as the one in Figure 97, obtained following oral administration of a drug that is represented by a one-compartment model. Under normal circumstances the method of Loo and Riegelman (Sec. V.A.) is employed to calculate the rate constant, k_a. It should be remembered that this method requires i.v. data. An example of Loo-Riegelman calculations is given in Sec. V.A.

Integration of Eq. (129) from time zero to infinity will lead to the area under the plasma concentration time curve. This is described by

$$\int_0^\infty C \, dt = \frac{N}{k_a} + \frac{L}{\alpha} + \frac{M}{\beta} \tag{135}$$

The area under the curve is important because it gives an indication of the extent of absorption, as shown in the section on bioabsorption.

The volume of distribution of a drug following oral administration and represented by a one-compartment model is given in Eq. (72). Similarly, the volume of distribution for a drug represented by a two-compartment model is given by Eq. (136).

$$V_d = \frac{FG_0}{\displaystyle\int_0^\infty C \, dt} \tag{136}$$

D. Two-Compartment Model: Multiple Oral Dosing

For a drug given by first-order input, a class in which most oral dosage regimens fall, the drug plasma concentration as a function of time can be readily obtained by multiplying each exponential term in Eq. (129) by the multiple-dosing function developed by Benet [392]. This leads to

$$C_n = N\left(\frac{1 - e^{-nk_a\tau}}{1 - e^{-k_a\tau}}\right)e^{-k_at} + L\left(\frac{1 - e^{-n\alpha\tau}}{1 - e^{-\alpha\tau}}\right)e^{-\alpha t} + M\left(\frac{1 - e^{-n\beta\tau}}{1 - e^{-\beta\tau}}\right)e^{-\beta t}$$

(137)

where N, L, and M have been previously defined. At steady-state levels the terms $e^{-n\alpha\tau}$, $e^{-nk_a\tau}$, and $e^{-n\beta\tau}$ will tend to zero and Eq. (137) reduces to

$$C_\infty = N\left(\frac{1}{1 - e^{-k_a\tau}}\right)e^{-k_at} + L\left(\frac{1}{1 - e^{-\alpha\tau}}\right)e^{-\alpha t} + M\left(\frac{1}{1 - e^{-\beta\tau}}\right)e^{-\beta\tau}$$

(138)

Equation (138) can be used to calculate the drug plasma concentration at any time during a dosing interval at steady state. Integration of Eq. (138) from time zero to infinity will give the area under the curve at steady state.

$$\int_0^\infty C_\infty\, dt = \frac{N}{k_a} + \frac{L}{\alpha} + \frac{M}{\beta}$$

(139)

It can be observed that Eq. (139) is identical to Eq. (135) obtained after single oral administration of a drug represented by a two-compartment model. The average drug plasma concentration at steady state is given by Eqs. (140) and (141).

$$\overline{C}_\infty = \frac{\int_0^\infty C\, dt}{\tau}$$

(140)

or

$$\overline{C}_\infty = \frac{\int_0^\infty C_\infty\, dt}{\tau}$$

(141)

These equations are the same as Eq (93) for a one-compartment model. Consequently,

$$\overline{C}_\infty = \frac{FG_0}{V_d\beta\tau}$$

(142)

Equations (140) to (142) hold as long as elimination of drug occurs only from the central compartment.

The minimum concentration of drug after the first dose can be obtained by setting n equal to unity in Eq. (137). Thus,

$$C_{min}^{1} = Ne^{-k_a t} + Le^{-\alpha t} + Me^{-\beta t} \tag{143}$$

Similarly, by setting n equal to 1 and t equal to τ in Eq. (138), the following equation results for the minimum plasma concentration C_{min}^{∞} at steady state.

$$C_{min}^{\infty} = N\left(\frac{1}{1 - e^{-k_a \tau}}\right)e^{-k_a \tau} + L\left(\frac{1}{1 - e^{-\alpha \tau}}\right)e^{-\alpha \tau} + M\left(\frac{1}{1 - e^{-\beta \tau}}\right)e^{-\beta \tau} \tag{144}$$

The loading dose A_0^* is calculated using the equation

$$A_0^* = A_0\left(\frac{1}{1 - e^{-\beta \tau}}\right) \tag{145}$$

as long as the maintenance dose A_0 is given in the postabsorptive, postdistributive phase of the loading dose.

Example 8 Sample Calculation of Pharmacokinetic Parameters Following Multiple Oral Administration of a Drug That Is Represented by a Two-Compartment Model

A subject received a tablet dosage form containing 100 mg of a drug every 4.5 hr for a period of 45 hr, and drug plasma concentrations were determined as a function of time. The graphical representation of the results is illustrated in Figure 103. Two weeks prior to this treatment the subject received a single oral dose of the tablet dosage form. Pharmacokinetic analysis of the drug plasma levels resulting from the single oral dose indicated that the data can be represented by a two-compartment model. The rate constant for absorption k_a was estimated using the method of Loo and Riegelman (see Sec. V.A) and was found to be 0.8 hr^{-1}. In addition, k_{12}, k_{21}, K, V_c, α, and β were calculated as 0.4 hr^{-1}, 0.6 hr^{-1}, 0.16 hr^{-1}, 10 liters, 1.14 hr^{-1}, and 0.09 hr^{-1}, respectively. The area under the plasma concentration-time curve after the single oral dose was found to be 58.5 μg ml^{-1} hr^{-1}. Assuming that the renal and metabolic functions of the subject remain the same in the multiple- as in the single-dose regimen, calculate (a) the drug plasma concentration 2 hr after the third dose was given, (b) the average drug plasma concentration at steady state, and (c) the drug plasma concentration 0.5 hr after the dose of 100 mg that will be given in the postabsorptive, postdistributive phase of the preceding dose.

Solution:

Step 1. The drug plasma concentration 2 hr after the third dose can be calculated using Eq. (137). However, to use this equation it is necessary to calculate the coefficients N, L, and M, given in Eqs. (130) to (132). Thus,

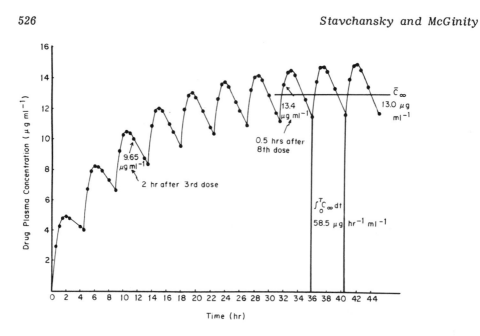

Figure 103 Two-compartment model of multiple-dose oral administration of equal doses of a drug at uniform time interval τ.

$$N = \frac{0.8 \times 1 \times 100(0.6 - 0.8)}{10(1.14 - 0.8)(0.09 - 0.8)} = 6.63 \ \mu g \ ml^{-1}$$

$$L = \frac{0.8 \times 1 \times 100(0.6 - 1.14)}{10(0.8 - 1.14)(0.09 - 1.14)} = 12.10 \ \mu g \ ml^{-1}$$

$$M = \frac{0.8 \times 1 \times 100(0.6 - 0.09)}{10(0.8 - 0.09)(1.14 - 0.09)} = 5.47 \ \mu g \ ml^{-1}$$

The drug concentration is given by

$$C = 6.63 \left(\frac{1 - e^{-3 \times 0.8 \times 4.5}}{1 - e^{-0.8 \times 4.5}} \right) e^{-0.8 \times 2}$$

$$- \ 12.10 \left(\frac{1 - e^{-3 \times 1.14 \times 4.5}}{1 - e^{-1.14 \times 4.5}} \right) e^{-1.14 \times 2}$$

$$+ \ 5.47 \left(\frac{1 - e^{-3 \times 0.09 \times 4.5}}{1 - e^{-0.09 \times 4.5}} \right) e^{-0.09 \times 2} = 9.65 \ \mu g \ ml^{-1}$$

See Figure 103 for comparison of results for drug plasma concentration 2 hr after administration of the third dose.

Step 2. The average plasma concentration at steady state $\overline{C}_\infty$ can be calculated using Eq. (141). However, knowledge of the area under the curve during a dosing interval at steady state is necessary. The area can be obtained using Eq. (139):

$$\int_0^\tau C \, dt = \frac{6.63}{0.8} - \frac{12.10}{1.14} + \frac{5.47}{0.09} + 58.5 \ \mu g \ ml^{-1}$$

Thus, $\overline{C}_\infty$ is given by

$$\overline{C}_\infty = \frac{58.5}{4.5} = 13.0 \ \mu g \ ml^{-1}$$

See Figure 103 for comparison of results.

Step 3. The drug plasma concentration 0.5 hr after the eighth dose was administered can be calculated using Eq. (138). This assumes that we are at steady state. Thus,

$$C = 6.63 \left(\frac{1}{1 - e^{-0.8 \times 4.5}} \right) e^{-0.8 \times 0.5}$$

$$- 12.10 \left(\frac{1}{1 - e^{-1.14 \times 4.5}} \right) e^{-1.14 \times 0.5}$$

$$+ 5.47 \left(\frac{1}{1 - e^{-0.09 \times 1.5}} \right) e^{-0.09 \times 0.5} = 13.4 \ \mu g \ ml^{-1}$$

Step 4. A loading dose can be calculated using Eq. (145). Thus,

$$A_0^* = 100 \left(\frac{1}{1 - e^{-0.09 \times 4.5}} \right) = 300 \ mg$$

V. KINETICS OF BIOABSORPTION

Perhaps the oldest published method for the estimation of the rate of absorption of a drug into the blood was developed by Dominguez and Pomerene [412]. This technique was based on the assumption that the body is a single compartment or reservoir from which the drug is eliminated by first-order processes. One of the pitfalls of the method is that estimates of the apparent volume of distribution must be employed. A number of other procedures using a one-compartment model have been proposed [4,13,414].

Wagner and Nelson [416, 445] published a method for estimating the relative absorption of drugs using a one-compartment model and collecting either urinary or blood data. This method has gained wide acceptance because it does not require prior estimate of the volume of distribution and places no limitations on the order of the absorption-rate constant.

Loo and Riegelman [417] published a second method for calculating the intrinsic absorption of drugs based on a two-compartment model. Let us

now examine these two methods, which yield graphs referred to as "percent unabsorbed-time plots." For a detailed treatment of the subject, the
reader should see Gibaldi and Perrier [418], Wagner [419], and Notari
[420].

A. Rate of Absorption: Percent-Unabsorbed-
Time Plots

One-Compartment Model: Wagner-Nelson Approach

Equation (146) derived by Wagner and Nelson [416] is useful for the determination of the fraction of drug absorbed to time T. We write it in the
form

$$\% \text{ absorbed} = \frac{A_T}{A_\infty} \times 100 = \frac{C_T + K \int_0^T C \, dt}{K \int_0^\infty C \, dt} \times 100 \qquad (146)$$

The one-compartment scheme on which the Wagner-Nelson method is based
can be depicted as follows:

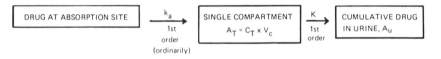

In this equation A_T is the cumulative amount of drug absorbed from time
zero to time T expressed in convenient units, A is the amount eventually
absorbed as expressed in the same units, K is the overall elimination-rate
constant given in the unit of reciprocal time, and C_T is blood, serum, or
plasma concentration at time T. From this equation, fraction-absorbed-
time data can be generated based on plasma concentration of drug and a
knowledge of the overall elimination-rate constant.

Example 9   Sample Calculation Illustrating the Wagner-Nelson Method

---

The following example illustrates the use of Eq. (146) for a drug whose
kinetics is represented by a one-compartment model. The plasma concentration-time data after oral administration, together with terms required
for an analysis of the data by the method of Wagner and Nelson, are
found in Table 27. A semilogarithmic plot of percent drug unabsorbed
[that is, $100 (1 - A_T/A_\infty)$] versus time is linear, with a slope equal to
$-k_a/2.303$. This graphical method yields the absorption-rate constant,
0.50 hr^{-1} (see Fig. 104). In some cases semilogarithmic plots are not
linear, and in those cases the rectilinear plot may yield a straight line
indicating that absorption is probably occurring by a zero-order process.
Examples of more complicated cases have been discussed by Wagner and
Nelson [416]. The illustration of Table 27 demonstrates the method of
calculating fractional (or percent) absorption of a drug from its oral
dosage form. The footnotes of Table 27 describe the steps for carrying
out the calculations.

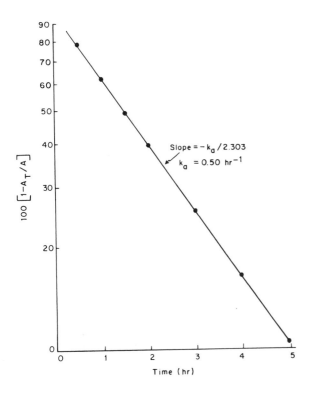

Figure 104 Semilogarithmic plot of percent drug remaining to be absorbed. Data from Table 27.

The relative efficiency of absorption of a drug from several tablet formulations can be estimated by this method. Thus, "percent-unabsorbed-time plots" are of use in the design of acceptable dosage forms or in the comparison of the relative bioavailability of marketed generic products. They also provide a means of calculating k_a, the rate of bioabsorption of drugs (see Fig. 104).

Wagner [421] has applied Eq. (146) to 12 separate studies with tetra-cycline combinations from 167 sets of serum tetracycline curves.

URINARY EXCRETION DATA. A method was also developed by Wagner and Nelson [416] in which urinary excretion data were used to obtain the percent of drug absorbed. The following equation is used:

$$\% \text{ absorbed} = \frac{A_T}{A_\infty} \times 100 = \frac{A_u + (1/K)(dA_u/dt)}{A_u^\infty} \times 100 \qquad (147)$$

where A_T is the cumulative amount of drug absorbed from time zero to time T given in convenient units; A_∞ the amount eventually absorbed expressed in the same units; K the overall rate constant for elimination from blood, plasma, or serum in units of reciprocal time; dA_u/dt the urinary excretion rate at time T; and A_u the cumulative amount excreted in the same period.

Table 27 Percent Unabsorbed Versus Time Data for a Drug that is Absorbed by an Apparent First-Order Process and Behaves According to a One-Compartment Model

1	2	3	4	5	6	7
T (hr)	C_T (µg ml^{-1})	$\int_0^T C\,dt$ (µg ml^{-1} hr^{-1})[a]	$K\int_0^T C\,dt$ (µg ml^{-1})[b]	$C_T = K\int_0^T C\,dt$ (µg ml^{-1})[c]	A_T/A_∞ (fraction absorbed)[d]	$100[1-(A_T/A_\infty)]$ (percent unabsorbed)[e]
0	0	0	0	0	0	100
0.5	2.16	0.54	0.049	2.21	0.212	78.8
1.0	3.75	2.01	0.181	3.93	0.378	62.2
1.5	4.89	4.18	0.376	5.27	0.506	49.4
2.0	5.69	6.82	0.614	6.30	0.606	39.3
3.0	6.59	12.96	1.17	7.76	0.746	25.4
4.0	6.86	19.68	1.77	8.63	0.830	17.0
5.0	6.77	26.50	2.39	9.16	0.880	11.95
6.0	6.50	33.14	2.98	9.48	0.912	8.80
7.0	6.13	39.45	3.55	9.68	0.931	6.89

8.0	5.71	45.37	4.08	9.79	0.942	5.80
12.0	4.11	65.01	5.85	9.96	0.958	4.19
24.0	1.40	98.07	8.83	10.23		
36.0	0.48	109.35	9.84	10.32		
48.0	0.16	113.19	10.19	10.35		
72.0	0.018	115.33	10.38	10.40		
∞	0	115.53	10.40	10.40		

[a]Cumulative areas under the curve are obtained by drawing trapezoids, calculating their areas, and summing the trapezoidal areas to each time T. See the text for use of the trapezoidal method.

[b]K is obtained from a plot of $\ln C_T$ versus T (use the data from columns 1 and 2) for times in the 12- to 72-hr range. The value obtained is K = 0.09 hr^{-1} (graph not shown).

[c]Values are obtained using K = 0.09 hr^{-1} and the values of columns 2 and 3. For example, for the 2.0-hr time, $C_T + K \int_0^T C\ dt = 5.69 + 0.09(6.82) = 6.30$.

[d]The values are obtained by dividing column 5 values by the column 4 value at T = ∞, that is, $K \int_0^\infty C\ dt = 10.40$. For example at time 2.0 hr, 6.30 ÷ 10.40 = 0.606. Either column 6 or column 7 may be used as a measure of absorption of a drug from its orally administered dosage form at various times.

[e]A plot of column 7 values on a log scale against time t in hours yields a line with a slope of $-k_a/2.303$, from which k_a, the rate of drug absorption, can be obtained. The value for k_a was found to be 0.5 hr^{-1}. See Figure 104.

The value (i.e., the value at $T = \infty$) of the numerator in Eq. (147) at times far beyond absorption (i.e., the value at $T \to \infty$) equals the denominator $(A_u)\infty$, and it is not necessary to determine $(A_u)\infty$ or to make a complete collection of the urine. There are no assumptions regarding the kinetic order of the absorption process. A semilogarithmic plot of the percent drug unabsorbed versus time will yield a straight line with a slope of $-k_a/2.303$ if absorption occurs by a first-order process. If a rectilinear plot results in a straight line, the absorption of drug may be a zero-order process.

Two-Compartment Model: Loo-Riegelman Approach

Loo and Riegelman [417] pointed out that methods based on the one-compartment model do not result in acceptable estimates of the absorption rates. These methods may yield an incorrect rate constant and occasionally lead to an erroneous assignment of the order of the process. Equation (148), derived by Loo and Riegelman, is useful for the determination of the fraction of drug absorbed to time T. This equation,

$$\% \text{ Absorbed to time } T = \frac{(A_1)_T}{(A_1)_\infty} \times 100$$

$$= \frac{(C_1)_T + (C_2)_T + K \int_0^T C_1 \, dt}{K \int_0^\infty C_1 \, dt} \times 100 \qquad (148)$$

is based on the assumption that a drug upon oral or intravenous administration confers upon the body the characteristics of a two-compartment model, which may be represented as

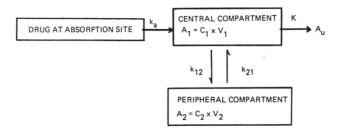

In Eq. (148), $(A_1)_T$ is the amount of drug absorbed to time T, $(A_1)_\infty$ the amount of drug absorbed to time ∞, $\int_0^T C \, dt$ the area under the plasma concentration-time curve from time zero to time T, V_1 the volume of the central compartment or compartment 1, $(A_2)_T$ the amount of drug in the peripheral compartment or compartment 2, and K the overall first-order rate constant for elimination of drug by all processes from the central compartment or compartment 1.

Gimbaldi and Perrier [418] and Wagner [422] show that the amount of drug in the peripheral compartment $(A_2)_T$ is

$$(A_2)_T = (A_2)_0 \, e^{-k_{21}t} + \frac{k_{12}(A_1)_0}{k_{21}} (1 - e^{-k_{21}t}) + \frac{k_{12}t^2}{2} \frac{\Delta A_1}{\Delta t} \qquad (149)$$

The time interval Δt is the time between two consecutive sampling periods. Division of Eq. (149) by V_1 (volume of central compartment) leads to the expression for $(C_2)_T$ required by Eq. (148). Thus,

$$(C_2)_T = \frac{(A_2)_T}{V_1} = \frac{(A_2)_0}{V_1} e^{-k_{21}t} + \frac{k_{12}(A_1)_0}{k_{21}V_1} (1 - e^{-k_{21}t}) + \frac{k_{12}t^2}{2} \frac{\Delta A_1}{V_1 \Delta t}$$

$$(150)$$

Letting $t = \Delta t$ reduces Eq. (150) to

$$(C_2)_T = \frac{(A_2)_T}{V_1} = \frac{(A_2)_0}{V_1} e^{-k_{21}\Delta t} + \frac{k_{12}(A_1)_0}{k_{21}V_1} (1 - e^{-k_{21}\Delta t}) + \frac{k_{12}\Delta t}{2} \Delta C_1$$

$$(151)$$

Criticisms that might be made against this equation are that the drug must be able to be given intravenously, so that an estimate of K and V_1 can be obtained. An estimate of the amount of drug in the peripheral compartment as a function of time after oral administration must also be made on the same subject under carefully replicated conditions. As shown in Eq. (161), this is indeed a complex calculation.

Equations (148) and (151) provide the data for calculating percent drug unabsorbed, $100[1 - (A_1)_T/(A_1)_\infty]$, versus time following oral or intramuscular administration. The estimates of K, k_{12}, k_{21}, and V_1 are obtained from intravenous administration of the drug.

Example 10   Sample Calculation Illustrating the Loo-Riegelman Method

The following example will illustrate the use of Eqs. (148) and (151). Consider a hypothetical drug that confers upon the body the characteristics of a two-compartment model, having a K of 0.16 hr^{-1}, a V_1 of 10 liters, a k_{12} of 0.4 hr^{-1}, and a k_{21} of 0.6 hr^{-1}. The plasma concentration-time data after oral administration is presented in Tables 28 and 29. These tables include the analysis of the data following the method of Loo and Riegelman.

Solution:

Using Eq. (151), with $(A_2)_0/V_1$ for time = 0.25 hr, one obtains from Table 25, column 10, for the first point,

$$(C_2)_T = 0.0 + 0.0 + \frac{(0.4)(1.69)(0.25)}{2} = 0.085$$

Table 28   Percent-Unabsorbed-Time Data for a Drug that is Absorbed by an Apparent First-Order Process and Behaves According to a Two-Compartment Model[a]

1	2	3	4	5	6
T (hr)	$(C_1)_T$ (μg ml^{-1})	ΔC_1 (μg ml^{-1})	Δt (hr)	$(A_1)_0$ (μg)	$(A_2)_0/V_1$ (μg ml^{-1})
0	0.0				
0.25	1.69	1.69	0.25	0.0	0.0
0.50	2.88	1.19	0.25	1.69	0.084
0.75	3.69	0.815	0.25	2.88	0.289
1.00	4.24	0.542	0.25	3.69	0.557
1.25	4.58	0.345	0.25	4.24	0.849
1.50	4.78	0.203	0.25	4.58	1.14
2.0	4.91	0.129	0.50	4.78	1.42
2.5	4.83	-0.078	0.50	4.91	1.89
3.0	4.66	-0.172	0.50	4.83	2.24
3.5	4.54	-0.208	0.50	4.66	2.48
4.0	4.24	-0.216	0.50	4.54	2.62
5.0	4.83	-0.410	1.00	4.24	2.69
6.0	3.47	-0.361	1.00	3.83	2.67
7.0	3.15	-0.316	1.00	3.47	2.54
8.0	2.87	-0.280	1.00	3.15	2.38
10.0	2.39	-0.478	2.00	2.87	2.20
12.0	2.00	-0.395	2.00	2.39	1.80
14.0	1.67	-0.328	2.00	2.00	1.50
16.0	1.39	-0.275	2.00	1.67	1.25
20.0	0.98	-0.420	4.00	1.40	1.05

[a] $V_1 = 10$ liters, $k_{12} = 0.4$ hr^{-1}, $k_{21} = 0.6$ hr^{-1}, and $K = 0.16$ hr^{-1}.

7	8	9	10
$\dfrac{(A_2)_0}{V_1}\, e^{-k_{21}\,\Delta t}$	$\dfrac{k_{12}(A_1)_0}{k_{21}\, V_1}\, (1 - e^{-k_{21}\,\Delta t})$	$\dfrac{k_{21}(\Delta t)}{2}\, \Delta C_1$	$(C_2)_T$
0.0	0.0	0.085	0.085
0.073	0.157	0.059	0.289
0.248	0.267	0.040	0.557
0.479	0.343	0.027	0.849
0.731	0.393	0.017	1.14
0.983	0.425	0.010	1.42
1.05	0.826	0.013	1.89
1.40	0.849	-0.008	2.24
1.66	0.835	-0.017	2.47
1.84	0.806	-0.021	2.62
1.94	0.769	-0.022	2.69
1.48	1.27	-0.082	2.67
1.46	1.15	-0.072	2.54
1.40	1.04	-0.063	2.38
1.30	0.947	-0.056	2.20
0.661	1.34	-0.191	1.80
0.544	1.11	-0.158	1.50
0.452	0.930	-0.131	1.25
0.377	0.778	-0.110	1.05
0.095	0.846	-0.336	0.604

Table 29 Percent-Unabsorbed-Time Data for a Drug that is Absorbed by an Apparent First-Order Process and Behaves According to a Two-Compartment Model[a]

1 T (hr)	2 $(C_1)_T$ (μg ml^{-1})	3 $k_{el} \int_0^T C\, dt$ (μg ml^{-1})	4 $(C_2)_T$ (μg ml^{-1})	5 % $(A_1)_T/(A_1)_\infty$ (% absorbed)	6 $100[1 - (A_1)_T/(A_1)_\infty]$ (% unabsorbed)
0	0.0	0.0	0.0		
0.25	1.69	0.0334	0.085	18.18	81.82
0.50	2.88	0.125	0.289	33.0	66.93
0.75	3.69	0.257	0.557	45.27	54.73
1.00	4.24	0.415	0.849	55.24	44.76
1.25	4.58	0.591	1.14	63.41	36.59
1.50	4.78	0.778	1.42	70.11	29.89
2.0	4.91	1.16	1.89	80.04	19.96

2.5	4.83	1.56	2.24	86.70	13.30
3.0	4.66	1.94	2.47	91.17	8.83
3.5	4.54	2.30	2.62	94.17	5.83
4.0	4.24	2.64	2.69	96.19	3.81
5.0	4.83	3.29	2.67	98.34	1.66
6.0	3.47	3.88	2.54	99.32	0.68
7.0	3.15	4.40	2.38	99.78	0.22
8.0	2.87	4.89	2.20	100.00	0.0
10.0	2.39	5.73	1.80		
12.0	2.00	6.43	1.50		
14.0	1.67	7.02	1.25		
16.0	1.39	7.51	1.05		
20.0	0.98	8.27	0.604		
	0.0	10.0			

[a]Continuation of data for Loo-Riegelman method.

Employing the data of Table 28 and Eq. (161), one obtains for the second point at 0.5 hr:

$$(C_2)_T = (0.084)e^{-(0.6)(0.25)} + \frac{(0.4)(0.2577)}{(0.6)} [1 - e^{-(0.6)(0.25)}]$$

$$+ \frac{(0.4)(1.19)(0.25)}{2} = 0.289$$

See column 10 of Table 28 for comparison.

Column 10 in Table 28 is obtained by adding columns 7, 8, and 9. The percent absorbed to time T of 0.5 hr is then obtained using columns 2, 3, and 4 of Table 29. Thus, for T = 0.5 hr and using Eq. (148), one obtains

$$\% \frac{(A_1)_T}{(A_1)_\infty} = \frac{2.88 + 0.289 + 0.25}{10.01} \times 100 = 33\%$$

See column 5 of Table 29 for comparison.

A semilogarithmic plot of percent drug unabsorbed [that is, $100 \times 1 - (A_1)_T/(A_1)_\infty$] (column 6, Table 29) is linear with a slope equal to $-k_a/2.303$. Figure 105 illustrates the semilogarithmic plot of percent drug remaining to be absorbed versus time. From its slope, one obtains a value for k_a of 0.8 hr^{-1}, the rate of absorption of the drug from the gastrointestinal tract or other site (such as intramuscular, rectal, etc.) of administration. Comparative bioavailability of a drug contained in various dosage forms can thus be assessed using percent rate of absorption.

B.   Extent of Absorption

Assessment of Bioavailability from Plasma Levels

By its definition, bioavailability includes both extent and rate of absorption. The questions to be answered are how fast and how much of an administered drug reaches the systemic circulation. In the preceding section we discussed the Wagner-Nelson and Loo-Riegelman methods to calculate the speed of absorption. Both of these methods are model-dependent. In the following section we discuss methods for estimating absorption *extent*, which are not model-dependent. It is generally well accepted that the absolute bioavailability of a drug can only be determined by comparison with an intravenous dose, and a widely used method to determine the absorption of a drug is to compare plasma level or urinary excretion following oral administration of a drug (also other routes) with that following intravenous administration of a solution of drug. Absorption extent following intravenous administration of a drug solution is equated to 100% availability.

In many instances intravenous administration is not possible. Examples are drugs that are damaging to the vessels when injected. Suspensions of highly insoluble drugs are not ordinarily administered by the i.v. route. In these cases, the bioavailability of a drug is established by comparing it to a secondary standard (oral solution). Thus, relative

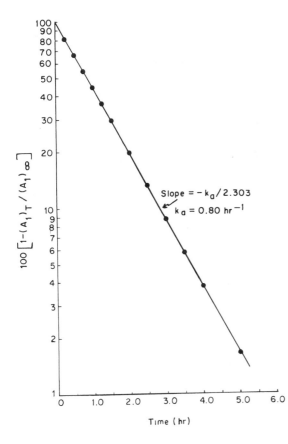

Figure 105 Semilogarithmic plot of percent drug remaining to be absorbed versus time. Data from Tables 28 and 29.

bioavailability is determined as opposed to absolute bioavailability, which is obtained when an i.v. dose is used. Lalka and Feldman suggested an approach for approximating the absolute bioavailability without the administration of an intravenous dose; the paper should be seen for details of the method [423].

In order to determine the absolute extent of bioavailability afforded by a drug dosage form, we compare the areas under the plasma concentration-time curve following oral (or other route, excluding i.v.) and intravenous administration of the same dose of drug. This is mathematically expressed as

$$\text{Absolute availability} = \frac{\left(\int_0^\infty C \, dt \right)_{\text{oral}}}{\left(\int_0^\infty C \, dt \right)_{\text{i.v.}}} \tag{152}$$

where $\left(\int_0^\infty C\ dt\right)_{\text{oral}}$ and $\left(\int_0^\infty C\ dt\right)_{\text{i.v.}}$ are the areas under the plasma concentration-time curves after oral and intravenous administration, respectively.

The area under the plasma concentration-time curve can be calculated with the trapezoidal rule:

$$\int_{t_1}^{t_2} C(t)\ dt = \frac{t_2 - t_1}{2}\ (C_1 + C_2)$$

Using this equation for the time interval 0 to 0.5 hr in Table 27, for example, one obtains for the second point in column 3.

$$\int_0^T C\ dt = \text{area} = \frac{0.5 - 0}{2}\ (0 + 2.16) = 0.54$$

Following oral administration, the fraction of the dose that is absorbed, or efficiently of absorption F, corrected for intrasubject and intersubject variability in half-life, can be expressed as

$$F = \frac{\left(\int_0^\infty C\ dt\right)_{\text{oral}} (t_{1/2})_{\text{i.v.}}}{\left(\int_0^\infty C\ dt\right)_{\text{i.v.}} (t_{1/2})_{\text{oral}}} \tag{153}$$

Equation (153) is valid regardless of the number of compartments describing the time course of drug in the body. If the half-life for elimination following i.v. injection $(t_{1/2})_{\text{i.v.}}$ is identical with the biological half-life following oral administration $(t_{1/2})_{\text{oral}}$, then the fraction of dose absorbed by the oral route F of Eq. (153) is exactly equal to absolute availability as defined by Eq. (152).

As discussed previously, in certain cases intravenous administration of the drug is not possible. In this case the relative bioavailability is given by Eq. (154):

$$\text{Relative availability} = \frac{\left(\int_0^\infty C\ dt\right)_{\text{oral}}}{\left(\int_0^\infty C\ dt\right)_{\text{oral standard}} (t_{1/2})_{\text{oral}}} \tag{154}$$

in which the standard is administered as an oral solution, suspension, or other form serving as the reference system. The fraction of dose absorbed, when relative availability is being determined, is given by

$$F_{relative} = \frac{\left(\int_0^\infty C\ dt\right)_{oral}(t_{1/2})_{oral\ standard}}{\left(\int_0^\infty C\ dt\right)_{oral\ standard}(t_{1/2})_{oral}} \qquad (155)$$

There are a number of cases in which the availability of a drug cannot be obtained after single administration. In these cases the availability of a drug may be determined using steady-state levels of drugs following multiple administration. The following equation is useful to determine a realistic estimate of the relative amount absorbed, under conditions of multiple dosing:

$$F_{rel(mult)} = \frac{\left(\int_0^\infty C(\tau)\ dt\right)_{oral}(t_{1/2})_{oral\ standard}}{\left(\int_0^\infty C(\tau)\ dt\right)_{oral\ standard}(t_{1/2})_{oral}} \qquad (156)$$

where $\left(\int_0^\infty C(\tau)\ dt\right)_{oral}$ and $\left(\int_0^\infty C(\tau)\ dt\right)_{oral\ standard}$ are the area under the plasma concentration-time curve during a dosing interval τ at steady state after oral administration of the test drug dosage form, and the corresponding area for the standard oral dosage form, respectively.

Equation (156) is a valid measure of absorption efficiency regardless of the number of compartments describing the time course of drug in the body. However, it requires that the dosing interval τ be sufficiently large to permit an estimate of half-life from the terminal linear segment. Wagner et al. applied this method for different dosage forms of indoxole [424].

Example 11   Sample Calculation of Relative Bioavailability Employing Extent of Absorption

A bioavailability study was conducted with the purpose of determining the relative availability (extent of absorption) of a tablet dosage form. A group of subjects received an oral standard preparation (oral solution, treatment A) and a test formulation (tablet, treatment B). On each study, drug plasma concentration was determined as a function of time. Plasma concentration-times curves were constructed and the elimination half-lives as well as the areas under the curves (AUC) were determined. The following table provides the result:

	Treatment A	Treatment B
Half-life (hr)	12	11
AUC ($\mu g\ ml^{-1}\ hr^{-1}$)	120	113

Calculate the relative bioavailability.

Step 1.   Equation (155) allows the calculation of the relative bioavailability. Thus,

$$F_{relative} = \frac{113 \times 12}{120 \times 11} = 1.03$$

It should be noted that $F_{relative}$ can be greater than unity, owing to the ratios of half-lives in Eq. (155).

Other Techniques for Assessing Bioavailability

Absolute and relative availability of a drug from various dosage forms and routes of administration may also be determined by analysis of unaltered drug in the urine.   In cases where the drug is eliminated almost totally by metabolism or where an assay for the metabolite is more adaptable than for the unchanged drug in plasma or urine, an index of comparative bio-availability may be better obtained by comparing areas under the plasma concentration-time curves for metabolites following oral and intravenous ad-ministration of the drug at identical dose levels.

Assessment of Bioavailability From Pharmacological Response

The use of pharmacological data as an alternative to direct assay data for performing bioavailability and pharmacokinetics analyses of drug has been examined by Smolen and co-workers [425].   Chlorpromazine was used as a model drug for the application of pharmacological data to the study of bio-availability.   The work consisted of monitoring changes in pupil size, intraocular pressure, heart rate, body temperature, blood pressure, drug-induced changes in ECG, and spontaneously and visually evoked response EEG.   Figure 106 illustrates the time variation of averaged miotic response

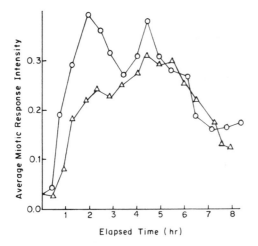

Figure 106   Time variation of average miotic response intensities observed in crossover experiments following oral dosing of nine normal human sub-jects with 100-mg oral doses of chlorpromazine syrup (○) and tablets (△). (From Ref. 425.)

intensities observed in crossover experiments following oral chlorpromazine syrup and tablets. The areas under the pharmacological intensity versus time curves have the same interpretation with regard to reflecting extent of bioavailability as areas under blood level versus time curves [426−429]. The results of these studies present the opportunity to further evaluate bioavailability from pharmacological response. This is a noninvasive method which deals not only with bioavailability but also with therapeutic equivalency.

As a result of some of these studies, the FDA has included in their regulations measurement of an appropriate acute pharmacological effect as a general approach for determining bioavailability [2].

VI. IN VITRO, IN SITU, AND IN VIVO METHODS TO STUDY PHYSIOLOGIC FACTORS AFFECTING DRUG ABSORPTION

As mentioned previously, various physiological factors may affect the absorption of drugs from the gastrointestinal tract. The characterization of the absorption behavior of a drug w.ll permit the development and/or improvement of drug dosage forms. In vitro, in situ, and more recently new in vivo techniques have assisted the investigator in examining absorption characteristics of drugs. Apparatus and techniques for studying in vitro dissolution have already been discussed (Sec. III.C). Absorption studies include examination of the region of the gastrointestinal tract for maximum absorption, investigation of the processes by which drugs are absorbed (i.e., passive diffusion and active transport), and elucidation of the physicochemical factors affecting dosage form behavior (i.e., active ingredient/excipient ratio, film versus coated tablets, and solubility parameters).

In vitro and in situ methods are simple and reproducible. In vivo animal models usually consist of lower experimental animals, such as rats, hamsters, rabbits, and sometimes dogs and monkeys. These provide clues to drug absorption and action but must be used with caution when comparison is made with clinical studies. In vivo human experimentation provides the most useful information, but the work is expensive, difficult to interpret, and limited by stringent restrictions, such as patient consent, particularly in the case of pediatric and geriatric subjects. In vitro and in situ studies are therefore of value as more direct and economical studies of drug absorption and action.

Table 30 summarizes some of the better known techniques available to the pharmaceutical scientist for the purpose of characterizing drug absorption. These are elaborated on in the following paragraphs.

A. Everted Sac Technique

The everted sac method, devised by Wilson and Wiseman [430], involves isolating a small segment of the intestine of a rat or hamster, inverting the intestine, and filling the sac with drug-buffered solution. Both ends of the segment are tied off and the sac is immersed in an Erlenmeyer flask containing a large volume of a buffer solution. The flask and its contents are oxygenated and agitated at 37°C for a specified period of time and the fluids are assayed for drug content. The major disadvantage of the

Table 30   In Vitro, In Situ, and In Vivo Methods to Study Physiological Factors Affecting Drug Absorption

In Vitro	In Situ	In Vivo
Everted sac (Weisman and Wilson [430])	Perfusion technique (Shanker et al. [45])	Direct methods: blood levels, urinary levels
Everted sac modification (Crane and Wilson [431])	Rat gut technique (Doluisio et al. [435])	Indirect methods: pharmacologic response (Irwin et al. [438], De Cato et al. [439], Levy [440])
Circulation technique (Fisher and Parsons [432], Wiseman [433], Darlington and Quastel [444])	Intestinal loop technique (Levine and Pelikan [436])	
Everted ring or slice technique (Crane and Mandelstam [434])	Rat stomach technique (Schanker et al. [437], Dolusio et al. [435])	Short-lived isotope methods (Digenis et al. [441])
Everted sac flow-through technique (Newburger and Stavchansky [443])		

method is the difficulty in obtaining more than one sample per intestinal segment.

B. Single-Segment Modification of the Everted Sac Method

A modification of the original everted sac technique was introduced by Crane and Wilson [431] to permit the testing of different solutions with a single intestinal segment. The major change from the original everted sac technique is the attachment of the intestine to a cannula from which frequent samples can be obtained. Several investigators have used this method to study active and passive transport processes [445–447].

C. Circulation Technique

The circulation method involves isolating the entire small intestine of a rat or hamster [432], or a segment [433,444] with circulation of oxygenated buffer through the lumen and serosal side of the intestinal membrane. Absorption rates are calculated after drug content is determined in the lumen and serosal solutions.

D. Everted Ring or Slice Technique

Crane and Mandelstam [434] devised an everted ring technique, which involves cutting the entire small intestine or a segment of the intestine into riglike slices 0.1 to 0.5 cm in length. The slices are oxygenated with Krebs buffer and dried with filter paper and placed in a flask containing

a drug in buffered solution at 37°C. At selected time intervals the slices
are assayed for drug content. This technique has been used by several
investigators to examine active and passive absorption processes [434,448,
449].

E. Everted Sac Flow-Through Technique

Newburger and Stavchansky [443] modified the Crane and Wilson method.
The major advantage of this technique is that solutions placed inside the
everted preparation can be removed by a simple flushing process. Other
techniques require a sampling device to be placed inside the intestine,
thereby possibly causing damage by "raking" the intestinal wall as the
sampling device is introduced or removed. Also, the orifice of the sampling device may become occluded against the intestinal wall, thus preventing withdrawal of the sample.

The apparatus is illustrated in Figure 107. It consists of a glass tube
permanently secured inside a plastic jacket through which water is circulated at 37°C. The top of the tube is closed with a rubber stopper which
supports a gas dispersion tube of medium porosity through which oxygen
is bubbled. Also supported in the stopper are a thermometer; a hypodermic needle, which acts as a pressure-relief valve for the escaping
oxygen; a polyethylene tube inserted through the hypodermic needle to

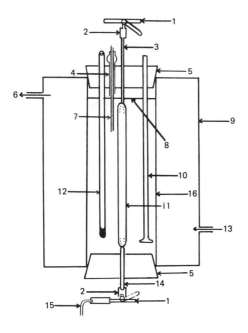

Figure 107 Everted intestinal segment flow through apparatus. 1, Three-
way valve; 2, Ttgon tubing; 3, beaded pipet; 4, hypodermic needle;
5, rubber stopper; 6, water outlet; 7, polyethylene tube; 8, drug solution
level; 9, constant-temperature jacket; 10, gas dispersion tube; 11, intestinal segment; 12, thermometer; 13, water inlet; 14, connecting tube;
15, glass L; 16, inside container. (From Ref. 443.)

allow the outside drug solution to be sampled; and a beaded pipet over
which the intestinal segment has been everted and secured with a silk
suture. A piece of Tygon tubing is connected to the top of the pipet to
which a three-way plastic valve is attached. The bottom of the glass tube
is closed with another rubber stopper which supports a constricted glass
connector. The other end of the everted intestinal segment is secured
with a silk suture to this connector. To the outside of the glass connector
a three-way plastic valve is connected by a piece of Tygon tubing. One
of the other ends of the three-way plastic valve is connected to a glass L
by a piece of Tygon tubing. The glass tube must be long enough to accommodate a 10-cm length of intestine which is completely immersed in the
drug solution, but leave an air space above the top of the solution to
prevent the bubbling of the solution up through the hypodermic needle
with the escaping oxygen. The oxygen flow rate is adjusted to a minimum
so that the bubbling of the solution can be observed. Distilled water is
circulated through the jacket by connecting hoses from the circulating pump
to the inlet and outlet ports of the container. A constant temperature of
37°C is attained before the animal surgery is started. The apparatus is
supported on a ring stand during the experiments.

Newburger [443] employed this technique to examine the metabolism of
quaternary ammonium compounds in the presence and absence of trichloro-
acetic acid.

F. Perfusion Technique

The perfusion method of Schanker et al. [45] involves anesthetizing the
animal with pentobarbital and then exposing small intestine by a midline
abdominal incision. The intestine is cannulated at the duodenal and ileal
ends with polyethylene cannulas having inside diameters of 2.5 mm and
outside diameters of 3.5 mm. The stomach and cecum are closed off by
ligatures, care being taken not to occlude major blood vessels. The bile
duct may or may not be ligated. The intestine is replaced in the abdomen,
the incision closed, and perfusion from pylorus to ileocecal junction is
started immediately. The small intestine is first cleared of particulate
matter by perfusion with a drug-free solution (buffer) for 30 min. The
solution containing drug is then perfused for 30 min to displace the previous wash, after which samples are collected at definite time periods from
the ileal outflow. The concentration of drug is measured in each of the
collected samples and the relative rate of absorption is calculated from the
difference in concentration of drug entering and leaving the intestine.

Recently, Sinko and Amidon [451] published an in situ rat perfusion
technique which gives reliable absorption permeability parameters.

G. Rat Gut Technique

In this method, introduced by Doluisio et al. [435], the small intestine is
exposed by a midline abdominal incision, and two L-shaped glass cannulas
are inserted through small slits at the duodenal and ileal ends. Care is
taken to handle the small intestine gently and to reduce surgery to a minimum to maintain an intact blood supply. The cannulas are secured by
ligation with silk suture, and the intestine is returned to the abdominal
cavity to aid in maintaining its integrity. Four-centimeter segments of

Tygon tubing are attached to the exposed ends of both cannulae, and a 30-ml hypodermic syringe fitted with a three-way stopcock and containing perfusion fluid warmed to 37°C is attached to the duodenal cannula. As a means of clearing the gut, perfusion fluid is then passed slowly through it and out the ileal cannula and discarded until the effluent is clear. The remaining perfusion solution is carefully expelled from the intestine by means of air pumped in from the syringe, and 10 ml of drug solution is immediately introduced into the intestine by means of the syringe. A stopwatch is started, and the ileal cannula is connected to another 30-ml syringe fitted with a three-way stopcock. This arrangement enables the operator to pump the lumen solution into either the ileal or the duodenal syringe, remove a 0.1-ml aliquot, and return the remaining solution to the intestine within 10 to 15 sec. To assure uniform drug solution concentrations throughout the gut segment, aliquots are removed from the two syringes alternately.

The Doluisio rat gut technique has been useful in examining the behavior of weakly acidic and basic drugs. In addition, the effects of membrane storage on the kinetics of drug absorption have been determined [450].

H. Intestinal Loop Technique

Levine and Pelikan [436] devised an intestinal loop procedure involving the formation of either single or multiple intestinal loops. The single-loop method consists of anesthetizing the animal under light ether anesthesia, then exposing the intestine and placing the proximal ligature about 6 in. from the pylorus. The length of the loop (about 4 in.) is determined in vivo by counting off four mesenteric blood vessels between the proximal and distal ligatures. No major blood vessels are occluded by these ties. After the drug solution is injected quantitatively into the loop (without puncturing the gut wall between ligatures), the proximal ligature is secured and the incision closed. The rat used in the study reported appeared fully recovered from the procedure within 5 min. After 3 hr, the animal is again anesthetized with ether and, before the animal is killed, the loop of the gut is removed for chemical analysis and determination of its quality of unabsorbed drug.

The multiple-loop procedure is similar to that for the single-loop preparation. The proximal ligature of the first loop is placed about 6 in. from the pylorus, four mesenteric blood vessels counted off, and the second ligature placed and secured. The second and third loops, each of which is about 4 in. long, are prepared similarly, leaving about 0.5 in. of intestine between loops. The appropriate solution is injected quantitavely into each loop. At the end of 3 hr, each loop is excised and analyzed separately. The portion of the gut used in the single-loop preparation is always found to be macroscopically free of food. In the multiple-loop preparation, the more distal portions of the gut have to be cleared of visible boluses of food; the boluses are removed by a gentle milking technique.

I. Rat Stomach Technique

There are two widely used rat stomach procedures: a method developed by Schanker et al. [437] and a modification introduced by Doluisio et al.

[435]. The latter allows a determination of the amount of drug absorbed as a function of time. The rat stomach is exposed, cannulated at the cardiac and duodenal ends, and washed from the cardiac end with perfusion solution until the effluent is clear. The perfusion solution is expelled with air, and 5 ml of drug solution is introduced through the cardiac cannula. A stopwatch is started and a 15-cm section of 0.011-cm-ID polyethylene tubing, connected to a 2-ml syringe and fitted with a three-way stopcock, is inserted through the duodenal cannula. At specified intervals the stomach contents are sampled by withdrawing about 0.5 ml of the solution into the syringe, removing a 0.1-ml aliquot, and returning the remainder.

J. In Vivo Methods

The methods described above were of the in vitro type. In vivo method have also been successfully employed to characterize the absorption characteristics of drugs. Direct methods employ blood or urine data to calculate absorption rates. Indirect methods use pharmacologic response data for the purpose of examining physiological and physicochemical factors influencing drug absorption. Irwin et al. [438] and Newburger [443] utilized mydriases to demonstrate gastrointestinal absorption of quaternary

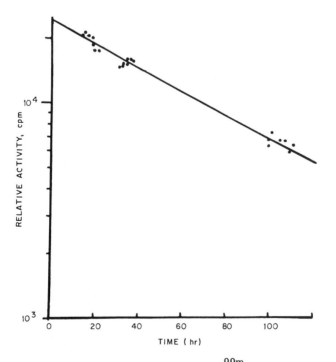

Figure 108 Rate of clearance of ^{99m}Tc-labeled polystyrene beads bearing triethylenetetramine functions from the stomach of a normal human male subject (half-time of gastric emptying = 51 min). (From Ref. 441; reproduced with permission of the copyright owner.)

ammonium compounds. DeCato [439] used blepharoptic assay procedures to study the absorption of reserpine. Smolen et al. [425] examined mydriasis response to determine the bioavailability of chlorpromazine preparations. Levy [440] has reviewed the methods for estimating absorption rates from pharmacologic response data.

Recently, Digenis et al. [441] used ^{99m}Tc-labeled triethylenetetramine-polystyrene resin for measuring gastric emptying in humans. Quantitative dynamic data were obtained with these radionucleides without physical or physiological influences on the gastrointestinal tract [442]. In addition, excellent scintigraphic images of the stomach, intestines, and colon were obtained with a low-target-organ, total-body-radiation dose. Figure 108 illustrates the rate of clearance of ^{99m}Tc-labeled polystyrene beads bearing triethylenetetramine functions from the stomach of a normal human subject. The authors reported a half-life time of gastric emptying of 51 min.

VII. SUSTAINED RELEASE MEDICATION

Sustained release dosage forms provide a prolonged dosing of the drug from the product by supplying an initial amount or loading dose, perhaps one-half of the total dose released, followed by a gradual and uniform release of the remainder of the drug over the desired time period.

It is not difficult to write equations that describe the release characteristics of sustained action tablet and capsule forms. It is another matter to formulate and manufacture products that faithfully deliver the drug uniformly under variable conditions of patient physiology and therapy and that reflect the desired plasma level profiles designed into the dosage form. Cabana and Kumkumian [452] outlined the position of the FDA regarding the design of controlled-release products for use in humans, and requirements for substantiating safety and efficacy and providing proper labeling of these products.

The formulation and manufacture of sustained-release products is the subject of another chapter in this series of monographs. It is our intention here only to introduce equations that describe the time course of drug in the body following administration of a sustained-action formulation.

Sustained-release forms are designed to provide adequate blood levels over a sufficient period of time at the pharmacological site so as to result in clinical advantages.

Antihistamines, sedatives, and tranquilizers are particularly well adapted to sustain action, as the blood levels in these cases are desired to be maintained over prolonged periods of time.

Time-release preparations have no rational for drugs with a long biologic half-life in the body ($t_{1/2} > 12$ hr). The half-life of some drugs are found in Table 31. Furthermore, highly potent drugs are not candidates for sustained release. It is desirable to be able to alter dosage or withhold the potent drug at will during the regimen, and such control is lost when the patient is under continuous medication with an 8- to 12-hr sustained-dose form.

Let us suppose that a new potent ephedrine-like tablet, 15 mg when taken four times during the day for its nasal decongestant effect, is found to be therapeutically effective. The daily dose is $4 \times 15 = 60$ mg. The dosing interval τ is 24 hr, although the drug is administered only during the waking hours of each day: 8 a.m., 12 p.m., 4 p.m., and 8 p.m.

Table 31   Biological Half-Lives of Drugs

Acetosal	20 min
Salicylic acid	4 – 4 1/2 hr
Phenacetine	45 – 90 min
Phenazone	10 – 15 hr
Phenylbutazone	3 days
Hydroxyphenylbutazone	3 days
Aminophenazone	3 hr
Paracetamol	95 – 170 min
Barbital	4 – 5 days
Phenobarbital	3-1/2 days
Butobarbital	30 – 45 hr
Pentobarbital	42 hr
Thiopental	16 hr
Hexobarbital	17 hr
Gluethimide	10 hr
Paraldehyde	7-1/2 hr
Diphenylhydantoin	9 hr
Meprobamate	11 – 14 hr
Diazepam	27 – 28 hr
Ethylbiscoumacetate	1 – 2 hr
Discoumarol	32 hr
Warfarine	30 – 40 hr
Heparine	60 – 90 min
Digitoxine	4 – 6 days
Digoxine	40 – 50 hr
Xylocaine	75 min
Pentazocine	2 hr
Norephedrine	4 hr
Ephedrine	3 – 4 hr
Methylephedrine	4 – 5 hr
Methoxyphenamine	8 – 15 hr
Dexamphetamine	6 – 7 hr
(+)-Methamphetamine	12 – 14 hr
(+)-Ethylamphetamine	13 – 17 hr

Table 31 (Continued)

(+)-Isopropylamphetamine	2 – 3 hr
(+)-Dimethylamphetamine	5 1/2 – 6 hr
Phentermine	19 – 24 hr
Mephentermine	17 – 18 hr
Chlorphentermine	37 – 38 hr
Pipradrol	22 – 27 hr
Fencamfamin	10 – 12 hr
Caffeine	3 1/2 – 6 hr
Lysergide (LSD)	3 hr
Imipramine	3 1/2 hr
Desipramine	30 – 35 hr
Mepacrine	5 days
Hexamethonium	1 1/2 hr
Tubocurarine	12 – 15 min
Succinylcholine	3 1/2 min
Noscapine	40 – 50 min

Source: From Ref. 453 and other sources.

The plasma levels fluctuate greatly as each dose is absorbed and eliminated, and it is desired to prepare a sustained release form that would allow administration only once or twice a day. It is expected that this would be more convenient for the patient and provide more uniform blood levels. Let us see how such a product might be formulated. In this example we follow the treatment of Notari [454].

The average steady-state plasma concentration for this drug, following the regimen above, is given by

$$\overline{C} = F \frac{A_0}{V_d K \tau} \tag{157}$$

for drug concentration at steady state following first-order absorption according to a one-compartment model. We obtain the result

$$\overline{C} = 0.86 \frac{60 \text{ mg}}{18,000 \text{ ml} \times 0.231/\text{hr} \times 24 \text{ hr}} = \frac{51.6}{99,792}$$

$$= 5.171 \times 10^{-4} \text{ mg ml}^{-1} = 0.517 \text{ } \mu\text{g ml}^{-1}$$

In this example we have assumed that the fraction of drug absorbed from the gastrointestinal tract into the systemic circulation, F, equals 0.86. The 24-hr dose (four doses × 15 mg) of the ephedrine tablet A_0 is 60 mg. The apparent volume of distribution V_d is 18,000 ml, and K, the elimination-rate constant, is 0.231 hr^{-1}.

To prepare a sustained-release product, we design it so that one 60-mg tablet is taken each 12 hr, or two tablets of 30 mg each are taken over 24 hr. It is assumed that the drug is absorbed orally and eliminated in the urine by first-order processes.

It would be more desirable to have the drug released from its preparation and absorbed from the gastrointestinal tract by zero-order kinetics, providing 60 mg/24 hr or a steady release of 2.5 mg of drug each hour. But true zero-order release products are not yet commercially available; we must therefore satisfy ourselves for the present with first-order release from the dosage form.

To overcome the time lag following administration before the drug reaches steady-state concentration in the body, as we noted earlier under intravenous administration, some sustained action products are currently formulated with a loading dose in the outer coating together with the sustained-release mass in the core of the tablet. Care must be taken, however, that this administration form does not lead to an accumulation of drug as each new dose is taken. Accumulation will occur if sufficient time is not allowed for all drug to be cleared from the body between doses. Gibaldi and Perrier [455] discuss this difficulty.

If, however, the sustained-release tablet is given in 30-mg dose twice a day (once each 12 hr), and if its first-order absorption half-life is, for example, 2 hr, then six half-lives transpire before the new dose is taken. This allows a sufficient washout period of the first dose so that only 1.5% of the drug remains in the gastrointestinal tract when the second dose is administered.

In the case of the product we are formulating, the tablet contains 30 mg of drug and for a first-order absorption process has a half-life of 2.0 hr. In the gut it is released over a period of 12 hr before the second dose is given, so that accumulation of drug does not occur in the body.

The equation used to describe the concentration of drug in the plasma over a 24-hr period is, according to Gibaldi and Perrier [455]:

$$C_n = F \frac{k_a A_0}{V_d(k_a - K)} \left[\left(\frac{1 - e^{-nK\tau}}{1 - e^{-k\tau}} \right) e^{-kt} - \left(\frac{1 - e^{-nk_a\tau}}{1 - e^{-k_a\tau}} \right) e^{-k_a t} \right] \quad (158)$$

where n is the dose number, 1 and 2. For our tablet A = 30 mg, K = 0.231 hr^{-1}, V_d = 18 liters, t = 12 hr, F is 0.86, and k_a = 0.693/2.0 = 0.347 hr^{-1}. Using this equation, we can evaluate C at 6 hr after the first tablet is administered:

$$C_1 = \frac{(0.86)(0.347)(30)}{18(0.347 - 0.231)} \left[\left(\frac{1 - e^{-(1)(0.231)(12)}}{1 - e^{-(0.231)(12)}} \right) e^{-(0.231)(6)} \right.$$

$$\left. - \left(\frac{1 - e^{-(1)(0.347)(12)}}{1 - e^{-(0.347)(12)}} \right) e^{-(0.347)(6)} \right] = 0.54 \ \mu g \ ml^{-1}$$

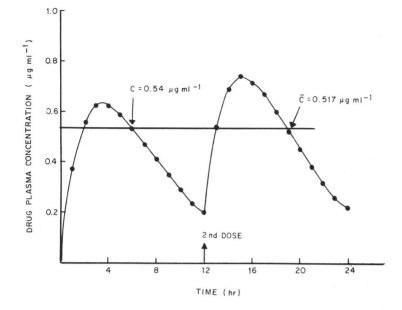

Figure 109 Plasma levels of a hypothetical ephedrine derivative resulting from the oral administration of a sustained-release tablet containing 30 mg of the drug. The drug is released at an apparent first-order rate with a half-life of 2 hr.

Thus, we see in Figure 109 that after 6 hr, the plasma concentration C_6 of the ephedrine derivative has risen to a concentration of 0.54 µg ml^{-1}. Calculating C_2 with n = 2 in Eq. (158) and letting t = 9 gives the computed point on C = 0.38 µg ml^{-1} at a 21-hr running time on the right-hand side of Figure 109. The horizontal line in the figure signifies the "average" steady-state plasma concentration $\bar{C}$. Instead, the profile for the two 30-mg tablets actually provides the body with periods of greater than and less than a uniform blood level. Nevertheless, the formulation of this product into sustained-action tablets provides convenience for the patient and relatively continuous blood levels over a 24-hr period, the peaks and valleys of which are probably in the range of therapeutic efficacy. Thus, pharmacokinetic modeling can assist the formulator to make a realistic appraisal of what can be expected at the present stage of technology in designing sustained-release dosage forms.

REFERENCES

1. Teorell, T., *Arch. Int. Pharmacodyn.*, *57*:205 (1937).
2. *Bioequivalence Requirements and In Vivo Bioavailability Procedures*, Fed. Regist., Jan. 7, 1977.
3. MacDonald, H., Pisano, F., Barger, J., Dornbush, A., and Pelcak, E., *Clin. Med.*, *76*:30 (1969).
4. Barr, W. H., Gerbracht, L. M., Letchen, K., Plant, M., and Strahl, N., *Clin. Pharmacol. Ther.*, *13*:97 (1972).

5. Glazko, A. J., Kinkel, A. W., Alegmani, W. C., and Holmes, E. L.,
    Clin. Pharmacol. Ther., *9*:472 (1968).
6. Wagner, J. G., Christensen, M., Sakmar, E., Blair, D., Yates,
    P. W., III, and Sedman, A. J., *J. Am. Med. Assoc.*, *224*:199 (1973).
7. Lindenbaum, J., *N. Engl. J. Med.*, *285*:1344 (1971).
8. Van Pettin, G., Feng, H., Withey, R. J., and Lettau, H. F.,
    J. Clin. Pharmacol., *11*:177 (1971).
9. Choiu, W. L., *J. Clin. Pharmacol.*, *12*:296 (1972).
10. Blair, D. C., Barnes, R. W., Wildner, E. L., and Murray, W. J.,
    J. Am. Med. Assoc., *215*:251 (1971).
11. Brice, G. W. and Hammer, H. F., *Drug Inf. Bull.*, *3*:112 (1969).
12. Catz, B., Ginsburg, E., and Salenger, S., *N. Engl. J. Med.*, *266*:
    136 (1962).
13. Sullivan, T. J., Sakmar, E., Albert, K. S., Blair, D. C., and
    Wagner, J. G., *J. Pharm. Sci.*, *64*:1723 (1975).
14. Aguiar, A. J., Wheeler, L. M., Fusari, S., and Zelmer, J. E.,
    J. Pharm. Sci., *57*:1844 (1968).
15. *Bioavailability Requirements for Prescription Drugs*, Fed. Regis.,
    Jan. 3, 1973.
16. *Drug Bioequivalence—A report of the Office of Technology Assess-
    ment Drug Bioequivalency Study Panel*, Superintendent of Docu-
    ments, U.S. Government Printing Office, Washington, D.C., 1974.
17. *Approved Drug Products with Therapeutic Equivalence Evaluation*,
    U.S. Department of Health and Human Services, Public Health
    Service, Food and Drug Administration, Center for Drug Evaluation
    and Research, 8th Edition, 1988.
18. Levy, G., Leonards, J. R., and Procknal, J. A., *J. Pharm. Sci.*,
    54:1719 (1965).
19. Wagner, J. G., Generic equivalence and inequivalence of oral prod-
    ucts, in *Biopharmaceutics and Relevant Pharmacokinetics*, Drug
    Intelligence Publications, Hamilton, Illinois, 1971, pp. 166–179.
20. Barr, W. H., *Pharmacology*, *8*:55 (1972).
21. Nelson, E., *J. Am. Pharm. Assoc., Sci. Ed.*, *47*:297 (1958).
22. Levy, G., *J. Pharm. Sci.*, *50*:388 (1961).
23. MacDonald, H., Pisano, F., Burger, J., Dornbush, A., and
    Pelcak, E., *Drug Inf. Bull.*, *3*:76 (1969).
24. Bergan, T., Oydvin, B., and Lundo, I., *Acta Pharmacol. Toxicol.*,
    33:138 (1973).
25. Bates, T. R., Lambert, D. A., and Johns, W. H., *J. Pharm. Sci.*,
    58:1468 (1969).
26. Gibaldi, M. and Weintraub, H., *J. Pharm. Sci.*, *59*:725 (1970).
27. *Guidelines for Biopharmaceutical Studies in Man*, American Pharma-
    ceutical Association, Academy of Pharmaceutical Sciences, Washington,
    D.C., 1972.
28. Calter, P., *Problem Solving with Computers*, McGraw-Hill, New York,
    1973; J. M. Smith, *Scientific Analysis on the Pocket Calculator*,
    Wiley, New York, 1975; R. Hamming, *Numerical Methods for Scientists
    and Engineers*, McGraw-Hill, New York, 1973.
29. Wagner, J. G., *Pharmacology*, *8*:102 (1972).
30. Skelly, J. R., Bioavailability policies and guidelines, in *Industrial
    Bioavailability and Pharmacokinetics: Guidelines, Regulations and*

Controls (A. Martin and J. T. Doluisio, eds.), Drug Dynamics Institute, College of Pharmacy, The University of Texas at Austin, Austin, Texas, 1977.

31. Schuirmann, D. J., *J. Pharmacokin. Biopharm.*, *15*(6):657 (1987).
32. Hauck, W. W. and Anderson, S., *J. Pharmacokin. Biophar.*, *12*:83 (1984).
33. Westlake, W. J., *Biometrics*, 37:589 (1981).
34. Dighé, S., *Clin. Res. Pract. Drug Reg. Affairs*, *2*(4):401 (1984).
35. Dittert, L. W. and DiSanto, R., *J. Am. Pharm. Assoc.*, *NS13*(8):421 (1973).
36. Levy, G. and Jusko, W., *J. Pharm. Sci.*, 55:285 (1966).
37. Schanker, L. S. and Tocco, D. J., *J. Pharmacol. Exp. Ther.*, *128*: 115 (1960).
38. Goldstein, A., Aronow, L., and Kalman, S. M., eds., *Principles of Drug Action*, 2nd Ed., Wiley, New York, 1974, p. 143.
39. Schanker, L. S. and Jeffrey, J. J., *Biochem. Pharmacol.*, *11*:961 (1962).
40. Evered, D. F. and Randall, H. G., *Biochem. Pharmacol.*, *11*:371 (1962).
41. Higuchi, T., Thermodynamics, Kinetics and Mechanisms of Interface Transport of Organic Ammonium Species, seminar presented at The Upjohn Company, July 12, 1967.
42. Boroujerdi, M., *Drug Develop. Indust. Pharm.*, *13*(1):181 (1987).
43. Shore, P. A., Brodie, B. B., and Hogben, C. A. M., *J. Pharmacol. Exp. Ther.*, *119*:361 (1957).
44. Hogben, C. A. M., Tocco, D. J., Brodie, B. B., and Schanker, L. S., *J. Pharmacol. Exp. Ther.*, *125*:275 (1959).
45. Schanker, L. S., Tocco, D. J., Brodie, B. B., and Hogben, C. A. M., *J. Pharmacol. Exp. Ther.*, *123*:81 (1958).
46. Brodie, B. B. and Hogben, C. A. M., *J. Pharm. Pharmacol.*, *9*:345 (1957).
47. Schanker, L. S., *J. Med. Chem.*, *2*:343 (1960).
48. Brodie, B. B., in *Absorption and Distribution of Drugs* (T. B. Binns, ed.), William & Wilkins, Baltimore, Maryland, 1964, p. 42.
49. Suzuki, A., Higuchi, W. I., and Ho, N. F. H., *J. Pharm. Sci.*, *59*: 644 (1970).
50. Suzuki, A., Higuchi, W. I., and Ho, N. F. H., *J. Pharm. Sci.*, *59*: 651 (1970).
51. Koizumi, T., Arita, T., and Kakemi, K., *Chem. Pharm. Bull.*, *12*:413 (1964).
52. Koizumi, T., Arita, T., and Kakemi, K., *Chem. Pharm. Bull.*, *12*:421 (1964).
53. Kakemi, K., Arita, T., and Muranishi, S., *Chem. Pharm. Bull.*, *13*: 861 (1965).
54. Kakemi, K., Arita, T., Hori, R., and Konishi, R., *Chem. Pharm. Bull.*, *15*:1534 (1967).
55. Davenport, H. W., *Physiology of the Digestive Tract*, 3rd ed., Year Book Medical Publ. is here, Chicago, 1971, Chap. 13.
56. Levy G. and Jusko, W., *J. Pharm. Sci.*, *54*:219 (1965).
57. Okuda, K., *Proc. Sco. Expl. Biol. Med.*, *103*:588 (1960).
58. Lish, P. M., *Gasteroenterology*, *41*:580 (1961).

59. Necheles, H. and Sporn, G., *Am. J. Gastroenterol.*, *41*:580 (1961).
60. Hawkins, G. K., Margolin, S., and Thompson, J. J., *Am. J. Gastroenterol.*, *24*:193 (1953).
61. Crone, R. S. and Aroran, G. M., *Am. J. Gastroenterol.*, *32*:88 (1957).
62. Weikel, J. H., Jr. and Lish, P. M., *Arch. Int. Pharmacodyn. Ther.*, *119*:398 (1959).
63. Consolo, S and Ledinsky, H., *Arch. Int. Pharmacodyn. Ther.*, *192*: 265 (1971).
64. Bianchine, J. R., Calimlin, L. R., Morgan, J. P., Dryurene, C. A., and Lasagna, L., *Ann. N.Y. Acad. Sci.*, *179*:126 (1971).
65. Beermann, B., Hellstrom, K., and Rosen, A., *Circulation*, *43*:852 (1971).
66. Jaffee, J. M., Colaizzi, J., and Barry, H., *J. Pharm. Sci.*, *60*: 1646 (1971).
67. Bates, T. R., Sequeira, J. A., and Tembo, A. V., *Clin. Pharmacol. Ther.*, *16*:63 (1974).
68. Conklin, J. D., in *Bioavailability of Drugs* (B. B. Brodie and W. H. Heller, eds.), S. Karger, New York, 1972, p. 178.
69. Klein, J. O. and Finland, M., *N. Engl. J. Med.*, *269*:1019 (1963).
70. Wagner, J. G., *Can. J. Pharm. Sci.*, *1*:55 (1966).
71. Rosenblatt, J. E., Barrett, J. E., Brodie, J. L., and Kirby, W. M. M., *Antimicrob. Agents Chemother.*, *1*:286 (1961).
72. Hirch, H. A. and Finland, M., *Am. J. Med. Sci.*, *237*:693 (1959).
73. Karim, A., *Clin. Pharmacol. Therap.*, *39*:598 (1986).
74. Crounse, R. G., *J. Invest. Dermatol.*, *37*:529 (1961).
75. Nogami, H., Fukuzawa, H., and Nakai, Y., *Chem. Pharm. Bull.*, *11*: 1389 (1963).
76. Koysooko, R. and Levy, G., *J. Pharm. Sci.*, *63*:829 (1974).
77. Koysooko, R., Ellis, E. F., and Levy, G., *J. Pharm. Sci.*, *64*:299 (1975).
78. Houston, J. B. and Levy, G., *J. Pharm. Sci.*, *64*:1504 (1975).
79. Marks, V. and Kelly, J. F., *Lancet*, *1*:827 (1973).
80. Elias, E., Gibson, G. J., Greenwood, L. F., Hunt, J. N., and Tripp, J. H., *J. Physiol.*, *194*:317 (1968).
81. Hunt, J. N. and Knox, M. T., *J. Physiol.*, *201*:161 (1969).
82. Wagner, J. G., *Am. J. Pharm.*, *141*:5 (1969).
83. Wilson, C. G. and Washington, N., *Drug Develop. Indust. Pharm.*, *14*(2&3):211 (1988).
84. Thebault, J. J., Aiache, J. M., Mazoyer, F., and Cardot, J. M., *Clin. Pharmacokin.*, *13*:267 (1987).
85. Gibaldi, M. and Feldman, S., *J. Pharm. Sci.*, *59*:579 (1970).
86. Bates, T., Gibaldi, M., and Kanig, J. L., *Nature (Lond.)*, *210*: 1331 (1966).
87. Faloon, W. W., Paes, I. C., Woolfolk, D., Nankin, H., Wallace, K., and Haro, E. N., *Ann. N.Y. Acad. Sci.*, *132*:879 (1966).
88. Thompson, G. R., Barowman, J., Gutierrez, L., and Dowling, R. H., *J. Clin. Invest.*, *50*:319 (1971).
89. Schneierson, S. S. and Amsterdam, D., *Nature (Lond.)*, *182*:56 (1958).
90. Glazko, A. J., Dill, W. A., and Wolf, L. M., *Fed. Proc.*, *9*:48 (1950).

91. Gibaldi, M. and Schwartz, M. A., *Br. J. Pharmacol. Chemother.*, 28:360 (1966).

92. Nelson, E., unpublished data.

93. Levine, R. R., Blair, M. R., and Clark, B. B., *J. Pharmacol. Exp. Ther.*, 114:78 (1955).

94. Fix, J. A., *J. Control. Release*, 6:151 (1987).

95. Boston Collaborative Drug Surveillance Program: Clinical depression of the central nervous system due to diazepam and chlordiazepoxide in relation to cigarette smoking and age, *N. Engl. J. Med.*, 288:277 (1973).

96. Boston Collaborative Drug Surveillance Program: Decreased clinical efficacy of propoxyphene in cigarette smokers, *Clin. Pharmacol. Ther.*, 14:259 (1973).

97. Boston Collaborative Drug Surveillance Program: Drowsiness due to chlorpromazine in relation to cigarette smoking, *Arch. Gen. Psychiatry*, 31:211 (1974).

98. Kerri-Szanto, M. and Pomeroy, J. R., *Lancet*, 1:947 (1971).

99. Pantuck, E. J., Hsiao, K. C., Maggio, A., Nakamura, K., Kuntzman, R., and Conney, A. H., *Clin. Pharmacol. Ther.*, 14:9 (1974).

100. Beckett, A. H. and Triggs, E. J., *Nature (Lond.)*, 216:587 (1967).

101. Hunt, S. N., Jusko, W. J., and Yarchak, A. M., *J. Clin. Pharm. Ther.*, 19:546 (1976).

102. Riegelman, S., *Pharmacology*, 8:118 (1972).

103. Levy, G., *Pharmacology*, 8:33 (1972).

104. Heizer, W. D., Smith, T. W., and Goldfinger, S. E., *N. Engl. J. Med.*, 285:257 (1971).

105. Beermann, B., Hellstrom, K., and Rosen, A., *Acta Med. Scand.*, 193:293 (1973).

106. Monkhouse, D. C. and Lach, J. L., *Can. J. Pharm. Sci.*, 7:29 (1972).

107. Wagner, J. G., *Drug Intell. Clin. Pharm.*, 3:189 (1969); 4:77 (1970).

108. Higuchi, W. I., *J. Pharm. Sci.*, 56:315 (1967).

109. Goyan, J. E., *J. Pharm. Sci.*, 54:645 (1965).

110. Noyes, A. A. and Whitney, W. R., *J. Am. Chem. Sco.*, 19:930 (1897).

111. Carstensen, J. T., *Pharmaceutics of Solids and Solid Dosage Forms*, Wiley, New York, 1977.

112. Higuchi, T., *J. Pharm. Sci.*, 52:1145 (1963).

113. Robinson, J. R. and Eriksen, S. P., *J. Pharm. Sci.*, 55:1254 (1966).

114. El-Fattah, S. A. and Khalil, A. H., *Int. J. Pharm.*, 18:225 (1984).

115. Goodhart, F. W., McCoy, R. H., and Ninger, F. C., *J. Pharm. Sci.*, 63:1748 (1974).

116. Parnarowski, M., in *Dissolution Technology* (L. Leeson and J. T. Carstensen, Eds.), Industrial Pharmaceutical Technology Section, Academy of Pharmaceutical Sciences, Washington, D.C., 1974, p. 58.

117. Lettir, A., *Abrégé de pharmacie galénique*, Masson et Cie., Paris, 1974, p. 109.

118. Hersey, J. A., *Manuf. Chem. Aerosol News*, 40:32 (1969).

119. Baun, C. D. and Walker, C. G., *J. Pharm. Sci.*, 58:611 (1969).

120. Swarbrick, J., in *Current Concepts in the Pharmaceutical Sciences: Biopharmaceutics* (J. Swarbrick, ed.), Lea & Febiger, Philadelphia, 1970, p. 276.

121. Stricker, H., In vitro studies on the dissolution and absorption behavior of orally administered drugs, and the connection to their bioavailability, in *The Quality Control of Medicines* (P. B. Deasy and R. F. Timoney, eds.), Elsevier, Ansterdam, 1976, Chap. 16.

122. Stavchansky, S., Dissolution — State of the Art 1982. Apparatus Designs, "Proceedings of the Second Wisconsin Update Conference," "Dissolution State of the Art, 1982," October 25–27, Extension Services in Pharmacy, Health and Human Services Area, University of Wisconsin, Extension, Madison, Wisconsin (1982).

123. Lathia, C. V. and Banakar, U. V., *Drug Devel. and Industrial Pharm.*, *12*(1):71 (1986).

124. Dakkuri, A. and Shah, A. C., *Pharmaceutical Technology*, pp. 28–28–86, (June 1982).

125. Wagner, G. J., *Biopharmaceutics and Relevant Pharmacokinetics*, Drug Intelligence Publications, Hamilton, Illinois, 1971, p. 110.

126. Shah, A. C., Peot, C. B., and Ochs, J. F., *J. Pharm. Sci.*, *62*: 671 (1973).

127. Hanson, W., personal communication.

128. Gershberg, S and Stoll, D. F., *J. Am. Pharm. Assoc.*, *Sci. Ed.*, *35*:284 (1946).

129. Huber, H. E., Dale, B. L., and Christenson, L. G., *J. Pharm. Sci.*, *55*:974 (1966).

130. Kaplan, L. L., *J. Pharm. Sci.*, *54*:457 (1965).

131. Schroeter, C. L. and Hamlin, J. W., *J. Pharm. Sci.*, *51*:957 (1962).

132. Schroeter, C. L. and Wagner, J. C., *J. Pharm. Sci.*, *51*:957 (1962).

133. Lazarus, J., Pagliery, M., and Lachman, L., *J. Pharm. Sci.*, *53*: 798 (1964).

134. Simoons, J. R. A., Drukkery Wed. G. Van Soeste N.V. Amst. (1962).

135. Parrott, E. L., Wurster, D. E., and Higuchi, T., *J. Am. Pharm. Assoc.*, *Sci. Ed.*, *44*:269 (1955).

136. Nelson, E., *J. Am. Pharm. Assoc.*, *Sci. Ed.*, *46*:607 (1957).

137. Levy, G. and Hayes, B., *N. Engl. J. Med.*, *262*:1053 (1960).

138. Levy, G., *J. Pharm. Sci.*, *52*:1039 (1963).

139. Levy, G. and Procknal, J. A., *J. Pharm. Sci.*, *53*:656 (1964).

140. Campagna, F. A., Cureton, G., Mirigian, R. A., and Nelson, E., *J. Pharm. Sci.*, *52*:605 (1963).

141. Niebergall, P. J. and Goyan, J. E., *J. Pharm. Sci.*, *52*:29 (1963).

142. Gibaldi, M. and Feldman, S., *J. Pharm. Sci.*, *56*:1238 (1967).

143. Castello, R. A., Jeelinek, G., Konieczny, J. M., Kwan, K. C., and Toberman, R. O., *J. Pharm. Sci.*, *57*:485 (1968).

144. Paikoff, M. and Drumm, G., *J. Pharm. Sci.*, *54*:1693 (1965).

145. Poole, J. W., *Drug Inf. Bull.*, *2*:8 (1968).

146. Pernarowski, M., Woo, W., and Searl, R. O., *J. Pharm. Sci.*, *57*: 1419 (1968).

147. Himmelfarb, P., Thayer, S. P., and Martin, E. H., *Science*, *164*: 555 (1969).

148. Shah, A. C. and Ochs, F. J., *J. Pharm. Sci.*, *63*:110 (1974).

149. Stricker, H., *Drugs Made in Ger.*, *14*:93 (1971).

150. Stricker, H., *Drugs Made in Ger.*, *14*:80 (1973).

151. Braybrooks, P. M., Barry, W. B., and Abbs, T. B., *J. Pharm. Pharmacol.*, *27*:508 (1975).

152. Nozaki, M., Hayashi, M., Shibuya, T., Tsurumi, K., and Fujimura, H., Proceedings of the 5th Symposium on Drug Metabolic Action, Shirvoka, Japan, Nov. 9–10, 1973.

153. Toverud, L. E., *Medd. Nor. Farm. Selsk.*, *36*:87 (1974).

154. Singh, P., Guillory, J. K., Sokoloski, T. D., Benet, L. Z., and Bhatia, V. N., *J. Pharm. Sci.*, *55*:63 (1966).

155. Solvang, S. and Finholt, P., *J. Pharm. Sci.*, *59*:49 (1970).

156. Smolen, V., Dissolution — State of the Art 1982. Apparatus Designs, "Proceedings of the Second Wisconsin Update Conference," "Dissolution State of the Art, 1982," October 25–27, Extension Services in Pharmacy, Health and Human Services Area, University of Wisconsin, Extension, Madison, Wisconsin (1982).

157. Nyberg, L., Andersson, K., and Bertier, A., *Acta Pharmaceutical Suecica.*, *2*:471 (1974).

158. Smolen, V. F., Practical pharmacodynamic engineering in the design, development, and evaluation of optimal drug products, in *Advances in Pharmaceutical Sciences* (H. S. Bean, A. H. Backett, and J. E. Canless, eds.), Vol. 5, Academic Press, London, pp. 115–198.

159. Smolen, V. F., Ball, L., and Scheffler, M., *Pharm. Tech.*, *3*:88 (1979).

160. Smolen, V. F., *Pharma. Tech.*, *1*:27 (1977).

161. Smolen, V. F. and Weigand, W. A., *Acta Pharmaceutica Suecica*, *15*:309 (1979).

162. Smolen, V. F. and Erb, R. K., *J. Pharm. Sci.*, *66*:297 (1977).

163. Smolen, V. F., *J. Pharm. Sci.*, *60*:878 (1971).

164. Smolen, V. F., *J. Pharmacokin. Biopharm.*, *4*:355 (1977).

165. Smolen, V. F., Kuehn, PP. B., and Williams, E., *J. Drug Dev. Commun.*, *1*:231 (1975).

166. Smolen, V. F., *Hospp. Pharm.*, *4*:14 (1969).

167. Smolen, V. F. and Ball, L., *BioPredictor: a microprocessor-controlled dissolution apparatus substitute for bioavailability testing of drug products*, Proceedings of Interphex '80 USA Instrumentation and Equipment Conference: Pharmaceutical Technology, Marina Del Rey, California, pp. 27–85 (1980).

168. Smolen, V. F. and Weigand, W. A., *J. Pharm. Sci.*, *65*:1718 (1976).

169. Smolen, V. F., A frequent response method for pharmacokinetic model identification, in *Kinetic Data Analysis* (L. Endrenyl, ed.), Plenum, New York, 1981, p. 209.

170. Smolen, V. F., A generalized numerical deconvolution procedure for computing absolute bioavailability-time profiles, in *Kinetic Data Analysis* (L. Endrenyl, ed.), Plenum, New York, 1981, p. 375.

171. Smolen, V. F., *Annual Reviews of Pharmacology and Toxicology 18*, p. 495 (1978).

172. Tuey, D. B., Cosgrove, R. J., Meyer, M. C., and Smolen, V. F., *Proceedings of the 129th AphA Annual Meeting*, Las Vegas, Nevada, 1982, p. 49.

173. Smolen, V. F., *J. Pharmacokinet. Biopharm.*, *4*:337 (1976).
174. Yau, M. D. T. and Meyer, M. D., In vivo–in vitro correlations with a commercial dissolution simulator. I: Methenamine, nitrofurantoin and chlorthiazide, *J. Pharm. Sci.*, *70*:1017 (1981).
175. Smolen, V. F., Method and Apparatus for Automatic Dissolution Testing of Products, U.S. Patent No. 4,335,438, June 15, 1982.
176. Smolen, V. F., Multiple Injector Flow Through Dissolution Cell for Dissolution Testing Apparatus, U.S. Patent No. 4,279,860, July 21, 1980.
177. PMA's Joint Committee on Bioavailability, *Pharmaceutical Technology*, pp. 63–66 (June 1985).
178. PMA's Joint Committee on Bioavailability, *Pharmaceutical Technology*, pp. 63–66 (June 1985).
179. Melikian, A. P., Straughn, A. B., Slywka, G. W. A., Whyatt, P. L., and Meyer, M. C., *J. Pharmacokinet. Biopharm.*, *5*:133 (1977).
180. Gollamundi, R., Straughn, A. B., and Meyer, M. C., *J. Pharm. Sci.*, *70*:596 (1981).
181. Yau, M. K. T. and Meyer, M. C., *J. Pharm. Sci.*, *72*:681–686 (1983).
182. Shah, V. P., *J. Pharm. Sci.*, *72*:306–308 (1983).
183. Yau, M. K. T. and Meyer, M. C., *Pharm. Sci.*, *70*:1017 (1981).
184. Meyer, M. C., Gollamudi, R., and Straughn, A. B., *J. Clin. Pharmacol.*, *19*:435 (1979).
185. Meyer, M. C., Straughn, A. B., Lieberman, P., and Jacob, J., *J. Clin. Pharmacol.*, *22*:131 (1982).
186. Prasad, V. K., *Int. J. Pharmac.*, *13*:1 (1983).
187. Lindenbaum, J., Mellow, M. H., Blackstone, M. O., and Butler, V. P., *N. Engl. J. Med.*, *285*:1344 (1971).
188. *FDA Drug Bull.*, *8*:27 (1978).
189. *The United States Pharmacopeia*, 20th Rev., United States Pharmacopial Convention, Rockville, Maryland, pp. 621–622 (1980).
190. *The Medical Letter*, *20*(12): 13 (June 1980).
191. Wagner, J. G., Wilkinson, P. K., Sedman, A. J., and Stoll, R. J., *J. Pharm. Sci.*, *62*:859 (1973).
192. Glazko, A. J., Kinkel, A. W., Alegnani, W. C., and Holmes, E. L., *Clin. Pharmacol. Therap.*, *9*:472 (1968).
193. Monroe, A. M. and Welling, P. G., *Wur. J. Clin. Pharmacol.*, *7*:47 (1974).
194. Berlin, A., Siwers, B., Agurell, S., Hiort, A., Sjoqvist, F., and Strom, J., *Clin. Pharmacol. Therap.*, *13*:733 (1972).
195. Lander, H., *Med. J. Aust.*, *2*:984 (1971).
196. Meyer, M. C., Slywka, G. W. A., Dann, R. E., and Whyatt, P. L., *J. Pharm. Sci.*, *63*:1693 (1974).
197. Blair, D. C., Banner, R. W., Wildner, E. L., and Murray, W. J., *JAMA*, *215*:251 (1971).
198. Searl, R. O. and Pernarowski, M., *Can. Med. Assoc. J.*, *96*:1513 (1967).
199. Sullivan, T. S., Sakmar, E., Albert, K. S., Blair, D. C., and Wagner, J. G., *J. Pharm. Sci.*, *64*:1723 (1975).

200. DeSante, K. A., DiSanto, A. R., Chodes, D. J., and Stoll, R. G., *JAMA*, *232*:1349 (1975).
201. Wagner, J. G., Welling, P. G., Kwang, P. L., and Walker, J. E., *J. Pharm. Sci.*, *60*:666 (1971).
202. Strom, B. L., *N. Engl. J. Med.*, *316*(23):1456 (1987).
203. Task Force on Prescription Drugs, Final Report, Washington, D.C., Government Printing Office, 36–37 (1969).
204. Barone, J. A. and Colaizzi, J. L., *Drug Intell. Clin. Pharm.*, *19*: 847–858 (1985).
205. Chien, C. P., *Integr. Psychiatr.*, *3(Suppl)*:58S (1985).
206. DeVeaugh-Geiss, J., *Clin. Ther.*, *7*:544 (1985).
207. Lamy, P. P., *J. Clin. Pharmacol.*, *26*:309 (1986).
208. Meyer, M. C., The Therapeutic Equivalence of Drug Products — A Second Look, Memphis, University of Tennessee Center for the Health Sciences, 1985.
209. Schwartz, L. L., *Am. J. Med.*, *79(Suppl 2B)*:38 (1985).
210. Generic drugs, *Med. Lett.*, *28*:1 (1986).
211. Young, M. J., Bresnitz, E. A., and Strom, B. L., *Ann. Intern. Med.*, *99*:248 (1983).
212. Strom, B. L., *Annu. Rev. Pharmacol. Toxicol.*, *27*:71 (1987).
213. Pharmacopeial Forum, p. 4160 (July–Aug. 1988).
214. Skelly, J. P., Yamamoto, L. A., Shah, V. P., Yau, M. K., and Barr, W. H., *Drug Develop. Ind. Pharm.*, *12*(8):1159 (1986).
215. Skelly, J. P., Yau, M. K., Elkins, J. S., Yamamoto, L. A., Shah, V. P., and Barr, W. H., *Drug Develop. Ind. Pharm.*, *12*(8): 1177 (1986).
216. Souder, J. C. and Ellenbogen, W. C., *Drug Stand.*, *26*:77 (1958).
217. Vleit, E. B., *Drug Stand.*, *27*:97 (1959).
218. Cook, D., Chang, H. S., and Mainville, C. A., *Can. J. Pharm. Sci.*, *1*:69 (1966).
219. Cook, D., *Can. J. Pharm. Sci.*, *2*:91 (1967).
220. Langenbucher, F., *Pharm. Acta Helv.*, *49*:187 (1974).
221. Marshall, K. and Book, D. B., *J. Pharm. Pharmacol.*, *21*:790 (1969).
222. Marlowe, E. and Shangraw, R. F., *J. Pharm. Sci.*, *56*:498 (1967).
223. Barzilay, R. B. and Hersey, J. A., *J. Pharm. Pharmacol.*, *20*:232S (1968).
224. Northern, R. E., Lach, J. L., and Fincher, J. H., *J. Am. Hosp. Pharm.*, *30*:622 (1975).
225. Goldberg, A. H., Gibaldi, M., Kanig, J. L., and Shanker, J., *J. Pharm. Sci.*, *54*:1722 (1965).
226. Edmunson, I. C. and Lees, K. A., *J. Pharm. Pharmacol.*, *17*:193 (1965).
227. Tingstad, J. E. and Riegelman, S., *J. Pharm. Sci.*, *59*:692 (1970).
228. Niebergall, P. J., Patel, M. Y., and Sugita, E. G., *J. Pharm. Sci.*, *56*:943 (1967).
229. Wurster, D. E. and Taylor, P. W., *J. Pharm. Sci.*, *54*:169 (1965).
230. Hamlin, W. E., Nelson, E., Ballard, B. E., and Wagner, J. G., *J. Pharm. Sci.*, *51*:432 (1962).
231. Levy, G., Antkowiak, J. M., Procknal, J. A., and White, D. C., *J. Pharm. Sci.*, *52*:1047 (1963).

232. Endicott, C. J., Lowenthall, and Gross, H. M., *J. Pharm. Sci.*, *50*:343 (1961).

233. Nelson, E., *Drug Stand.*, *24*:1 (1956).

234. McCallam, A., Butcher, J., and Albrecht, R., *J. Am. Pharm. Assoc.*

235. Huber, H. E. and Christenson, G. C., *J. Pharm. Sci.*, *57*:164 (1968).

236. Jacob, J. T. and Plein, E. M., *J. Pharm. Sci.*, *57*:802 (1968).

237. Stern, P. W., *J. Pharm. Sci.*, *65*:1291 (1976).

238. Lachman, L., *J. Pharm. Sci.*, *54*:1519 (1965).

239. Alam, A. S. and Parrott, E. L., *J. Pharm. Sci.*, *60*:263 (1971).

240. Kornblum, S. S. and Hirschorn, J. O., *J. Pharm. Sci.*, *60*:445 (1971).

241. Johnsgard, M. and Wahlgren, S., *Medd. Nor. Farm. Selsk.*, *32*:25 (1971).

242. Shotten, E. and Leonard, G. S., *J. Pharm. Pharmacol.*, *24*:798 (1972).

243. Ganderton, D., *J. Pharm. Pharmacol.*, *21*:9S (1969).

244. Finholt, P., in *Dissolution Technology* (L. J. Leeson and J. T. Carstensen, eds.), Industrial Pharmaceutical Technology Section, Academy of Pharmaceutical Sciences, Washington, D.C., 1976, p. 119.

245. Khalil, S. A. H., *J. Pharm. Pharmacol.*, *26*:961 (1974).

246. Loo, J. C. K., Rowe, M., and McGilveray, I. J., *J. Pharm. Sci.*, *64*:1728 (1975).

247. Nyqvist, H., Lundgren, P., and Nystrom, C., *Acta Pharm. Suec.*, *15*:150 (1978).

248. Frantz, R. M. and Peck, G. E., *J. Pharm. Sci.*, *17*:1193 (1982).

249. Okada, S., Nakahara, H., and Isaka, H., *Chem. Pharm. Bull.*, *35*(2):761 (1987).

250. Khalil, S. A. H., Mortada, L. M., Shams-Eldeen, M. A., and El-Khawas, M. M., *Drug Develop. Indust. Pharm.*, *13*(2):369 (1987).

251. Singh, G. N. and Gupta, R. P., *Drug Develop. Indust. Pharm.*, *14*(13):1845 (1988).

252. Monkhouse, D. C., Ph.D. Thesis, University of Iowa, Iowa City, Iowa, 1970.

253. Levy, G., *J. Pharm. Sci.*, *50*:388 (1961).

254. Higuchi, W. I., Parrott, E. L., Wurster, D. E., and Higuchi, T., *J. Am. Pharm. Assoc.*, *Sci. Ed.*, *47*:376 (1958).

255. Anderson, R. A. and Sneddon, W., *Med. J. Aust.*, *1*:585 (1972).

256. Finholt, P. and Solvang, S., *J. Pharm. Sci.*, *57*:1322 (1968).

257. Vivino, E. A., *J. Pharm. Sci.*, *43*:234 (1954).

258. Gagliani, J., DeGraff, A. C., and Kupperman, H. S., *Int. Rec. Med. Gen. Prac. Clin.*, *167*:251 (1954).

259. Nelson, E., *J. Am. Pharm. Assoc.*, *Sci. Ed.*, *48*:96 (1959).

260. Juncher, H. and Raaschov, F., *Antibiot. Med. Clin. Ther.*, *4*:497 (1957).

261. Levy, G. and Procknal, J. A., *Antibiot. Med. Clin. Ther.*, *51*:294 (1962).

262. O'Reilly, R. A., Nelson, E., and Levy, G., *Antibiot. Med. Clin. Ther.*, *55*:435 (1966).

263. Higuchi, W. I. and Hamlin, W. E., *Antibiot. Med. Clin. Ther.*, *52*: 575 (1963).

264. Griffith, R. S. and Black, H. R., *Antibiot. Chemother.*, *12*:398 (1962).

265. Griffith, R. S. and Black, H. R., *Am. J. Med. Sci.*, *247*:69 (1964).

266. Bell, S. M., *Med. J. Aust.*, *2*:1280 (1971).

267. Wan, S. H., Pentikainen, P. J., and Azarnoff, D. L., *J. Pharm. Sci.*, *63*:708 (1974).

268. Berge, S. H., Bighley, L. D., and Monkhouse, D. C., *J. Pharm. Sci.*, *66*:1 (1977).

269. Miyazaki, S., Oshiba, M., and Nadai, T., *J. Pharm. Sci.*, *70*(6): 594 (1981).

270. Dittert, L. W., Higuchi, T., and Reese, D. R., *J. Pharm. Sci.*, *53*: 1325 (1964).

271. Miyazaki, S., Oshiba, M., and Nadai, T., *Chem. Pharm. Bull.*, *29*(3):883 (1981).

272. Walkling, W. D., Reynolds, B. E., Fegely, B. J., and Janicki, C. A., *Drug Develop. Indust. Pharm.*, *9*(5):809 (1983).

273. Benjamin, E. J. and Lin, L.-H., *Drug Develop. Indust. Pharm.*, *11*(4):771 (1985).

274. Serajuddin, A. T. M., Sheen, P. C., and Augustine, M. A., *J. Pharm. Pharmacol.*, *39*:587 (1987).

275. Bedford, C., Busfield, D., Child, K. J., MacGregor, I., Sutherland, P., and Tomich, E. G., *Arch. Dermatol.*, *81*:735 (1960).

276. Atkinson, R., Bedford, C., Child, K. J., and Tomich, E. G., *Nature (Lond.)*, *193*:588 (1962).

277. Shaw, T. R. D. and Carless, J. E., *Eur. J. Clin. Pharmacol.*, *7*: 269 (1974).

278. Jounela, A. J., Pentikainen, P. J., and Sothmann, A., *Eur. J. Clin. Pharmacol.*, *8*:365 (1975).

279. Strickland, W. A., Nelson, E., Busse, L. W., and Higuchi, T., *J. Am. Pharm. Assoc., Sci. Ed.*, *45*:51 (1956).

280. Armstrong, A. and Haines-Natt, R. F., *J. Pharm. Pharmacol.*, *22*: 85 (1970).

281. Kornblum, S. S. and Hirschorn, J. O., *J. Pharm. Sci.*, *59*:606 (1970).

282. Paul, H. E., Hayes, K. J., Paul, M. F., and Borgmann, A. R., *J. Pharm. Sci.*, *56*:882 (1967).

283. Monkhouse, D. C. and Lach, J. L., *J. Pharm. Sci.*, *61*:1430 (1972).

284. Abdallah, H. Y., Khalafallah, N., and Khalil, S. A., *Drug Develop. Indust. Pharm.*, *9*(5):795 (1983).

285. Yang, K. Y., Glemza, R., and Jarowski, C. I., *J. Pharm. Sci.*, *68*:560 (1979).

286. McGinity, J. W. and Harris, M. R., *Drug Develop. Indust. Pharm.*, *6*(1):35 (1980).

287. Eckert-Lill, C., Lill, N. A., Endres, W., and Rupprecht, H., *Drug Develop. Indust. Pharm.*, *13*(9−11):1511 (1987).

288. Munzel, K., *Arch. Pharm.*, *293*(65):766 (1967).
289. Narurkar, A., Sheen, P. C., Hurwitz, L. E., and Augustine, M. A., *Drug Develop. Indust. Pharm.*, *13*(12):319 (1987).
290. Harper, N. J., *Prog. Drug Res.*, *4*:221 (1962).
291. Kupchan, S. M. and Isenberg, A. C., *J. Med. Chem.*, *10*:960 (1967).
292. Higuchi, T., *Acta Pharm. Suec.*, *13*(*Suppl*):3 (1976).
293. Stella, V. J., *Aust. J. Pharm. Sci.*, *NS2*:57 (1973).
294. Sinkula, A. A., *Acta Pharm. Suec.*, *13*(*Suppl*):4 (1976).
295. Daehne, W. V., Frederiksen, E., Gundersen, E., Lund, F., Morch, P., Peterson, H. J., Roholt, K., Tybring, L., and Godtfredsen, W. O., *J. Med. Chem.*, *13*:607 (1970).
296. Schwartz, M. A. and Hayton, W. L., *J. Pharm. Sci.*, *61*:906 (1972).
297. Butter, K., English, A. R., Knirsch, A. K., and Korst, J. J., *Del. Med. J.*, *43*:366 (1971).
298. Sinkula, A. A. and Lewis, C., *J. Pharm. Sci.*, *62*:1757 (1973).
299. Sinkula, A. A., *Acta Pharm. Suec.*, *13*(*Suppl*):7 (1976).
300. Bundgaard, H., *Design of Prodrugs*, Elsevier, New York, 1985.
301. Sekiguchi, K. and Obi, N., *Chem. Pharm. Bull.*, *9*:866 (1961).
302. Sekiguchi, K., Obi, N., and Ueda, Y., *Chem. Pharm. Bull.*, *12*:134 (1964).
303. Goldberg, A. H., Gibaldi, M., and Kanig, J. L., *J. Pharm. Sci.*, *54*:1145 (1965).
304. Goldberg, A. H., Gibaldi, M., and Kanig, J. L., *J. Pharm. Sci.*, *55*:482 (1966).
305. Goldberg, A. H., Gibaldi, M., and Kanig, J. L., *J. Pharm. Sci.*, *55*:487 (1966).
306. Goldberg, A. H., Gibaldi, M., Kanig, J. L., and Mayersohn, M., *J. Pharm. Sci.*, *55*:581 (1966).
307. Chiou, W. L. and Riegelman, S., *J. Pharm. Sci.*, *58*:1505 (1969).
308. Chiou, W. L. and Riegelman, S., *J. Pharm. Sci.*, *60*:1281 (1971).
309. Chiou, W. L. and Riegelman, S., *J. Pharm. Sci.*, *60*:1569 (1971).
310. Chio, W. L. and Niazi, S., *J. Pharm. Sci.*, *60*:1333 (1971).
311. Chiou, W. L. and Smith L. D., *J. Pharm. Sci.*, *60*:125 (1971).
312. McGinity, J. W., Maness, D. D., and Yakatan, G. J., *Drug Dev. Commun.*, *1*:369 (1975).
313. Svoboda, G. H., Sweeney, M. J., and Walkling, W. D., *J. Pharm. Sci.*, *60*:333 (1971).
314. Stoll, R. G., Bates, T. R., Nieforth, K. A., and Swarbrick, J., *J. Pharm. Sci.*, *58*:1457 (1969).
315. Stoll, R. G., Bates, T. R., and Swarbrick, J., *J. Pharm. Sci.*, *62*:65 (1973).
316. Stupak, E. I. and Bates, T. R., *J. Pharm. Sci.*, *61*:400 (1972).
317. Aguiar, A. J., Krc, J., Jr., Kinkel, A. W., and Samyn, J. C., *J. Pharm. Sci.*, *56*:847 (1967).
318. Corrigan, O. I., *Drug Develop. Indust. Pharm.*, *11*(203):697 (1985).
319. Ford, J. L., *Drug Develop. Indust. Pharm.*, *13*(9-11):1741 (1987).
320. McGinity, J. W., Maincent, P., and Steinfink, H., *J. Pharm. Sci.*, *73*:1441 (1984).

321. Khalil, S. A. H., El-Fattah, S. A., and Mortada, L. M., *Drug Develop. Indust. Pharm.*, *10*(5):771 (1984).
322. Hamburger, R., Azaz, E., and Donbrow, M., *Pharm. Acta Helv.*, *50*:10 (1975).
323. Coates, L. V., Pashley, M. M., and Tattersall, K., *J. Pharm. Pharmacol.*, *13*:620 (1961).
324. Asker, A., E.-Nakeeb, M., Motawi, M., and El-Gindy, N., *Pharmazie*, *27*:600 (1972).
325. McGinity, J. W., Hill, J. A., and La Via, A. L., *J. Pharm. Sci.*, *64*:357 (1975).
326. Deshpande, A. V. and Agrawal, D. K., *Drug Develop. Indust. Pharm.*, *8*(6):883 (1982).
327. Sumnu, M., *S.T.P. Pharm.*, *2*(15):299 (1986).
328. Haleblian, J. K., *J. Pharm. Sci.*, *64*:1269 (1975).
329. Armour Research Foundation of Illinois Institute of Technology, *Anal. Chem.*, *21*:1293 (1949); through *Chem. Abstr.*, *44*:13003 (1950).
330. Shefter, E. and Higuchi, T., *J. Pharm. Sci.*, *52*:781 (1963).
331. Mesley, R. J. and Houghton, E. E., *J. Pharm. Pharmacol.*, *19*:295 (1967).
332. Moustafa, M. A., Khalil, S. A., Ebian, A. R., and Motawi, M. M., *J. Pharm. Sci.*, *63*:1103 (1974).
333. Moustafa, M. A., Khalil, S. A., Ebian, A. R., and Motawi, M. M., *J. Pharm. Sci.*, *64*:1481 (1975).
334. Moustafa, M. A., Khalil, S. A., Ebian, A. R., and Motawi, M. M., *J. Pharm. Sci.*, *64*:1485 (1975).
335. Gibbs, I. S., Heald, A., Hacobson, H., Wadke, D., and Weliky, I., *J. Pharm. Sci.*, *65*:1380 (1976).
336. Macek, T. J., *Am. J. Pharm.*, *137*:217 (1965).
337. Sokoloski, T. D., *Hosp. Pharm.*, *3*:15 (1968).
338. Ueda, H., Nambu, N., and Nagai, T., *Chem. Pharm. Bull.*, *30*: 2618 (1982).
339. Ueda, H., Nambu, N., and Nagai, T., *Chem. Pharm. Bull.*, *32*(1): 244 (1984).
340. Takahashi, Y., Nakashima, K., Ishihara, T., Nakagawa, H., and Sugimoto, I., *Drug Develop. Indust. Pharm.*, *11*(8):1543 (1985).
341. Lefebvre, C. and Guyot-Hermann, A. M., *Drug Develop. Indust. Pharm.*, *12*(11−13):1913 (1986).
342. Narurkar, A., Purkaystha, R., Sheen, P.-C., and Augustine, M. A., *Drug Develop. Indust. Pharm.*, *14*(4):465 (1988).
343. Ballard, B. E. and Biles, J. A., *Steroids*, *4*:273 (1964).
344. Lin, S. L. and Lachman, L., *J. Pharm. Sci.*, *58*:377 (1969).
345. Fukumori, Y., Fukuda, T., Yamamoto, Y., Shigitani, Y., Hanyu, Y., Takeuchi, Y., and Sato, N., *Chem. Pharm. Bull.*, *31*(11):4029 (1983).
346. Flynn, E. H., Sigal, M. V., Wiley, P. F., and Gerzon, K., *J. Am. Chem. Soc.*, *76*:3121 (1954).
347. Allen, P. V., Rahn, P. D., Sarapu, A. C., and Vanderwielen, A. J., *J. Pharm. Sci.*, *67*:1087 (1978).
348. Higuchi, T. and Lach, J. L., *J. Am. Pharm. Assoc.*, *Sci. Ed.*, *43*:524 (1954).

349. Bettis, J., Hood, J., and Lach, J. L., *Am. J. Hosp. Pharm.*, *30*: 240 (1973).
350. Higuchi, W. I., Nir, N. A.. and Desai, S. J., *J. Pharm. Sci.*, *54*: 1405 (1965).
351. Zoglio, M. A., Maulding, H. V., and Windheuser, J. J., *J. Pharm. Sci.*, *58*:222 (1969).
352. Higuchi, T. and Ikeda, M., *J. Pharm. Sci.*, *63*:809 (1974).
353. Kaplan, S. A., in *Dissolution Technology* (L. Leeson and J. T. Carstensen, eds.), Industrial Pharmaceutical Technology Section, Academy of Pharmaceutical Sciences, Washington, D.C., 1974, pp. 183−185.
354. Duchene, D., Vaution, C., and Glomot, F., *Drug Develop. Indust. Pharm.*, *12*(11−13):2193 (1986).
355. Szeman, J., Ueda, H., Szejtli, J., Fenyvesi, E., Machida, Y., and Nagai, T., *Chem. Pharm. Bull.*, *35*(1):282 (1987).
356. Akers, M. J., Lach, J. L., and Fischer, L. J., *J. Pharm. Sci.*, *62*: 391 (1973).
357. Akers, M. J., Lach, J. L., and Fischer, L. J., *J. Pharm. Sci.*, *62*: 1192 (1973).
358. Spivey, R., Ph.D. Thesis, University of Iowa, Iowa City, Iowa, 1976.
359. McGinity, J. W. and Lach, J. L., *J. Pharm. Sci.*, *65*:896 (1976).
360. McGinity, J. W. and Lach, J. L., *J. Pharm. Sci.*, *66*:63 (1977).
361. Sorby, D. L., *J. Pharm. Sci.*, *54*:677 (1965).
362. Tsuchiya, T. and Levy, G., *J. Pharm. Sci.*, *61*:587 (1972).
363. Chowhan, Z. T. and Chi, L.-H., *J. Pharm. Sci.*, *75*:534 (1986).
364. Chowhan, Z. T. and Chi, L.-H., *Pharm. Tech.*, *9*:84 (1985).
365. Chowhan, Z. T. and Chi, L.-H., *Pharm. Tech.*, *9*:28 (1985).
366. Signoretti, E. C., Dell-Utri, A., De Salvo, A., and Donini, L., *Drug Develop. Indust. Pharm.*, *12*(4):603 (1986).
367. Chrzanowski, F. A., Ulissi, L. A., Fegely, B. J., and Newman, A. C., *Drug Develop. Indust. Pharm.*, *12*(6):783 (1986).
368. Jacobs, A. L., *Pharm. Manufac.*, *6*:43 (1985).
369. Hollenbeck, R. G., *Int. J. Pharm.*, *47*:89 (1988).
370. Chien, Y. W., Van Nostrand, P., Hurwitz, A. R., and Shami, E. G., *J. Pharm. Sci.*, *70*:709 (1981).
371. Hollenbeck, R. G., Mitrevej, K. T., and Fan, A. C., *J. Pharm. Sci.*, *72*:325 (1983).
372. Nogami, H., Nagai, T., and Uchida, H., *Chem. Pharm. Bull.*, *14*: 152 (1966).
373. Nagami, H., Hasegawn, J., and Miyamoto, W., *Chem. Pharm. Bull.*, *15*:279 (1967).
374. Ganderton, D., *Pharm. Acta Helv.*, *42*:152 (1967).
375. Gouda, M. W., Malik, S. N., and Khalil, S. A., *Can. J. Pharm. Sci.*, *10*:24 (1975).
376. Khalafallah, N., Gouda, M. W., and Khalil, S. A., *J. Pharm. Sci.*, *64*:991 (1975).
377. Reddy, R. K., Khalil, S. A., and Gouda, M. W., *J. Pharm. Sci.*, *65*:115 (1976).
378. Levy, G. and Gumtow, R. H., *J. Pharm. Sci.*, *52*:1139 (1963).
379. Weintraub, H. and Gibaldi, M., *J. Pharm. Sci.*, *58*:1368 (1969).

380. Lim, J. K. and Chen, C. C., *J. Pharm. Sci.*, *63*:559 (1974).

381. Chiou, W. L., Chen, S. J., and Athanikar, N., *J. Pharm. Sci.*, *65*:1702 (1976).

382. Parrott, E. L. and Sharma, V. K., *J. Pharm. Sci.*, *56*:1341 (1967).

383. Braun, R. J. and Parrott, E. L., *J. Pharm. Sci.*, *61*:175 (1972).

384. Elworthy, P. H. and Lipscomb, F. J., *J. Pharm. Pharmacol.*, *20*: 923 (1968).

385. Fatmi, A. A., Hickson, E. A., and Williams, G. V., *Drug Develop. Indust. Pharm.*, *14*(5):711 (1988).

386. Pandit, N. K., Strykowski, J. M., McNally, E. J., and Waldbillig, A. M., *Drug Develop. Indust. Pharm.*, *11*(9&10):1797 (1985).

387. Itai, S., Nemoto, M., Kouchiwa, S., Murayama, H., and Nagai, T., *Chem. Pharm. Bull.*, *33*(12):5464 (1985).

388. Feely, L. C. and Davis, S. S., *Int. J. Pharm.*, *41*:83 (1988).

389. Daly, P. B., Davis, S. S., and Kennerley, J. W., *Int. J. Pharm.*, *18*:201 (1984).

390. Mayersohn, M. and Gibaldi, M., *Am. J. Pharm. Ed.*, *34*:608 (1970).

391. Benet, L. Z. and Turi, J. S., *J. Pharm. Sci.*, *60*:1593 (1971).

392. Benet, L. A., *J. Pharm. Sci.*, *61*:536 (1972).

393. Swintosky, J. V., *Nature (Lond.)*, *179*:98 (1957).

394. Martin, B. K., *Br. J. Pharmacol. Chemother.*, *29*:181 (1967).

395. Wilkinson, G. R. and Beckett, A. H., *J. Pharmacol. Exp. Ther.*, *162*:139 (1968).

396. Taylor, J. A., *Clin. Pharmacol. Ther.*, *13*:710 (1972).

397. Bray, H. G., Thorpe, W. V., and White, K., *Biochem. J.*, *48*:88 (1951).

398. Gibaldi, M. and Perrier, D., *Pharmacokinetics*, Marcel Dekker, New York, 1975, Chap. 1.

399. Wagner, J. G., *Fundamentals of Clinical Pharmacokinetics*, Drug Intelligence Publications, Hamilton, Illinois, 1975, Chap. 3.

400. Doluisio, J. T., LaPiana, C. J., and Dittert, L. W., *J. Pharm. Sci.*, *60*:715 (1971).

401. Krüger-Thiemer, E., *J. Am. Pharm. Assoc., Sci. Ed.*, *49*:311 (1960).

402. Krüger-Thiemer, E., *J. Theor. Biol.*, *13*:212 (1966).

403. Krüger-Thiemer, E. and Bünger, P., *Chemotherapia*, *10*:61 (1965/1966).

404. Krüger-Thiemer, E. and Bünger, P., *Chemotherapia*, *10*:129 (1965/1966).

405. Krüger-Thiemer, E., Bünger, P., Dettli, L., Spring, P., and Wempe, E., *Chemotherapia*, *10*:325 (1965/1966).

406. Krüger-Thiemer, E., *J. Theor. Biol.*, *23*:169 (1969).

407. Wagner, J. G., *Biopharmaceutics and Relevant Pharmacokinetics*, Drug Intelligence Publications, Hamilton, Illinois, 1971, pp. 272, 292.

408. Wagner, J. G., *Fundamentals of Clinical Pharmacokinetics*, Drug Intelligence Publications, Hamilton, Illinois, 1975, pp. 144−148.

409. Gibaldi, M. and Perrier, D., *Pharmacokinetics*, Marcel Dekker, New Yorl, 1975, Chap. 2.

410. Krüger-Thiemer, E., Berlin, H., Brante, G., Bünger, P., Dettli, L., Spring, P., and Wempe, E., *Chemotherapia*, *14*:273 (1969).

411. Gibaldi, M. and Perrier, D., *Pharmacokinetics*, Marcel Dekker, New York, 1975, p. 63.

412. Dominguez, R. and Pomerene, B., *Proc. Soc. Exp. Biol. Med., 60*: 173 (1945).

413. Dost, F. H., *Der Blutspiegel*, Georg. Thieme Verlag, Leipzig, East Germany, 1953.

414. Diller, W., *Antibiot. Chemother., 12*:85 (1964).

415. Wagner, J. G. and Nelson, E., *J. Pharm. Sci., 52*:610 (1963).

416. Wagner, J. G. and Nelson, E., *J. Pharm. Sci., 53*:1392 (1964).

417. Loo, J. C. K. and Riegelman, S., *J. Pharm. Sci., 57*:918 (1968).

418. Gibaldi, M. and Perrier, D., *Pharmacokinetics*, Marcel Dekker, New York, 1975, pp. 130−145.

419. Wagner, J. G., *Fundamentals of Clinical Pharmacokinetics*, Drug Intelligence Publications, Hamilton, Illinois, 1975, pp. 174−184, 185−201.

420. Notari, R. E., *Biopharmaceutics and Pharmacokinetics*, Marcel Dekker, New York, 1975, pp. 89, 93.

421. Wagner, J. G., *J. Clin. Pharmacol., 7*:89 (1967).

422. Wagner, J. G., *Fundamentals of Clinical Pharmacokinetics*, Drug Intelligence Publications, Hamilton, Illinois, 1975, pp. 185−187.

423. Lalka, D. and Feldman, H., *J. Pharm. Sci., 63*:1812 (1974).

424. Wagner, J. G., Gerard, E. S., and Kaiser, D. G., *Clin. Pharmacol. Ther., 7*:610 (1966).

425. Smolen, V. F., Murdock, H. R., Stoltman, W. P., Clevenger, J. W., Combs, L. W., and Williams, E. J., *J. Clin. Pharmacol., 15*: 734 (1975).

426. Smolen, V. F., Barile, R. D., and Teophamous, T. G., *J. Pharm. Sci., 61*:467 (1972).

427. Smolen, V. F., Turrie, D. B., and Weigand, W. A., *J. Pharm. Sci., 61*:1941 (1972).

428. Smolen, V. G., *J. Pharm. Sci., 60*:354 (1971).

429. Smolen, V. F. and Wiegand, W. A., *J. Pharmacokinet., Biopharm., 1*:329 (1973).

430. Wilson, T. H. and Wiseman, G., *J. Physiol., 123*:116 (1954).

431. Crane, R. K. and Wilson, T. H., *J. Appl. Physiol., 12*:145 (1958).

432. Fisher, R. B. and Parsons, D. S., *J. Physiol. (Lond.), 110*:36 (1949).

433. Wiseman, G., in *Methods in Medical Research*, Vol. 9 (J. H. Quastel, ed.), Year Book Medical Publishers, Chicago, p. 287.

434. Crane, R. K. and Mandelstam, P., *Biochim. Biophys. Acta, 45*:460 (1960).

435. Doluisio, T. J., Billups, F. N., Dittert, L. W., Sugita, E. G., and Swintosky, V. J., *J. Pharm. Sci., 58*:1196 (1969).

436. Levine, R. R. and Pelikan, W. E., *J. Pharmacol. Exp. Ther., 131*: 319 (1961).

437. Schanker, L. S., Shone, B. A., Brodie, B. B., and Hogben, M. A., *J. Pharmacol. Exp. Ther., 120*:528 (1957).

438. Irwin, G. M., Kostenbauder, H. B., Dittert, L. W., Staples, R., Misher, A., and Swintosky, J. B., *J. Pharm. Sci., 58*:313 (1969).

439. De Cato, L., Malone, M. H., Stoll, R., and Nieforth, D. A., *J. Pharm. Sci., 58*:273 (1969).

440. Levy, G., *Clin. Pharmacol. Ther.*, 7:362 (1966).
441. Digenis, A. G., Beihn, M. R., Theodorakis, C. M., and Shambhu, B. M., *J. Pharm. Sci.*, 66:442 (1977).
442. Harvey, F. R., Brown, J. N., Machie, D. B., Kelling, H. D., and Davies, T. W., *Lancet*, 1:16 (1970).
443. Newburger, J., Ph.D. Thesis, University of Kentucky, Lexington, 1974; J. Newburger and S. Stavchansky, unpublished data.
444. Darlington, W. A. and Quastel, J. H., *Arch. Biochem.*, 43:194 (1953).
445. Aguiar, A. J. and Fifelski, R. J., *J. Pharm. Sci.*, 55:1387 (1966).
446. Taraszka, M. J., *J. Pharm. Sci.*, 60:946 (1971).
447. Reunig, R. and Levy, G., *J. Pharm. Sci.*, 57:1355 (1968).
448. Agar, W. T., Herd, F. J. R., and Sidhu, G. S., *Biochim, Biophys. Acta*, 14:80 (1954).
449. Finch, L. R. and Herd, F. J. R., *Biochim. Biophys. Acta*, 43:278 (1960).
450. Doluisio, J. T., Crouthamel, G. W., Tan, H. G., Swintosky, J. V., and Dittert, L. W., *J. Pharm. Sci.*, 59:72 (1970).
451. Sinko, H. P. M., deMeere, A., Johnson, D. A., and Amidon, G. L., *J. Theor. Biol.*, 131:107 (1988).
452. Cabana, B. E. and Kumkumian, C. S., A view of controlled release dosage forms, in *Industrial Bioavailability and Pharmacokinetics* (A. Martin and J. T. Doluisio, eds.), Drug Dynamics Institute, The University of Texas at Austin, Austin, Texas, 1977, p. 51.
453. Van Rossum, J. M., Significance of pharmacokinetics for drug design and the planning of dosage regimens, in *Medical Chemistry*, Vol. 1 (E. J. Ariens, ed.), Academic Press, New York, 1971, p. 470.
454. Notari, R. E., *Biopharmaceutics and Pharmacokinetics: An Introduction*, Marcel Dekker, New York, 1975, p. 163.
455. Gibaldi, M. and Perrier, D., *Pharmacokinetics*, Marcel Dekker, New York, 1975, p. 172.

7

Pharmaceutical Tablet Compression Tooling

George F. Loeffler and Glen C. Ebey

Thomas Engineering Incorporated, Hoffman Estates, Illinois

I. INTRODUCTION

The compaction tooling involved in the manufacture of the tablet is as critical as the formulation or the tablet press if a quality product is to result. It must meet many requirements to satisfy the needs of dosage uniformity, production efficiency, and aesthetic standards. A basic knowledge of the subject will be of assistance in eliminating unnecessary delays in vendor communication and "starting off on the wrong track" with a proposed novel tablet design. An added plus would be lengthening the service life of the tooling involved.

The intention of this chapter is not to make the pharmacist a tool designer or a line mechanic, but rather to give sufficient background on the subject so that possible production pitfalls (unfortunately inherent in many new products) can be avoided or at least reduced in magnitude.

II. TERMINOLOGY

To best understand the following material, it is necessary to be familiar with the commonly accepted terminology (see Fig. 1). The tooling depicted is for the most popular single-stroke and rotary machines.

<u>Punch land</u>	Area between the edge of the punch cup and the outside diameter of the punch tip
Head	End of the punch that is controlled by the machine camming
Head flat	Area receiving the force of the compression rolls at the time that the tablet is being formed

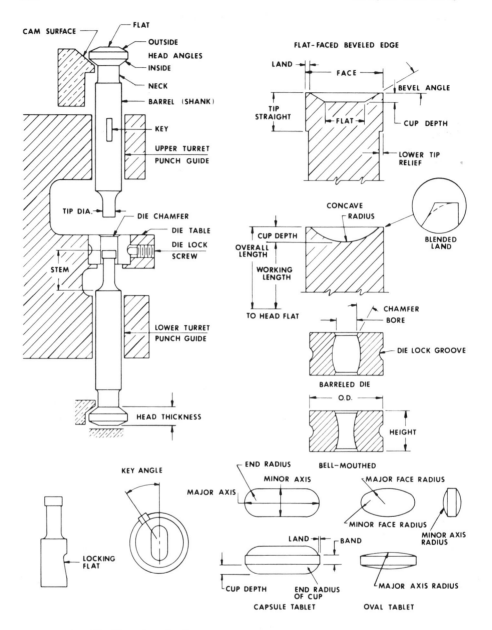

Figure 1   Tooling terminology.

Head angles	"Inside" and "outside" are the contact areas with the machine cams
Neck	Clearance provided for the cams
Barrel	(Shank) Vertical guiding surface for the tool in the machine
Tip straight	Axial section of the punch, upper or lower, that maintains the exact contour of the punch face
Overall length	Total length of the punch
Working length	Length of the punch from the bottom of the cup to the head flat (critical length)
Bakelite relief	Extra-deep undercut below the lower punch tip straight
Key angle	Relationship of the punch key to the tablet shape
Galling	Roughly worn areas on the metal surfaces
Core rod	Special punch configuration to produce a tablet with a center hole
"Rockwell"	Hardness of the tool
Fluting	Vertical grooves in the punch barrel
Die groove	Accepts the press locking screw
Chamfer	Entry angle on the die bore
Taper	Gradual increase in the die bore diameter from the point of compaction to the die chamfer area
Barreled bore	Diameter at the center is larger than at either or both of the ends
Bell-mouthed bore	Converse of the above
Ring	Eroded area in the die bore at the point of compaction
Carbide insert	High-wear lining for the die bore
Tablet flash	Semicompressed material formed on the perimeter of the tablet due to the punch tip to die bore clearance
Capping	Laminar separation
Picking	Granulation adherance to the punch face
Compaction ratio	Thickness of uncompressed material relative to compacted tablet
Punch face embossing	
Stroke	Width and depth of the engraving cut
Islands	Isolated "mesa" formed by certain letters or numbers, such as "B" and "8"

Striking   (Slug) Formed metal pressing of the punch face
design; used for approval of the punch face design

Overlay   Outline of the tablet face on a glass or plastic
film; used for checking the tablet monogram with
the aid of an optical comparitor

The most common tools employed in the industry are referred to as BB
tools. These are 5 1/4 in. long and have a nominal 3/4-in. barrel diameter with a 1-in. head diameter. The tablet machines that employ these
punches usually are available with either of two die sizes: 0.945 in. outside diameter to accept up to a 7/16-in. round or 9/16-in. capsule tablet,
and a 1 3/16-in.-OD die, which can make a tablet up to 9/16 in. round or
3/4-in. capsule, all with a maximum depth of fill of 11/16 in.

B tool machines are identical to the above except that the lower
punches are only 3 9/16 in. long.

The next most popular machines use D tools. These are also 5 1/4 in.
long, but have a 1-in. barrel diameter with a 1 1/4-in. head diameter.
The two standard die sizes available are a 1 1/2 in. OD, to accept up to a
1-in. round or capsule tablet, and a 1 3/16-in. OD die, which can make up
to a 3/4-in.-major-axis tablet. The maximum depth of fill is 13/16 in.

III. TABLET DESIGN

The tools must mold the granulation or powder to the required shape and
face design, while minimizing the possibility of adherence of the product
to the punch face. Consideration must be given to the compaction forces
that will be required, potential packaging problems, and possible limitations to the tableting machine output. Selecting the proper tablet design
is very critical to the performance of the tools in the machine. Round
tablets usually run best on the highest-speed rotary machines since they
do not normally require keying to maintain orientation of the upper punch
while out of the die. This permits them to rotate, presenting a better
distribution of the lubrication.

Dosage size or marketing requirements, however, may dictate an irregular shape, such as capsules, ovals, triangles, or squares. Although
these shapes require a little more attention to the mechanical lubrication
of the tooling, they can be operated at the higher machine output speeds
more readily if severe "self-locking" shapes are avoided.

A. Punch-to-Die Binding

One of the more important pitfalls to avoid in the design of the tablet is to
introduce the possibility of a self-locking effect between the lower punch
tip and the die bore. This is the result of peculiar radii combinations of
the tablet perimeter that permit a wedging action between the punch tip
and the die wall as the punch rotates through its available clearance.

The rotation is due to the inside head angle of the punch contacting
only one side of the fill cam in the machine. The resultant rotational
force or torque on the punch is increased as the punch is pulled down by
the cam, causing an increase in the tip to bore binding, which in turn
causes an increase in the applied torque, etc. The result can be severe

enough to twist the lower punch stem, damage the cam contact areas, or even to the extent of pulling the tips off the smaller tools.

The fill cams are normally double-sided; that is, they have contact lips on both sides of the inside head angle of the punch for theoretical even pulldown to eliminate the adverse rotational effect. Unfortunately, there are a number of machining tolerances that are required for the manufacture of the various involved press components that can negate the probability of absolute even pulldown.

The severity of the self-locking effect will be dependent on several factors: (a) the angle formed between the two tablet face radii and the rotational radius of the punch (keep the angle as large as possible; Fig. 2); (b) the coefficients of friction between the punch tip/die bore and between the punch inside head angle/cam lip (good lubrication is a major factor); (c) the size of the tablet relative to the punch head diameter (if the tablet is small, it would be better to run it on a machine that employs BB size tooling rather than the larger "D" tooling); (d) the degree of misalignment of the cam with the punch flight; (e) the concentricity of the punch head with its barrel; and (f) the slope of the weight cam.

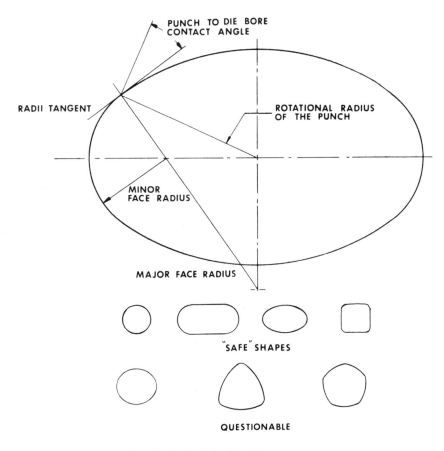

Figure 2   Punch tip "self-locking" shapes.

To be on the safe side, it would be best to avoid any shape that approaches this hazardous condition (see Fig. 2). If in doubt on a selected shape, it would be advisable to submit the tablet proposal to the tooling manufacturer for his advice. The involved forces can be calculated to a degree and a reasonable prognosis can be given.

B. Die Fracture

The increased emphasis on product recognition by pharmaceutical companies has given rise to a great deal of interest in unique or unusual tablet shapes. Polygonal designs such as triangles, squares, and pentagons (see Fig. 2) are just a few of the variations possible. Since it is not feasible to manufacture tools with perfectly sharp corners, a compromise is made by the addition of small radii in these locations. Tablet designers will normally want to keep all corner radii as small as possible in order to maintain the original shape selected.

Corner radii that are too small can, however, lead to a number of problems: (a) honing and polishing the die bore is more difficult; (b) punch tips will wear prematurely; and (c) stress concentrations in the die may result in fracture during use. Although there really is not an ideal radius for all applications, a good rule is to use a 0.050 in. radius as a minimum and a larger radius, if possible.

Of the three problems created by small corner radii, the last one is of the greatest concern since it renders the dies unusable and can result in damage to the tablet press. The mechanism by which failure can occur is illustrated in Figure 3. Normal tablet compaction forces tend to expand dies in a radial direction. For tablet shapes where the length is significantly different than the width, the resulting radial expansion forces are greater in one direction than the other. This imbalance creates local areas of high stress in the die wall. Sharp radii serve to concentrate these stresses which ultimately leads to crack formation and propagation.

If die fracture does become a problem and tablet shape redesign is not an option, the use of insert dies should be considered. Insert dies are comprised of an inner part which contains the bore and an outer shell (see Fig. 4). By shrink fitting the outer shell onto the insert a determinant amount of compressive pre-stress can be introduced in the insert piece, thereby reducing the tensile stress in the die wall during tablet

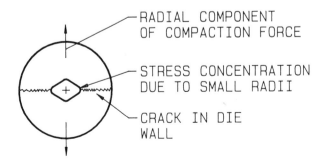

Figure 3   Die fracture due to sharp corners in bore.

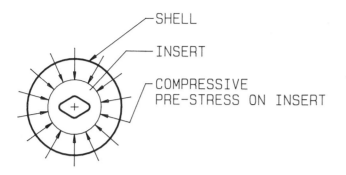

Figure 4   Insert die configuration.

compaction. The end result is that cracks which lead to die fracture do not form.

C. Punch Cup Contour

Next in importance is the proper selection of the punch cup contour. If heavy compaction forces are anticipated, the sturdier shapes should be selected, if possible. For example, shallow or standard concave cups are preferable to the flat-face beveled edge, deep, and modified ball shapes.

The pressure required to compress the tablet (which can range up to 150,000 lb/in.^{2}) has a lateral-force component that tends to bend the punch cup edge outward each time a tablet is made (Fig. 5). This continued flexing can cause premature failure if excessive. The degree of this flexing pressure is a function of the angle between the cup and the tip straight for a given compaction force. The more acute the angle, the greater the relative bending force.

There are several ways to strengthen the selected cup shape if the problem is anticipated: (a) increase the width of the land to permit more metal in this more fragile area (this can be "blended" to reduce the visual effect and aid in coating if involved; see Fig. 1), (b) alter the steel and heat-treating specifications for greater ductility, (c) increase the radius between the flat and the bevel on flat-faced beveled-edge tooling to better distribute the stresses, and (d) specify that the tooling be kept at minimum cup depth to reduce the area that the bending force can act on. Deep punch cup contours should be avoided if the granulation has a tendency to cap because of air entrapment.

Once the compression force necessary to produce tablets having the desired hardness has been experimentally determined, it is good practice to check for safe punch-tip stress levels. Unless tools are excessively overloaded, cracks leading to catastrophic failure may not occur until thousands or even millions of compression cycles have been logged on each station of tooling. Thus, tooling that may have been performed without incident during limited research and development tablet-making studies could conceivably fail prematurely during production runs. By the time the problem is recognized it may be difficult, if not impossible, to implement design changes without drastically altering the appearance of the

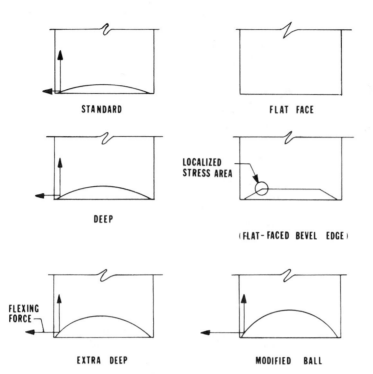

Figure 5   Punch tip shapes.

tablet.   In many cases, granulations still under development are compressed using round tooling and are later introduced into the marketplace
in an entirely different form.   Doing a preproduction stress check can
save a great deal of time and money later on.

A tabulation of maximum recommended compression forces as a function of punch-tip diameter for standard steel (AISI S5) punches appears in
Table 1.   Note that shallow and standard concave punch tips which have
relatively small lateral flexing loads can tolerate much higher operating
forces than can deep and flat faced bevel edge tips.   Granulations that
require high compaction pressures (>40,000 pounds per square inch)
should therefore be limited to those punch tip contours, if possible.

D. Engraving

The third major concern in the design of the tablet is the engraving.   It
must avoid any tendency of the granulation to adhere to the punch face
(pick) and must have the mechanical strength to withstand the tumbling
action involved in dedusting, film coating, and packaging.   Above all,
it must be legible on the tablet.

Often, the company involved has an excellent trademark or monogram
they would like to reproduce on their new products.   This design, as it
appears on their stationery or in their advertising, might be an inch in
height with considerable fine detail.   In reducing this logo to fit on a

Table 1   Maximum Recommended Compression Force Versus
Punch Tip Diameter for Standard Steel (S5) Punches

Diameter (in.)	Maximum force lb (KN)			
	Flat faced, shallow, standard concave		Deep, extra deep, flat-faced bevel edge	
3/32	700	(3.1)	275	(1.2)
1/8	1225	(5.5)	500	(2.2)
5/32	1925	(8.5)	775	(3.4)
3/16	2750	(12.3)	1100	(4.9)
7/32	3750	(16.7)	1500	(6.7)
1/4	4900	(21.5)	1975	(8.7)
9/32	6200	(27.5)	2475	(11.1)
5/16	7700	(34.0)	3075	(13.6)
11/32	9300	(41.0)	3700	(16.5)
3/8	11000	(49.0)	4400	(19.5)
13/32	13000	(57.5)	5200	(23.0)
7/16	15000	(67.0)	6000	(26.5)
15/32	17300	(77.0)	6900	(30.5)
1/2	19600	(87.0)	7900	(35.0)
17/32	22200	(98.5)	8900	(39.5)
9/16	24900	(110.5)	9900	(44.0)
5/8	30700	(136.5)	12300	(54.5)
11/16	37100	(165.0)	14800	(66.0)
3/4	44200	(196.5)	17700	(78.5)
13/16	51800	(230.5)	20700	(92.0)
7/8	60100	(267.5)	24100	(107.0)
1	78500	(349.0)	31400	(139.5)
1 1/8	99400	(442.0)	39800	(177.0)
1 1/4	122700	(546.0)	49100	(218.5)

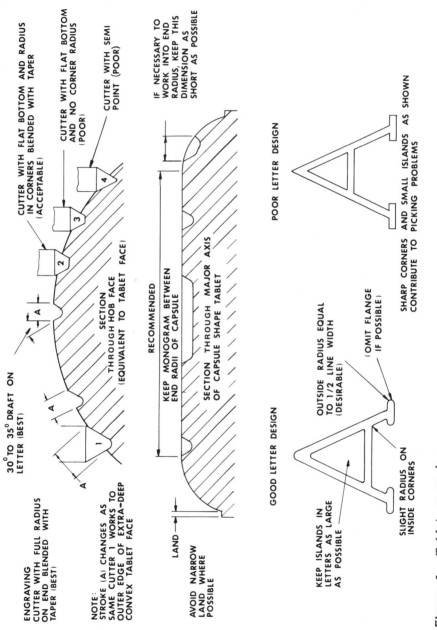

Figure 6 Tablet engraving.

small tablet, most of the fine lines must be sacrificed. Sometimes this detail is so important that the reduced design becomes a meaningless blob.

Broad, simple block letters and numbers should be selected whenever possible (Fig. 6). Script letters and fine lines, which may present a beautiful appearance on a letterhead, can cause problems with all of the foregoing requirements. "Fine lines" on the punch also will not withstand as much wear because of granulation abrasion and therefore will reduce the usable life of the tool. The design should be recessed in the tablet face, as raised letters with not withstand tumbling action. Square corners and small "islands" in the engraving are apt to cause picking. Where islands are necessary, as in "B" and "8," the tendency for the granulation to stick in these areas can be reduced by reducing their height and/or making them as large as possible (e.g., make them equal in size, dropping the cross bar in the "A" or opening the "4," as shown). The height in the island area can also be reduced (or eliminated).

Some design rules of thumb are as follows:

1. Stroke width = 1/5 letter height.
2. Stroke depth = 1/2 stroke width.
3. Space between letters = stroke width.
4. Space between letter and edge of bevel on flat-faced beveled-edge tablets = stroke width (minimum).
5. Monogram should not exceed 75% of face width of tablet.
6. Avoid sharp outside corners, if possible. Use 1/2 of the stroke width for outside radii.
7. 30° draft angle on uncoated tablets; 35° draft angle for film-coated tablets.
8. Place deepest embossing on the upper punch face (aids in tablet take-off from the machine).
9. When designing a new logo intended for a range of tablet sizes, work with the smallest tablet on which it will be employed. Significant detail may have to be sacrificed if proportioning down is required.

Following these suggestions does not guarantee success, but it will increase the probability of a good legible debossing, while decreasing the chances of "picking" or tool breakage due to the weakening effect of the grooving.

E. Keying Angle

All tablets, other than rounds, require a device on the upper punch to keep it aligned when the punch tip is out of the die bore to permit proper reentry. This device is customarily a projection or key on the barrel. This key rides in a vertical groove in the turret bore, thereby providing vertical travel freedom but preventing rotation of the punch.

The turret keyway is normally located in the line of travel of the compressing station, so the angle between the punch key and the major axis of the tablet will determine where the tablet take-off blade will strike the periphery of the tablet.

It is usually best to have the largest flat (or if no flat is available, such as on an oval tablet, the largest radius) make the initial contact with the take-off blade. This becomes more critical when friable tablets are compacted at the higher machine speeds and where heavy lower punch embossing is present.

The conventional angle between the punch key and the major axis of the tablet is 35°; that is, when facing the upper punch cup with the key at 12 o'clock, the major tablet axis would be at approximately 1 o'clock.

Although the conventional manufacturing angle is 35°, many presses do not have their take-off blade mounted at this angle. So if a take-off problem is anticipated, it would be best to measure the required angle on the press to be employed and transmit this information with the tooling order.

IV. SPECIFICATIONS AND INFORMATION
REQUIRED BY THE VENDOR

One major problem that a vendor has is that of communication. The time spent in clarifying the requirements on a new project unfortunately often exceeds the actual manufacturing time for the tooling. To initiate and preserve a position of confidence with the customer, a vendor must know what the customer wants and needs. This, coupled with the "state of the art" in manufacturing, can produce the best tooling for the particular application in the shortest period of time.

A good drawing of the tablet with accurate dimensioning and compatible tolerances will greatly reduce the overall time involved in completing a set of tools. Any information available on the proposed product, such as abrasiveness, required compaction pressure, excessive ejection pressures, tendency to cap or laminate, and previous tooling problems, is very helpful in the design of the new tooling. Adverse effects, if present, can often be alleviated or eliminated entirely in the design of the new tooling so that problems in production can be minimized.

Very often with older products, a good drawing is not available. The vendor can copy an existing punch or tablet and will prepare a proper drawing. However, its accuracy will be dependent on the condition of the sample furnished and where it fell within the original manufacturing tolerance. This may result in slight appearance deviations in the tablets produced from the new tooling. Reputable tooling manufacturers will supply a drawing as part of their services.

Additional information that is required with the request for a quotation or an order is (a) the tablet press to be employed (if the press has been modified to accept other than standard tooling, this should be noted); (b) "standard" or "premium" steel (this may be questioned by a vendor if it is felt that it is not compatible with other information received); and (c) the quantity of tools needed and whether overruns will be accepted.

Overruns are a necessary evil with a manufacturer. Because of the number of close-tolerance machining operations involved in producing a tool, a number of tools may be discarded during the course of their manufacturing cycle. This "shrinkage" can account for up to 10% of the order. As a consequence, it is customary to start out with approximately 10% more tools than the customer requested.

Since the loss is not always as severe, the quantity of completed tools may exceed that called for on the order. These overruns are priced at the full set rate. Accepting these tools has an advantage to the supplier

OVAL TABLET

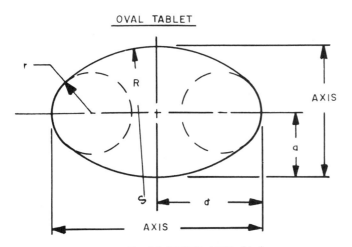

a = HALF THE LENGTH OF SHORT AXIS (in)
d = HALF THE LENGTH OF LONG AXIS (in)
R = RADIUS OF LONG SIDE (in)
r = RADIUS OF SMALL END (in)

$$R = \frac{a^2 + d^2 - 2rd}{2(a - r)}$$

$$d = r + (r^2 - 2Rr + 2Ra - a^2)^{1/2}$$

$$a = R - (R^2 - 2Rr + 2dr - d^2)^{1/2}$$

$$r = \frac{a^2 - 2aR + d^2}{2(d - R)}$$

FLAT FACED BEVEL EDGED CUP

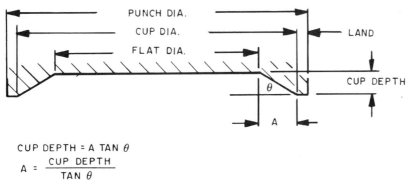

$$\text{CUP DEPTH} = A \, \tan \theta$$

$$A = \frac{\text{CUP DEPTH}}{\tan \theta}$$

(a)

Figure 7 Tablet calculations.

ENGRAVING CUT RADIUS

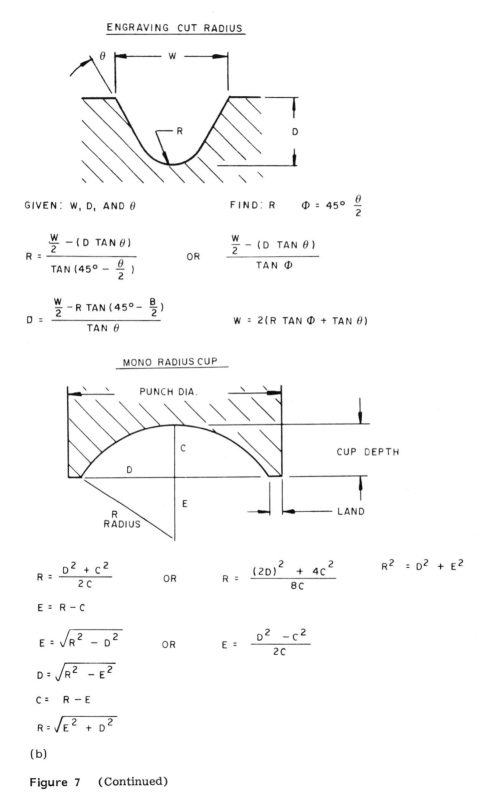

GIVEN: W, D, AND θ FIND: R $\Phi = 45° \dfrac{\theta}{2}$

$$R = \frac{\dfrac{W}{2} - (D \ TAN \ \theta)}{TAN \left(45° - \dfrac{\theta}{2}\right)}$$ OR $$\frac{\dfrac{W}{2} - (D \ TAN \ \theta)}{TAN \ \Phi}$$

$$D = \frac{\dfrac{W}{2} - R \ TAN \left(45° - \dfrac{B}{2}\right)}{TAN \ \theta}$$ $$W = 2(R \ TAN \ \Phi + TAN \ \theta)$$

MONO RADIUS CUP

$$R = \frac{D^2 + C^2}{2C}$$ OR $$R = \frac{(2D)^2 + 4C^2}{8C}$$ $$R^2 = D^2 + E^2$$

$$E = R - C$$

$$E = \sqrt{R^2 - D^2}$$ OR $$E = \frac{D^2 - C^2}{2C}$$

$$D = \sqrt{R^2 - E^2}$$

$$C = R - E$$

$$R = \sqrt{E^2 + D^2}$$

(b)

Figure 7   (Continued)

in keeping overall costs down (and therefore, ultimately, the customer's) and to the user as spares to replace the inevitable handling accident.

A. Steel and Hardness Section

Several types of tool steel are normally used in the fabrication of compression tooling. Since each has its advantages and disadvantages relative to a particular compressing application, the proper selection becomes critical to a successful overall operation.

The steel characteristics to be looked for in descending order of importance are:

1. Toughness to withstand the cyclic compacting forces
2. Wear resistance
3. Cost

The latter is not necessarily the initial cost but rather the cost per tablet produced.

The industry-accepted terminology groups the steels used into a standard or premium category. The former is usually an S5-classified, shock-resistant silicone steel which has good ductility and toughness after hardening. Occasionally, when a very fragile cup shape is involved, the vendor may recommend a 3% nickel steel, which has greater ductility but is less resistant to abrasion than the S5.

The premium steels are usually high carbon/high chrome alloys classified as D2 or D3. These steels have a much greater resistance to wear but have considerably less ductility and therefore are more subject to breakage when fragile cup shapes are involved. They should not be specified for deep punch cups or flat-faced beveled-edge tools unless relatively light compaction forces are anticipated.

The steel numbers S5, D2, and so on, are formulae designations by the American Institute of Steel Industries (AISI). They are adhered to by the various tool steel manufacturers to a close degree; however, slight variation can exist.

Unfortunately, there is no single steel available that combines the quality of high wear resistance with high ductility and toughness. The selection of the best steel for the job must be based on experience and the accumulated history of the product being tableted.

Figure 8 is an empirically derived chart depicting the relation of wear to "breakage" resistance for the more common steels employed. The S7 steel shown is an intermediate premium grade, employed where the punch cup geometry and required compation pressure would not tolerate the more fragile D2 steel. The relationship shown can be altered to some degree by variations in the heat treatment.

In order for the vendor to make the most intelligent steel selection, the following information must be available: (a) the shape of the punch tip (tablet face), (b) the compressing force required to form the tablet to the acceptable weight and thickness, (c) whether the material being compressed is abrasive, and (d) if the compressed material is corrosive in nature. Generally, with a new product, where sufficient background is not available, the steel and its hardness should be selected for the best ductility. Failure due to premature wear is certainly to be preferred over failure by cup breakage, with its associated possibility of metal contamination of the product.

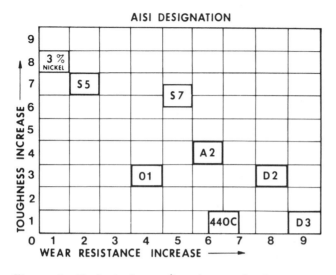

Figure 8   Tool steel-wear/toughness chart.

Stainless steel tools are recommended when resistance to corrosion is a major consideration. The absolute need should be well evaluated before specifying because of the negative aspects involved:

1. Higher initial cost and less wear resistance than premium steel tools
2. Relatively poor ductility compared with standard steel punches (see Fig. 8)

Often, a corrosive product can be successfully tableted without recourse to stainless steel by maintaining proper room humidity levels and by not allowing the material to remain on the press overnight.

The stainless steel that is normally employed in the manufacture of the majority of pharmaceutical and chemical equipment can be divided into two basic categories: austenitic and martensitic.

The former encompasses the Series 300 steels, which contain nickel-stabilized austenite. This is the type most widely used in tanks, sinks, sterile equipment, and so on. These steels will not accept heat treatment to achieve the proper qualities required for punches and dies.

The martensitic or Series 400 steels, containing little or no nickel, can be properly heat-treated by quenching and tempering. The 400C grade is the type that meets the requirements of concern here. It has very little corrosion resistance in the unhardened state and must be heat-treated to produce a hardness of at least 56 Rc to achieve a good degree of resistance to chemical attack. (Rc is a measure of hardness; it refers to a Rockwell hardness level in the C range. Hardness and its method of measurement are explained in Section VI.A.) Optimum hardness for the best strength of the 400C would be 58 Rc.

Standard steel dies are normally made from a 5% carbon, air-hardening material, designated A2. Premium steel dies are made from D2 or D3 steel. Ductility is not a critical factor in the selection of die steels, and therefore premium steel, although more expensive, is usually the wisest choice. Because of its greater ability to resist wear, its life will be several times that of a standard steel die for the same application.

Where an extremely abrasive material is being compacted, it may be advantageous to specify carbide-lined dies. Although the initial cost is much higher, the increased production life usually more than justifies the expenditure. Bear in mind, when making the decision, that these dies require more careful handling. Improper insertion techniques or dropping on a concrete floor may wipe out part or all of your investment.

Carbide is not a panacea to all die-wear problems. Several other negative aspects must be considered before selection. Carbide is a sintered material and as such it is more porous than tool steel. These microscopic pores can minutely add to a tablet ejection problem. They also form an excellent lapping surface that can wear away the punch tips more rapidly. This may in some instances create a false economy. The die life may be extended many times, but the cost savings in the dies by the selection of carbide can be more than offset by the possibility of shortened punch life. Carbide should be specified only when sufficient production history has been established for the particular product using premium steel dies as a basis.

Heat treatment of the tools in manufacturing is, of course, extremely important. The life of the tooling can be severely reduced by improper procedures. Excess carbon can be introduced or lost from the surface of the tool at the elevated temperatures required. Introducing carbon can create a brittle outer structure that can start cracks in the punch cup edges. The loss of carbon will leave the tool with a soft outer surface that will rapidly wear away in use, together with any delicate engraving. The usual heat-treatment systems employed for pharmaceutical tooling are: (a) molten salt baths, (b) electrically heated ovens where the steel is heated and quenched under a vacuum, and (c) electrically heated ovens where the carbon balance of the furnace atmosphere is carefully controlled.

The degree of hardness employed in the tool must be correlated to the application. As a general rule, an increase in hardness increases wear resistance but decreases ductility and toughness, all within the limits of the particular steel involved.

The higher-speed compressing machines should employ punches with a shank and head hardness of at least 54/56 Rc, preferably 58/59. This may be too hard to provide the needed ductility for a fragile punch tip. To overcome this problem, a selective heat-treatment procedure is employed known as tip drawing. This involves the timed immersion of the punch tips in molten lead held to a critical temperature. The punch tip hardness is thereby drawn down to the required level without affecting the rest of the tool.

Proper heat treatment of the tools is one of the important areas where great dependence must be made on the reliability of the vendor. There is no good nondestructive metallurgical test available that will assure you that the incoming tools have received the correct treatment for the application.

The Rockwell hardness check is an indication but in no way is it the complete story. Tools with the correct specified hardness could still have problems. For instance:

1. During the heat-treatment stage of the punch, it has approximately 0.012 in. of excess material over all its surfaces, with the exception of the punch cup. This material will be removed in subsequent grinding operations. The punch cup, however, will receive only a light polishing. Consequently, any carbon exchange, with its detrimental effect as mentioned previously, will be removed with the grinding stock on any measurable surface, but not in the most delicate part of the punch.

2. An adverse grain structure can be created by improper overheating of the steel in the austenizing step.

3. To achieve the optimum metallurgical structure for the steels involved, it is important that both the initial and tempering temperatures be properly established. Various combinations can often be employed to achieve the same hardness, but with varying effects on the toughness of the tool.

B. Tooling Tolerances and Clearances

This subject can be divided into two categories. The first consists of those dimensional variations permitted the manufacturer for the most economical construction of the tooling and machine, commensurate with the required tablet quality; and second, the permissible wear on the tool before it need be discarded. The former can be further separated into the tolerances that affect the machine operation and the flight and centering of the tooling and those that affect the actual tablet being compacted.

Figure 9 depicts a typical station of upper punch and die in a rotary tablet press. The upper punch has the minimum nominal clearance to its guiding surface in the turret that is commensurate with the lubrication film requirements. The involved machining tolerance would permit this clearance to vary from 0.00175 to 0.00275 in.

The die should be a snug fit in the die pocket to minimize its centerline shift due to the radial pressure of the die locking screw. This shift, up to 0.00025 in., is due to the required manufacturing tolerances on the die outside diameter and the turret die pocket. The combination of these two adverse effects can permit the punch tip to strike the die surface as it enters the bore.

The degree of interference is reduced by the punch tip-to-die bore clearance, which will range from approximately 0.001 in. to 0.005 in., dependent on the tablet size. It can be increased by the concentricity tolerance between the punch tip-to-barrel and die bore-to-die outside diameter, which can add up to 0.0005 in. to the effect. The sum of all the tolerances and clearances involved could add up to as much as 0.005 in. overlap of the punch tip as it tries to enter the die bore. This could even be true on a *new* machine. Although the probability of all these tolerances being in the adverse mode is very small, the die must accept the punch tip under all conditions or a smash-up in the machine would be inevitable.

The die bore must have an entry angle or chamfer that will direct an offset tip into the bore. The accepted American standard of a 30° angle on this chamfer (Fig. 10) does an effective job, so the negative effect on the punch tip life is small. However, the European standard of 20° should be considered to further reduce the deflection forces involved.

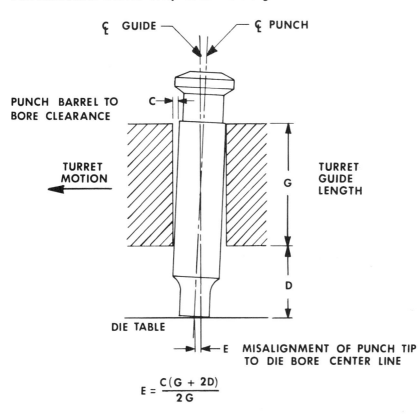

$$E = \frac{C(G + 2D)}{2G}$$

Figure 9   Punch-to-die misalignment.

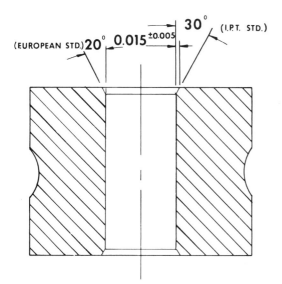

Figure 10   Die chamber.

Wear on the guiding surfaces, turret guide, and punch barrel will add
to the interference problem. Older machines should be checked periodically
for excessive upper punch "play" to avert unnecessary wear on an expensive set of tools. To measure the play, drop the punch tip down until it
is just above the die surface. Using a dial indicator, measure the total
amount of tip movement in the direction of travel of the punch. It should
not exceed 0.010 to 0.012 in.

The bore in the die should be straight and square with the die faces.
A barreled die (Fig. 1) is very detrimental to good tablet production, in
that the tablet would be formed at one diameter and then constricted as it
leaves the die on ejection. This can cause excessively heavy ejection pressures and/or fracture of the tablet. Bell mouthing is not as serious (within limits); in fact, it can be of aid in air relief and ejection.

The dimensions that most seriously affect the geometry and compaction
of the finished tablet are the punch length from the bottom of the cup to
the head flat and, to a lesser degree, the die bore diameter. In any one
set of tooling, these dimensions should be held as uniform as possible.

The American Pharmaceutical Association, Industrial Pharmaceutical
Technology (IPT) Section Committee on Specifications, in cooperation with
the leading tooling manufacturers, has established the maximum dimensional
variations permissible. Study of their published material is recommended in
conjunction with this chapter. The tolerances involved permit proper mechanical tooling performance in the tablet press and a good-quality tablet at
a reasonable cost for the tools. The dimensions we will be concerned with
in the following exercise are: Bottom of cup to head flat ±0.001 in. and
the die bore −0.0000 + 0.0005 in.

The effect of these allowable dimensional differences between the tools
in any one set will depend greatly on the size of the tablet being produced. To illustrate this, we will compare a small, thin tablet and a relatively larger tablet as follows:

Tablet A: 1/4-in. diameter × 0.090-in. thick, flat faced (FF)
           1.75:1 compaction ratio
Tablet B: 7/16-in. diameter × 0.200-in. thick (FF)
           1.75:1 compaction ratio

The term "compaction ratio" as employed here refers to the volume of
the uncompressed granulation at the weight adjustment point to the volume
of the finished tablet. This will vary with different granulations and will
be affected by the speed and filling efficiency of the tablet press.

The tolerance on the die bore (+0.0005 −0.0000 in.) will permit a 0.40%
total volume change for tablet A but only 0.23% variation in tablet B, the
larger-diameter tablet.

The most adverse tolerance combinations of the punches would be to
match a short lower with a short upper punch (−0.001 in. each) and a long
lower and upper (+0.001 in. each). These extremes would result in a
0.002 in. variation in the uncompressed fill depth and a 0.004 in. variation
in the compacted tablet thickness.

The ±0.001 in. tolerance on the lower punch working length can affect
the die fill of the thinner tablet, A, by ±0.68%, and the thicker tablet, B,
by ±0.28%. The resultant weight variation could be cumulative with the

variation due to die bore diameter. The compression ratio will be affected by both the upper and lower punch working lengths and is independent of the die bore variation. The percentage change due to the 0.004-in. difference in tablet thickness that could occur between any two press stations is partially offset by their respective die fill (the short lower accepts more material than the long lower punch). But again this density variation would be more serious with the thinner tablet: tablet A, 3.18%; and tablet B, 1.43%.

It can be concluded from the above that a possibly significant variation in tablet geometry could be caused by the industry-accepted standards for the punch length tolerances, the effect being more pronounced with thinner tablets.

The calculations are based on the tooling being matched in their most adverse relationship. The probability of this occurring in actual practice and the real need for increased accuracy for the product involved must be considered before specifying tighter (and more costly) tooling tolerances. It may be desirable in some situations to actually match the punches for length in each station of the turret (i.e., a short lower with a long upper, and vice versa). This would have the major corrective effect on the variation of the tablet density without resorting to more expensive tool construction.

C. Check List

The following information would aid in expediting a tooling order and also permit possible construction criticism by the vendor.

1. Size and shape of tablet.
2. Design drawing (or drawing number if repeat order).
3. Hob number if a repeat order.
4. Any problems experienced with the previous tooling (or if a new product, any anticipated difficulties: e.g., heavy compaction required, tendency for air entrapment, etc.).
5. Number of tools required (are overruns accepted?).
6. Tableting machine to be employed (manufacturer and number of stations). Is it a standard or a special model? If the latter, a tool drawing or sample tool(s) are required.
7. Steel to be used and required hardness.
8. Any special features required (e.g., chrome plating, special keying, fluting, non-IPT specifications, etc.).
9. Is the striking of a new face design or sample station required?
10. When the tools will be needed.
11. Any special shipping instructions.

V. HOBBING

This is the procedure in which a hardened steel form (hob), having a mirror image of the required punch face, is pressed with heavy tonnage into a soft steel punch blank.

The procedure of preparing the hob is as follows:

1. A mutually accepted and approved drawing at approximately 10:1 magnification is reproduced on a dimensionally stable film, usually a polyester.
2. The film is used to make a contact print on a photosensitized plate.
3. The plate is chemically etched to produce a relieved outline of the required engraving.
4. The plate is then used as a template on an engraving machine (pantograph).
5. Employing a cutter very accurately ground to the required draft and tip radius, the pantograph operator reproduces the design to the required size on the face of the soft hob blank (Fig. 6).
6. The hob is then checked for dimensional accuracy, heat-treated to produce the proper hardness, and polished.
7. When requested, a sample striking made from the hob will be furnished to the customer for approval.

The life of the hob is limited by the number of punches produced, the degree of pressure required to bring up the engraving detail, and the punch steel employed. The original cost of the hob is borne by the customer, but all maintenance and replacement costs are absorbed by the manufacturer.

VI. USE AND CARE OF THE TOOLING

A. Incoming and Routine Inspection

Pharmaceutical punches and dies are precision tools that require dozens of different machining operations to complete. The manufacturer performs inspection checks after each operation to ensure that the final product will be to specification. On completion, the tool is given a full 100% inspection before shipment.

In spite of all the checks and double checks, mistakes and errors can be made and, therefore, pharmaceutical companies should have an incoming inspection procedure to check the vendor's product. It is suggested that at least a spot check of critical dimensions be made on all tools received to ensure good tablet production capability.

The basic equipment required for an inspection facility is:

1. A clean, well-lighted area with a wood- or Masonite-covered benchtop
2. Surface plate (approximately 12 × 12 in.)
3. Dial indicator (0.0005-in. increments, 0.500 travel) with stand
4. Accurate (hardened and ground) V block
5. Micrometers 0−1 and 1−2 in.
6. Set of length standards or JO blocks
7. Set of ball and telescope gages to measure die bores
8. Illuminated magnifying glass.

This list can be expanded to the limit of any budget with equipment such as optical comparators, air gages for die bores, Magnaflux equipment,

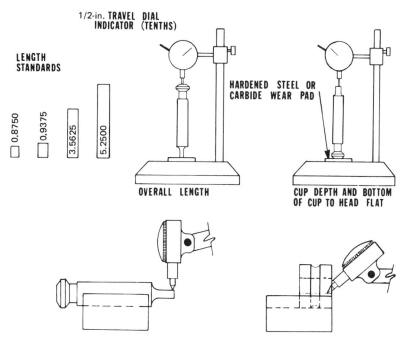

Figure 11 Punch and die inspection equipment.

digital-readout height gages, a steel hardness-checking device, and a tool-maker's microscope. Although these devices are all quite useful and will speed up and/or expand the quality assurances, the return on the invest-ment becomes more marginal. The basic equipment outlined, however, will permit confirmation of the essential measurements.

The dial indicator is used to check the overall length of the punch and the length of the punch to the bottom of the cup. It would be set up using the length standards or gage blocks (dimensionally precise hardened steel blocks that are combined to produce the desired dimension). It is also used for checking the punch tip to barrel and the die bore concen-tricity by rotating the punch or die in the V block (Fig. 11).

The micrometers are used to check the barrel, tip, head, and neck diameters of the punch and the height and outside diameter of the die.

The die bore would be checked with the ball or telescope gages or plug gages can be employed.

A magnifying glass can be used to detect possible rough spots in the punch face embossing. However, if a precise dimensional check of the logo is needed, it would require the use of a toolmaker's microscope.

An optical comparator is often used for the dimensional measurement since it is much faster than the microscope. This could be used in con-junction with an overlay, an accurately drawn outline of the design on glass or dimensionally stable plastic film. Caution must be used with an overlay system to avoid measurement errors. The embossing ridges composing the design are all radiused. As a consequence, the reflected light from the punch face that produces the image is dependent on its angle of incidence as it bounces off these curved surfaces. Both the comparator and the microscope are affected. However, the available depth perception on the microscope permits a much better judgment of the correct measuring points. If a comparator is employed, it should have the light source as parallel as possible with the viewing line of sight to minimize the possibility of error. ("Through the lens" lighting is best.)

The most popular device for measuring the steel hardness is a Rockwell Hardness Checker. This unit forces a diamond stylus into the steel with a fixed pressure. The amount of penetration is related to the hardness and appears on a dial indicator on the machine.

The normal Rockwell range for the steels used in pharmaceutical tooling is the C scale. It will be specified as a double number, which indicates the accepted tolerance (e.g., a punch barrel hardness would be specified as 56/58 Rc). Since the accepted practice is to round off the reading to the closest whole number, the actual acceptance level for this hardness would be 55.5/58.5 Rc. The slight ridge around the indentations caused by this measurement device must be stoned flush before using the tool.

When measuring, it is important to note that anything but an absolutely firm or rigid support of the test piece will introduce an error in the reading. Measurement on a curved surface such as a punch barrel or tip creates an error due to the unequal resistance of the metal flow at the penetration point. The smaller the diameter, the greater the deviation from the true hardness. The manufacturer of the instrument supplies a compensation chart for correcting the reading. Three readings should be taken: the first is discarded and the second and third are averaged.

Magnaflux equipment is used to check for minute cracks or flaws that are not readily apparent. These faults are not usually present in new tools, but can appear in the life cycle of the tool as it fatigues. This equipment is not too useful as an incoming checking device, but is helpful when running routine checks on used tools.

Each time a set of tooling is removed from the machine, it should be immediately checked for signs of cam wear before the tablet machine is set up for its next production run. Badly worn or "galled" areas on the punch heads would indicate rough spots on the cams and/or pressure roll faces which, if not corrected, will cause unnecessary abuse to the next set of tooling.

The tools should be checked for other visual indications and dimensional variations calling for rework or replacement (e.g., curled cup edges, worn logo design, die bore "rings"). Periodic length checks on the critical cup bottom-to-head flat dimension should be made to see if length resizing is required (see Sec. VI.E).

B. Handling and Storage of Tooling

The hard steel structure of tooling often creates a feeling of indestructibility to the uniniated. This, of course, is not true, as attested by the number of tools that are ruined by careless handling and storage. The cup edges on the punches are especially delicate. Contact of these areas with another punch or the press turret when inserting or removing the tools can cause them to crack or chip. A slight crack can result in

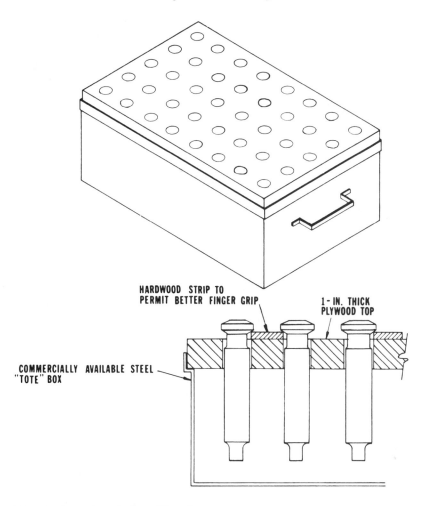

HARDWOOD STRIP TO
PERMIT BETTER FINGER GRIP

1- IN. THICK
PLYWOOD TOP

COMMERCIALLY AVAILABLE STEEL
"TOTE" BOX

Figure 12   Punch handling box.

chipping during the production run, with a possible serious contamination
of the latter.

A good procedure to follow is to make punch handling boxes (Fig. 12).
The box should be large enough to hold a full set of tools or of a size
that meets "in-plant" weight limits. A wooden or metal tray with a perforated wooden top to accept the punches works quite well. The dies,
which are much less subject to damage, can be handled in a smaller tray.

When removing the punches from the tablet press, each punch should
be wiped and dropped into a hole in the tray top as it is removed. Do
not accumulate and clean these as a group, since possible rolling on a
cart top can damage the tips. The trays should be brought to a cleaning
and inspection area, where the tools can be thoroughly cleaned, inspected
for abnormal wear, and a rustproof oil applied.

If rework or replacement is indicated, this should be inaugurated.
Rough areas on the punch heads would indicate that some attention should

be given to the press cams before resuming the operation of the machine.
If the tools are acceptable for their next production run, they can be returned to the handling boxes; or, to save the cost of the number of boxes
required for storage, a more compact procedure is to return the tools to
their protective cardboard sleeves and store in metal file drawers. Never
store any tools unless they have been adequately cleaned and have a good
application of rust-preventive oil.

Rust is very detrimental to the tool. Obviously, rust and its accompanying pitting on the punch cup could result in picking and obliteration of any
delicate engraving. However, corrosion on the remainder of the tool surface can result in a problem that is just as serious. It can adversely
affect the fatigue resistance of the tool. Although the general loss of
section due to corrosion is negligible, the stress concentration effect of
the corrosion pits formed can result in punches failing at the key insert or
at the punch neck.

C. Tool and Die Control

A good tooling program should include an accurate recording of the history
of each set of tools employed. The advantage of this, once established, is
that future tooling requirements can be better forecast. The information
is of further value for possible upgrading of the life of new tool sets (e.g.,
better steel for the application and/or heat treatment). It is also a good
check on the reliability of the vendor since, as mentioned previously, some
tooling quality must be accepted "on faith." The information that should be
included in the record is shown on a typical 5- × 8-in. file card (Fig. 13).

Product: _GUMBUT_   NDA# _XYZ_   Hob # _1592_
Tool: UP LP Die Size/Shape: _3/8 STD. CONC._ Steel: _S-5_ Rc BBL/Tip: _56/52_
Vendor: _BEST MFG._   P.O.# _6295_   Date: _7/17/75_ Qty: _61_

Date	No. Tablets Produced	Press Employed	Condition and/or Needs	Set Ready for Reuse
10/18/75	73 M	RP MII	—	10/12 GM
1/7/76	18 M	"	REPOLISH FACE (ONE DROPPED)	1/9 GM
2/20/76	54 M	"	RESIZE LENGTH	2/25 GM
5/4/76	60 M	"	MONOGRAM WORN – DISCARD —	GM

Spares on Hand: _X   10/18/75_
                 _5   1/9/76_

Figure 13   Tool record card.

The tools should be kept in sets. An inexpensive electric pencil can be used to put a code number on the neck of the punch to avoid mix-ups.

D. Punch Lubrication

A good film of lubricant on the punch contact areas of the turret would theoretically eliminate any possibility of metal abrasion, and would therefore prolong indefinitely this factor in the wear life of the tool. Unfortunately, this protective barrier between the metal surfaces cannot always be maintained. Free-flowing oils will "heal" worn spots in the film; however, their very ability to flow permits possible product contamination and requires constant replenishment. Greases, which are more apt to stay in place, flow and "heal" only when the film is broken to the degree where metal-to-metal contact is made, which in turn causes sufficient frictional heat to melt the grease.

The lubricant should meet several requirements: (a) it must have the film strength to resist the contact pressures involved, (b) it should not be easily contaminated by the dust from the granulation such as occurs with sugar and mineral oil, (c) it must adhere well to the metal surfaces to minimize any tendency to run off, and (d) it should be "edible" when used on the upper punches, where the possibility of product contamination exists.

Upper punch barrels and heads present the greatest problem. Approved (edible) lubricants have adequate film strength to work reasonably well in the punch barrel guide and upper cam area. However, they must be applied very sparingly. The possibility exists of forming black specks, which are a combination of lubricant, dust, and worn-off metal. These can drop into the product. The relatively poor film strength of these lubricants will break down in the head/cam contact area unless the punches remain free in their guides.

Normal practice is to apply a few drops of light mineral oil (approximately 10W) in the palm of the hand and rub sparingly on the punch barrel before inserting it in the turret. Grease would be applied to the punch heads using a small paint brush at periodic intervals during the production run. (The brush should be examined regularly and discarded if there are any indications of loose bristles.) The frequency of application would be dependent on the operating conditions (i.e., press speed, dust conditions, and round or irregularly shaped tools). Because irregularly shaped tools cannot rotate to better distribute the available lubricant, they will require considerably more attention than will round tools.

Teflon, which is gaining in popularity, reduces the possibility of the formation of the black specks. However, it does not always withstand the extra demand placed on the lubricant at the higher machine speeds that are available today.

Since the normally used Teflon is not miscible with oil (the combination will form a binding substance), it is imperative that all traces of oil be removed from the guides before applying. Teflon powder mixed with a volatile solvent would be brushed or sprayed on the punch barrel before insertion in the turret. This material does not usually have sufficient strength to enable its use on the cam tracks; therefore, grease must be employed on the punch heads. Careful application of the grease would be required to prevent it from coming in contact with the barrel lubricant.

The use of plastic dust cups on the upper punch tips is strongly recommended to trap possible falling particles. When employing unkeyed punches

in turrets that have keyways, a further precaution is to employ inserts to
fill these unused channels.

The lubrication of the lower punches presents a different problem than
that of the uppers. In this case it is a matter of the product contaminating the lubricant. Material sifting through the clearance between the
lower punch tip and die bore drops down along the punch barrel to the
lower cam track. This sifted material rapidly blots up the applied lubricant, causing the need for more frequent replenishment. The demand on
the lubricant film is usually much higher than with the upper punch,
owing to the heavier ejection and punch pulldown forces that are encountered.

Oil spray mist systems, with their coalescing nozzles aimed at the
ejection cam surfaces, can be employed. High film-strength grease applied periodically during the production run is also effective. A light oil
would be applied to the barrels.

The more recently designed presses employ stripper seals at the top
of the lower punch guides. These prevent the sifted tableting material
from reaching the cam area and, therefore, greatly reduce the lubrication
problem.

The cutting or grinding action employed to machine the turret, cams,
or tools leaves microscopic sharp ridges that can puncture the best lubrication film. It is advisable when starting up a new press or installing any
new "wear" components that the press be operated under very light loading, with more than normal lubrication, until these sharp surfaces are
lapped down. This greatly reduces the demand on the lubrication and
permits the use of the poorer film-strength approved lubricants.

Good dust control is important to the proper lubrication of a tablet
press. The vacuum nozzles furnished as standard on the machine are
usually adequate. However, improvements based on the actual operating
conditions and granulation employed often can be made. Care must be
exercised to avoid pulling granulation out of the die cavity prior to compaction by too much or misdirected air flow.

E. Refinishing

The good working life of the tooling can be extended to a degree by the
careful reworking of certain critical areas.

The erosion inherent in the compacting process can start small pits in
the punch face. Unless smoothed out in time, these areas will enlarge and
get rougher, resulting in granulation adherence or picking. Judicious application of a fine diamond paste with a small, soft, rotary-end bristle
brush will usually be very effective.

Plain cupped punches can be reground with a wheel dressed to the
required radius; however, this requires more extensive equipment (i.e.,
chucking lathe and tool post grinder). A chucking lathe can also be employed to correct curled-in punch cup edges. A fine abrasive stone
would be applied to the curled edge as the punch rotates. Care must be
exercised in this operation to avoid contacting any embossing present.

The punch head, which is subject to cam and pressure roll wear,
should be carefully checked each time the tools are removed from the
machine. Any rough areas should be smoothed with a fine-grit emery
cloth, or the angles can be reground. The marks need not be removed

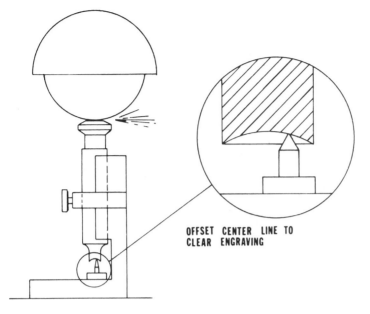

OFFSET CENTER LINE TO
CLEAR ENGRAVING

Figure 14 Punch length sizing on a surface grinder.

entirely. In fact, with irregularly shaped tools, which do not rotate in
their turret guides, the angular wear flats created convert the original
line contact with the cam to an area contact. The latter decreases the
unit contact pressure, resulting in a decelerated wear rate (providing that
they are smoothed).

It is usually advisable to periodically check the critical length of the
punch (the dimension from the bottom of the cup to the head flat). This
length can be resized to uniformity within the set, when required, through
use of a simple fixture, shown in Figure 14, used in conjunction with a
small surface grinder. The V block holds the punch in a vertical position.
The center of the cup rests on a pointed brass or nylon plug. (If embossing is present in the cup center, it will be necessary to offset the
plug.)

The tools should all be at uniform temperature before any measurements are made. This could become critical when sizing the length, owing
to the coefficient of expansion of the steel. This factor is 6.3×10^{-6} in.$^{-1}$
$°F^{-1}$. For example, if the tools were cleaned in a hot bath, it is con-
ceivable that the last out could be 30°F warmer than the first ones cleaned.
This 30° temperature difference would cause a 5 1/4-in. long punch to
grow in length by 0.001 in. If sized at this length, it would become too
short when it cooled down (0.0000063 in. $\times 5.25$ in. $\times 30°F = 0.00099$ in.).

Before grinding, check all the punches to find the shortest. Set this
one up first and bring the grinding wheel down so that it barely touches
and just begins to spark. Then grind all of the other punches to this
length.

One word of caution: The diameter of the head flat must not exceed
the neck diameter of the punch or the compression roll force on the punch

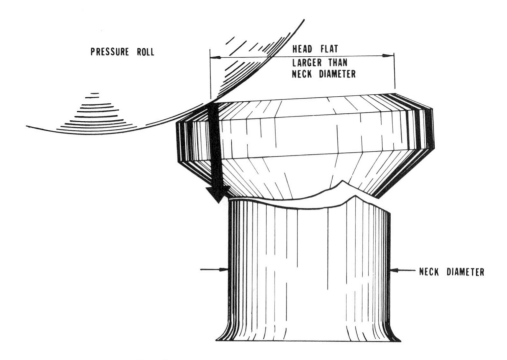

Figure 15 Punch head.

head may cause the punch head to break off as the tablet is formed
(Fig. 15). If the head flat gets too large, the outside head angle will require regrinding. However, care must be exercised not to get the heads
too thin for fear of breakage in use.

Because of the cyclic pressure to which the punch is subject in its operation to compact the tablet, fatigue due to the constant flexing may
cause premature failure. It is advisable when the more fragile punch cup
shapes are employed to periodically stress-relieve the tools. This is a
simple operation that involves baking the tools in an oven for several
hours at a temperature approximately 30 to 50°F below their original tempering temperature. This value for the particular set of tools involved can
be obtained from the supplier.

The reworking of the dies is limited to the enlarging of the bore to
the "die ring" diameter. The "ring" is an eroded band in the die bore
located in the final compaction area of the tablet. This worn section permits a tablet to be formed that is larger in diameter than the mouth of the
bore that it must pass in ejection.

Polishing will not be effective in this case. It will require enlargement
of the entire bore to the diameter of the worn area. This can be accomplished through use of a honing machine. However, a wooden dowel rod
wrapped with fine emery cloth used in the chuck of a drill press will suffice. Obviously, there is a limit to how far the bore can be enlarged,
since excessive sifting and tablet "flash" will result.

VII. PROBLEM SOLVING

A. Special Tooling Features

Problems that arise when employing a more difficult granulation can sometimes be alleviated or eliminated by design changes in the tooling.

The tendency of the tablet to "cap" or delaminate as it is ejected can
be reduced by tapering the die bore (Fig. 16). This not only permits
better air escapement during compression, but also permits the tablet to
expand at a more gradual rate as it leaves the die bore. It also has an
advantage in that it reduces the required ejection force.

Its disadvantage is that it raises the initial cost of the die and pro-
hibits "turning over" the die for extended die life, since a taper on the
lower end of the die would permit excessive escape ("sifting") of the granulation if deep-fill cams are employed.

If material has a tendency to adhere to the die bore wall, causing the
lower punch tip to bind, a Bakelite relief would be helpful. This is a
method of obtaining a sharp lower edge on the tip straight, which tends to
scrape the die bore clean as the punch lowers (Fig. 16).

Chrome plating can be used to alleviate a tendency of product adherence to the punch face or die bore. The plating, as employed on
pharmaceutical tooling, is referred to as hard chrome, differing from the
normal decorative plating in that a thickness of only 0.0001 to 0.0002 in.
is applied directly to the steel surface. This is to assure the best bonding. Although some additional wear and slight corrosion resistance is also
gained by this form of plating, the possible adverse effects must be considered before selection.

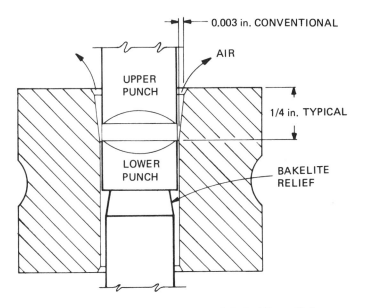

Figure 16 Tapered die bore and Bakelite relief.

If the entrapped hydrogen, a normal consequence of plating, is not completely baked out by the plater (not always possible), the resultant hydrogen embrittlement can cause premature punch cup failure. Further, the added chrome layer does not have the same flexural aspect as the parent steel and therefore could start cracks that can progress to punch cup failure or possibly spall (flake) off and contaminate the product.

The dust of some materials tends to combine with the lubrication and cause binding of the punches in their turret guides. This can be helped by machining vertical grooves in the punch barrels to reduce their contact area and to give them a self-cleaning action as they rotate with round tools. This is called fluting. This is not recommended except as a last resort, because it can cause product contamination if used on upper punch barrels and excess lower cam lubrication problems due to the sifted granulation if used on the lowers. It is far better to increase the exhaust system on the press, try for more compatible barrel lubrication, or run the product on one of the new-design presses that employ seals on the lower punch guides.

Worn upper punch turret guides can cause excessive contact of the punch tip with the die chamfer as it enters the die. This causes the edges of the cup to curl in, creating a problem as the tablet separates from the upper punch face. Although this hooked edge can be stoned out, it leaves a slight radius on the outside of the cup lip. This radius permits a firm ridge or "flash" on the tablet to be formed that is difficult to remove in the dedusting operation. It would be wiser to specify a smaller upper punch tip diameter, which would create a larger tip-to-bore clearance. The flash would not be any smaller, but it would be considerably softer and more apt to be completely removed in the cleaning operation.

Two or more tablets can be made at each station of the press through use of multiple-insert tooling (Fig. 17A). This can greatly increase the production output of the machine. However, it has several negative aspects that must be considered before investing in this higher-cost tooling: (a) since the punch length would be composed of two components, the length variation due to the required tolerance of both could be cumulative and thereby add to the nonuniformity of the tablets; (b) since the die bores do not all have exactly the same relationship to the powder feeding area, the die fill uniformity may be affected; (c) the setup of the press is more involved and time consuming; and (d) since it will probably require a slower turret rpm the increase in the press output rate will not be directly in proportion to the number of inserts/stations.

Core rod tooling (Fig. 17B) can be employed on most standard presses to make tablets that have a hole through their center (Fig. 17). Although this tablet configuration has an advantage where the need for more tablet surface area is indicated, it does require a considerably lower press output speed and much more expensive tooling.

B. Compressing Problems

Compressing problems may be caused by the granulation, the tablet press, or the compaction tooling. This chapter was to be concerned only with the latter; however, since many problems are interrelated, it was felt that sufficient interest and help would be gained by including the following troubleshooting list (starred items indicate features not available on all model machines).

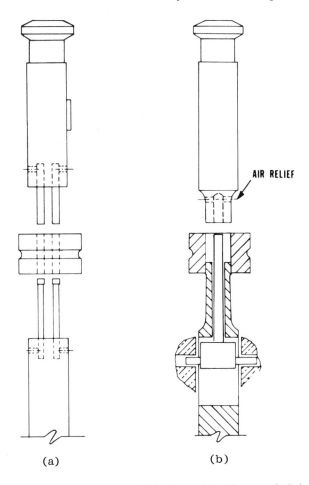

AIR RELIEF

(a)   (b)

Figure 17   (a) Multiple insert tooling and (b) core rod tooling.

	Problem		Possible cause		Check for
A.	Nonuniform tablet weight	1.	Erratic punch flight	a.	Freedom of punch barrels in guides (must be clean and well lubricated)
				b.	Excess machine vibration
				c.	Worn or loose weight adjustment ramp
				*d.	Proper operation of lower punch control devices
				*e.	Limit cam on weight adjustment head is missing or worn

Problem	Possible cause		Check for
	2. Material loss or gain after proper die fill	*a.	Tail over die missing or not lying flat on die table
		*b.	Recirculation band leaking
		c.	Excessive vacuum or nozzle improperly located
	3. Feeders "starved" or "choked"	a.	Wrong setting of hopper spout adjustment
		b.	Material bridging in hopper
		c.	Wrong fill cam
		d.	Too much recirculation
	4. Dies not filling	a.	Press running too fast
		b.	See A3 and A5
		*c.	Wrong feeder paddle speed or shape
	5. Lower punch starts pulling down without material coverage	a.	Inadequate recirculation
		b.	Recirculation scraper missing or bent
	6. Bad scrape-off	a.	Scraper blade bent, worn, or bad spring action
	7. Nonuniform punch length	a.	Punch cup bottom to head flats to be ±0.001 in., per IPT standards
	8. Die(s) projecting above die table	a.	Clean die pocket or check die dimension
B. Nonuniform tablet thickness	1. Nonuniform tablet weight	a.	See A above
	2. Pressure roll bounce	a.	Overload release improperly set
		b.	Operation near maximum density point of granulation (within allowable tablet tolerances, increase thickness and/or reduce weight)

Problem	Possible cause	Check for
		c. Pressure roll freedom and face condition
		*d. Air entrapment in hydraulic overload system
		e. Worn roll carrier pivot pins
	3. Nonuniform punch lengths	a. Punch cup bottom to head flats to be ±0.001 in., per IPT standards
C. Nonuniform density (friability)	1. Uniform tablet weight and thickness	a. See above.
		b. See "capping" (H)
	2. Unequal granule distribution in die cavities	a. Stratification or separation in hopper
		*b. Excess recriculation (causes classification of granulation since only the finer mesh material escapes the rotary feeders)
D. Excess machine vibration	1. Worn drive belt	
	2. Mismatched punch lengths	See A-7
	3. Operating near maximum density point of granulation	a. Increase tablet thickness and/or reduce weight within allowable tablet tolerances
	4. Heavy ejection pressure	a. Worn ejection cam
		b. Need for more lube in granulation or tapered dies
		c. Barreled dies
	5. Improper pressure-release setting	a. Increase to limit of tools
E. Excess punch head and cam wear	1. Binding punches	a. Dirty punch guides
		b. Inadequate and improper lubrication
		c. Inadequate exhaust

Problem	Possible cause		Check for
	2. Rough spots on surfaces from previous operation	a.	Not polishing off rough spots caused by normal wear or accidents
F. Dirt in product (black specks)		a.	Need for more frequent cleaning
		b.	Excess or wrong lubrication
		c.	Proper punch dust cups and keyway fillers
		d.	Feeder components rubbing
		e.	Punch-to-die binding
G. Excessive material loss	1. Incorrect feeder fit to die table	a.	Feeder bases incorrectly set (too high or not level)
		*b.	Feeder pan bottoms worn due to previous incorrect setting (relap if necessary)
	*2. Incorrect action on recirculation band	a.	Gaps between bottom edge and die table
		b.	Binding in mounting screw
		c.	Too little holddown spring pressure
	3. Die table scraper action insufficient	a.	Scraper blade worn or binding
		b.	Outboard edge permitting material to escape
	4. Loss out of die prior to upper punch entry	*a.	Tail over die not lying on die table
	5. Loss at compression point	a.	Compressing too high in the die
		b.	Excessive or misdirected suction on exhaust nozzle
	6. Excessive "sifting"	a.	Excessive lower tip-to-die bore clearance

Problem	Possible cause	Check for
		b. Excessive fines in the granulation
		c. Tapered dies installed upside down
H. "Capping"	1. Air entrapment	a. Compress higher in the die
		b. Reduce press speed
		*c. Employ precompression
		d. Reduce quantity of fines in the granulation
		e. Reduce cup depth on punches
		f. Taper dies
	2. Excess pressure	a. Reduce weight and/or increase thickness within allowable tolerances
	3. "Ringed" or barreled die bore	a. Reverse dies
		b. Hone or lap bores
		c. Compress higher in the die
	4. Too rapid expansion	a. Taper dies
I. Punch face "picking"	1. Excess moisture	a. Moisture content of granulation
		b. Room humidity condition
	2. Punch face condition	a. Punch face pits and/or improper draft on embossing (try repolishing)
		b. Try chrome-plating the punch faces
	3. Insufficient compaction force	a. Increase weight and/or reduce thickness within allowable tolerances

VIII.   SUMMARY

Careful consideration and implementation of the many factors involved in a good workable tooling program will reap benefits in many ways.

A well-thought-out design that satisfies the needs of production, packaging, and marketing, coupled with the manufacture of the tools to the exacting specifications required, are necessary to produce the highest quality product at the lowest overall cost.

The number of tablets that these tools will produce during their useful life and the resultant tooling costs per tablet will be a function of their design, the steel and hardness selected, and the quality of the maintenance and handling program employed.

The time required to implement the tooling for a new tablet design will be a function of the correctness and completeness of the information supplied to the tooling manufacturer.

Tooling suppliers have gained a wealth of experience in dealing with many compressing problems through the years. Do not hesitate to draw on this information if the need arises. They will be pleased to help where they can in the solution of any tablet compressing problem.

Index